P9-DUE-252

Preface

The practice of gastroenterology has evolved dramatically over the past two decades as the science of the alimentary canal has advanced rapidly and new diagnostic and therapeutic modalities have been added to our clinical armamentarium on an almost daily basis. In recognition of the need to advance current teaching materials on the subject of gastroenterology with the aim of incorporating this new knowledge, we undertook the editing of *Handbook of Gastroenterology*. The success of the first and second editions of *Textbook of Gastroenterology* attests to the demand for information on the practice of gastroenterology in the modern era. Recognizing the encyclopedic nature of the *Textbook* and the increasing demand for new knowledge in gastroenterology among trainees and medical students at the earliest level, we developed this handbook. Our aim was to present the quality and depth of the *Textbook* in a more concise and portable form. The *Handbook* focuses on the practical clinical aspects of the *Textbook*, making it particularly useful to the medical student, house officer, and advanced trainee. Of course, we hope that its clarity and completeness will also make it a useful resource for all physicians who treat patients with gastrointestinal disorders.

The associate editors and I are greatly indebted to William Hasler, William Tierney, and Peter Traber, who served as the special editors of the handbook. Their careful editing and attention to detail, as well as their obvious mastery of the practice of gastroenterology, have made the *Handbook* the useful guide to the discipline that we hope it will be to our readers.

Tadataka Yamada, M.D.

ix

Handbook of
Gastroenterology

46

Handbook of
Gastroenterology

EDITOR
Tadataka Yamada, M.D.
Adjunct Professor of Internal Medicine
University of Michigan Medical Center
Ann Arbor, Michigan

ASSOCIATE EDITORS

David H. Alpers, M.D.
William Kountz Professor of Medicine
Washington University School of
    Medicine
St. Louis, Missouri

Don W. Powell, M.D.
The Edward Randall and Edward Randall, Jr.,
    Distinguished Chair and Professor of
    Internal Medicine
Professor of Internal Medicine
Professor of Physiology and Biophysics
The University of Texas Medical Branch
    at Galveston
Galveston, Texas

Chung Owyang, M.D.
The H. Marvin Pollard Professor of
    Gastroenterology
Chief, Division of Gastroenterology
University of Michigan Medical Center
Ann Arbor, Michigan

Fred E. Silverstein, M.D.
Clinical Professor of Medicine
University of Washington School of Medicine
Partner, Frazier and Company
Seattle, Washington

SPECIAL EDITORS

William L. Hasler, M.D.
Associate Professor of Internal Medicine
Division of Gastroenterology
University of Michigan Medical Center
Ann Arbor, Michigan

Peter G. Traber, M.D.
Frank Wister Thomas Professor and Chair
Department of Medicine
University of Pennsylvania School of
    Medicine
Philadelphia, Pennsylvania

ASSISTANT SPECIAL EDITOR

William M. Tierney, M.D.
Assistant Professor of Medicine
University of Oklahoma Health Sciences Center
Oklahoma City, Oklahoma

Library Resource Center
Renton Technical College
3000 N.E. 4th St.
Renton, WA 98056

LIPPINCOTT WILLIAMS & WILKINS
A **Wolters Kluwer** Company
Philadelphia · Baltimore · New York · London
Buenos Aires · Hong Kong · Sydney · Tokyo

616
. 33
HANDBOO
1998g

Acquisitions Editors: Beth Barry, Joyce-Rachel John
Manufacturing Manager: Dennis Teston
Supervising Editor: Kimberly Swan
Production Editor: Dana L. Tackett, Silverchair Science + Communications
Cover Designer: Patricia Gast
Indexer: Linda Herr Hallinger, Herr's Indexing Service
Compositor: Tracy Eagan, Silverchair Science + Communications
Printer: Maple Press

© 1998, by Lippincott–Raven Publishers. All rights reserved. This book is protected by copyright. No part of it may be reproduced, stored in a retrieval system, or transmitted, in any form or by any means—electronic, mechanical, photocopy, recording, or otherwise—without the prior written consent of the publisher, except for brief quotations embodied in critical articles and reviews. For information write **Lippincott Williams & Wilkins, 227 East Washington Square, Philadelphia, Pennsylvania 19106-3780.**

Materials appearing in this book prepared by individuals as part of their official duties as U.S. Government employees are not covered by the above-mentioned copyright.

Printed in the United States of America

9 8 7 6 5 4 3 2

Library of Congress Cataloging-in-Publication Data

Handbook of gastroenterology / editor, Tadataka Yamada ; associate
   editors, David H. Alpers . . . [et al.] ; special editor, William L.
   Hasler, Peter G. Traber ; assistant special editor, William M.
   Tierney.
      p.   cm.
   Includes index.
   ISBN 0-397-51427-1
      1. Gastroenterology--Handbooks, manuals, etc. 2. Gastrointestinal
   system--Diseases--Handbooks, manuals, etc.   I. Yamada, Tadataka.
      [DNLM: 1.   Gastrointestinal Diseases--handbooks. WI 39 H2354
   1998]
   RC801.H28   1998
   616.3'3--dc21
   DNLM/DLC
   for Library of Congress   98-12187
                                                                     CIP

Care has been taken to confirm the accuracy of the information presented and to describe generally accepted practices. However, the authors, editors, and publisher are not responsible for errors or omissions or for any consequences from application of the information in this book and make no warranty, express or implied, with respect to the contents of the publication.

The authors, editors, and publisher have exerted every effort to ensure that drug selection and dosages set forth in this text are in accordance with current recommendations and practice at the time of publication. However, in view of ongoing research, changes in government regulations, and the constant flow of information relating to drug therapy and drug reactions, the reader is urged to check the package insert for each drug for any change in indications and dosage and for added warnings and precautions. This is particularly important when the recommended agent is a new or infrequently employed drug.

Some drugs and medical devices presented in this publication have Food and Drug Administration (FDA) clearance for limited use in restricted research settings. It is the responsibility of the health care provider to ascertain the FDA status of each drug or device planned for use in their clinical practice.

Contents

CHAPTER 1

Psychosocial Factors in the Care of Patients with Gastrointestinal Disorders

MULTIFACTORIAL MODEL OF DISEASE

Human illness results from a complex interplay of clinical, biological, psychological, and sociologic variables. The clinician's understanding of these diverse yet interacting variables is critical for adequate diagnosis and treatment of gastrointestinal disease. Much of this handbook deals with the biological aspects of clinical disorders of the gastrointestinal and hepatic systems. Compared with the biological factors, the data derived from psychosocial investigations are more variable and therefore more difficult to interpret.

Psychophysiologic Factors

It is well described that previously healthy persons experience abdominal discomfort and altered bowel patterns during periods of emotional distress. This correlates with experimental models that show altered intestinal vascularity, secretion, motor activity, and pain perception as a result of stressful stimulation. These stressors can modify a person's actions, evoking striking autonomic responses and emotional changes (e.g., increased anxiety). Conversely, primary alterations in bowel function can affect the central nervous system structures that regulate human emotion, such as the locus caeruleus. Various stressors modify humoral and cellular immunity, including delayed responsiveness to mitogens and antigens, reduced lymphocyte-mediated cytotoxicity, and reduced delayed hypersensitivity, potentially increasing a person's susceptibility to inflammatory or infectious disease.

These effects are mediated by bidirectional interconnecting pathways linking the cognitive and emotional centers in the brain with the neuroendocrine axis, the enteric nervous system, and the immune system by specific brain-gut neurotransmitters. It has been hypothesized that the functional bowel disorders (e.g., irritable bowel syndrome [IBS]) result from dysregulation of these brain-gut neuroenteric systems. For example, patients with IBS exhibit exaggerated responsiveness to meal ingestion, hormonal stimulation, and lumenal distention. A role for the central nervous system in IBS is supported by the disappearance of symptoms during sleep. It has been speculated that psychoimmune factors modify the clinical features of inflammatory bowel disease. Although not initiated by psychosocial stressors, dysregulation of immune function can prolong or exacerbate inflammatory and infectious conditions, producing an inability to clear or suppress the agent or stimulus that activated the immune response.

The Illness Experience

After an illness is established, cultural norms, family beliefs, personality, prior history of abuse or stress, and previous illness experiences affect a patient's reaction to the new illness and have an impact on symptom severity, psychological distress, quality of life, and health care use. The physician's attention to these psychosocial variables will probably improve the patient's clinical response to appropriate treatment directed at the biological illness. Therefore, assessment of the nonbiological factors should be a priority for the clinician.

INTERVIEWING A PATIENT WITH GASTROINTESTINAL OR HEPATIC DISEASE

The medical interview is the process by which the clinician obtains initial data with which to diagnose, direct management of, and determine the prognosis of an illness of the gastrointestinal tract and liver. The physician should strive to understand the illness from the patient's perspective and then generate a medical knowledge base organized into disease-related and behavioral categories. In the medical interview, the physician must employ flexible techniques, provide questions in an open-ended format, especially for patients with unexplained or chronic symptoms, and reserve directed queries to clarify answers or to be used in emergency situations when timely intervention is critical. It is more efficient to obtain psychosocial and biomedical data concurrently, because the patient often cannot separate an emotional response to illness from the strict biological factors that produce clinical disease. Moreover, addressing the patient's emotional state and underlying concerns facilitates a positive therapeutic relationship with the caregiver.

Once the medical and social data are obtained, their contribution to biological illness must be determined. Patients with long-standing, unexplained symptoms are less likely to be given a specific medical diagnosis, and thus psychosocial factors are likely to be major contributors to disease expression. The frequency of extraintestinal complaints from a patient with gastrointestinal disease and the number of health care visits are important prognostic indicators of the probability of diagnosis of organic illness and the response to specific medical or surgical therapy. The presence of an unresolved loss or a history of physical or sexual trauma in the recent or distant past can affect the timing of presentation and the severity of clinical symptoms. As part of the interview process, the physician must understand the expectations of the patient. Many patients with chronic illness have unrealistic expectations of cure. Some persons with persistent, unresolved symptoms acquire abnormal illness behaviors that prolong and embellish the symptom constellation (e.g., disability disproportionate to detectable disease, placement of responsibility on the physician, a sense of entitlement to be cared for by others, avoidance of health-promoting activities, and behavior that sustains the sick role).

For any illness, the clinician must decide if and when behavior intervention is required. For patients with chronic disease, this issue is best addressed in the context of the effect on daily life. It is important to consider the possibility of concurrent psychiatric diagnoses because these conditions are often subtle in presentation. Because psychiatric disease can modify the patient's experience of medical illness, proper treatment of the biological condition may include psychopharmacologic agents (e.g., antidepressant drugs) or behavior interventions and should take into account cultural and ethnic influences, family support, and psychosocial coping mechanisms that are unique to each patient.

PSYCHOSOCIAL TREATMENT

The initial step in any psychosocial intervention is to establish a therapeutic physician-patient relationship. This is accomplished when the physician elicits and validates the patient's beliefs, concerns, and expectations; offers empathy when needed; provides education; clarifies misconceptions; and, finally, develops a treatment plan with the patient's active involvement. A diagnostic plan, skillfully designed by the clinician, should exclude or detect organic disease without the performance of superfluous investigations, which can undermine patient confidence in physician competence. When appropriate to both the patient and the physician, the issue of psychosocial intervention may be raised.

Pharmacotherapy

The tricyclic antidepressants and serotonin reuptake inhibitors, in addition to treating major depression, are useful for treating chronic pain syndromes and associated vegetative symptoms (i.e., sleep disturbances, anorexia, weight loss, and decreased activity level). Tricyclic agents (e.g., amitriptyline and doxepin) control pain and have the added benefit of promoting sleep if given at bedtime. Desipramine and nortriptyline have fewer sedating and anticholinergic side effects but still provide relief of chronic pain. The serotonin reuptake inhibitors fluoxetine and sertraline have fewer side effects than the tricyclic agents, but their efficacy in treating gastrointestinal pain syndromes is less well established. Doses of these agents should be increased to therapeutic levels over 2 to 3 weeks and then maintained at these levels for at least 3 to 6 months. Poor clinical responses can result from inadequate dosing.

Other psychopharmacologic agents have been used for gastrointestinal disorders. Benzodiazepines and newer drugs (e.g., buspirone) have anxiolytic properties, but their utility is unproved. They can cause drug dependence behavior, and they may actually worsen underlying depression. Major tranquilizers or neuroleptics (e.g., the phenothiazines or butyrophenones) usually are of use only when disordered thought is present. Opiate agents have little or no role in treating chronic abdominal pain because of their abuse potential.

Behavior Treatments

Behavior treatments performed by psychologists, social workers, nurses, or physicians can reduce anxiety and pain levels, teach patients to promote their own health, and give them control over their treatment programs. Relaxation techniques, including biofeedback, meditation, and autogenic training, can alleviate stressors that contribute to biological illness. Biofeedback involves patient monitoring of physiologic activity, which may then be modified using visual or auditory cues. This technique has proved especially useful for bowel disturbances such as fecal incontinence or refractory constipation. Behavior modification may be used for patients with long-standing, maladaptive illness behavior. It may be used in withdrawal programs for narcotics addiction and in bowel retraining programs for severe constipation.

Psychotherapy

Psychotherapy should be considered if the patient has a treatable psychiatric disorder or an illness that impairs daily functioning or if the patient is motivated to address psychological functioning. The form of therapy is individualized: insight-oriented therapy for psychologically minded patients, group therapy for those who benefit from working on interpersonal issues, crisis intervention for persons with discrete recent stressors, and counseling for patients whose biological illness is affected by family or marital problems.

CHAPTER 2

Approach to the Patient with Dysphagia

DIFFERENTIAL DIAGNOSIS

Dysphagia refers to the sensation of food being hindered in its passage from the mouth to the stomach. The act of swallowing has four components—the oral preparation phase, the oral transfer phase, the pharyngeal phase, and the esophageal phase—all of which are mediated by a complex interplay of cranial nerves and motor and sensory pathways. An abnormality of any of the components can result in dysphagia. Dysphagia must be differentiated from odynophagia (pain on swallowing) and from globus sensation (perception of a lump, tightness, or fullness in the throat that is temporarily relieved by swallowing). Dysphagia is usually divided into two distinct categories: (1) those illnesses involving the oral preparation, oral transfer, or pharyngeal phases of swallowing, and (2) those conditions involving dysfunction of the esophageal phase (Table 2-1).

Oropharyngeal Dysphagia

Oral Preparation Defects

The oral preparation phase consists of the coordinated action of the lips, jaw, buccal and facial muscles, tongue, and soft palate that breaks down the food and mixes it with saliva to obtain a particle size and consistency appropriate for swallowing. Neurologic diseases that impair orofacial coordination, oral tumors that physically block food breakdown, poor dentition, and poor salivary output can affect the oral preparation phase of swallowing.

Oral Transfer Defects

The oral transfer phase is initiated by the movement of the tongue upward and backward against the palate, propelling the food bolus into the pharynx in a rapid symmetrical action that lasts <1 second. Neurologic diseases and tumors can cause incomplete bolus clearance from the mouth, delayed oral transit, and can require increased effort to swallow.

Pharyngeal Disorders

The pharyngeal phase coordinates pharynx and tongue movements to deliver the ingested bolus through an open cricopharyngeus (upper esophageal sphincter [UES]) into the esophagus in a rapid response that lasts <1 second. This process requires respiratory cessation, velopharyngeal and laryngeal closure, pharyngeal peristalsis, and elevation and anterior movement of the larynx. Pharyngeal phase defects that result in dysphagia include neurologic or structural diseases of the pharynx, many of which result in the filling of an inactive pharynx against a closed UES, and specific disorders of the UES, which are rare. Hypertensive UES syndrome is found in some patients with globus or with gastroesophageal reflux. Primary cricopharyngeal achalasia is characterized by the impaired transfer of barium from the pharynx to the upper esophagus. However, most cases of failure of UES relaxation result from central nervous system lymphoma and oculopharyngeal dystrophy. Zenker's diverticulum is an outpouching of one or more layers of the esophagus above the UES, which produces pharyngeal dysphagia as well as coughing, regurgitation, and aspiration. Radiographic and manometric studies suggest that Zenker's diverticulum may result from UES inelasticity.

Esophageal Dysphagia

The esophageal phase of swallowing involves the coordinated peristalsis of the esophageal body with the simultaneous relaxation of the lower esophageal sphincter (LES), a phenomenon that requires 7 to 15 seconds. This pattern,

---

TABLE 2-1
Causes of Dysphagia

Oropharyngeal dysphagia
    Neuromuscular diseases
        Cerebrovascular accident
        Parkinson's disease
        Wilson's disease
        Amyotrophic lateral sclerosis
        Brain stem tumors
        Bulbar poliomyelitis
        Peripheral neuropathy
        Myasthenia gravis
        Muscular dystrophies
        Polymyositis
        Metabolic myopathy
        Amyloidosis
        Systemic lupus erythematosus
    Local mechanical lesions
        Inflammation (pharyngitis, abscess, tuberculosis, radiation, syphilis)
        Neoplasm
        Congenital webs
        Plummer-Vinson syndrome
        Extrinsic compression (thyromegaly, cervical spine hyperostosis, adenopathy)
        Oropharyngeal resection
    Upper esophageal sphincter (UES) disorders
        Hypertensive UES
        Hypotensive UES
        Abnormal UES relaxation (cricopharyngeal achalasia, central nervous system
            lymphoma, oculopharyngeal muscular dystrophy, cricopharyngeal bar, Zenker's
            diverticulum, familial dysautonomia)
Esophageal dysphagia
    Motility disorders
        Achalasia
        Scleroderma
        Diffuse esophageal spasm
        Nutcracker esophagus
        Hypertensive lower esophageal sphincter
        Nonspecific esophageal dysmotility
        Other rheumatologic conditions
        Chagas' disease
    Intrinsic mechanical lesions
        Benign stricture (peptic, lye, radiation)
        Schatzki's ring
        Carcinoma
        Esophageal webs
        Esophageal diverticula
        Benign tumors
        Foreign bodies
    Extrinsic mechanical lesions
        Vascular compression
        Mediastinal abnormalities
        Cervical osteoarthritis

known as *primary peristalsis*, milks the food bolus into the stomach with little resistance. Secondary peristalsis refers to propulsive contractions of the esophageal body generated in response to retained food within the esophagus, and tertiary contractions signify uncoordinated, nonpropulsive motor activity, which may be observed in neuromuscular disease of the esophagus.

Obstructive Esophageal Lesions

The most prevalent causes of esophageal dysphagia are structural lesions that physically impede bolus passage into the stomach. Patients with esophageal strictures secondary to acid-peptic damage may have a long history of heartburn and present with progressive dysphagia. Peptic strictures are usually located in the distal esophagus; more proximal strictures suggest Barrett's esophagus, with metaplastic mucosal changes distal to the stricture. In contrast, patients with Schatzki's ring, which is a thin, circumferential mucosal structure at the gastroesophageal junction, present with episodic and nonprogressive dysphagia, which often occurs during rushed ingestion of poorly chewed meat. Patients with squamous cell carcinoma may present with progressive dysphagia, similar to peptic disease, but affected patients often are older with histories of long-standing tobacco or alcohol use and no prior pyrosis. Esophageal adenocarcinoma develops in areas of Barrett's metaplasia resulting from prolonged gastroesophageal reflux. Other mechanical lesions (e.g., abnormal great vessel anatomy, mediastinal lymphadenopathy, and cervical vertebral spurs) can rarely cause dysphagia.

Functional Esophageal Disease

The other major illness category responsible for esophageal dysphagia includes primary and secondary disorders of esophageal motor activity. Primary achalasia is an idiopathic disorder characterized by esophageal body aperistalsis and failure of the LES to relax on swallowing. Some patients have associated LES hypertension. Conditions that mimic the clinical presentation of primary achalasia include secondary achalasia, which is a disorder with identical radiographic and manometric characteristics resulting from malignancy at the gastroesophageal junction or from the paraneoplastic effects of a distant tumor, and Chagas' disease, resulting from an infection with *Trypanosoma cruzi*. Systemic diseases (e.g., scleroderma and other rheumatologic diseases) also can cause dysphagia because of effects on esophageal motor function. Other primary esophageal dysmotilities (i.e., nutcracker esophagus, diffuse esophageal spasm, vigorous achalasia, hypertensive LES, and nonspecific esophageal dysmotility) have also been associated with dysphagia.

WORKUP

History

The history should establish whether the dysphagia is oropharyngeal or esophageal in location and if it is structural or neuromuscular in origin. If dysphagia occurs during the act of swallowing and is associated with drooling, choking, coughing, nasal aspiration, or tossing movements of the head, then an oropharyngeal process is probable. Conversely, an esophageal cause is likely if dysphagia occurs seconds after swallowing, if there is associated retrosternal pain, and if regurgitation occurs some time after ingestion. Dysphagia perceived in the retrosternal or subxiphoid area is most consistent with an esophageal source, whereas in cervical dysphagia it is difficult to discriminate between oropharyngeal and esophageal causes. Structural disorders of the esophagus usually cause dysphagia to solids initially, with progression to liquid dysphagia only if lumenal narrowing becomes severe. In contrast, patients with neuromuscular disorders of the esophagus usually complain of both liquid and solid dysphagia from the onset of symptoms.

Physical Examination

The head and neck must be examined for sensory and motor function of the cranial nerves, masses, adenopathy, or spinal deformity. The patient is observed swallowing water so that the coordinated symmetrical action of the facial and cervical musculature can be visualized. The clinician should examine the patient for systemic disease, including the presence of sclerodactyly, telangiectasias, and calcinosis seen in scleroderma; neuropathies or muscle weakness characteristic of generalized neuromuscular disease; and hepatomegaly or adenopathy symptomatic of esophageal malignancy.

Additional Testing

The preferred diagnostic test for patients with oropharyngeal dysphagia is barium swallow radiography, which may require special techniques to assess the rapid changes in anatomy on swallowing (Fig. 2-1). If a structural lesion of the oropharynx is seen, upper endoscopy with biopsy is indicated to evaluate the underlying cause. Upper endoscopy may also identify vocal cord paralysis in neuromuscular disease. Videotaping of the patient swallowing barium preparations of different consistencies (i.e., thin liquid, thick liquid, barium cookie) can identify abnormalities of muscle action and direct therapies aimed at modifying meal composition and ingestion techniques. The development of improved UES manometry catheters has enhanced the ability to detect and characterize disorders of UES relaxation.

For dysphagia of presumed esophageal origin, barium swallow radiography may reveal occlusive lesions (e.g., carcinomas, strictures, rings, webs, or the characteristic bird's beak deformity of achalasia). The addition of a solid bolus (e.g., a marshmallow or barium pill) can increase the detection of subtle abnormalities. Upper endoscopy and possibly a biopsy should be performed to confirm any suggestive structural finding. If structural studies are nondiagnostic, manometry of the esophageal body and LES may assist in the diagnosis of achalasia and scleroderma as well as other primary and secondary esophageal motor disorders.

PRINCIPLES OF MANAGEMENT

Some patients with oropharyngeal dysphagia have treatable conditions, including Parkinson's disease, hypothyroidism, polymyositis, and myasthenia gravis. For untreatable neuromuscular conditions, consultation with a speech pathologist may afford development of a rehabilitation program to modify swallowing techniques. Surgical myotomy can benefit patients with Zenker's diverticulum

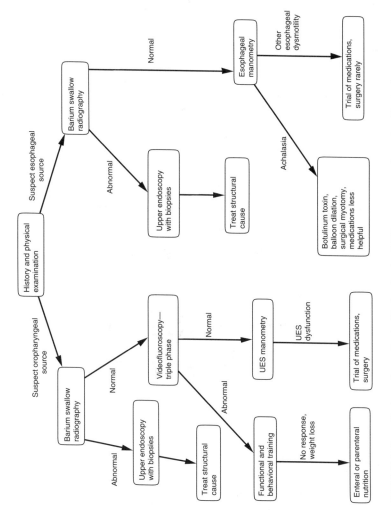

FIGURE 2-1. Workup of a patient with dysphagia. (UES = upper esophageal sphincter.)

or cricopharyngeal achalasia. A few limited studies suggest that myotomy may also be useful in the treatment of selected patients with neuromuscular disease.

Management of esophageal dysphagia is dependent on its cause. Benign strictures, webs, and rings can be dilated by bougienage. Early malignancies may be surgically resected, whereas dilation, cautery, laser, or stenting may be used for unresectable lesions. Achalasia can be treated with medications (e.g., calcium channel antagonists), with botulinum toxin injection into the LES, by endoscopic dilation, and by surgical myotomy. Other primary esophageal dysmotilities may respond to nitrates, calcium channel antagonists, and, in rare instances, surgical myotomy.

COMPLICATIONS

The most serious complication of oropharyngeal dysphagia is tracheal aspiration, with development of cough, asthma, or pneumonia. Esophageal dysphagia results in a failure to thrive because of reduced oral intake.

CHAPTER 3

Approach to the Patient with Chest Pain

DIFFERENTIAL DIAGNOSIS

Noncardiac chest pain is prevalent in the United States, with 180,000 new cases of chest pain occurring annually in patients who have patent coronary arteries on cardiac catheterization studies. Although these patients usually have a favorable prognosis, they represent a significant cost to the medical system because of physician visits, patient hospitalizations, and medication use. The differential diagnosis of noncardiac chest pain includes cardiac causes, musculoskeletal pain, psychiatric disease, and esophageal disorders (Table 3-1). Less common causes include peptic ulcer, biliary tract disease, pleuropul-

TABLE 3-1
Causes of Chest Pain

Cardiac disease
    Coronary artery disease
    Coronary artery spasm
    Microvascular angina
    Mitral valve prolapse
Musculoskeletal causes
    Costochondritis
    Fibromyalgia
    Inflammatory arthritis
    Osteoarthritis
    Thoracic spinal disease
    Nerve entrapment or compression
    Varicella-zoster virus reactivation
Esophageal disease
    Gastroesophageal reflux
    Nutcracker esophagus
    Diffuse esophageal spasm
    Hypertensive lower esophageal sphincter
    Achalasia
    Nonspecific esophageal dysmotility
    Infectious or pill-induced esophagitis
    Food impaction
Neuropsychiatric causes
    Panic disorder
    Anxiety disorder
    Depression
    Somatization

monary disease, mediastinitis, dissecting aortic aneurysm, and varicella-zoster virus infection of the chest wall.

Library Resource Center
Renton Technical College
3000 N.E. 4th St.
Renton, WA 98056

Cardiac Disease

Even if the coronary arteries are normal, cardiac sources need to be considered in a patient with chest pain. Coronary artery spasm in response to ergonovine infusion has been reported in subsets of patients with chest pain. Some patients with exertional chest pain have abnormalities of the smaller endocardial vasculature without evidence of fixed lesions or spasm of the epicardial vessels, a condition termed *microvascular angina*. Diagnosis of this disorder requires measurement of cardiac lactate production and coronary sinus blood flow during fasting and after rapid atrial pacing followed by intravenous ergonovine challenge. This condition should be considered in patients with ischemic ST segment changes on electrocardiographic examination or if left ventricular ejection fractions decrease in response to exercise on echocardiographic or radionuclide ventriculographic studies. The relationship of chest pain to mitral valve prolapse is controversial. Further confusing these issues are reports that document the coexistence of esophageal motor abnormalities with both microvascular angina and mitral valve prolapse.

Musculoskeletal Causes

Patients with chest pain from musculoskeletal sources (e.g., costochondritis [Tietze's syndrome], fibromyalgia, inflammatory arthritis, osteoarthritis, thoracic spinal disease) may have localized chest wall tenderness, definable trigger points, and pain at rest, with movement, or during sleep.

Neuropsychiatric Causes

Panic disorder, the most recognized psychiatric condition that presents with chest pain, is characterized by at least three attacks in as many weeks of intense fear or discomfort accompanied by at least four of the following symptoms: chest pain, restlessness, choking, palpitations, sweating, dizziness, nausea or abdominal distress, paresthesia, flushing, trembling, and a sense of impending doom. It has been reported that 34% to 59% of patients with noncardiac chest pain have panic disorder. Investigation of these patients demonstrates an increased prevalence of anxiety disorders, depression, and somatization.

Esophageal Disease

There are several distinct esophageal causes of noncardiac chest pain. Gastroesophageal reflux of acid produces chest pain in many patients; a small percentage exhibit altered esophageal motor patterns on acid perfusion. In most patients, however, there is a poor correlation between chest pain and acid reflux episodes. Primary esophageal motor disorders, including nutcracker esophagus, diffuse esophageal spasm, hypertensive lower esophageal sphincter (LES), achalasia, and nonspecific esophageal dysmotilities, are found in <50% of patients with noncardiac chest pain, although the causal nature of the dysmotilities is controversial. Studies indicating that many patients with noncardiac chest pain exhibit hypersensitivity to balloon distention of the esophagus suggest a defect in afferent neural function. Miscellaneous esophageal sources of chest pain include infectious or pill-induced esophagitis, which produces odynophagia, and food impaction.

WORKUP

History

Intermittent anterior chest pain is the basis of the esophageal chest pain syndrome and usually is described as squeezing or burning in character and substernal in location. The pain can radiate in a pattern indistinguishable from angina, and it may not be related to swallowing. Chest pain can be exacerbated by ingestion of cold or hot liquids or by stress, and it can awaken the patient from sleep. Esophageal chest pain can be severe, lasting from minutes to hours. If carefully questioned, the majority of persons with esophageal sources of pain report heartburn, regurgitation, dysphagia, or odynophagia. Despite this, it is often difficult to distinguish esophageal pain from cardiac chest pain based on the clinical history, although pain that persists for hours, pain without lateral radiation, pain that interrupts sleep or occurs with meals, pain that is relieved by antacids, and the presence of other esophageal symptoms suggest an esophageal focus.

Physical Examination

The physical examination rarely helps in diagnosing a patient with noncardiac chest pain. Reproduction of the presenting pain by chest wall palpation suggests a musculoskeletal source. Detection of pleural rubs or changes in breath sounds infers pleuropulmonary disease, and cutaneous eruptions in a dermatomal pattern indicate probable varicella-zoster virus reactivation as the cause of pain. The characteristic midsystolic click and murmur of mitral valve prolapse may be heard on cardiac auscultation. Abdominal tenderness should suggest peptic or biliary tract disease.

Additional Testing

The examination of a patient with chest pain must begin with the careful exclusion of cardiac disease, which in most cases will include negative findings on an electrocardiogram during chest pain, normal findings on an echocardiogram, and negative findings on exercise stress testing (Fig. 3-1). In older patients or patients with more difficult cases, cardiac catheterization with possible ergonovine testing may be required. Once cardiac disease is excluded, other noncardiac sources for chest pain may be evaluated. Musculoskeletal causes are usually detected on physical examination, whereas psychiatric causes may require referral for psychometric testing and for consideration of specific psychopharmacologic and behavior treatment.

Evaluation for esophageal disorders begins with barium swallow radiography or upper endoscopy, which may reveal esophageal or gastric ulcerations to be the cause of the pain. If structural studies produce normal results, gastroesophageal reflux should be excluded because this is the most common esophageal source of chest pain. Alternate approaches include an empirical trial with a proton pump inhibitor (e.g., omeprazole) or diagnostic confirmation of acid reflux with 24-hour ambulatory esophageal pH monitoring using a probe placed 5 cm above the LES. An esophageal pH of <4 for >5% of the total exposure time infers a diagnosis of gastroesophageal reflux with a sensitivity of 85% and a specificity of 95%. If ambulatory pH testing is unavailable, acid perfusion testing can be performed. With this technique, alternating infusions of 0.1 normal hydrochloric acid and normal saline should reproduce and then relieve the patient's chest pain.

If these tests are unrevealing, esophageal manometry with provocative testing may define an underlying esophageal dysmotility syndrome. Alone, manometry will detect potentially pathogenic motor abnormalities in only a minority of patients with noncardiac chest pain. Challenge with ergonovine, an α-adrenergic stimulant, reproduces chest pain in 22% to 48% of patients. However, this agent also evokes chest pain in 20% of asymptomatic volunteers and may induce cardiac arrhythmias in patients with underlying cardiac disease. Bethanechol is a cholinergic agonist that, in high doses, can produce chest pain and nonspecific motility changes in two-thirds of patients, although undesirable side effects are often observed. The cholinesterase inhibitor, edrophonium, is the most popular provocative test because of its safety profile. Edrophonium evokes chest pain and esophageal motor disturbances in 18% to 55% of patients referred for testing. Nonpharmacologic means of assessing primary esophageal dysmotilities as causes of chest pain (i.e., 24-hour ambulatory

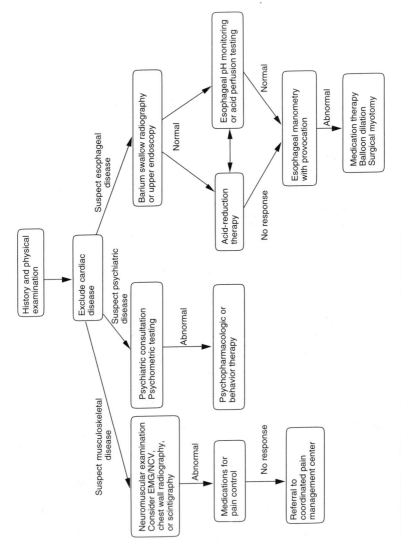

FIGURE 3-1. Workup of a patient with chest pain. (EMG/NCV = electromyogram/nerve conduction velocity test.)

esophageal manometry and provocative balloon distention of the esophagus) have given encouraging results but have not yet been widely used.

PRINCIPLES OF MANAGEMENT

Satisfactory treatment of esophageal chest pain traditionally has been difficult because of diagnostic uncertainties, the intermittent nature of symptoms, the side effect profiles of available pharmaceutical agents, and the awareness that many of these conditions improve spontaneously without treatment. If they are given a careful diagnostic examination, many patients respond to confident physician reassurance that no dangerous condition exists. In patients with underlying gastroesophageal reflux, a trial of aggressive antireflux therapy for 2 months is indicated. If a therapeutic response is achieved, long-term antireflux medical therapy may be needed. Alternatively, antireflux surgery should be considered in patients with severe pain secondary to gastroesophageal reflux that is poorly responsive to appropriate medical therapy. For painful esophageal dysmotility, nitrates and calcium channel blockers may be considered, although response rates for these agents often are low. Investigations suggest that many of these patients respond instead to antidepressant agents (e.g., trazodone or imipramine) at doses lower than those used to treat endogenous depression. For panic disorders, anxiolytics (e.g., benzodiazepines or buspirone) may be effective; however, these agents have abuse potential, may induce tolerance, and may exacerbate underlying depression. In refractory esophageal motor disorders, esophageal dilation or surgical myotomy may relieve symptoms in rare cases. Studies suggest a role for cognitive or behavioral therapy, which produces significant improvements in chest pain, functional disability, and psychological distress in selected patient populations.

COMPLICATIONS

Chest pain of esophageal origin rarely has long-term sequelae. The major risk in the evaluation of a patient with chest pain is the premature exclusion of coronary ischemia, which may have life-threatening consequences.

CHAPTER 4

Approach to the Patient with Gross Gastrointestinal Bleeding

Gastrointestinal (GI) bleeding is a common problem that varies in severity from life-threatening hemorrhage to insidious blood loss that produces iron deficiency anemia. It is therefore important to assess both the severity and the site of blood loss in a patient with GI hemorrhage. Hematemesis (vomiting of bright-red blood or coffee ground–colored matter) indicates an acute upper GI source, proximal to the ligament of Treitz. Melena (black, malodorous, tarry stools that indicate intestinal degradation of blood) usually results from acute upper GI bleeding, although bleeding from the small intestine and the right colon may produce melena. Hematochezia (bright-red rectal bleeding) usually indicates a colonic source; however, if an upper GI site bleeds briskly enough, hematochezia or maroon-colored stools can result. Because the evaluation and management of gross upper and lower GI bleeding are so different, they are addressed separately.

ACUTE UPPER GASTROINTESTINAL BLEEDING

Differential Diagnosis

The major causes of gross upper GI bleeding are peptic ulcer disease, gastritis, and sequelae of portal hypertension (i.e., esophageal and gastric varices, portal gastropathy), although other causes should be considered (Table 4-1). The distribution of these causes depends on the patient population studied.

Peptic Ulcer Disease

Duodenal, gastric, and stomal ulcers account for one-half of upper GI bleeding episodes. Despite effective therapy for chronic peptic ulcers, the rates of hospitalization of patients with bleeding ulcers have remained constant because many patients with ulcer hemorrhage present without a prior history of peptic ulcer disease and because of the increased use of NSAIDs in elderly populations. Bleeding occurs if an ulcer erodes into the lateral wall of a vessel, which may loop into the floor of the ulcer crater, forming an aneurysmal dilation. The most com-

---

TABLE 4-1
Causes of Gross Gastrointestinal Hemorrhage

Upper gastrointestinal sources
   Peptic ulcer disease (duodenal, gastric, stomal)
   Gastritis (NSAID-, stress-, chemotherapy-induced)
   Varices (esophageal, gastric, duodenal)
   Portal gastropathy
   Mallory-Weiss tear
   Esophagitis and esophageal ulcers (acid reflux, infection, pill-induced, sclerotherapy, radiation-induced)
   Neoplasms
   Vascular ectasias and angiodysplasias
   Watermelon stomach
   Aortoenteric fistula
   Hematobilia
   Hemosuccus pancreaticus
   Dieulafoy's erosion
Lower gastrointestinal sources
   Diverticulosis
   Angiodysplasia
   Hemorrhoids
   Anal fissures
   Neoplasms
   Inflammatory bowel disease
   Ischemic colitis
   Infectious colitis
   Radiation-induced colitis
   Meckel's diverticulum
   Intussusception
   Aortoenteric fistula
   Solitary rectal ulcers
   NSAID-induced cecal ulcers

---

mon causes of gastroduodenal ulcer disease are infection with *Helicobacter pylori* and ingestion of NSAIDs.

Gastritis

Endoscopically, gastritis is defined by the presence of mucosal hemorrhages, erythema, and erosions. An erosion, in contrast to an ulcer, represents a break in the mucosa of <5 mm that does not traverse the muscularis mucosae. Common causes of gastritis include NSAID ingestion and stress. NSAID gastritis or ulcer disease develops in a small percentage of patients chronically using the drugs, usually involves the antrum, and may quickly resolve if the medication can be discontinued. Stress gastritis most commonly occurs in patients in the intensive care unit who have respiratory failure, hypotension, sepsis, renal failure, burns, peritonitis, jaundice, or neurologic trauma. Of these patients, 2% to 10% exhibit gross hemorrhage. The hallmark of stress gastritis is the presence of multiple bleeding sites, which limits the therapeutic options. A rare cause of gastritis is chemotherapy delivered through the hepatic artery, which may induce mucosal necrosis of the stomach and duodenum.

Hemorrhage Secondary to Portal Hypertension

The common causes of upper GI hemorrhage in patients with portal hypertension include esophageal and gastric varices and portal gastropathy. Approximately one-fourth to one-third of patients with cirrhosis experience variceal hemorrhage on at least one occasion. This is significant because 30% to 50% of patients die of their initial esophageal variceal hemorrhage, and two-thirds die within one year. A portal pressure of 12 mm Hg or more must be present for varices to develop, although above this level the absolute pressure correlates poorly with the propensity for bleeding. The best predictor of esophageal variceal hemorrhage is variceal size, because wall tension is determined by the diameter of a hollow vessel. Other predictors of esophageal variceal bleeding include the red color sign, which is the result of microtelangiectasia; red wale marks, which appear as whip marks; hemocystic spots, which appear as blood blisters; and diffuse redness. The white nipple sign, a platelet-fibrin plug, is diagnostic of previous hemorrhage but is not predictive of rebleeding.

Gastric varices, usually in the fundus and cardia, are present in 20% of patients with portal hypertension and develop in another 8% after esophageal variceal obliteration. Most gastric varices span the gastroesophageal junction, merging with esophageal columns. The presence of isolated gastric varices suggests splenic vein thrombosis, which often is secondary to pancreatic disease and is treated by splenectomy. Patients with ectopic varices elsewhere in the stomach and duodenum may rarely present with hemorrhage. Portal gastropathy appears endoscopically as a mosaic, snakeskin-like mucosa that is caused by engorged vessels, which may bleed briskly or, alternatively, produce insidious iron deficiency anemia. Note that the presence of cirrhosis does not mean that varices or gastropathy are the source of hemorrhage, as ulcers and other bleeding sites are found in up to 50% of cases.

Miscellaneous Causes of Upper Gastrointestinal Bleeding

Mallory-Weiss tears are linear breaks in the mucosa of the gastroesophageal junction that are caused by retching, perhaps with forceful gastric mucosal prolapse. They often occur after alcohol ingestion. Most Mallory-Weiss tears resolve spontaneously with conservative management. Esophagitis and esophageal ulcers result from acid reflux, radiation therapy, infections with *Candida albicans* and herpes simplex virus, pill-induced damage, or iatrogenic sources (e.g., sclerotherapy). Because the lesions are shallower, hemorrhage from erosive duodenitis usually is less severe than that from a duodenal ulcer. Neoplasms most often exhibit slow blood loss but rarely may exhibit massive hemorrhage. Vascular ectasia and angiodysplasia are associated with advanced age, chronic renal failure, aortic valve disease, and prior radiation therapy. Hereditary hemorrhagic telangiectasia, or Osler-Weber-Rendu syndrome, is an autosomal dominant disorder characterized by telangiectasia of the tongue; lips; conjunctiva; skin; and mucosa of the gut, bladder, and nasopharynx. The watermelon stomach, or gastric arteriovenous ectasia, is a variant of gastric ectasia that endoscopically appears as columns of vessels along the tops of the antral longitudinal rugae. Biopsy specimens show dilated mucosal capillaries with focal thrombosis and fibromuscular hyperplasia of the vessels of the lamina propria. An aortoenteric fistula is a rare cause of massive upper GI hemorrhage, occurring most commonly after aortic graft surgery. This entity often exhibits a minor "herald" hemorrhage from the third portion of the duodenum before fatal exsanguination; therefore, immediate diagnosis is mandatory. Hemobilia and hemosuccus pancreaticus are complications of liver trauma or biopsy, malignancy, hepatic artery aneurysm, hepatic abscess, gallstones, and pancreatic pseudocyst and are characterized by rapid blood loss from the ampulla of Vater. A Dieulafoy's erosion is defined as a ruptured thick-walled artery that is larger than surrounding submucosal vessels, with little or no mucosal ulceration. Bleeding from a Dieulafoy's erosion is believed to result from pressure erosion of the overlying mucosa. Some patients present with upper GI bleeding from epistaxis, hemoptysis, oral lesions, or factitious blood ingestion.

Workup

Resuscitation

The first step in the assessment of a patient with upper GI bleeding is to determine the urgency of the clinical condition (Fig. 4-1). Hematemesis, melena, or hematochezia usually suggest a major hemorrhage. Pallor, hypotension, and tachycardia are evidence of substantial blood volume loss (>40%) and mandate immediate volume replacement. Postural hypotension of >10 mm Hg indicates a 20% blood volume reduction, which usually must be replaced immediately. Intravenous access should be obtained with two large-bore catheters, and, if the patient is in shock, a central venous line should be used. A nasogastric tube is placed. A bright-red aspirate that does not clear with lavage is an indication for emergency upper endoscopy, as this situation is associated with a 30% mortality, whereas coffee ground–colored material that clears permits further assessment in a hemodynamically stable patient. A clear aspirate is found in some patients with duodenal bleeding; therefore, the upper gut is not precluded as a source of hemorrhage. Blood samples are sent to the laboratory for measurement of hematocrit, platelets, and coagulation factors and for blood typing and crossmatching. Significant intravascular volume losses should be immediately replaced with normal saline while awaiting the arrival of blood products. Hemodynamically unstable patients should be admitted to an intensive care unit.

History

While resuscitation is under way, a directed history usually can be obtained. Prior histories of peptic disease and dyspeptic symptoms suggest ulcer bleeding. It is important to inquire about ingestion of NSAIDs, alcohol, or caustic substances. Patients with suspected liver disease are treated aggressively, usually undergoing urgent upper endoscopy because of the risk of varices. Other historical elements (e.g., prior aortic surgery, coagulopathies, known or suspected neoplasm, or recent nosebleeds) may suggest specific diagnoses.

Physical Examination

Careful physical examination can provide diagnostic clues. Cutaneous stigmata of cirrhosis or malignancy may be present. Multiple cutaneous telangiectases suggest possible hereditary hemorrhagic telangiectasia. Lymphadenopathy, hepatosplenomegaly,

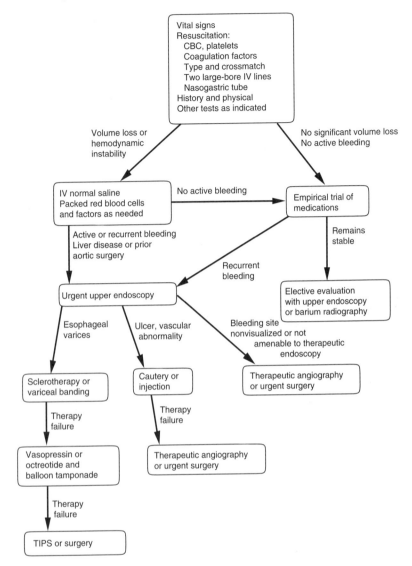

FIGURE 4-1. Workup of a patient with acute upper gastrointestinal bleeding. (CBC = complete blood count; IV = intravenous; TIPS = transjugular intrahepatic portosystemic shunt.)

and abdominal masses raise the possibility of neoplasm; splenomegaly, ascites, or dilated abdominal wall vessels suggest portal hypertension.

Additional Testing

Laboratory Studies. A hematocrit platelet count, and coagulation studies should be part of the initial workup. The first hematocrit determination may not reflect the degree of blood loss because acute hemorrhage produces loss of both red cells and volume, and therefore the ratio of the two variables does not change. As intravascular volume is replenished by endogenous and exogenous fluids, the hematocrit decreases gradually to a stable level over 24 to 48 hours. A low hematocrit or microcytic indices may indicate chronic blood loss, which can be confirmed with iron studies or ferritin measurement. Thrombocytopenia results from bone marrow disease, autoimmune disorders, or portal hypertension with splenomegaly. Prolongation of the prothrombin time is seen with liver disease, warfarin use, or malnutrition. In massive upper GI bleeding, azotemia reflects intestinal absorption of the nitrogenous breakdown products of blood coupled with hypovolemic effects, whereas azotemia with elevations in creatinine concentrations suggests renal insufficiency. Abnormal liver chemistry findings should raise concern about the possibility of cirrhosis with portal hypertension.

Upper Endoscopy.   Urgent upper endoscopy is indicated in patients with bleeding that does not stop spontaneously or in those patients suspected of having cirrhosis or aortoenteric fistulae. If bleeding has stopped, endoscopy may be postponed without compromising care. Some patients with uncomplicated courses of illness may be given empirical therapy for presumed peptic disease if both the physician and patient are comfortable without a specific diagnosis. Upper endoscopy is absolutely contraindicated in cases in which perforation is suspected and is relatively contraindicated in patients with compromised cardiopulmonary status or depressed levels of consciousness. In these circumstances, endotracheal intubation with mechanical ventilation may enhance the safety of the technique. Upper GI barium radiography is not performed in the acute setting with a potentially unstable patient.

Scintigraphy and Angiography.   When hemorrhage is so brisk that it obscures endoscopic visualization, studies to assess lumenal blood loss are indicated. Scintigraphic ^{99m}Tc-sulfur colloid– or ^{99m}Tc-pertechnetate–labeled erythrocyte scans can localize bleeding to an area of the abdomen if the rate of blood loss exceeds 0.5 ml per minute. Scintigraphy is most commonly used to determine if angiography is feasible and to direct the angiographic search while minimizing the dye load. Angiography is used in cases when endoscopy cannot visualize the lumen because of massive hemorrhage. However, to detect a source of bleeding, the rate of blood loss must exceed 0.5 ml per minute as well. Angiography also may detect vascular ectasia in patients with intermittent hemorrhage who have normal findings on upper endoscopy, and also is useful in identifying the bleeding source with hemobilia or hemosuccus pancreaticus.

Other Radiographic Studies.   If an aortoenteric fistula is suspected, a vigorous diagnostic approach including abdominal computed tomographic or magnetic resonance imaging studies should be pursued after endoscopy has excluded other bleeding sources.

Principles of Management

Transfusion of Blood Products

Volume replacement should begin with intravenous administration of normal saline, but transfusions of blood products may be needed to treat significant hemorrhage. The need for transfusion is influenced by patient age, coexistent cardiovascular disease, and persistent hemorrhage. In general, the hematocrit should be maintained above 30% in elderly patients and above 20% in younger patients. Packed red cells are preferred for blood transfusion to minimize the fluid load. If the findings of coagulation studies are abnormal, as in cirrhosis, fresh frozen plasma or platelets may be required to control ongoing hemorrhage. Even patients without coagulopathy may need fresh frozen plasma if multiple transfusions are given, as transfused blood is deficient in some clotting factors. Patients with massive blood loss (>3 liters) should receive warmed blood to prevent hypothermia; some of these patients receiving massive transfusions also require supplemental calcium to counter the calcium-binding effects of preserved blood.

Medications

Empirical medical treatment is often begun in a patient with upper GI hemorrhage before the diagnostic examination is completed; however, multiple trials of pharmacologic agents have not shown improved survival. For presumed peptic disease or stress gastritis, intravenous histamine H_2-receptor antagonists may be given, although meta-analyses demonstrate only marginally reduced rates of surgery or mortality. For presumed varices or portal gastropathy, intravenous vasopressin is given at a dose of 0.2 to 0.4 units per minute in patients without cardiovascular contraindications, although placebo-controlled trials do not reliably demonstrate the efficacy of this agent. Intravenous or transdermal nitroglycerin may enhance the reduction in portal pressures and reduce the complication rate of intravenous vasopressin. A synthetic analog of vasopressin, terlipressin, exhibits increased efficacy compared with vasopressin itself. Investigations suggest that intravenous somatostatin and its octapeptide analog, octreotide (25 to 50 µg per hour), reduce variceal bleeding more effectively than vasopressin, and many centers are using these agents in lieu of vasopressin. Intravenous or oral estrogens with or without progesterone can be of benefit in treating recurrent bleeding from angiodysplastic lesions, although they are unlikely to be effective in the acute setting.

Therapeutic Endoscopy

Urgent upper endoscopy is performed for acute upper GI hemorrhage in the setting of presumed liver disease, aortoenteric fistula, or bleeding that does not stop. Before endoscopy, the stomach should be lavaged through a large-bore orogastric tube with room temperature saline or water to enhance mucosal visualization. There are no advantages to chilled lavage solutions or preparations containing vasoconstricting agents such as levarterenol. If an actively bleeding ulcer is observed, endoscopic therapy may be provided using thermal and nonthermal methods, which are efficacious both in the initial control of hemorrhage and in the prevention of rebleeding. Additional meta-analyses also suggest reductions in mortality with endoscopic therapy. Thermal methods include bipolar electrocautery, heater probe application, and Nd:YAG laser therapy. Nonthermal injection techniques with vasoconstrictors (e.g., epinephrine), sclerosants (e.g., alcohol and ethanolamine), or even saline provide comparable control of upper GI hemorrhage to thermal methods. Stigmata of recent hemorrhage that significantly increase the risk of rebleeding in an ulcer patient who has stopped bleeding include a nonbleeding visible vessel and an adherent clot. In a patient who has had a major hemorrhage, thermal or injection therapy should be considered for visible vessels or for adherent clots, which, when washed off, reveal visible vessels or active bleeding. Other sources amenable to endoscopic therapy include refractory Mallory-Weiss tears, neoplasms, angiodysplastic lesions, or Dieulafoy's erosions. Conversely, patients with stress gastritis, NSAID-induced gastritis, and portal gastropathy usually present with multiple bleeding sites that cannot be controlled endoscopically.

Emergency upper endoscopy is indicated for management of esophageal variceal hemorrhage. Injection sclerotherapy (e.g., using sodium morrhuate, ethanolamine) into or adjacent to the bleeding varix has a success rate of 85% to 95% in controlling the initial hemorrhage. Variceal band ligation appears to be as effective as sclerotherapy and may reduce the development of complications (e.g., esophageal ulcers or stricturing). In contrast, gastric varices usually are not amenable to sclerotherapy or banding and require nonendoscopic control.

Mechanical Compression

For patients who fail to respond to endoscopic therapy of variceal hemorrhage, balloon tamponade with a Sengstaken-Blakemore or Linton-Nachlas tube achieves initial hemostasis in up to 90% of cases; however, rebleeding rates are high after removal of the device. Most patients benefit from prophylactic endotracheal intubation before balloon tamponade. Initial inflation of the gastric balloon controls hemorrhage in some patients, but many require controlled inflation of both the gastric and esophageal balloons for optimal hemostasis.

Therapeutic Angiography

In peptic ulcer hemorrhage refractory to endoscopic control, angiographic embolization with absorbable gelatin sponge (Gelfoam) or an autologous clot may be attempted, but these treatments are best reserved for patients who are not candidates for surgery. Intra-arterial vasopressin or embolization may be useful in some patients with stress gastritis bleeding, as well as in those with bleeding from esophageal sources, refractory Mallory-Weiss tears, neoplasms, hemobilia, and hemosuccus pancreaticus.

Patients with esophageal variceal hemorrhage refractory to endoscopic management or with bleeding from gastric varices or portal gastropathy may benefit from angiographic placement of a transjugular intrahepatic portosystemic shunt (TIPS). With TIPS, an expandable metal stent is placed between the hepatic and portal veins to reduce portal pressure. TIPS has been considered a bridge to more definitive treatment (i.e., hepatic transplantation or surgical portosystemic shunting) because the shunt tends to occlude over time. Other angiographic methods to control variceal hemorrhage are available but are not commonly used because of their technical difficulty and complication rates.

Surgery

In cases where upper endoscopy or angiography fails to control the source of bleeding, emergency surgery may be required. Early surgical intervention is indicated for persistent or recurrent bleeding from ulcers, Mallory-Weiss tears, Dieulafoy's erosions, or for "herald" bleeding from aortoenteric fistulae. Antrectomy may be required for watermelon stomach. Urgent portocaval shunting or esophageal devascularization may be required for hemorrhage in patients with portal hypertension, although the mortality rate for these procedures exceeds 50%. Moreover, many patients experience worsening liver function or hepatic encephalopathy after portocaval shunts. Recurrent variceal hemorrhage is considered an indication for hepatic transplantation in patients with advanced liver disease. In contrast, splenectomy is the procedure of choice for hemorrhage from isolated gastric varices secondary to splenic vein thrombosis.

Complications

The most serious complication of upper GI bleeding is exsanguination and death. Mortality is 8% to 10% for upper GI hemorrhage and increases to 30% to 40% for patients with persistent or recurrent bleeding. Therefore, a major focus of research has been on means to prevent initial or recurrent hemorrhage. For bleeding from ulcers, directed treatments at causes such as *H pylori* are indicated. Prostaglandin analogs (e.g., misoprostol) have demonstrated efficacy in preventing NSAID-induced gastritis and ulcers. H_2-receptor antagonists appear to prevent duodenal, but not gastric, mucosal lesions resulting from NSAID use. Stress gastritis prophylaxis includes H_2-receptor antagonists, high-dose antacids, or sucralfate, all of which have demonstrated efficacy. Sucralfate therapy may be associated with lower rates of nosocomial pneumonias in mechanically ventilated patients. Chronic estrogen-progesterone therapy may reduce transfusion requirements in patients with angiodysplasia, either with or without concomitant renal insufficiency.

Because of the high mortality of hemorrhage in patients with portal hypertension, prevention of rebleeding is crucial. Obliteration of varices with multiple courses of endoscopic sclerotherapy or variceal band ligation reduces rebleeding rates, although the effects on mortality are less certain. Meta-analyses suggest that propranolol therapy to reduce portal pressures reduces the probability of initial and recurrent hemorrhage from esophageal varices. Propranolol has also shown efficacy in preventing rebleeding from portal gastropathy.

ACUTE LOWER GASTROINTESTINAL BLEEDING

Differential Diagnosis

The two most common causes of acute lower GI bleeding are diverticulosis and angiodysplasia (see Table 4-1). Chronic or recurrent lower GI hemorrhage is most often caused by hemorrhoids and colonic neoplasia. Unlike most upper GI bleeding, most lower GI bleeding is slow and intermittent and does not require hospitalization.

Diverticulosis

Diverticular bleeding, which occurs in 3% of patients with diverticulosis, usually is associated with acute, painless passage of red or maroon stool, although melena may occur. Despite the preponderance of diverticula in the sigmoid colon, many bleeding diverticula are right-sided. Most cases spontaneously resolve and do not recur; therefore, no specific therapy is indicated for the majority of patients.

Angiodysplasia

Twenty percent to 40% of acute lower GI bleeding episodes result from vascular ectasia or angiodysplasia. Angiodysplastic lesions are also common causes of chronic blood loss. Colonic angiodysplastic lesions are usually multiple, small (<5 mm in diameter), and localized to the right colon and cecum. As with gastroduodenal vascular ectasia, colonic lesions are associated with advanced age and aortic valve disease, although the latter association has been questioned.

Perianal Disease

Hemorrhoids and anal fissures usually cause minor lower GI bleeding, most commonly observed in the form of spots of blood on the toilet tissue after a bowel movement. In contrast, hemorrhage from rectal varices in patients with portal hypertension may be life-threatening. Because patients with polyps and carcinoma may present in similar fashion to patients with hemorrhoids or fissures, these causes need to be excluded in the appropriate populations.

Colonic Neoplasia

Benign and malignant colonic neoplasms are common in elderly patients and usually associated with small degrees of intermittent bleeding or occult blood loss. In contrast, small intestinal neoplasms are rare disorders that have increased incidence in inflammatory conditions (e.g., Crohn's disease or celiac sprue).

Miscellaneous Causes of Lower Gastrointestinal Bleeding

The degree of bleeding from inflammatory bowel disease (IBD) is usually small to moderate, but rarely it may be massive. Blood is usually mixed with diarrheal stool in patients with IBD and is associated with tenesmus and pain. Colitis also may be produced by ischemia (most commonly with low-flow states), infection (*Campylobacter jejuni*, *Salmonella* species, *Shigella* species, *Escherichia coli*), and radiation therapy (acute or chronic). Meckel's diverticulum is the most prevalent congenital abnormality of the GI tract, being characterized as an ileal diverticulum resulting from incomplete obliteration of the vitelline duct. One-half of these lesions contain gastric mucosa that produces acid, resulting in ulceration of the adjacent ileal mucosa. Patients usually present in childhood with painless red or melenic bleeding, which has been described as having a "currant jelly" appearance. Patients with intussusception present with maroon stools and crampy pain; the intussusception usually occurs at the site of a polyp or malignancy in adults. Other rare causes of lower GI bleeding in adults include aortoenteric fistulae, solitary rectal ulcers (caused by constipation-induced rectal prolapse), and cecal ulcers (most often caused by NSAIDs).

Workup

Resuscitation

Resuscitation of acute lower GI bleeding follows similar protocols to those for upper GI hemorrhage, with prompt correction of volume deficits and stabilization of hemodynamic variables (Fig. 4-2). Although most sources of bright-red rectal bleeding are colonic, extremely brisk upper GI hemorrhage may rarely be associated with hematochezia. If there is any doubt about the location of bleeding, a nasogastric tube should be placed and upper endoscopy performed. Laboratory studies provide the same information as with upper GI sources,

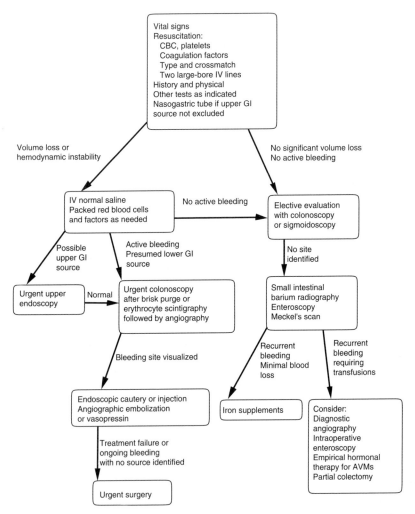

FIGURE 4-2. Workup of a patient with acute lower gastrointestinal bleeding. (CBC = complete blood count; IV = intravenous; AVMs = arteriovenous malformations.)

although azotemia resulting from intralumenal blood degradation usually does not occur.

History and Physical Examination

Prior histories of GI disease (e.g., hemorrhoids or IBD) may suggest specific diagnoses. Coexistent symptoms (e.g., diarrhea or pain) raise the possibility of colitis or malignancy. Malignancy is also indicated by other findings (e.g., weight loss, anorexia, lymphadenopathy, or palpable masses).

Additional Testing

Endoscopy.   In cases of lower GI bleeding that is slow or stopped, colonoscopy is the diagnostic procedure of choice and is capable of detecting nearly all potential colonic sources of blood loss, including angiodysplasia, perianal disease, neoplasms, colitis, and colorectal ulcers. Colonoscopy will document the presence of diverticula; however, in many instances it will not identify the actual bleeding site. In contrast, barium enema radiography may miss up to 20% of endoscopically identifiable lesions, especially angiodysplastic lesions, and is less useful. With brisk, ongoing bleeding, colonoscopy may be attempted after a rapid purge, providing a diagnostic accuracy similar to angiography in such settings. In patients with presumed GI bleeding distal to the ligament of Treitz who have undergone a colonoscopy with negative results, peroral enteroscopy may detect small intestinal angiodysplastic lesions or other subtle lesions. Sonde enteroscopy involves passage of a thin, nonsteerable enteroscope into the distal ileum over several hours. This technique can visualize the entire length of the small intestine, although some intestinal segments may not be seen because of the lack of operator control. The other disadvantage of sonde enteroscopy is the inability to perform cautery or injection control of hemorrhage. Conversely, push enteroscopy uses a steerable endoscope that is limited to visualizing the jejunum; therefore, distal sites will not be visualized. The push enteroscope has a central channel that permits passage of thermal devices or injection needles.

Scintigraphy and Angiography.   In patients with rapid bleeding, angiography can provide important diagnostic information. With hemorrhage of >0.5 ml per minute, lumenal blood extravasation from diverticula, angiodysplastic lesions, neoplasms, Meckel's diverticula, and aortoenteric fistulae may be observed. In rare cases, angiodysplastic lesions or neoplasms in the small intestine and colon may be detected from the angiographic blush pattern in the absence of active bleeding. Before angiography, most radiologists recommend performance of a scintigraphic bleeding scan in an attempt to localize the site of hemorrhage, thus minimizing the angiographic dye load. The other important scintigraphic study to consider in appropriate patients is the Meckel's scan, which uses a radiolabeled technetium compound that accumulates in acid-producing mucosa in the diverticulum.

Other Radiographic Studies.   Barium enema radiography may be useful for both diagnosis and treatment of intussusception. Barium radiography dedicated to the small intestine may detect a Meckel's diverticulum. Selected rare cases of bleeding sites in the small intestine may require enteroclysis, a barium study of the small intestine that involves perfusion of barium, water, and methylcellulose through a tube fluoroscopically advanced to the ligament of Treitz to create a double-contrast image. If enteroscopy, colonoscopy, and barium radiography do not identify the source in such a case but iron supplementation compensates for the blood loss, no further intervention is required.

Principles of Management

Medications

Certain lower GI bleeding sources are amenable to specific medication therapy. Hemorrhoids, anal fissures, and solitary rectal ulcers will benefit from bulk-forming agents, sitz baths, and avoidance of straining. Steroid-containing ointments and suppositories are used in many cases, but their efficacy is questioned. Estrogen-progesterone combinations may reduce bleeding in some patients with angiodysplasia. IBD usually responds to specific anti-inflammatory drug therapy. Recent reports suggest that intrarectal formalin may reduce bleeding secondary to radiation proctitis. Similar responses to hyperbaric oxygen have been anecdotally noted.

Therapeutic Endoscopy

Colonoscopic bipolar cautery, monopolar cautery, heater probe application, and Nd:YAG laser have all been used to successfully treat angiodysplasia and the vascular changes seen with chronic radiation proctocolitis. Colonoscopy also may be used to ablate or resect bleeding polyps or reduce hemorrhage associated with colonic malignancy. Sigmoidoscopy may be used to treat bleeding internal hemorrhoids, with banding or thermal techniques.

Therapeutic Angiography

Patients with extensive bleeding may be treated angiographically. Intra-arterial vasopressin controls 90% of hemorrhages secondary to diverticula and angiodysplasia; however, this agent has significant cardiovascular toxicity. Angiographic embolization is considered a last resort procedure because of the 13% to 18% risk of bowel infarction.

Surgery

For individual cases of lower GI bleeding (e.g., Meckel's diverticulum or some malignancies), surgery is the appropriate initial therapy after stabilization of the patient. Emergency surgery carries a high morbidity and mortality that increase as the clinical condition deteriorates. For those difficult cases of recurrent significant bleeding without a defined source of hemorrhage, right hemicolectomy or subtotal colectomy may be indicated in patients with good overall prognoses. In cases of suspected angiodysplasia in the small intestine, intraoperative enteroscopy may localize the bleeding site.

Complications

As with upper GI sources, massive lower GI bleeding can have profound sequelae. Chronic or recurrent lower GI bleeding can be associated with significant morbidity, subjecting the patient to the risks of frequent transfusions. It can also use significant health care resources. The failure to determine a diagnosis in difficult cases most often reflects the relative inaccessibility of the small intestine to direct visualization.

CHAPTER 5

Approach to the Patient with Occult Gastrointestinal Hemorrhage

DIFFERENTIAL DIAGNOSIS

Occult gastrointestinal (GI) hemorrhage is by definition bleeding that is not apparent on examination of the stool. It has a prevalence as high as 1 in 20 adults. Up to 200 ml of blood may be lost in the proximal gut without reliably producing melena, whereas smaller losses produce visible bleeding from the lower GI tract. Most occult GI bleeding is chronic and, if significant, can produce profound iron deficiency anemia. An extensive list of disorders, including inflammatory disorders, infectious causes, vascular diseases, neoplasms, and other conditions, may produce occult bleeding with and without iron deficiency anemia (Table 5-1).

Inflammatory Causes

Acid-peptic diseases, including erosions or ulcers of the esophagus, stomach, and duodenum, are the most common causes of occult GI bleeding and are associated with iron deficiency in 30% to 70% of cases. Longitudinal erosions within the large hiatal hernia sac, known as Cameron's erosions, may cause up to 10% of the cases of iron deficiency anemia. Other inflammatory causes of occult bleeding include inflammatory bowel disease, celiac sprue, Meckel's diverticulum, eosinophilic gastroenteritis, radiation enteritis, colorectal ulcers, and Whipple's disease.

TABLE 5-1
Causes of Occult Gastrointestinal Blood Loss

Tumors and neoplasms
    Primary adenocarcinoma
    Metastases
    Large polyps
    Lymphoma
    Leiomyoma
    Leiomyosarcoma
    Lipoma
Infectious causes
    Hookworm
    Strongyloidiasis
    Ascariasis
    Tuberculous enterocolitis
    Amebiasis
Miscellaneous causes
    Medications (NSAIDs)
    Long-distance running
    Gastrostomy tubes and other appliances
Vascular causes
    Angiodysplasias and vascular ectasias
    Portal gastropathy
    Hemangiomas
    Blue rubber bleb nevus syndrome
    Watermelon stomach
Inflammatory disorders
    Acid peptic disease
    Hiatal hernia (Cameron's erosions)
    Inflammatory bowel disease
    Celiac sprue
    Whipple's disease
    Eosinophilic gastroenteritis
    Meckel's diverticulum
    Solitary rectal ulcer
    Cecal ulcer

Infectious Causes

In the United States, infectious causes of occult GI bleeding are uncommon, but organisms such as hookworms, *Mycobacterium tuberculosis*, amebae, and *Ascaris* species cause chronic blood loss in several hundred million people worldwide.

Vascular Causes

Vascular ectasias may cause up to 6% of all cases of occult bleeding. Some of these are acquired lesions, such as sporadic telangiectasia, postradiation telangiectasia, scleroderma, and the watermelon stomach (a vascular ectasia that appears as jagged stripes and is due to longitudinal vessels on the tops of antral rugae). Alternatively, inherited conditions of vascular ectasia (e.g., hereditary hemorrhagic telangiectasia [Osler-Weber-Rendu disease], Turner's syndrome, and Klippel-Trénaunay syndrome) can bleed in occult fashion. In patients with portal hypertension, portal gastropathy is a common cause of occult blood loss and iron deficiency.

Neoplasms

GI tumors are the second most prevalent cause of occult bleeding in the United States after acid-peptic disease. Colorectal carcinoma and adenomatous polyps are the most common neoplasms, followed by gastric, esophageal, and ampullary malignancies. Other tumors, such as lymphomas, metastases, leiomyomas and leiomyosarcomas, and juvenile polyps, also produce occult blood loss.

Other Causes of Occult Gastrointestinal Bleeding

Drugs should be considered in the differential diagnosis of occult bleeding. Ulcerations and erosions of the stomach, small intestine, and colon can result from therapeutic doses of NSAIDs. Other medications that cause occult bleeding include potassium preparations, certain antibiotics, and antimetabolites. Use of anticoagulants (e.g., warfarin) is associated with an increased incidence of occult blood loss, although anticoagulants more commonly reveal bleeding from other sources. Esophageal webs may be associated with iron deficiency, as in the Plummer-Vinson or Paterson-Kelly syndrome. Iron deficiency anemia may develop in long-distance runners, possibly secondary to mechanical jarring or to subclinical mesenteric ischemia. Non-GI causes such as hemoptysis, oral bleeding, epistaxis, and factitious blood ingestion can mimic occult GI blood loss.

WORKUP

History

The history should attempt to elicit the severity of blood loss as well as its cause. Fatigue, palpitations, postural lightheadedness, and exertional dyspnea suggest significant anemia. Some women and children exhibit pica, or compulsive eating behavior, with iron deficiency. Dyspepsia, abdominal pain, heartburn, or regurgitation suggest possible peptic causes, whereas weight loss and anorexia raise concern about malignancy. Recurrent episodes of occult blood loss in elderly patients without other symptoms are consistent with angiodysplasia or other vascular ectasias.

Physical Examination

Profound iron deficiency may present with pallor, tachycardia, postural or supine hypotension, and a hyperdynamic heart caused by high cardiac output. Other rare findings include papilledema, hearing loss, cranial nerve palsies, retinal hemorrhages, as well as koilonychia (brittle, furrowed, and spooned nails), glossitis, and cheilosis. The presence of lymphadenopathy, masses, hepatosplenomegaly, or jaundice is suggestive of malignancy, whereas epigastric tenderness may be seen with peptic disease. Splenomegaly, jaundice, or spider angiomata raise the possibility of blood loss secondary to portal hypertension. Cutaneous telangiectasias are suggestive of possible hereditary hemorrhagic telangiectasia.

Additional Testing

Tests for Iron Deficiency

Hypochromic, microcytic anemia, determined by visual or automated peripheral smear analysis, is often the first clue to occult GI blood loss, although it is a late manifestation. Anisocytosis, or variability of cell size reflected by the red cell distribution width, is also often increased with iron deficiency. In addition to these measured variables of complete blood count analysis, values of serum iron and transferrin may be obtained. With iron deficiency, the iron level is low with a compensatory increase in transferrin concentration, resulting in a reduced percentage of saturation of transferrin by iron. Low values for serum iron and transferrin saturation also may be seen in the anemia of chronic disease. Serum ferritin levels correlate better with tissue iron stores and may fall before anemia develops, although inflammatory conditions may falsely elevate ferritin levels, as this marker is an acute phase reactant. In questionable cases, determination of bone marrow iron stores remains the gold standard for diagnosis of iron deficiency anemia.

Fecal Blood Testing

Guaiac preparations, such as Hemoccult cards, are the most widely used fecal blood tests because of their simplicity and portability. The leuco-dye guaiac is a colorless compound that turns blue on exposure to blood. However, other peroxidase compounds, such as radishes, turnips, cantaloupe, bean sprouts, cauliflower, broccoli, and grapes may also cause the color change. Color changes to blue have been reported with sucralfate, cimetidine, halogens, and toilet bowl sanitizers. Iron, however, causes a green, not a blue, color change. Conversely, ascorbic acid, antacids, heat, and acid pH can inhibit guaiac reactivity. In general, fecal blood loss must exceed 10 ml per day (normal <2 ml per day) for Hemoccult cards to produce positive findings 50% of the time. Guaiac testing should be performed on a diet low in red meats and devoid of NSAIDs to prevent false-positive results. Wetting the card before addition of the peroxide catalyst may increase the sensitivity of Hemoccult testing but raises false positivity rates to levels considered unacceptable by some.

Other methods of fecal blood testing are available but have not achieved widespread use. Immunochemical detection of fecal blood has been tested and is very sensitive for fresh blood; however, the metabolism of globin during gut transit compromises the immunologic detection, rendering the techniques less useful for upper GI sources. Fluorometric assays of heme and heme-derived porphyrin, such as HemoQuant, are quite sensitive for both upper and lower GI bleeding sources, but the need to send out stool samples for reference laboratory measurement is a distinct disincentive for physicians. Fecal recovery of intravenously injected ^{51}Cr-labeled erythrocytes is the standard for quantifying enteric blood loss, but it is impractical in most clinical settings.

Proposed clinical roles for fecal occult blood testing include colorectal cancer screening in persons older than 50 years and verifying a GI source for iron deficiency anemia in children, menstruating women, strict vegetarians, postgastrectomy patients, immigrants from underdeveloped countries, and patients with steatorrhea. With the application of annual fecal blood testing in appropriate populations, 30% reductions in colorectal cancer mortality have been achieved, validating this screening protocol.

Endoscopy and Radiography

For a patient with asymptomatic guaiac-positive stools, colonoscopy is the appropriate diagnostic procedure, as most studies show little risk of upper GI malignancies in this setting. In large, population-based screening studies, 2% to 10% of patients with guaiac-positive stools will be found to have colorectal cancer, although a much higher percentage will have nonmalignant polyps. Use of sigmoidoscopy plus barium enema radiography is advocated by some clinicians as an alternate approach, although many studies document a significantly lower sensitivity for detection of colonic neoplasia using this protocol.

With iron deficiency anemia and occult GI bleeding, the approach shown in Fig. 5-1 is recommended. Using this protocol, a GI lesion will be found in 66% to 97% of men and postmenopausal women. An initial colonoscopy is performed. If no lesion is detected, upper endoscopy is immediately performed. If both endoscopic investigations fail to reveal a bleeding source, barium radiography of the small intestine is performed. In patients with specific GI symptoms, the sequence of diagnostic testing should be directed to the anatomic site from which symptoms appear to arise. If no lesion is found using this protocol, further evaluation is indicated only if oral iron fails to correct the patient's anemia. Enteroclysis, a double-contrast radiography technique for the small intestine involving fluoroscopic infusion of barium, methylcellulose, and water, provides greater mucosal detail than standard single-contrast procedures but it is technically demanding. Enteroscopy may provide direct visualization of the mucosa of the small intestine. Sonde enteroscopy uses a thin endoscope that is passed into the distal ileum over several hours and is then slowly withdrawn. With this method, up to 70% of the mucosa is observed; however, sonde enteroscopy offers no therapeutic capability. Push enteroscopy offers steerability and a central channel for therapeutic options, but the enteroscope usually cannot be passed beyond the mid-jejunum. Angiography may in rare instances demonstrate mucosal blush patterns in patients with occult angiodysplasia. Abdominal computed tomographic scanning may define intra-abdominal disease not detected by lumenal investigations.

PRINCIPLES OF MANAGEMENT

Treatment of occult GI bleeding is dictated by the findings of the diagnostic evaluation. Peptic disease is managed according to its cause, but usually involves short-term or long-term courses of acid-suppressive medications. Many premalignant colon polyps and some pedunculated malignant polyps can be removed colonoscopically. Angiodysplasia may be cauterized endoscopically or treated medically with estrogen-progesterone preparations if the lesions are the source of significant anemia. Portal gastropathy may respond to measures designed to reduce portal hypertension. If medications are the cause of occult blood loss, their withdrawal may correct the problem.

Some conditions of chronic blood loss require long-term iron supplementation. Oral ferrous sulfate, at a dose of 325 mg three times daily, is preferred in most patients because it is inexpensive, effective, and well tolerated. Other oral

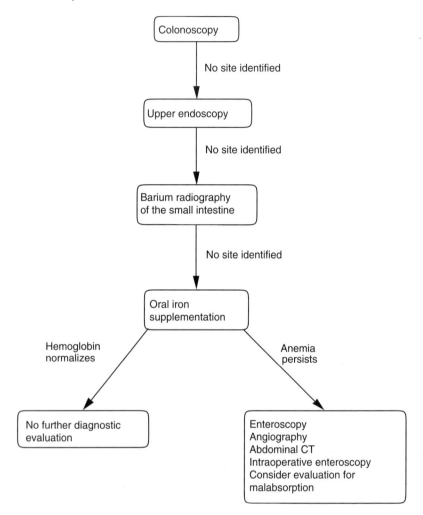

FIGURE 5-1. Workup of a patient with occult gastrointestinal bleeding. (CT = computed tomography.)

preparations include ferrous fumarate, ferrous gluconate, and preparations with added ascorbic acid to enhance absorption. Repletion of iron stores may take 3 to 6 months, although reticulocytosis peaks within 10 days and the hemoglobin level normalizes within 2 months. Parenteral iron, in complexed form, is indicated for patients who cannot absorb or do not tolerate oral iron. Usually 7 to 10 intramuscular injections of 250 mg elemental iron are required for moderate anemia. In some instances, iron may be administered intravenously. Parenteral preparations may result in rare anaphylaxis, and 10% of patients develop serum sickness–like reactions.

COMPLICATIONS

Chronic occult GI blood loss usually is well tolerated in young individuals; however, older patients or those with underlying cardiorespiratory disease may note symptomatic deterioration because of the reduction in the oxygen-carrying capacity of their blood.

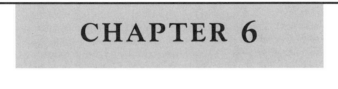

CHAPTER 6

Approach to the Patient with Unexplained Weight Loss

DIFFERENTIAL DIAGNOSIS

The occurrence of unexplained weight loss results from combinations of biological and behavioral factors. Hunger results from physiologic mechanisms, whereas appetite is more heavily influenced by environmental and psychological input, including the aroma and appearance of the food and the underlying mood of the person. In general, a person's weight can fluctuate by as much as 1.5% per day, thus a sustained weight loss of >5% of body weight warrants concern and possible investigation. In addition to anorexia, other symptom complexes contribute to the development of weight loss, including nausea, vomiting, postprandial abdominal pain, and altered consciousness. A number of general medical, gastrointestinal (GI), and behavioral illnesses produce unexplained weight loss (Table 6-1).

General Medical Disorders

Endocrinopathies such as thyrotoxicosis, diabetes, and Addison's disease may produce weight loss by varying mechanisms. Chronic infections (e.g., tubercu-

TABLE 6-1
Causes of Weight Loss

General medical disorders
  Endocrinopathies (thyrotoxicosis, diabetes mellitus, Addison's disease)
  Chronic infections (tuberculosis, fungal infections, endocarditis, acquired immuno-deficiency syndrome)
  Malignancy (carcinoma, lymphoma, leukemia)
  Medications
  Inadequate intake (immobility, impaired consciousness, dementia)
Behavior disorders
  Depression
  Schizophrenia
  Anorexia nervosa
  Bulimia nervosa
  Adult rumination syndrome
Gastrointestinal disease
  Gastrointestinal obstruction (stricture, adhesions, neoplasm)
  Motility disorders (achalasia, gastroparesis, intestinal pseudo-obstruction)
  Pancreaticobiliary disease (biliary colic, chronic pancreatitis, pancreatic carcinoma)
  Chronic hepatitis
  Malabsorption in the small intestine
  Bacterial overgrowth
  Chronic mesenteric ischemia

losis, fungal diseases, subacute bacterial endocarditis, and the acquired immuno-deficiency syndrome [AIDS]) and occult malignancies (e.g., carcinomas, lymphomas, and leukemias) can cause weight loss. In elderly patients, weight loss results from physiologic changes, neuropsychiatric syndromes, medication effects, and lack of available food.

Gastrointestinal Disorders

GI obstruction usually is associated with exacerbation of symptoms on meal ingestion, either immediately (esophageal stricture or cancer, achalasia), 1 to 3 hours postprandially (gastric or proximal intestinal blockage), or several hours later (distal ileitis, colon cancer). Similarly, pain from pancreaticobiliary sources may worsen after food ingestion, thus reducing intake. Malabsorption with steatorrhea may result from disease of the small intestine or pancreas.

Behavior Disorders

Weight loss from behavioral causes results from decreased food intake and can be determined by a careful interview or psychological testing. The most common behavior disorder that produces decreased food intake is depression, which is also characterized by mood changes, sleep disruption, anhedonia, and low self-esteem. Weight loss may also occur with thought disorders (e.g., schizophrenia) because of a distorted perception about food or eating. Eating disorders such as anorexia nervosa, bulimia nervosa, both of which may affect 5% to 10% of young women, and adult rumination syndrome are distinguished by the patient's desire to maintain thinness in association with an altered body image.

Anorexia Nervosa

Anorexia nervosa predominantly affects young, affluent, white women. More than 80% of patients develop the disorder within 7 years of menarche, indicative of the psychosocial distress associated with puberty. There is a 6% prevalence of anorexia nervosa in siblings and significant concordance in identical twins, which suggest biological factors as well. Patients are not truly anorectic but struggle against hunger to achieve an unrealistic degree of weight loss through dietary restriction and exercise as well as self-induced vomiting or laxative abuse. Major affective disorders (e.g., depression) may be present in up to 50% of cases.

Bulimia Nervosa

Bulimia nervosa is characterized by episodes of overeating followed by acts to avert weight gain (e.g., self-induced emesis, laxative or diuretic abuse, excessive exercise) and occurs almost exclusively in women younger than 30 years of age, with a prevalence of about 1%. Partial syndromes with occasional binge-eating behavior followed by self-induced vomiting or laxative abuse are considerably more common. Patients commonly report a past history of childhood obesity that has resolved; later in life they begin to compulsively eat large amounts of food that they have denied themselves for years. These episodes may be secretive and precipitated by frustration, loneliness, or the sight of tempting food. In contrast to anorectics, bulimics generally appear healthy and are more outgoing, although depression with suicidal ideation is not uncommon.

Adult Rumination Syndrome

Rumination syndrome, or merycism, is an eating disorder in which the patient repetitively regurgitates food from the stomach, rechews it, and then reswallows it. Adult patients generally report weight loss, regurgitation, and vomiting and are concerned about medical rather than psychiatric causes. The episodes are initiated by belching or swallowing, with creation of a common esophageal and gastric channel through reduction of lower esophageal sphincter pressure. Diaphragmatic and rectus abdominis muscle contraction produces regurgitation, expelling gastric contents into the mouth, where they are rechewed and ingested. The differential diagnosis includes esophageal strictures, gastroesophageal reflux or dysmotilities, and GI obstruction. Characteristic manometric patterns are seen in patients with rumination syndrome.

WORKUP

History

The history can provide important etiologic clues. Endocrinologic disease can be suggested by agitation and palpitations in hyperthyroidism; polydipsia and nocturia with diabetes; or skin pigmentation, fatigue, and lightheadedness with Addison's disease. Medications (e.g., procainamide, theophylline, thyroxin, and nitrofurantoin) may be factors in causing weight loss in older patients. Fever or chills may suggest infectious causes, whereas risk factors such as intravenous drug abuse or sexual exposure raise the possibility of AIDS. The presence of nausea or pain may be consistent with GI obstruction, whereas masses or jaundice suggest underlying malignancy. Bulky, foul-smelling, greasy stools indicate probable malabsorption.

A careful mental history can suggest possible behavioral causes. Psychomotor retardation or lack of interest in daily activities is consistent with depression. A denial of significant weight loss is common in anorexia nervosa, whereas secretive purging is classic in bulimia. Anorexia nervosa may also be associated with symptoms of altered gut function (e.g., early satiety, bloating, vomiting, constipation) and endocrine activity (e.g., amenorrhea, loss of libido, symptoms of hypothyroidism).

Physical Examination

The physical findings of weight loss relate to the underlying cause and degree of malnutrition. Cutaneous examination may suggest findings compatible with endocrine disease or AIDS (Kaposi's sarcoma). Jaundice reflects hepatic disease caused by inflammation or malignancy. Malignancy is suggested by lymphadenopathy, occult fecal blood, or masses, whereas obstruction produces abdominal distention and high-pitched bowel sounds. Demonstrably impaired mental function may be an underlying cause of weight loss in older patients. Gross GI bleeding may be seen as a result of emesis-induced esophageal damage.

Severe malnutrition can be reflected by bradycardia, arrhythmias, hypotension, hypothermia, and signs of dehydration. Emetics (e.g., ipecac) may produce cardiac arrhythmias. Brittle hair or nails, decreased fat stores, acrocyanosis, downy hair, yellow discoloration (from hypercarotenemia), and loss of secondary sexual characteristics may be seen, especially in a young patient with anorexia nervosa. Patients with self-induced vomiting or regurgitation exhibit halitosis, pharyngitis, and gingival or dental erosions from reflux of gastric acid. Self-induced vomiting also produces parotid swelling and abrasion of the knuckles from inserting the fingers into the mouth.

Additional Testing

Laboratory, radiologic, and endoscopic evaluations are guided by factors found in the history and the physical examination, including associated symptoms, patient age, symptom duration, prior medical conditions, degree of malnutrition, cost, and risk to the patient (Fig. 6-1). Laboratory studies should include a complete blood count; a measurement of the sedimentation rate, electrolytes, blood urea nitrogen, creatinine, total protein, and albumin; a urinalysis; and liver chemistry studies. Radiography of the chest and abdomen can detect malignancy or obstruction. Specific blood testing can screen for thyroid disease, and human immunodeficiency virus assays or placement of a purified protein derivative can test for infectious causes (e.g., AIDS and tuberculosis).

If malabsorption is suspected, screening tests such as qualitative fecal fat, serum carotene, and prothrombin time are obtained. Specific testing for causes of malabsorption that originates in the small intestine includes D-xylose absorption, bentiromide testing for pancreatic insufficiency, and breath tests for bacterial overgrowth or ileal disease. Schilling's tests can be used to document vitamin B_{12} malabsorption, and aspirates from the small intestine can be cultured if bacterial

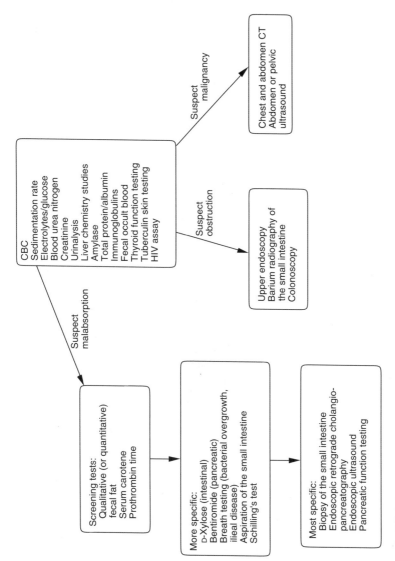

FIGURE 6-1. Workup of a patient with unexplained weight loss. (CBC = complete blood count; HIV = human immunodeficiency virus; CT = computed tomography.)

overgrowth is suspected. The most specific tests for malabsorption, however, are mucosal biopsies of the small intestine and endoscopic retrograde pancreatography, exocrine pancreatic function testing after cholecystokinin or secretin infusion, and endoscopic ultrasonography for pancreatic insufficiency.

If structural disease is suspected, abdominal computed tomographic or ultrasound scanning may detect underlying malignancies, whereas barium radiography and endoscopic evaluation may define sites of obstruction. A young patient suspected of having anorexia nervosa should be considered for structural evaluation of the GI tract, as Crohn's disease is an important condition in the differential diagnosis. Upper endoscopic or barium radiographic studies should also be performed with suspected rumination, because esophageal disease can mimic the clinical presentation in this disorder.

When biological disease has been excluded, referral to a psychiatrist, psychologist, or social worker is contemplated to exclude psychiatric causes of weight loss. Establishment of a specific diagnosis using strict criteria (e.g., *Diagnostic and Statistical Manual [of Mental Disorders]-IV*) benefits the patient by directing psychosocial treatment of the underlying condition.

PRINCIPLES OF MANAGEMENT

The management of the patient with unexplained weight loss is directed by the responsible disorder. Specific therapies are used for inflammatory conditions, endocrinopathies, malabsorption, gut obstruction, and some malignancies. With severe malnutrition (<65% of ideal body weight), hospitalization is necessary. Enteral refeeding may be attempted and should be delivered at 1680 to 2520 kcal above daily caloric needs to gain 1 to 2 kg per week. If feedings are poorly tolerated or refused by the patient, central or peripheral parenteral nutrition may be required. In the patient with anorexia nervosa, continuation of nutritional intervention after achieving 80% of ideal body weight is not recommended, as this is psychologically invasive and increases patient anxiety and resistance. In any condition of severe malnutrition, including anorexia nervosa, rapid refeeding should be avoided because of potential gastroduodenal dilation and refeeding pancreatitis or diarrhea.

Medical and psychological management of patients with behavioral disease should be initiated immediately to prevent complications of malnutrition. Tricyclic or serotonin reuptake-inhibiting antidepressant medications may produce striking weight gain in depressed patients. A short course of chlorpromazine, lithium, and cyproheptadine are effective in some patients with anorexia nervosa. Use of prokinetic medications (e.g., cisapride) may reduce GI symptoms in anorexia nervosa, thus aiding the overall treatment plan. Antidepressants may reduce binge episodes and impulsive behavior in some patients with bulimia nervosa. Behavior therapy may achieve short-term weight gain in anorexia nervosa; family therapy may have long-term benefits, especially in young patients. Cognitive-behavior therapy, in which the patient identifies aberrant behaviors and then extinguishes them, is recommended for patients with bulimia nervosa. For patients with adult rumination syndrome, behavior modification and biofeedback appear to be the most effective approaches.

COMPLICATIONS

Profound weight loss has significant complications regardless of its cause. Cardiac complications include arrhythmias and sudden death, caused by either the primary disorder or by metabolic consequences secondary to purgation. Electrocardiographic changes include bradycardia, decreased QRS amplitude, QT prolongation, ST segment changes, and U waves. Death from cardiomyopathy caused by taking ipecac has been reported. Liver chemistry abnormalities result from hepatic steatosis. Fecal impaction can result from many of the causes of weight loss as well as from decreased oral intake and dehydration. Clinical features of hypothyroidism may develop, although free thyroxin levels are usually normal. Leukopenia and hypocomplementemia can occur, although susceptibility to infection usually does not increase.

The prognosis of a patient with unexplained weight loss depends on the cause. Many conditions ultimately prove to be fatal. For patients for whom a cause cannot be diagnosed and whose weight loss stabilizes, the prognosis is usually excellent, and multiple invasive diagnostic evaluations are discouraged. For patients with anorexia nervosa, the short-term prognosis is good, with >75% of patients achieving significant weight gain; however, many patients suffer long-term relapses. The degree of social integration is the best predictor of prolonged improvement with anorexia nervosa.

CHAPTER 7

Approach to the Patient with Nausea and Vomiting

DIFFERENTIAL DIAGNOSIS

Nausea, the subjective sensation of an impending urge to vomit, and vomiting, the forceful ejection of gastrointestinal contents, are nonspecific, symptomatic responses to conditions. Although usually preceded by nausea, vomiting can occur independently in some clinical settings. Retching involves the coordinated action of thoracoabdominal striated musculature but does not produce oral discharge of lumenal contents. Other symptoms may be reported by a patient as nausea, but they are distinct from nausea. Regurgitation is the effortless return of gastric or esophageal contents in the absence of nausea or spasmodic muscular contractions. Rumination is the regurgitation of food into the mouth, where it is rechewed and reswallowed. Anorexia refers to a loss of appetite and may not be associated with nausea. Early satiety is the sensation of gastric fullness before the completion of a meal. Nausea may be part of a general complaint of indigestion that includes abdominal discomfort, heartburn, anorexia, and bloating. The differential diagnosis of nausea and vomiting includes the effect of medications; infections; disorders of the gastrointestinal tract, peritoneal cavity, and central nervous system; and endocrine and metabolic activities (Table 7-1).

Medications

The most common causes of nausea and vomiting are adverse medication responses, which usually present early in the course of their administration. Chemotherapeutic agents such as cisplatin and cyclophosphamide are potent emetic stimuli that act on the central nervous system. In contrast, analgesics such as aspirin or NSAIDs induce nausea by direct gastrointestinal mucosal irritation. Other classes of medications that produce nausea include cardiovascular drugs (e.g., digoxin, antiarrhythmics, antihypertensives), diuretics, hormonal agents (e.g., oral antidiabetics, contraceptives), antibiotics (e.g., erythromycin), and gastrointestinal medications (e.g., sulfasalazine).

Disorders of the Gastrointestinal Tract and Peritoneum

Gut and peritoneal disorders constitute the second most common cause of nausea and vomiting. Gastric outlet obstruction may produce intermittent symptoms, whereas obstruction of the small intestine is usually acute and associated with abdominal pain. Superior mesenteric artery syndrome, a condition that manifests rarely in patients who have had severe weight loss, recent surgery, or prolonged bedrest, occurs when the duodenum is compressed by the overlying superior mesenteric artery as it originates from the aorta, producing an anatomic obstruction. Functional disorders of gut motility (e.g., gastroparesis and chronic intestinal pseudo-obstruction) evoke nausea because of an inability to clear retained food and secretions. Gastroparesis may occur with systemic diseases (e.g., diabetes, scleroderma, lupus, amyloidosis) or it may be idiopathic, occurring after a viral prodrome in some cases. Chronic intestinal pseudo-obstruction may be hereditary, result from systemic disease, or occur as a paraneoplastic response to malignancy (most commonly, small cell lung carcinoma). Other intra-abdominal disorders produce nausea and vomiting, with and without associated complaints of pain. Inflammatory conditions (e.g., pancreatitis, appendicitis, and cholecystitis) irritate the peritoneal surface, whereas biliary colic produces nausea by activating the afferent neural pathways. Fulminant hepatitis causes nausea, presumably because of the accumulation of emetic toxins and the increased intracranial pressure. Pancreatic adenocarcinoma produces gastroparesis by unknown mechanisms.

Disorders of the Central Nervous System

Conditions associated with increased intracranial pressure, such as tumors, infarction, hemorrhage, infections, or congenital abnormalities, produce emesis

TABLE 7-1
Causes of Nausea and Vomiting

Medications
  NSAIDs
  Cardiovascular drugs (e.g., digoxin, antiarrhythmics, antihypertensives)
  Diuretics
  Hormonal agents (e.g., oral antidiabetics, contraceptives)
  Antibiotics (e.g., erythromycin)
  Gastrointestinal drugs (e.g., sulfasalazine)
Central nervous system disorders
  Tumors
  Cerebrovascular accident
  Intracranial hemorrhage
  Infections
  Congenital abnormalities
  Psychiatric disease (e.g., anxiety, depression, anorexia nervosa, bulimia nervosa, psychogenic vomiting)
  Motion sickness
  Labyrinthine causes (e.g., tumors, labyrinthitis, Ménière's disease)
Miscellaneous causes
  Posterior myocardial infarction
  Congestive heart failure
  Excess ethanol ingestion
  Jamaican vomiting sickness
  Prolonged starvation
  Cyclic vomiting
Gastrointestinal and peritoneal disorders
  Gastric outlet obstruction
  Obstruction of the small intestine
  Superior mesenteric artery syndrome
  Gastroparesis
  Chronic intestinal pseudo-obstruction
  Pancreatitis
  Appendicitis
  Cholecystitis
  Acute hepatitis
  Pancreatic carcinoma
Endocrinologic and metabolic conditions
  Nausea of pregnancy
  Uremia
  Diabetic ketoacidosis
  Thyroid disease
  Addison's disease
Infectious disease
  Viral gastroenteritis (e.g., Hawaii agent, rotavirus, reovirus, adenovirus, Snow Mountain agent, Norwalk agent)
  Bacterial causes (e.g., *Staphylococcus* spp., *Salmonella* spp., *Bacillus cereus, Clostridium perfringens*)
  Opportunistic infection (e.g., cytomegalovirus, herpes simplex virus)
  Otitis media

with and without concomitant nausea. Emotional responses to unpleasant smells or tastes can induce vomiting, as can anticipation of cancer chemotherapy. Psychiatric conditions such as anxiety, depression, anorexia nervosa, and bulimia nervosa cause nausea. Young women with histories of psychiatric illness or social difficulty often present with psychogenic vomiting. Labyrinthine causes of nausea include labyrinthitis, tumors, and Ménière's disease. Motion sickness is induced by repetitive movements that result in vestibular nuclei activation.

Endocrinologic and Metabolic Conditions

Nausea in the first trimester of pregnancy is the most common endocrinologic emetic condition, occurring in 70% of pregnancies. This condition usually is transitory and is not associated with poor fetal or maternal outcome; however, 1% to 5% progress to hyperemesis gravidarum, which may produce dangerous fluid losses and electrolyte disturbances. Other endocrinologic and metabolic conditions characterized by vomiting include uremia, diabetic ketoacidosis, thyroid and parathyroid disease, and Addison's disease.

Infectious Causes

Viral gastroenteritis, secondary to the Hawaii agent, rotaviruses, reoviruses, adenoviruses, the Snow Mountain agent, and the Norwalk agent, can cause nausea, as can bacterial infection with *Staphylococcus* or *Salmonella* organisms, *Bacillus cereus*, and *Clostridium perfringens*. In many instances, nausea results from the effects of toxins produced by the infectious agents. Nausea in immunosuppressed patients may result from gastrointestinal cytomegalovirus or herpes simplex infections. Infections not involving the gastrointestinal tract, such as hepatitis, otitis media, and meningitis, may also manifest themselves as nausea.

Miscellaneous Causes of Nausea and Vomiting

Nausea may be a manifestation of posterior wall myocardial infarction as well as of congestive heart failure. Excess ethanol intake evokes nausea by acting on the central nervous system. Jamaican vomiting sickness results from ingestion of unripe akee fruit. Excess vitamin intake and prolonged starvation also cause nausea. Cyclic vomiting is a condition of unknown etiology characterized by episodes of emesis with intervening asymptomatic periods.

WORKUP

History

Acute vomiting (lasting 1 to 2 days) usually results from infections, medications, ingested toxins, or endogenous toxins (as produced in uremia and diabetic ketoacidosis). Chronic vomiting (lasting 1 week) usually results from long-standing medical or psychiatric conditions. Vomiting soon after meals suggests gastric outlet obstruction or inflammatory conditions (e.g., cholecystitis and pancreatitis), whereas delayed vomiting is characteristic of gastroparesis or more distal obstruction. Psychogenic vomiting may occur soon after eating, but most patients control their emesis until the gastric contents can be expelled into a toilet or other receptacle. Early morning nausea characterizes endocrine conditions, such as in the first trimester of pregnancy. Meals may relieve the nausea associated with peptic ulcer or esophagitis.

The character of the vomitus can provide diagnostic clues. The vomiting of undigested food is seen with Zenker's diverticulum and achalasia; partial digestion is observed with gastric obstruction and gastroparesis. The vomiting of bile excludes the possibility of a proximal obstruction, and the vomiting of blood suggests mucosal damage (as occurs with ulcers and malignancy). Voluminous acidic emesis is observed with gastrinomas, whereas feculent emesis occurs in distal obstructions, bacterial overgrowth, and gastrocolic fistulae.

The presence of associated symptoms should be determined. Pain is reported with ulcer disease, obstruction, or inflammatory disorders. Diarrhea, fever, or myalgias suggest possible infection. Weight loss occurs in many patients with chronic nausea, but those who have a psychogenic cause for their vomiting often maintain stable weight. Headaches, visual changes, altered mentation, and neck stiffness raise the possibility of central nervous system lesions. Reports of lightheadedness, palpitations, and dry mucous membranes suggest severe dehydration.

Physical Examination

Careful examination can assess the severity of the illness and provide diagnostic information. Fever is noted with inflammation or infection. Dehydration is suggested by orthostatic tachycardia or hypotension and loss of skin turgor. Sclerodactyly and jaundice are characteristic skin findings in scleroderma and hepatobiliary disease, respectively. A loss of dental enamel is seen in chronic vomiting conditions (e.g., bulimia nervosa). Adenopathy and masses suggest malignancy; hepatomegaly is also found in malignancy and in benign hepatic disease. Ileus is indicated by an absence of bowel sounds, whereas hyperactive bowel sounds characterize intestinal obstruction. A succussion splash may be found in gastric obstruction and gastroparesis. Abdominal tenderness is noted with inflammation, infection, and lumenal distention, whereas gross or occult fecal blood should prompt evaluation for ulcer, inflammation, or malignancy. Focal neurologic signs and papilledema suggest central nervous system disease, whereas nuchal rigidity is consistent with meningitis. Asterixis is noted with uremia and hepatic failure. Gastroparesis and pseudo-obstruction may be associated with peripheral and autonomic neuropathy.

Additional Testing

Laboratory Studies

The blood tests that are used are based on the history and the physical examination findings (Fig. 7-1). Serum electrolyte determinations are used to screen for hypokalemia and contraction alkalosis; a complete blood count tests for anemia, leukocytosis, and leukopenia. Blood loss may be further suggested by a low serum iron level and iron saturation of transferrin and by a low ferritin level. Hypoalbuminemia results from chronic disease and gut protein loss. Amylase, lipase, and liver chemistry determinations are obtained when pancreaticobiliary or hepatic disease is suspected. If indicated, a serum pregnancy test and thyroid func-

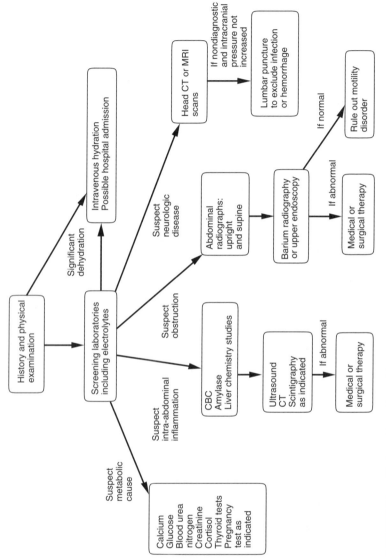

FIGURE 7-1. Workup of a patient with nausea and vomiting. (CT = computed tomography; MRI = magnetic resonance imaging; CBC = complete blood count.)

tion tests may be performed, and values for blood urea nitrogen and creatinine, glucose, ketones, calcium, and plasma cortisol concentrations may be obtained. Specific serologic markers are used to evaluate for collagen vascular diseases, and myenteric neuronal antibody determinations are used to screen for paraneoplastic pseudo-obstruction. Meningitis may be confirmed by lumbar puncture.

Structural Studies

Anatomic evaluation may be indicated in some cases of nausea. Abdominal radiography may show air-fluid levels, an ileus, or subdiaphragmatic free air. Partial obstruction may be revealed by upper gastrointestinal barium radiography, whereas upper endoscopy can be used to assess for ulcer disease or gastric outlet narrowing. Retained food in the absence of obstruction is seen in gastroparesis. Ultrasound, computed tomography, and biliary scintigraphy can be used to detect pancreaticobiliary sources, and angiography can detect mesenteric ischemia. Computed tomographic and magnetic resonance imaging scans of the head are used to evaluate possible central nervous system sources.

Functional Studies

Gastric emptying of liquids (^{111}In-DTPA in water) and solids (^{99m}Tc-sulfur colloid in a solid meal) can be used to test for gastroparesis after the possibility of obstruction is excluded. Gastroparesis usually affects solid phase emptying more severely than liquid emptying. In difficult cases, specialized centers have the capability of performing manometry of the stomach and duodenum, which measures motor activity under fasting and fed conditions. Manometry should be considered in patients with nausea and negative evaluation findings and in patients with nausea and delayed gastric emptying who do not respond to prokinetic medications. Manometry should be performed to detect concomitant dysmotility of the small intestine if surgery or jejunostomy is being considered. A new technique, electrogastrography (EGG), measures electrical pacemaker activity that regulates gastric contractions. The clinical role of EGG is being defined, but disturbances of pacemaker frequency and amplitude are well described in large subsets of patients with unexplained nausea and vomiting. In chronic intestinal pseudo-obstruction, barium radiography of the small intestine may reveal dilation and delayed transit. Esophageal or gastroduodenal manometry may reveal specific patterns consistent with visceral myopathic or neuropathic disease, providing supportive evidence for the diagnosis of pseudo-obstruction. In many cases, a full-thickness biopsy specimen of the small intestine is obtained to document nerve and smooth muscle degeneration.

PRINCIPLES OF MANAGEMENT

The severity of the clinical condition must initially be ascertained. Poor skin turgor and changes in orthostatic pulse rate and blood pressure are indications for the administration of intravenous fluids, usually normal saline. Potassium may be given for hypokalemia if urine output is normal. Nasogastric suction may benefit patients with obstruction or ileus. The threshold for hospitalization is lower for diabetics, patients with concurrent diarrhea, persons with other chronic debilitating diseases, and very young and very old patients. If the patient can return home, frequent small liquid meals in the form of carbohydrates, not fats, are recommended.

Medications may be prescribed to treat specific conditions (e.g., cortico-steroids for Addison's disease and acid-suppressing drugs for peptic disease). Alternatively, surgery is indicated for certain inflammatory conditions and for obstruction. If a specific therapy cannot provide rapid symptom control, antiemetic medications can be given. Antihistamines (e.g., meclizine, dimen-hydrinate) are used for motion sickness, labyrinthitis, postoperative nausea, and nausea with uremia. Anticholinergics (e.g., scopolamine) are most effec-tive in treating motion sickness. Sedation and dry mouth are side effects of antihistamines and anticholinergics. Antidopaminergics (e.g., phenothiazines, butyrophenones) are the most commonly prescribed drugs for chronic nau-sea and are active against gastroenteritis, the effects of medication and radia-tion, and postoperative nausea. Because of their effect on the central nervous system, antidopaminergics have a number of side effects, including mood changes, sleep disruption, dystonic reactions, parkinsonian symptoms, and galactorrhea.

Patients with gastrointestinal motility disorders may benefit from prokinetic agents that promote gastric emptying and intestinal transit if they are given before meals. The agent used most often is metoclopramide, given in 5-mg to 20-mg doses. It acts as a dopamine antagonist as well as a cholinergic nerve stim-ulant in the stomach, using serotonin $5\text{-}HT_4$ pathways. Because of central anti-dopaminergic effects as described above, metoclopramide is poorly tolerated in 20% of patients. Newer antidopaminergic prokinetic agents, such as domperi-done, are being tested for the U.S. market. Cisapride exhibits prokinetic effects at doses of 5 to 20 mg by stimulating gastric cholinergic pathways using $5\text{-}HT_4$ receptors and by directly affecting gut smooth muscle but without exhibiting antidopaminergic properties. The main side effects of cisapride are diarrhea and cramping caused by prokinetic effects in the colon. The macrolide antibiotic erythromycin, which acts on gut motilin receptors, is the most potent available prokinetic agent. It has a narrow dose range of efficacy; low doses (125 to 250 mg) produce a beneficial prokinetic effect and only slightly higher doses cause abdominal pain, nausea, and diarrhea.

The treatment of nausea induced by cancer chemotherapy may be chal-lenging. Most antiemetic regimens used by oncologists consist of multiple agents that act at different sites. Serotonin $5\text{-}HT_3$ antagonists, such as ondansetron and granisetron, have become mainstays in regimens that use potent emetic stimulants (e.g., cisplatin and radiation therapy). The side effects of $5\text{-}HT_3$ antagonists include headache, constipation, and rare eleva-tions in liver chemistry values. High-dose metoclopramide may also be useful, perhaps because of weak $5\text{-}HT_3$ antagonist effects. Other antidopaminergics are also used. Combination regimens often include corticosteroids, which act through unknown mechanisms, and benzodiazepines (e.g., lorazepam), which reduce anticipatory nausea. Cannabinoids (e.g., tetrahydrocannabinol, nabilone) are no more efficacious than antidopaminergics and are poorly tol-erated, producing somnolence, ataxia, syncope, seizures, and hallucinations, especially in elderly patients.

Certain therapies have efficacy in selected settings. Tricyclic antidepres-sants reduce nausea in patients with depression, whereas naloxone reduces nausea in patients withdrawing from opium. Some female patients with nau-sea and functional bowel disease respond to the gonadotropin-releasing hor-mone analog leuprolide. Acupuncture and acustimulation may be used to treat the nausea of pregnancy and motion sickness. Reports suggest that elec-trical pacing of the gastric wall may be a feasible treatment for severe gastro-paresis in the future.

COMPLICATIONS

Chronic nausea and vomiting can produce dehydration, weight loss, and electrolyte abnormalities (e.g., hypokalemia and metabolic alkalosis), which may be life-threatening in certain patient populations. Increased intrathoracic pressure during vomiting produces purpura on the face and neck, whereas a patient with gastroesophageal mucosal tears (Mallory-Weiss tears) may present with upper gastrointestinal hemorrhage. A more severe complication, Boerhaave's syndrome, results if vomiting ruptures the esophagus, leading to mediastinitis or peritonitis. In patients with impaired mentation, emesis may cause pulmonary aspiration, producing chemical pneumonitis.

CHAPTER 8

Approach to the Patient with Abdominal Pain

DIFFERENTIAL DIAGNOSIS

Abdominal pain is caused by conditions that range from being trivial to being life-threatening. Two types of nerve fibers carry pain impulses: rapidly conducting A-delta fibers, which yield a well-localized sensation, and slowly conducting C fibers, which yield a dull, poorly localized pain. Most abdominal visceral fibers responsive to mechanical (e.g., stretch, spasm) or chemical (e.g., inflammation, ischemia) stimuli are of the C type; therefore, pain from these organs is dull, gnawing, burning, and poorly localized. The parietal peritoneum has both A and C fibers; thus, pain is better localized and sharper. Nociceptive nerve endings in solid organs such as the liver and kidney are limited to the capsule; therefore, pain from disease of these organs results only with capsular stretching. Referred pain is explained by the convergence of visceral pain fibers and fibers from peripheral somatic sites at the level of the spinal cord. An intact cerebral cortex is required for appropriate pain perception. Impaired consciousness blunts pain perception, whereas psychological conditions (e.g., severe anxiety) can amplify the level of discomfort.

The differential diagnosis of abdominal pain includes pathologic processes within and outside the abdomen (Table 8-1). In general, obstruction, ulceration, inflammation, perforation, or ischemia of any hollow organ (e.g., gastrointestinal tract, urinary tract, pancreaticobiliary tree) has the potential to produce pain. Conversely, in solid organs (e.g., liver, kidneys, spleen) pain is only evoked by capsular distention resulting from infection, obstruction to drainage, vascular congestion, and some disorders with rapid mesenchymal infiltration. The adnexa and uterus are additional sources of pain in women. Lung or cardiac abnormalities may produce referred pain in the upper abdomen. Metabolic conditions (e.g., lead poisoning and diabetic ketoacidosis) can cause diffuse and localized abdominal pain. Acute intermittent porphyria is a disorder of heme biosynthesis that results in the accumulation of toxic intermediates that cause colicky abdominal pain, ileus, and psychiatric disturbances. Familial Mediterranean fever induces painful inflammation of the abdominal and thoracic serosa as well as the joints and skin. Degenerative disk disease, tabes dorsalis, and herpes zoster reactivation may produce severe superficial abdominal wall pain, as can thoracic and abdominal trauma.

The acuteness of the patient presentation affects the differential diagnostic possibilities the clinician must consider. With acute abdominal pain, the central task is to establish an accurate diagnosis as efficiently as possible and then to implement specific measures to reduce pain perception and treat the underlying cause. Diagnosis and management of the various causes responsible for production of the acute abdomen are discussed in Chapter 9. Patients with recurrent pain that lasts hours to days with asymptomatic intervals represent a subset in whom a diagnosis may be particularly difficult. Many of these patients are dismissed as having "functional" disease; however, it is vital to ascertain the cause of this type of chronic pain because specific and often curative treatment may be available. Chronic, continuous abdominal pain often has an obvious cause. Disorders in this category include disseminated malignancies, chronic pancreatitis, or less serious illnesses with concurrent depression. Chronic intractable abdominal pain (CIAP) is defined as pain that lasts for at least 6 months and remains undiagnosed after an appropriate history, physical examination, and laboratory investigation. Patients with CIAP are predominantly women; have a history of childhood abdominal pain; often report prior physical or sexual abuse; and exhibit global disability with compromised work, family, and social functioning. Features of hypochondriasis and somatization disorder are prevalent in CIAP, as are abnormal illness behavior and a constellation of personality characteristics that has been termed the *pain-prone disorder*. Extensive diagnostic testing usually has been performed for vague and inconsistent symptoms including abdominal pain and somatic complaints.

WORKUP

History

Pain Localization

Pain from esophageal disease usually presents substernally, although some lower esophageal obstructions may refer pain to the suprasternal region. Esophageal dysmotilities produce dull substernal pressure that may radiate to the back, jaw, and left arm, mimicking the symptoms of myocardial infarction. The usual pain of peptic ulcer is epigastric; that from duodenal ulceration may be perceived to the right of the midline, and that from gastric body ulceration to the left of the midline.

TABLE 8-1
Causes of Abdominal Pain

Intra-abdominal
    Parietal inflammation
        Perforated viscus
        Spontaneous bacterial peritonitis
        Appendicitis
        Diverticulitis
        Pancreatitis
        Cholecystitis/cholangitis
        Pelvic inflammatory disease
        Familial Mediterranean fever
    Visceral mucosal disorders
        Peptic ulcer disease
        Inflammatory bowel disease
        Infectious colitis
        Esophagitis
    Visceral obstruction
        Intestinal obstruction (adhesions, hernia, volvulus, intussusception, malignancy)
        Biliary obstruction (stone, tumor, stricture)
        Renal colic (stone, tumor)
    Capsular distention
        Hepatitis
        Budd-Chiari syndrome
        Pyelonephritis
        Tubo-ovarian abscess
        Ovarian cyst
        Endometritis
        Ectopic pregnancy
    Vascular disorders
        Intestinal ischemia
        Abdominal aortic aneurysm
        Splenic infarction
        Tumor necrosis
    Visceral motility disorders
        Irritable bowel syndrome
        Nonulcer dyspepsia
        Esophageal dysmotility
        Viral gastroenteritis
Extra-abdominal
    Neurologic
        Radiculopathy
        Herpes zoster reactivation
    Musculoskeletal
        Trauma
        Fibromyalgia
    Cardiothoracic
        Pneumonia
        Myocardial infarction
        Pneumothorax

(continued)

TABLE 8-1   *(Continued)*

Empyema
Pulmonary infarction
Toxic/metabolic
  Uremia
  Diabetic ketoacidosis
  Porphyria
  Lead poisoning
  Reptile venom, insect bite
  Addison's disease

Patients with posterior penetrating duodenal ulcer as well as an obstruction of the small intestine may have pain that radiates to the back. More distal lesions of the small intestine evoke periumbilical pain, although ileal disease may cause hypogastric referral. Pain from the colon may be perceived in any site in the abdomen and back. Liver capsular distention produces right upper quadrant pain. Gallbladder and bile duct pain may initially be localized in the middle epigastrium or in the right upper quadrant, but with parietal peritoneal inflammation, right upper quadrant symptoms predominate. Pain from the head, body, and tail of the pancreas is felt in the right, middle, and left epigastrium, respectively. Left upper quadrant pain may result from pancreatic disease, ulcers of the greater curvature of the stomach, splenic lesions, perinephric disease, and colonic splenic flexure lesions. Acute pyelonephritis and ureteropelvic junction obstruction produce costovertebral, flank, or upper abdominal pain. Ureteral pain may radiate to the testes or thigh, leading the patient to believe that the problem originates in the groin. Uterine lesions evoke midline lower abdominal pain, whereas ovarian or tubal pain is ipsilaterally localized. Pelvic pain may radiate to the back.

Pain Quality

Specific terminology must be used when characterizing pain quality. Sharp pain should be limited to symptoms with a sticking or cutting quality. Crampy pain is a squeezing pain that waxes and wanes rhythmically. Certain clinical conditions are associated with specific pain qualities. Esophagitis produces burning or warm pain, whereas peptic ulcer pain is dull and gnawing. Intestinal pain from obstruction or inflammation is colicky or crampy, with distention and gurgling. Pain from appendicitis may be colicky, but usually it is dull, constant, and achy. Despite use of the terms biliary colic and renal colic, obstruction of these organs yields pain of a steady rather than colicky character. Acute cholecystitis leads to squeezing pain, whereas acute pancreatitis results in penetrating or boring pain. Nephrolithiasis evokes a sharp or cutting pain.

Pain Intensity

Intensity of acute abdominal pain is easily assessed. Pain intensity with common disorders is as follows: extremely severe—ulcer perforation, acute pancreatitis, renal stone; severe—intestinal obstruction, cholecystitis, appendicitis; moderate—peptic ulcer, gastroenteritis, esophagitis. Chronic abdominal pain is more difficult to assess because psychological factors can modify pain perception; therefore, indirect questions may provide useful information about pain intensity. For example, pain that does not interfere with sleep or daily function probably is not severe.

Pain Chronology

Ulcer pain may be intermittent, occurring daily at specific times in the early morning or before meals. Posterior penetration should be considered if peptic ulcer pain becomes constant. Cholecystitis commonly develops during sleep, not after meals. Appendicitis typically manifests progressive pain without remission for a period of 10 to 15 hours. Pain that reaches peak intensity within minutes characterizes ulcer perforation, abdominal aortic aneurysm, renal stones, and ruptured ectopic pregnancy, whereas peak pain intensity is reached in 10 to 60 minutes with acute pancreatitis, intestinal obstruction, cholecystitis, and mesenteric arterial occlusion. A gradual onset of pain for a period of several hours is reported in appendicitis, some cases of cholecystitis, diverticulitis, and mesenteric venous occlusion. The pain of irritable bowel syndrome is chronic and may be most intense after meals and in the evening. Pain occurring at monthly intervals in a woman suggests endometriosis or is related to ovulation. Pain that occurs after medication ingestion raises the possibility of acute intermittent porphyria (barbiturates) or pancreatitis (steroids, tetracycline, thiazides).

Alleviating and Aggravating Factors

Acid-suppressive or neutralizing agents may relieve pain from esophagitis or ulcer disease, although diagnosis based on response to therapy may be inaccurate. Food ingestion can relieve duodenal ulcer discomfort, but it may aggravate gastric body ulcer pain, providing a possible explanation for the weight loss that is common in patients with gastric ulcers. The pain of pancreatic disease is nearly always intensified by meal ingestion, as is discomfort from intestinal obstruction or mesenteric ischemia. Pain from duodenal obstruction may present within minutes of eating, whereas pain from ileal blockage may occur 1 to 2 hours postprandially. Lactase deficiency may produce discomfort that is specific to ingestion of dairy products. Certain body positions modify pain intensity in different diseases. The pain of nerve root compressions and other musculoskeletal conditions may worsen with some movements. Heartburn is aggravated by reclining or straining, whereas pancreatic pain is exacerbated in the supine position and lessened by leaning forward. Back pain in irritable bowel syndrome may be relieved by spine hyperextension, and abdominal pain in this condition is improved by passage of flatus or stool. Defecation may also relieve pain caused by other colonic disorders.

Other Symptoms

Nausea and vomiting are associated with pain in many conditions. Pain usually precedes nausea in surgical conditions but occurs afterward in nonsurgical disorders. Diarrhea typically indicates nonsurgical disease, although appendicitis is an exception to this rule. Ischemic colitis is considered in elderly patients with acute left-sided pain and bloody stools, whereas colonic neoplasm or inflammatory bowel disease is considered in patients with chronic pain and rectal bleeding. Acute abdominal pain with acute constipation raises the possibility of intestinal obstruction; chronic pain with constipation suggests irritable bowel syndrome. Anorexia and weight loss may indicate underlying malignancy. High fevers (>39.5°C) early in the course of a painful condition suggest cholangitis, urinary tract infection, infectious enteritis, or pneumonia. Fevers that occur later in the course of the disease, however, are more common with diverticulitis, appendicitis, and cholecystitis. Jaundice suggests hepatic or pancreaticobiliary disease. Patients with familial Mediterranean fever usually have arthritis or pleuritic pain.

Associated Conditions

Predisposing factors for specific conditions must be ascertained. Heavy, prolonged ethanol intake may cause pancreatitis, whereas analgesic intake predisposes a person to ulcer disease. Cardiovascular disease can be associated with mesenteric ischemia. Prior abdominal surgery increases the likelihood of intestinal obstruction. Coexistent perianal disease suggests Crohn's disease. Pathologic bone fractures are most common with disseminated malignancy. Many conditions produce recurrent pain attacks—for example, pancreatitis, peptic ulcer, cholecystitis, renal stones, pyelonephritis, and intestinal obstruction. In contrast, acute pain with no predisposing medical conditions and with no consistent localized pain or aggravating or relieving factors is observed in rare conditions (e.g., acute intermittent porphyria, tabes dorsalis, lead or arsenic poisoning, and black widow spider bite). Similar pain over several weeks characterizes mesenteric venous thrombosis, which may not be definitively diagnosed until gangrene appears. Long-standing atypical pain is most characteristic of CIAP.

Physical Examination

General Appearance

The first part of the examination begins during the history, with an assessment of the patient's general appearance. Severe pain is almost always reflected in the face, even when the patient describes pain that is no longer present. A writhing, diaphoretic patient usually is more ill than one who is resting comfortably; however, some patients with peritonitis may lie motionless to avoid abdominal irritation.

Abdominal Examination

The critical signs of an acute abdomen are those that indicate peritonitis or obstruction. Pain elicited by pressure over the inflamed peritoneum causes reflexive or involuntary guarding. With generalized peritonitis, rigidity may be present. A means of distinguishing voluntary from involuntary guarding is to forcibly compress the abdomen with the pressure of a stethoscope while distracting the patient. Another way to look for peritonitis is to jar the bed while the patient is in the supine position. In contrast, documentation of rebound tenderness has no predictive value in assessing peritonitis. Reports of severe pain with little tenderness on examination are consistent with intestinal infarction or early pancreatitis. Carnett's test may determine if chronic intermittent pain arises from the abdominal wall or if it has an intraabdominal origin. When the site of maximal tenderness is located, the patient sits up with arms crossed, thereby tensing the abdominal wall. A positive result, signified by increased tenderness, is found with nerve entrapment, abdominal wall hernia, myofascial pain, rectus sheath hematoma, and the rib tip syndrome.

Bowel sound auscultation is crucial. Bowel sounds are absent with ileus, whereas high-pitched, hyperactive bowel sounds suggest intestinal obstruction. If surges of peristalsis are powerful enough, visible peristaltic waves may be observed with obstruction. A succussion splash, elicited by an abrupt, lateral movement of the patient, is heard with gastric obstruction or gastroparesis. Examination of the abdomen should include inspection for scars and palpation for hernias.

The examination of a patient with CIAP is characterized by abdominal tenderness without signs of surgery and an absence of autonomic activation (i.e., no tachycardia or diaphoresis). Distraction of the patient can reduce tenderness. Often, a patient with CIAP will keep the eyes closed and have a fixed, placid smile during the abdominal examination.

Other Examinations

Any part of the physical examination can elicit diagnostic information from the patient with abdominal pain. Scleral icterus and jaundiced skin suggest hepatic or pancreaticobiliary disease or hemolysis, whereas purpura is observed with autoimmune diseases (e.g., Henoch-Schönlein purpura). Adenopathy, masses, and hepatomegaly suggest malignancy. A chest examination may reveal pneumonia as the cause of pain, whereas an irregular heart rhythm might suggest new-onset atrial fibrillation as a source of mesenteric arterial embolism. Patients with diabetes or those with possible disease of the spine should be assessed for radiculopathy, which might be accompanied by asymmetrical strength or sensation. Peripheral or autonomic neuropathies are found in some patients with gastrointestinal dysmotility. The presence of occult fecal blood on rectal examination raises the possibility of malignancy, ischemia, ulcer disease, and inflammation. Right-sided tenderness on rectal examination may also be found with appendicitis. Perianal fistulae, fissures, and abscesses suggest Crohn's disease. In women, a pelvic examination is used to evaluate possible adnexal or uterine causes of abdominal pain.

Additional Testing

Confirmation of the suspected diagnosis may require appropriate laboratory, radiographic, and endoscopic studies (Fig. 8-1). A complete blood count may show leukocytosis with inflammation or leukopenia in viral infection. Microcytic anemia is found with mucosal blood loss. Urinalysis may show red cells, white cells, and bilirubin, suggesting renal calculi, urinary infection, and hepatic or pancreaticobiliary disease, respectively. Elevated amylase and lipase levels are seen in early acute pancreatitis. Perforated ulcers, diabetic ketoacidosis, and mesenteric infarction also may cause hyperamylasemia. Elevated levels of bilirubin or alkaline phosphatase suggest cholestasis, whereas aminotransferase elevations indicate hepatocellular disease. The sedimentation rate may be elevated in inflammatory conditions. Metabolic conditions (e.g., acute porphyria and heavy metal intoxication) require specific testing. Chest radiographs can eliminate pulmonary sources of acute abdominal pain. Supine and upright (or decubitus) abdominal radiography can confirm the presence of pneumoperitoneum, calcified gallstones or renal stones, and distended bowel loops with or without air-fluid levels, especially if performed during the actual pain attacks. Symptoms and findings suggestive of obstruction and ulcer disease should be further evaluated with barium radiographic studies or endoscopy. Patients with colicky pain should undergo radiographic studies of the intestinal tract, not the biliary tree. In contrast, attacks of severe epigastric or right upper quadrant pain lasting hours should direct the evaluation to the gallbladder and pancreas. The presence of diarrhea, constipation, and rectal bleeding suggests a colonic source, which is best evaluated by colonoscopy or barium enema radiography. The specifics of diagnostic testing for var-

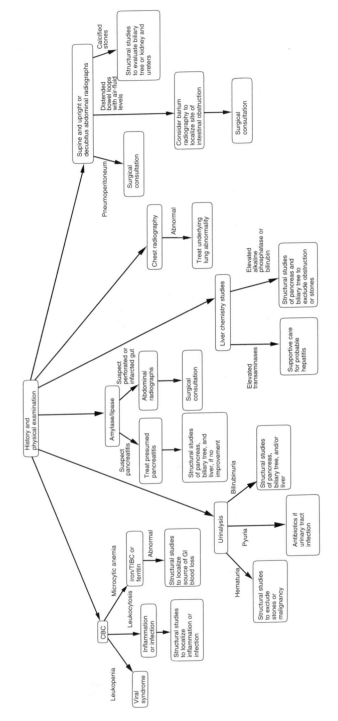

FIGURE 8-1. Workup of a patient with abdominal pain. (CBC = complete blood count; TIBC = total iron-binding capacity.)

ious abdominal conditions are covered in chapters dealing with those disorders. For a patient with CIAP of unknown cause, the physician should resist the temptation to pursue extended and repetitive invasive evaluations in the absence of objective abnormalities on screening tests, because these may divert the attention of the physician and the patient from appropriate treatment.

PRINCIPLES OF MANAGEMENT

An important goal in treating abdominal pain of any cause is to reduce pain. For many conditions that produce acute or chronic intermittent abdominal pain, specific therapy exists that relieves pain and resolves the underlying condition. This includes specific medication regimens for disorders such as peptic ulcer disease and esophagitis, and curative surgical procedures for appendicitis, biliary colic, cholecystitis, and ulcer perforation.

The best symptomatic treatment for patients with chronic, continuous abdominal pain for which there is no cure is an individualized blend of therapeutic approaches. Drugs are the most commonly used form of therapy; unfortunately, their efficacy in the treatment of chronic pain may be limited. NSAIDs are often prescribed for chronic pain. However, because many chronic conditions have little tissue damage or inflammation, it is not surprising that NSAIDs are often ineffective. Opioid agents are useful in the management of pain that is secondary to unresectable malignancy; however, their prescription for chronic nonmalignant states is more controversial. Regardless of the indication, narcotics are best administered within the context of an integrated treatment program. The use of opioids at regular intervals, rather than on an as-needed basis, is often more effective for treating severe pain. Pain cocktails that incorporate opioids, acetaminophen, and antiemetics allow flexible dosing that prevents opioid side effects such as mental clouding, respiratory depression, nausea, and constipation. Tricyclic antidepressants have analgesic effects that are independent of their mood-elevating effects. Agents with serotonergic and noradrenergic activity (e.g., amitriptyline, doxepin) appear to exhibit the greatest effects, often at lower doses than is required for the treatment of depression. A meta-analysis of tricyclic agents used to treat irritable bowel syndrome showed significant therapeutic benefits compared with the placebo. Conversely, although anxiolytics may reduce anxiety, they have little long-term efficacy in managing chronic abdominal pain and may actually worsen symptoms because of depletion of brain serotonin levels.

Nonmedical treatments may also be useful in treating chronic pain syndromes. Celiac plexus blockade is effective therapy for selected patients with pancreatic adenocarcinoma, but it is less likely to control the pain from chronic pancreatitis. Rhizotomy and cordotomy involve severing the neural pathways that sense pain and are indicated only for conditions in which the life expectancy does not exceed 6 months because of significant complications, including bowel and bladder dysfunction, dysesthesias, and exacerbation of the pain. Transcutaneous electrical nerve stimulation and dorsal column stimulation reduce pain in some chronic conditions, presumably because of stimulation of pain inhibitory nerve fibers and activation of endogenous opioid production. Acupuncture may work by similar mechanisms. Unfortunately, these techniques have not shown significant efficacy in treating chronic pain that is secondary to intra-abdominal causes.

Like most chronic illnesses, CIAP has no cure; therefore, efforts should be directed to enhancing the functional quality of the patient's life. It is essential for the physician to establish a good working relationship with the patient and to acknowledge the reality of the pain and the suffering that it causes. Scheduling of frequent brief visits and directed appropriate diagnostic evaluation is important. Afterward, the emphasis must shift from diagnosis to treatment with a realization by the patient that a cure is not possible and an understanding that a major part of the treatment process will be to minimize the impact of the pain on daily life. Psychological or psychiatric consultation is appropriate when the clinician suspects a concurrent, major affective or personality disorder. With the possible exception of antidepressants, medications play little role in the management of CIAP. Opioid agents should be strictly avoided in these patients because of drug dependency. Relaxation training, biofeedback, and hypnosis have been proposed, but evidence of their efficacy is limited. Behavior therapy reduces chronic pain behavior by rewarding the patient's expression of well behavior. Cognitive therapies promote healthy behavior by increasing the patient's awareness of situations that increase pain, with the goal of increasing the patient's control over these situations. Subsets of patients with CIAP may benefit from formal psychotherapy.

COMPLICATIONS

The potential for complications depends on the cause of the pain. Failure to diagnose peritonitis, a ruptured ectopic pregnancy, or an aortic aneurysm could have fatal consequences. Other inflammatory conditions (e.g., pancreatitis, inflammatory bowel disease, or pelvic inflammatory disease) may require prolonged courses of treatment, producing debilitating symptoms and loss of productivity at home and work. Renal stones may lead to infection and renal insufficiency. The prognosis is excellent for many patients with chronic noninflammatory abdominal pain, including those with irritable bowel syndrome, endometriosis, and nerve root compression syndromes.

CHAPTER 9

Approach to the Patient with Acute Abdomen

DIFFERENTIAL DIAGNOSIS

The differential diagnosis of the acute abdomen is nearly as extensive as for abdominal pain itself and includes intra- and extra-abdominal disease processes. Many cases require urgent surgical management, although some can be managed nonsurgically (Table 9-1). The physician must consider all possible causes and be prepared to perform emergency surgery, as a delay invites a cascade of complications.

Acute Appendicitis

Acute appendicitis is the most common cause of the acute abdomen in the United States and must be in the differential diagnosis of every patient with acute abdominal pain. The disorder results from obstruction of the appendiceal lumen by a fecalith, appendiceal calculus, or hyperplastic submucosal lymphatic tissue. Typically, the patient presents with periumbilical pain, low-grade fever, and anorexia with or without vomiting. Over several hours, this is followed by movement of the pain into the right lower quadrant as the inflamed serosal surface of the appendix contacts the overlying parietal peritoneum. Classically, tenderness is elicited at McBurney's point, which is located one-third of the distance from the anterior-superior iliac spine to the umbilicus, although the point of maximal tenderness is variable depending on the location of the appendix. If the appendix is in the pelvis, tenderness may be best appreciated on rectal examination, whereas retrocecal appendicitis produces flank tenderness. A medial appendix may evoke psoas muscle inflammation, resulting in pain on hip flexion (psoas sign). Two percent to 3% of patients with appendicitis present with an abdominal mass, which signifies phlegmon or abscess development secondary to perforation. This complication should be suspected if the pain has lasted >24 hours, the patient's temperature is >38°C, and if the leukocyte count is >15,000 per μl.

TABLE 9-1
Causes of Acute Abdomen That May Require Surgical Intervention

Gastrointestinal
  Appendicitis
  Perforated peptic ulcer
  Intestinal obstruction
  Intestinal ischemia
  Diverticulitis
  Inflammatory bowel disease
  Meckel's diverticulitis
Pancreaticobiliary tract, liver, spleen
  Acute pancreatitis
  Calculous cholecystitis
  Acalculous cholecystitis
  Acute cholangitis
  Hepatic abscess
  Ruptured hepatic tumor
  Splenic rupture
Urinary tract
  Renal/ureteral stone
Gynecologic
  Ectopic pregnancy
  Tubo-ovarian abscess
  Ovarian torsion
  Uterine rupture
  Ruptured ovarian cyst or follicle
Retroperitoneum
  Abdominal aortic aneurysm
Supradiaphragmatic
  Pneumothorax
  Pulmonary embolus
  Acute pericarditis
  Empyema

Perforated Duodenal Ulcer

Patients with a perforated ulcer commonly present with sudden, severe upper abdominal pain, with or without radiation to the shoulders. This is followed by diffuse pain that is exacerbated by respiration or movement because of gastric acid irritation of the peritoneum. Because gastric secretions are nearly sterile, the risk of peritoneal infection depends on the length of time that elapses before definitive treatment; less than one-half of the cases exhibit positive findings on peritoneal fluid cultures within 12 hours of perforation. Two-thirds of the patients report prior dyspepsia or a history of ulcer disease. The physical examination may reveal fasting tachycardia and fever. Bowel sounds are usually absent, and the liver span may not be detectable by percussion because of air interposed between the liver and the abdominal wall. Rigidity and involuntary guarding signify peritonitis.

Obstruction of the Small Intestine

In the United States, 70% to 80% of the cases of obstruction of the small intestine result from postoperative adhesions. Other causes include primary and metastatic carcinoma, external and internal hernias, Crohn's disease, prior radiation therapy, intussusception, endometriosis, volvulus, and congenital abnormalities. Patients with obstruction present with periodic crampy pain centered in the midabdomen, interspersed with nearly asymptomatic intervals, which may progress to unrelenting pain. Vomiting is progressive and may provide transient relief of symptoms; with prolonged obstruction, bacterial overgrowth develops and leads to feculent emesis. Complete obstruction produces constipation or obstipation. In cases of bowel strangulation, signs of peritonitis, an abdominal mass, tachycardia, and fever may be observed.

Colonic Diverticulitis

Although colonic diverticula are common in the United States, symptomatic diverticulitis is rare, with a lifetime risk of approximately 5%. Diverticulitis occurs when the ostia of one or more diverticula, usually in the sigmoid colon, are obstructed with feces. The signs and symptoms depend on the involved colonic segment, the degree of pericolonic inflammation, and the development of extracolonic complications. Most patients present with lower abdominal pain, fever, and obstipation with minimal nausea. Distention is variable, and examination may reveal a palpable, tender mass in the lower abdomen. Leukocytosis is so common that the diagnosis should be questioned in its absence. If colonic rupture occurs, peritonitis may result. In complicated cases, a peridiverticular abscess can extend into an adjacent organ (e.g., the bladder) and cause recurrent urinary infections and pneumaturia.

Acute Cholecystitis

Impaction of a gallstone in the cystic duct causes biliary colic, characterized by epigastric or right upper quadrant pain. Continued cystic duct obstruction initiates an inflammatory response in the gallbladder wall, which distinguishes acute cholecystitis from biliary colic. Although 95% of patients with acute cholecystitis have gallstones, some patients with severe systemic disease develop acalculous cholecystitis. The pain of acute cholecystitis may occur after a meal and is often accompanied by nausea and vomiting, reaching maximum intensity quickly and persisting until medical or surgical therapy is provided. Patients may report prior histories of biliary colic and fatty food intolerance. The physical examination reveals tenderness and guarding in the right upper quadrant. Movement of the inflamed gallbladder against the parietal peritoneum may inhibit deep inspiration, producing Murphy's sign. Low-grade fever is common and jaundice occurs in 10% of cases.

Mesenteric Ischemia

The four major ischemic syndromes are mesenteric embolism, acute mesenteric thrombosis, low-flow mesenteric ischemia, and iatrogenic mesenteric ischemia. Each may produce life-threatening disease. Mesenteric embolism, which accounts for 50% of cases of mesenteric ischemia, often derives from cardiac sources (e.g., mural thrombi associated with myocardial infarction or atrial fibrillation), usually with lodging of the embolus at branch points of the superior mesenteric artery (SMA) distal to its origin. Patients with a mesenteric embolism have sudden, severe epigastric and midabdominal pain with forceful vomiting and defecation. The classic early presentation of a patient with a mesenteric embolism is severe abdominal pain with an unremarkable abdominal examination; distention, guarding, and the absence of bowel sounds imply intestinal infarction. Laboratory findings in advanced disease include hemoconcentration, leukocytosis, and acidosis. Mesenteric thrombosis occurs if atherosclerotic narrowing of the SMA, usually at its origin from the aorta, exceeds a critical level. Many patients have histories of postprandial abdominal pain and weight loss consistent with chronic intestinal angina. Nonocclusive visceral ischemia with intestinal vasoconstriction occurs in low-flow states such as shock, reduced cardiac output, and dehydration and is usually responsive to measures that restore intravascular volume and hemodynamic stability. Iatrogenic mesenteric ischemia most commonly occurs after angiographic dislodgment of an atheroma or induction of vascular dissection.

Abdominal Aortic Aneurysm

Acute symptoms may result from expansion, rupture, dissection, distal embolism, and thrombosis of an abdominal aortic aneurysm. Severe pain in the back, flank, or abdomen occurs with aneurysmal expansion or small tears. Hypotension or shock implies free intraperitoneal blood loss. Physical examination reveals a pulsatile abdominal mass.

Other Causes of Acute Abdomen

Many other conditions produce the clinical presentation of acute abdomen. Acute pancreatitis evokes epigastric and left upper quadrant pain with radiation to the back. Abdominal tenderness often is out of proportion to the physical findings of rigidity or rebound. In severe cases, hypovolemia, hypotension, and respiratory distress may complicate the course of this disorder. If a peripancreatic phlegmon dissects down either paracolic gutter, the presentation may be confused with that of acute appendicitis or diverticulitis. Charcot's triad of right upper quadrant pain, jaundice, and fever is classic for acute cholangitis secondary to choledocholithiasis or bile duct obstruction, although the triad is present in only 60% of cases. Esophageal rupture from instrumentation or forceful vomiting (Boerhaave's syndrome) produces pneumomediastinum or pneumoperitoneum and peritonitis. The diagnosis is suggested by subcutaneous emphysema, pleural effusions, friction rubs, and pneumothorax. An intra-abdominal catastrophe occurs when a tubal pregnancy ruptures into the peritoneum. Sudden lower abdominal pain is followed by generalized peritonitis and hypovolemic shock as a result of intra-abdominal hemorrhage. Pelvic examination may reveal a blue-colored cervix or blood at the cervical os as well as uterine enlargement or a palpable hematoma in the cul-de-sac. A syndrome of diffuse pain, fever, and diarrhea has been reported by patients with severe neutropenia. The pathologic entity, termed *neutropenic colitis*, is characterized by mucosal ulceration, invasive infection with enteric organisms, and sepsis.

WORKUP

History

A detailed approach to taking a history from a patient with abdominal pain is provided in Chapter 8. This section focuses on historical features that help to determine the need for surgical intervention. The potential for rapid disease progression and for adverse consequences of a delay in specific therapeutic intervention places time constraints on diagnosis and treatment. Initially, the nature and timing of pain should be addressed. The pain of ulcer perforation or rupture of an abdominal aortic aneurysm is sudden and incapacitating. The pain reaches an early maximal intensity in contrast to the pain of appendicitis, which may increase over hours. Pain duration can assist with diagnosis; biliary colic lasts for hours before resolving, whereas pancreatitis pain is unrelenting. Pain perception results from stimulation of the visceral or parietal peritoneum. Visceral pain is perceived in patterns corresponding to the embryologic origin of the diseased organ and is sensed as a vague midline discomfort. Ulceration of the duodenum, an embryologic foregut structure, is experienced as epigastric discomfort, whereas early appendicitis produces periumbilical pain that corresponds to the embryologic midgut origin of the appendix. With progressive inflammation, the adjacent parietal peritoneum may become irritated, resulting in a shift in the region where the pain is most intense. With progressive appendicitis, the location of the pain moves from the periumbilical region to the right lower quadrant. Parietal pain is sharp, well localized, and easily described. Pain may also be referred to anatomically distant sites—for example, the right scapula in gallbladder disease, the back in pancreatic disease, and the groin or testicle in renal colic.

Symptoms other than pain may provide useful diagnostic clues. The diagnosis of appendicitis should be questioned in the absence of anorexia. With mechanical obstruction, vomiting is progressive and may relieve the pain resulting from lumenal distention, whereas in inflammatory conditions, vomiting is not progressive and does not reduce abdominal discomfort. Constipation is reported in obstructive conditions and with inflammatory disorders that produce ileus, although some partial obstructions may permit some passage of intestinal contents. Watery diarrhea suggests gastroenteritis, whereas bloody diarrhea results from infectious colitis, inflammatory bowel disease, and mesenteric ischemia. Jaundice occurs with hepatic and pancreaticobiliary disease and with generalized sepsis. Urinary frequency, dysuria, hematuria, and suprapubic or flank pain suggest urologic disease.

Confounding factors can limit the list of diagnostic possibilities in a given patient. Most studies of surgically treated patients with abdominal pain report high levels of diagnostic inaccuracy in young women; therefore, careful detailed sexual and menstrual histories must be taken and the patient must be examined for possible ectopic pregnancy, ovarian cyst, salpingitis, and tubo-ovarian abscess. Pregnancy is rarely complicated by acute abdomen; the most common complication is appendicitis. Diagnosis is more difficult in pregnant women because of uterine displacement of intraperitoneal structures. The diagnosis of the acute abdomen is most difficult at extreme ages. Infants cannot adequately communicate their symptoms, and their abdominal walls are poorly developed, thus reducing manifestations of peritonitis. Elderly patients exhibit reduced febrile and inflammatory responses, which also may falsely reassure the clinician about the severity of the underlying condition. Similarly, patients who are immunosuppressed (e.g., by corticosteroid use or with Cushing's syndrome) may not demonstrate the appropriate clinical responses to acute intraperitoneal inflammatory processes. Diabetics have less pain and tenderness with acute abdominal conditions than do nondiabetics. Reliable abdominal symptoms and signs may not develop in patients with impaired mentation or spinal cord injury. In such patients, fever, leukocytosis, and hypotension may be the only presenting findings of an acute abdomen. A complete record of surgical procedures is necessary to confirm or exclude certain causes. Prior laparotomy increases the risk of obstruction, whereas prior cholecystectomy and appendectomy eliminate the possibility of cholecystitis and appendicitis, respectively. Abdominal pain in the acute postoperative period should suggest prolonged ileus, abscess, acalculous cholecystitis, and anastomotic dehiscence. A family history may suggest sickle cell anemia or familial Mediterranean fever. Certain medications can produce acute abdomen— for example, hepatic adenoma rupture secondary to oral contraceptive use.

Physical Examination

Observation of a patient with acute abdomen reveals anxiety, with a pale, diaphoretic face, dilated pupils, and shallow respirations. Parietal peritoneal inflammation causes the patient to lie quietly, often with flexed knees. In contrast, renal colic or mesenteric ischemia may produce restless behavior. Determination of vital signs may detect fever, tachypnea, tachycardia, and hypotension. The abdomen should be carefully inspected for surgical scars. Distention suggests obstruction, ileus, and ascites. Bluish discoloration of the flanks or periumbilical regions provides evidence for retroperitoneal or intra-abdominal hemorrhage. An absence of bowel sounds after 2 minutes of auscultation suggests ileus, whereas high-pitched, hyperactive bowel sounds suggest obstruction. Bruits are found in some patients with mesenteric thrombosis. The abdomen is gently percussed beginning in the quadrant farthest from the site of the pain. Gentle palpation is performed last to assess for mass lesions or fullness as well as point tenderness, rigidity, and involuntary guarding. Point tenderness, as seen in parietal peritoneal inflammatory processes (e.g., appendicitis), is elicited by one-finger palpation. Rebound tenderness is nonspecific and is not useful in diagnosing the source of an acute abdomen. Every patient must undergo a rectal examination, which may detect pelvic inflammatory processes or occult fecal blood. In women, manual and speculum pelvic examinations are required. Ectopic pregnancy may present as a unilateral adnexal mass with blue cervical discoloration, whereas inflammation of the fallopian tubes or uterus may manifest as cervical tenderness, cervical displacement, adnexal mass, and cervical discharge.

Additional Testing

Initial Studies

Blood testing should be performed in all patients (Fig. 9-1). A complete blood count is used to detect anemia, leukocytosis, or leukopenia, whereas levels of serum electrolytes, blood urea nitrogen, and creatinine indicate the metabolic effects of vomiting or diarrhea. Urinalysis provides useful information in diabetic ketoacidosis, urinary infection, or nephrolithiasis. If pancreatitis is a diagnostic possibility, measurements of serum amylase or lipase are ordered; in uncomplicated pancreatitis, no further invasive investigation is needed. Liver chemistry values may be abnormal in hepatic and pancreaticobiliary disease. A pregnancy test

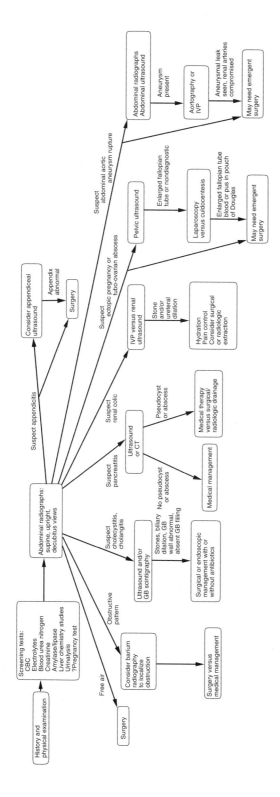

FIGURE 9-1. Workup of a patient with acute abdomen. (CBC = complete blood count; CT = computed tomography; GB = gallbladder; IVP = intravenous pyelography.)

is mandatory in every woman of child-bearing potential with acute abdomen. Microscopic examination of cervical discharge in addition to aerobic and anaerobic cultures can direct the treatment of women with certain gynecologic causes of acute abdomen. If peritonitis is present or if obstruction or infarction is suspected, abdominal radiographs obtained with the patient supine, upright, or decubitus provide important information. Free subdiaphragmatic air is observed in 75% of patients with ulcer perforation; pneumoperitoneum may be more pronounced with colonic perforation. Ileus manifests as diffusely dilated loops of the small intestine and colon, whereas obstruction is characterized by proximal distention and air-fluid levels with little or no air distal to the blockage. Gas in the biliary tree is found with fistulae or cholangitis secondary to gas-forming organisms, whereas gas in the intestinal wall or portal vein is seen with intestinal infarction. Abdominal radiography may also demonstrate localized ileus in patients with pancreatitis or abdominal aortic aneurysmal calcification.

Decision to Operate Immediately

After the initial history and physical examination, with or without selected screening tests, a decision to proceed immediately to laparotomy must be made. Immediate surgery is indicated if the suspected pathologic process is rapidly progressive and potentially fatal—for example, a ruptured abdominal aortic aneurysm or an ectopic pregnancy. If pneumoperitoneum is found, the source can be determined at the time of laparotomy.

Imaging Studies

A large fraction of cases of acute abdomen will afford time to complete a diagnostic evaluation with selected imaging techniques. Although appendicitis is usually a clinical diagnosis, ultrasound may be useful with atypical presentations, and computed tomographic (CT) scanning may distinguish periappendiceal phlegmon from abscess. In cases of mechanical obstruction, barium-enhanced radiographic and endoscopic evaluation may be indicated depending on the suspected site of blockage. As with appendicitis, the diagnosis of acute diverticulitis is primarily clinical, although CT scanning in difficult cases may show colonic thickening, mesenteric edema, abscesses, and phlegmon formation. Barium radiography and colonoscopy are generally contraindicated for suspected acute diverticulitis. Ultrasound is the preferred modality for examining a patient for gallstones, gallbladder wall inflammation, biliary dilation, or liver lesions. If cholecystitis is suspected, biliary scintigraphy may reveal cystic duct obstruction. Subsequent evaluation can be performed with endoscopic retrograde cholangiopancreatography (ERCP) or percutaneous transhepatic cholangiography. Mesenteric angiography is diagnostic in patients with mesenteric embolism or thrombosis. In cases in which bleeding from an abdominal aortic aneurysm is suspected, ultrasound and aortography may detect the aneurysm; however, these procedures should be performed in an operating room because of the risk of exsanguination. A CT scan can exclude abscess, hemorrhage, and pseudocyst in complicated pancreatitis, whereas ERCP can exclude gallstones. Renal ultrasound or intravenous pyelography may reveal ureteral stones that cause renal colic, whereas pelvic ultrasound can provide images of the adnexa in women with suspected tubo-ovarian abscess or ectopic pregnancy. Other useful studies include laparoscopy, which can visualize abdominal or pelvic structures (e.g., the uterus and adnexa), or culdocentesis, which aids in the assessment of intraperitoneal hemorrhage. In some cases of acute abdomen, no combination of laboratory or imaging studies can provide the information on which to confidently base the diagnosis. In such a setting, the importance of using laparotomy in establishing a diagnosis should not be overlooked.

PRINCIPLES OF MANAGEMENT

After conditions that require immediate surgery have been excluded and an appropriate diagnostic evaluation has been completed, it must be determined if surgical intervention is required and when it should be performed. Urgent surgery is required to treat most cases of perforated viscus, appendicitis, and intestinal obstruction, but diagnostic testing usually can be completed before operative intervention. In cholecystitis or cholangitis, definitive surgery usually is not performed until after the repletion of intravascular fluids and the administration of systemic antibiotics. However, some unstable patients may need an operation more urgently. Some appendiceal masses or abscesses initially may be treated nonsurgically with percutaneous drainage and intravenous antibiotics, with appendectomy reserved until a later date. Before surgical management of intestinal obstruction, abdominal decompression with nasogastric suction is instituted. In contrast to appendicitis, many cases of mild diverticulitis are managed with intravenous antibiotics, bowel rest, and intravenous fluids. Control of mesenteric ischemia resulting from embolism and thrombosis may be achieved operatively and with angiographic angioplasty techniques. Nonocclusive mesenteric ischemia usually responds to hemodynamic stabilization. Acute pancreatitis usually responds to intravenous hydration, parenteral narcotics, and restriction of oral intake. Surgery for neutropenic colitis is indicated if perforation is suspected; however, recovery correlates more closely with recovery of the neutrophil count.

COMPLICATIONS

Complications of acute abdomen depend on the cause. In extreme circumstances—for example, the rupture of an aortic aneurysm or an ectopic pregnancy—brisk exsanguination and death are possible. In visceral perforation, the probable outcome is generalized peritonitis followed by systemic infection and death if surgery is not performed. In inflammatory conditions (e.g., appendicitis, diverticulitis, and cholecystitis), the major risk is the spread of infection resulting in intra-abdominal or hepatic abscess, followed by sepsis. Complications of acute pancreatitis include hypocalcemia, acidosis, and respiratory problems as well as structural abnormalities of the pancreas (e.g., pseudocyst). Intestinal obstruction may result in pulmonary aspiration as a result of intractable nausea and vomiting. Renal calculi may be complicated by pyelonephritis or renal failure.

CHAPTER 10

Approach to the Patient with Gas and Bloating

DIFFERENTIAL DIAGNOSIS

The intestine of a normal person typically contains >200 ml of gas, and gas expulsion averages 600 ml per day. The principal gases in flatus include nitrogen, oxygen, carbon dioxide, hydrogen, and methane. Nitrogen, which usually represents 90% of expelled gas, and oxygen result primarily from swallowed air. Mammalian tissues do not produce hydrogen; therefore, expelled hydrogen results from bacterial fermentation of dietary carbohydrates and endogenous glycoproteins. Methane is a highly volatile metabolite produced by anaerobic methanogenic bacteria (e.g., *Methanobrevibacter smithii*). Carbon dioxide in expelled flatus derives from bacterial fermentation of dietary carbohydrates, fats, and proteins. Various clinical syndromes are associated with complaints of gas and bloating (Table 10-1).

Eructation

Eructation, or belching, is the retrograde expulsion of esophageal and gastric gas from the mouth. Involuntary belching after eating is a normal phenomenon caused by the release of swallowed air after gastric distention, which may be exacerbated by foods that reduce lower esophageal sphincter tone. The Magenblase syndrome is defined as epigastric fullness and bloating relieved by belching. The bulk of upper gastrointestinal air accumulates because of aerophagia, which is worsened by stimuli that evoke hypersalivation, including gum chewing, smoking, and oral irritation. Patients with ulcer disease, gastroesophageal reflux, or biliary colic often exhibit aerophagia and chronically belch in an effort to reduce their symptoms.

Flatulence

Frequent flatulence, although disturbing to the patient, is rarely an indicator of serious disease. Therefore, in the absence of objective indicators of organic dis-

TABLE 10-1
Causes of Gas and Bloating

Eructation
    Involuntary postprandial belching
    Magenblase syndrome
    Aerophagia (e.g., as from gum chewing, smoking, oral irritation)
    Gastroesophageal reflux
    Biliary colic
Bacterial overgrowth
    Intestinal or colonic obstruction
    Diverticula of the small intestine
    Hypochlorhydria
    Chronic intestinal pseudo-obstruction
    Cologastric fistula
    Coprophagia
Functional bowel disorders
    Irritable bowel syndrome
    Nonulcer dyspepsia
    Idiopathic constipation
    Functional diarrhea
Carbohydrate malabsorption
    Lactase deficiency
    Fructose, sorbitol, and starch intolerance
    Bean and legume ingestion
Gas-bloat syndrome
    Postfundoplication
Miscellaneous causes
    Hypothyroidism
    Medications (e.g., anticholinergics, opiates, calcium channel antagonists,
        antidepressants)

ease, endoscopic or barium radiographic evaluation of the gut is usually not warranted. Studies have reported that, on average, healthy young men pass flatus 14 times per day, with normal persons experiencing up to 25 daily gas expulsions. Common dietary causes of increased flatulence include maldigestion and malabsorption of poorly absorbed carbohydrates (see section on carbohydrate malabsorption). Disorders that alter colonic transit (e.g., irritable bowel syndrome) may modify colonic bacterial gas production, as can changes in colonic pH, antibiotic use, and bowel cleansing.

Functional Bowel Disorders

Many patients with functional bowel disease (e.g., irritable bowel syndrome) complain of excess gas. Using careful argon washout techniques, however, these patients have been demonstrated to retain normal volumes of intralumenal gas. The patients with functional bowel disease were distinguished by the development of severe abdominal discomfort with intestinal gas perfusion and by the presence of retrograde air flow from the small intestine to the stomach. These findings are consistent with the recent hypothesis that functional abdominal pain results from hyperalgesia to visceral distending stimuli. Historical diagnoses of hepatic and splenic flexure syndromes in patients with purported gas trapping in these sites probably represent subsets of functional bowel disorders.

Carbohydrate Malabsorption

Hydrogen breath testing has provided evidence that malabsorption of small amounts of carbohydrates may produce eructation, bloating, abdominal pain, and flatulence. Clinically inapparent malabsorption of lactose, fructose, sorbitol, and starch have been reported. In children with unexplained chronic abdominal pain, lactose intolerance may be present in 40% of the cases. Of the complex carbohydrates, only rice and gluten-free wheat are completely absorbed in healthy individuals, whereas up to 20% of the carbohydrates from whole wheat, oat, potato, and corn flour are not absorbed. Nondigestible oligosaccharides (e.g., stachyose, raffinose, and verbascose) are abundant in beans and legumes. Fructose is naturally found in honey and fruits as well as in onions, asparagus, and wheat and is used as a sweetener for many commercial soft drinks. Sorbitol is also present in fruits and is used as a sweetener for dietetic candies and chewing gum. Malabsorption of as little as 25 g of fructose and 2.5 g of sorbitol has been reported. Although the symptoms may be similar, there is no increased prevalence of carbohydrate malabsorption in irritable bowel syndrome.

Bacterial Overgrowth

The stomach and small intestine are relatively sterile compared with the colon. Gastrointestinal bacterial overgrowth may complicate several structurally obstructive disorders of the gut, including postoperative adhesions, Crohn's disease, radiation enteritis, ulcer disease, and malignancy. Other anatomic abnormalities that predispose to bacterial overgrowth include diverticula of the small intestine and postvagotomy changes (which produce hypochlorhydria). Functional disorders of the gut, most commonly those conditions that produce intestinal pseudo-obstruction, are associated with overgrowth because of an impaired ability to clear organisms from the gut. Disorders that increase bacterial delivery to the upper gut (e.g., cologastric fistulae and coprophagia) can overwhelm normal defenses against infection.

Gas-Bloat Syndrome

Many fundoplication procedures for gastroesophageal reflux involve wrapping the gastric fundus around the lower esophagus, thus reducing the ability to belch or vomit. In the initial postoperative months, 25% to 50% of patients experience bloating, upper abdominal cramping, and flatulence—a constellation of symptoms known as *gas-bloat syndrome*. Surgical revision is rarely necessary because most patients improve with time.

Other Causes of Gas and Bloating

Rarely, patients with intestinal obstructions present only with gas and bloating, although other symptoms are usually present. Patients with endocrinopathies (e.g., hypothyroidism) may complain of gaseousness as part of a broader symptom presentation. Many medications (e.g., anticholinergics, opiates, calcium channel antagonists, and antidepressants) produce gas by affecting gut motility.

WORKUP

History

Patients with complaints of excess gas may have a myriad of symptoms, including pain, bloating, halitosis, anorexia, early satiety, nausea, belching, loud borborygmi, constipation, and flatulence, all of which suggest functional bowel disease. The clinician must search for clues that exclude or suggest an organic cause. Relief of symptoms with defecation or passage of flatus is consistent with a functional disorder, as is the absence of symptoms that awaken the patient from deep sleep. Conversely, the presence of associated vomiting, fever, weight loss, nocturnal diarrhea, steatorrhea, and rectal bleeding indicate probable organic disease. Other medical conditions that predispose to bacterial overgrowth should be determined from the patient's history. The use of medications that delay gastrointestinal transit should be questioned. Certain carbohydrate malabsorptive conditions are hereditary and are more prevalent in some ethnic groups (e.g., lactase deficiency). A history of anxiety or psychiatric disease raises the possibility of chronic aerophagia or functional bowel disease.

A precise dietary history may correlate specific foods with symptoms. Ingestion of legumes, beans, apples, prunes, raisins, and unrefined starches should be addressed, as should consumption of diet foods and candies and soft drinks containing fructose. Gum chewing, smoking, and chewing tobacco predispose to aerophagia.

Physical Examination

Physical examination findings are usually normal in patients with complaints of excess gas; however, anxiety, hyperventilation, and air swallowing may be evident in patients with functional disease. Certain findings may suggest organic disease, including sclerodactyly with scleroderma, peripheral or autonomic neuropathy with dysmotility syndromes, and cachexia, jaundice, and palpable masses with malignant intestinal obstruction. Abdominal inspection may reveal scars indicative of prior fundoplication and vagotomy and other operations that might predispose to adhesions. Auscultation should be used to assess for absent bowel sounds with ileus or myopathic dysmotility, high-pitched bowel sounds with intestinal obstruction, or a succussion splash with gastric obstruction or gastroparesis. Abdominal percussion and palpation may reveal tympany and distention in mechanical obstruction and intestinal dysmotility. The presence of ascites should be assessed because patients will occasionally misinterpret the fluid accumulation as excess gas. Occult fecal blood on rectal examination is indicative of mucosal damage, as occurs with ulceration, inflammation, and neoplasm.

Additional Testing

Laboratory Studies

Screening laboratory tests are of use in excluding organic disease (Fig. 10-1). Normal values for a complete blood count, electrolytes, glucose, albumin, total protein, and sedimentation rate exclude most inflammatory and neoplastic conditions. In selected patients, calcium and phosphate levels, renal function, liver chemistry values, and thyroid function tests may be needed. Patients with diarrhea should undergo stool examination for ova and parasites to rule out giardiasis.

Structural Studies

Abdominal radiographs with the patient flat and upright can reveal diffuse distention consistent with ileus, diffuse haziness in ascites, and air-fluid levels consistent with mechanical obstruction. Barium radiography and endoscopy should be considered in a patient with suspected obstruction, pseudo-obstruction, and an intralumenal inflammatory or neoplastic process. Other tests such as ultrasound and computed tomography can be used to assess the patient for other intra-abdominal disorders that might predispose the patient to complaints of excess gas.

Functional Studies

In patients with suspected motility disorders, gastric emptying scintigraphy and manometry of the esophagus, stomach, and small intestine may be considered. Hydrogen breath testing to detect monosaccharide or disaccharide malabsorption confirms associations between symptoms and specific foods. Conceptually, this technique relies on the ability of lumenal bacteria to produce hydrogen gas during metabolism of ingested substrates and the concurrent inability of human tissue to use similar metabolic pathways. Expired breath samples are obtained before and for 2 hours after ingestion of an aqueous solution of the sugar that is presumed to be malabsorbed. Breath hydrogen measurements may need to be extended for up to 10 hours if the test is for the malabsorption of complex carbohydrates (e.g., starch). An increase in breath hydrogen of >20 parts per million within 120 minutes of lactose ingestion distinguishes biopsy-proven, lactase-deficient persons from lactase-sufficient persons with a sensitivity of approximately 90%. Elevations in fasting breath hydrogen before substrate ingestion and early rises (i.e., within 30 minutes of ingestion) raise the possibility of bacterial overgrowth. Glucose is the most commonly used sugar for breath hydrogen testing in suspected bacterial overgrowth; this test has a diagnostic sensitivity of 70% to 90%. Other centers have relied on ^{14}C- or ^{13}C-labeled substrates, with measurement of expired $^{14}CO_2$ or $^{13}CO_2$; however, special facilities are necessary for these analyses. Some patients may be tested for fructose or sorbitol malabsorption using hydrogen breath testing, but the normal values of these tests are less well characterized.

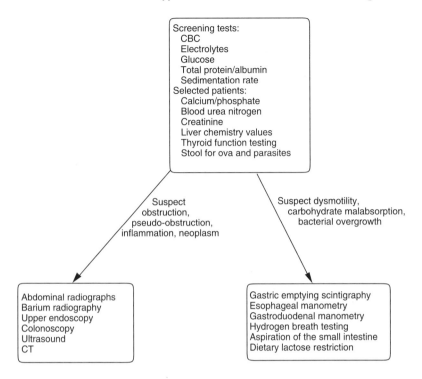

FIGURE 10-1.   Workup of a patient with gas and bloating. (CBC = complete blood count; CT = computed tomography.)

PRINCIPLES OF MANAGEMENT

Any underlying disorder responsible for symptoms of excess gas should be specifically managed, if possible. Obstructions are usually managed surgically, whereas some motility disorders respond to prokinetic medications. Lactase deficiency is controlled by excluding lactose from the diet or by supplementing the diet with exogenous lactase. Belching often occurs with gastroesophageal reflux disease; therefore patients with concomitant pyrosis should be given acid-suppressive medications. If bacterial overgrowth is documented, oral antibiotics are indicated.

For patients with complaints of excess gas who exhibit no definable disorder after appropriate diagnostic testing, attempts should be made to decrease intestinal gas and to regulate bowel function. Aerophagia may be controlled by cessation of gum chewing and smoking and improving oral hygiene. The chronic belcher may be aided by self-observation in a mirror to demonstrate aerophagia. Dietary restriction of legumes, beans, fruits, soft drinks, dietetic candies and gums, and complex carbohydrates may be of benefit in some persons. Patients with constipation may note fewer gaseous symptoms when on an osmotic laxative regimen, with or without fiber supplementation; ingestion of poorly absorbable sugars (e.g., lactulose and sorbitol) is probably not wise in this setting. Simethicone alters the elasticity of mucus-covered intralumenal gas bubbles, which leads to their coalescence; however, there are few data to support its use in a patient who complains of excess gas. Activated charcoal reduces breath hydrogen and the symptoms caused by ingestion of indigestible carbohydrates, although the mechanism of its action is uncertain. Bacterial α-galactosidase (Beano) has been marketed to reduce symptoms after ingestion of legumes high in indigestible oligosaccharides, presumably by hydrolyzing these sugars in the lumen of the small intestine, thereby decreasing their fermentation by colonic bacteria; however, its efficacy in clinical conditions of excess gas is unproved.

COMPLICATIONS

Few complications occur in patients with gas and bloating caused by functional disease. However, complications from organic disease do occur, and usually they are manifestations of the underlying disease rather than of the gas itself. There have been rare case reports of explosions resulting from ignition by tobacco smoking of feculent gas expelled by eructation in patients with gastrointestinal obstruction and proximal bacterial overgrowth, signifying the most serious consequence of excess gas production. Similarly, colonic explosions with perforation have been reported in patients undergoing colonoscopy with intracolonic cautery. In general, these rare complications result from inadequate bowel cleansing or the use of mannitol or sorbitol purging solutions, both of which generate hydrogen gas.

CHAPTER 11

Approach to the Patient with Ileus or Obstruction

DIFFERENTIAL DIAGNOSIS

Ileus is a potentially reversible, pathophysiologic state of inhibited motor activity in the gastrointestinal tract. Pseudo-obstruction describes a chronic abnormality of function that simulates mechanical obstruction, but it has no anatomic cause and may exhibit clinical manifestations similar to ileus. Obstruction implies complete or partial blockage of the gut at one or more levels. Ileus, pseudo-obstruction, and mechanical obstruction have numerous causes (Table 11-1).

Ileus and Pseudo-Obstruction

Acute Ileus

Although the conditions associated with acute motor paralysis of the gut can be defined, the underlying responsible mechanisms often are not known. Ileus is a normal physiologic response to laparotomy. Gastric and small intestinal motility recover in the first postoperative day, and colonic contractions return in 3 to 5 days. Postoperative ileus beyond that time is pathologic and warrants a search for complications. Other intra-abdominal causes of acute ileus include abdominal trauma and inflammatory gut disorders (e.g., ulcer perforation, bile or chemical peritonitis, toxic megacolon, pancreatitis, cholecystitis, appendicitis, diverticulitis, and inflammatory bowel disease). Noninflammatory processes include radiation damage and mesenteric ischemia. Retroperitoneal disorders (e.g., renal calculi, pyelonephritis, renal transplantation, and retroperitoneal hemorrhage) can also produce acute ileus. Extra-abdominal causes of ileus include reflex inhibition of gut motility by craniotomy, fractures, myocardial infarction, heart surgery, pneumonia, pulmonary embolus, and burns. Medications (e.g., anticholinergics, opiates, calcium channel antagonists, chemotherapeutic agents, and antidepressants) may inhibit motor activity, as may metabolic abnormalities, including electrolyte disturbances, sepsis, uremia, diabetic ketoacidosis, sickle cell anemia, respiratory insufficiency, porphyria, and heavy metal intoxication.

TABLE 11-1
Causes of Ileus and Obstruction

Acute ileus
  Postoperative ileus
  Abdominal trauma
  Ulcer perforation
  Bile or chemical peritonitis
  Toxic megacolon
  Pancreatitis
  Cholecystitis
  Appendicitis
  Diverticulitis
  Inflammatory bowel disease
  Radiation therapy
  Mesenteric ischemia
  Retroperitoneal disorders (e.g., renal calculi, pyelonephritis, renal transplant,
    hemorrhage)
  Extra-abdominal sources (e.g., craniotomy, fractures, myocardial infarction, cardiac
    surgery, pneumonia, pulmonary embolus, burns)
  Metabolic disorders (e.g., electrolyte abnormalities, uremia, sepsis, diabetic ketoacidosis,
    sickle cell anemia, respiratory insufficiency, porphyria, heavy metal toxicity)
  Medications (e.g., anticholinergics, opiates, calcium channel antagonists,
    chemotherapy, antidepressants)
Intestinal pseudo-obstruction
  Hereditary diseases (e.g., familial visceral neuropathy, familial visceral myopathy)
  Diabetes mellitus
  Rheumatologic disorders (e.g., scleroderma, systemic lupus erythematosus,
    amyloidosis)
  Endocrinopathies (e.g., hypothyroidism, hyperparathyroid disease or hypoparathyroid
    disease, Addison's disease)
  Neuromuscular diseases (e.g., muscular dystrophy, myotonic dystrophy)
  Chagas' disease
  Infectious pseudo-obstruction
  Pheochromocytoma
  Paraneoplastic pseudo-obstruction
Mechanical obstruction
  Adhesions
  Congenital bands (e.g., Ladd's bands)
  Hernias (e.g., external, internal, diaphragmatic, pelvic)
  Volvulus (e.g., colon, small intestine, stomach)
  Obstructive lumenal tumors
  Inflammatory bowel disease
  Mesenteric ischemia
  Intussusception
  Fecal impaction
  Gallstone ileus
  Retained barium
  Gastric bezoars

Chronic Intestinal Pseudo-Obstruction

Chronic intestinal pseudo-obstruction may be idiopathic, often occurring after a viral prodrome, thereby suggesting a possible infectious etiology. In rare cases, hereditary conditions (e.g., familial visceral myopathies and neuropathies) produce pseudo-obstruction at early ages. Certain systemic disorders have chronic effects on gastrointestinal motor function. Advanced diabetes mellitus may result in the inhibition of motility in the small intestine, in addition to gastroparesis. Rheumatologic disorders (e.g., scleroderma, systemic lupus erythematosus, and amyloidosis) produce pseudo-obstruction, as do endocrinopathies (e.g., hypothyroidism, hyper- or hypoparathyroidism, and Addison's disease). Neuromuscular diseases (e.g., myotonic dystrophy or muscular dystrophy) chronically disrupt motor activity. In selected geographic locations, Chagas' disease, which results from exposure to *Trypanosoma cruzi*, represents an infectious cause of pseudo-obstruction. Infectious pseudo-obstruction in immunosuppressed patients has been reported with cytomegalovirus and other agents. Pheochromocytoma produces chronic intestinal hypomotility, probably because of the motor inhibitory effects of the circulating catecholamines. Chronic intestinal pseudo-obstruction can be a paraneoplastic manifestation of malignancy, usually small cell lung carcinoma, a condition first described by Ogilvie. It may result from malignant invasion of the celiac axis or, alternatively, from a plasma cell infiltration of the myenteric plexus, leading to the loss of enteric neural function.

Mechanical Obstruction

Extrinsic Lesions

The causes of mechanical intestinal obstruction may be divided into extrinsic lesions, intrinsic lesions, and intralumenal objects. Extrinsic adhesions are the most common cause of obstruction of the small intestine in adults, but they rarely occlude the colon. Adhesions may become clinically apparent a few days to 20 years postoperatively and they may occur in nonoperative conditions, usually after intra-abdominal infection or radiation. The adhesive bands constrict the bowel over time and may lead to intestinal strangulation. Congenital bands behave similarly and may occur in association with malrotation (Ladd's bands). Hernias represent another extrinsic cause of obstruction that may be external (protruding through the abdominal wall), internal, diaphragmatic (usually paraesophageal), or pelvic. Internal and pelvic hernias usually are identified at the time of surgery. Volvulus is an abnormal torsion of bowel that produces a closed and obstructed loop of bowel, associated with an impairment of blood flow. It involves the cecum in 10% to 20% and the sigmoid colon in 70% to 80% of cases and manifests as sudden abdominal pain followed by distention. Cecal and sigmoid volvulus are rare in adults; gastric volvulus occurs with diaphragmatic defects, congenital malformations, and large paraesophageal hernias.

Intrinsic Lesions

Intrinsic lesions are less common causes of mechanical obstruction. Benign and malignant tumors can obstruct the lumen or provide a leading point for intussusception. Primary malignancies of the small intestine are rare but include lymphoma, adenocarcinoma, or carcinoids, whereas adenocarcinoma represents the most common obstructing colonic neoplasm. Metastatic tumors usually tether and fix the bowel rather than obstruct the lumen. Inflammatory processes and ischemia cause obstructing strictures, whereas blunt trauma may produce an intramural hematoma. In addition to neoplasm, a Meckel's diverticulum may initiate intussusception; in children, there usually is no predisposing lesion with intussusception.

Intralumenal Objects

Intralumenal objects represent the least common causes of mechanical obstruction. Fecal impaction may produce colonic obstruction in patients who are dehydrated or immobile, who have underlying constipation, and who are taking medications that slow colonic transit. Rarely, large gallstones erode through the gallbladder into the gut lumen, where they migrate to obstruct the intestine, usually at the level of the distal ileum. Barium from radiographic procedures may obstruct the colon in patients with underlying colonic motility disorders. Gastric bezoars and ingested foreign bodies may occlude the gut lumen in select cases.

WORKUP

History

Patients with ileus and obstruction may present with similar symptoms (e.g., pain, nausea, vomiting, abdominal distention, and obstipation). These symptoms may develop acutely or over a period of several hours, or they may be persistent, as in chronic intestinal pseudo-obstruction. Abdominal pain is usually minimal with adynamic ileus as well and gastric or duodenal obstruction, whereas distal intestinal and colonic obstruction produce greater discomfort. Upper and midabdominal pain are characteristic of obstruction proximal to the transverse colon, whereas left colonic blockage produces lower abdominal discomfort. The pain of mechanical obstruction is dull, ill-defined, or squeezing in character; intermittent waves of pain signify true colic.

Distention may be severe in ileus as well as with distal obstruction, whereas gastric obstruction produces little distention. Audible bowel sounds may be present with intestinal obstruction. Copious vomiting of clear liquid characterizes gastric obstruction, and copious vomiting of bile occurs with duodenal blockage. Distal obstruction and ileus produce only mild nausea and vomiting. The pain of proximal, not distal, obstruction is often relieved by vomiting. If mechanical obstruction is incomplete or if ileus is mild, pain and distention may be intermittent and aggravated by fiber-rich, poorly digestible foods. Complete obstruction usually produces obstipation and the inability to expel flatus. Conversely, watery diarrhea is noted with partial obstruction and fecal impaction. Children with intussusception may pass bloody mucus that resembles red currant jelly.

Clues about the cause of ileus or obstruction can be determined from the history. Careful family, medication, endocrine, immunologic, and metabolic histories should be obtained from a patient with ileus, and the clinician should be alert to thyroid and parathyroid disorders, diabetes, scleroderma, heavy metal intoxication, and porphyria. Prior surgery raises the possibility of adhesions, and known abdominal wall bulging suggests hernias as a possible cause of obstruction. Prior histories of malignancy, radiation, inflammatory bowel disease, ulcer disease, gallstones, diverticular disease, pancreatitis, motility disorders, and foreign body ingestion suggest specific causes. Exacerbation of pain with menses is consistent with endometriosis.

Before making management decisions, it is important to determine if complications such as peritonitis, perforation, sepsis, or strangulation have occurred. Constant localized pain, fever, rigors, and a sudden clinical deterioration suggest bowel ischemia and infarction, although strangulation with necrosis may be present before these symptoms develop. Therefore, a high degree of suspicion must be maintained and the clinician must be ready to intervene if the status of the patient changes.

Physical Examination

Careful examination of the patient is necessary before determining the appropriate diagnostic and therapeutic course. A patient with obstruction usually appears to be in great distress, whereas a patient with ileus may be more comfortable despite the presence of obvious distention. Cutaneous findings in selected causes of obstruction include pyoderma gangrenosum and erythema nodosum with inflammatory bowel disease, Cullen's sign or Grey-Turner's sign with pancreatitis, vesicles and bullae with select forms of porphyria, acanthosis nigricans with gastrointestinal malignancy, butterfly dermatitis with systemic lupus erythematosus, and sclerodactyly and telangiectasias with scleroderma.

The most important portion of the examination of a patient with ileus or obstruction is the abdominal examination. Inspection may reveal scars and visible distention. Gentle palpation may detect subtle hernias that are not obvious on inspection. Hepatosplenomegaly, lymphadenopathy, and masses raise concern for malignancy, although tender masses may be palpable in inflammatory diseases (e.g., Crohn's disease). Tympany accompanies both ileus and obstruction, whereas shifting dullness and a fluid wave characterize ascites. Auscultation usually reveals hypoactive or absent bowel sounds with ileus, whereas obstruction produces louder, high-pitched, hyperactive bowel sounds that may have a musical or tinkling quality. Shaking of the abdomen while listening through a stethoscope may reveal a succussion splash, which is rarely found with gastric obstruction and gastroparesis. Rectal examination may detect occult fecal blood with inflammatory, neoplastic, infectious, or ischemic disease. Digital rectal and pelvic examinations may also detect subtle masses not found on abdominal palpation and may reveal obturator or sciatic hernias.

Repeated abdominal examinations are essential for surveillance for complications. If fever, hypotension, or signs of sepsis or peritonitis develop or if bowel sounds disappear, the viscus may be ischemic and operative intervention may be urgently indicated.

Additional Testing

Laboratory Studies

Biochemical and hematologic tests aid in establishing the cause of mechanical obstruction only rarely, as with inflammation, infection, and neoplasm. In contrast, laboratory studies are essential in discovering the cause of ileus (Fig. 11-1). Measurement of electrolytes (including calcium, phosphate, and magnesium), blood urea nitrogen, and creatinine is used to detect dehydration. With progressive dehydration, hemoconcentration develops, as indicated by increases in hemoglobin and albumin levels. Leukocytosis may be present with inflammation or infection. Measurement of arterial blood gases may be necessary to evaluate acid-

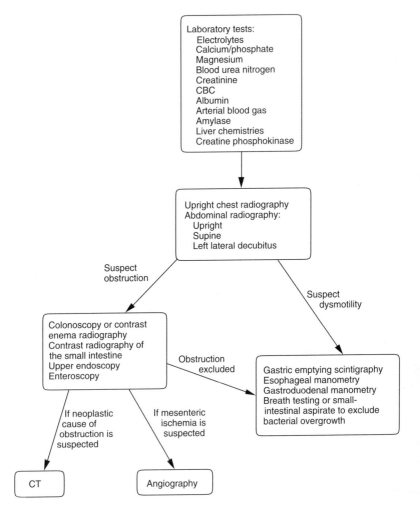

FIGURE 11-1. Workup of a patient with ileus or obstruction. (CBC = complete blood count; CT = computed tomography.)

base balance. With an ischemic or infarcted bowel, elevations in amylase, alkaline phosphatase, creatine phosphokinase, aspartate and alanine aminotransferase, and lactate dehydrogenase may be evident, although these enzymes also increase with hepatic and pancreaticobiliary disease.

Plain Radiographic Studies

The initial studies that should be obtained on a patient with suspected ileus or obstruction are chest radiographs, which can be used to detect pneumonia, evaluate cardiorespiratory status, and detect free subdiaphragmatic air, and radiographs of the abdomen with the patient upright and supine, which show intra-abdominal gas distribution. Left lateral decubitus abdominal radiographs may be obtained on patients who cannot assume an upright position. In general, the jejunum lies in the left upper and central abdomen, the ileum in the right central and lower abdomen, and the colon in the flanks and right iliac fossa. In early or partial obstruction, lumenal distention occurs, but air may still be present in sites distal to the blockage. With total obstruction of the small intestine, the lumen is widely distended with the characteristic spanning of the lumenal diameter by the valvulae conniventes. Upright or decubitus views will demonstrate air-fluid levels in a stepladder configuration. With distal to complete obstruction, the colon empties and collapses within 12 to 24 hours and no colonic air is radiographically visible. With colonic obstruction, the colon proximal to the blockage dilates and the characteristic incomplete and scalloped indentations of the haustra are visible. With advanced strangulation, the bowel wall becomes edematous, exhibiting a thumbprinting pattern on radiographs, and air in the intestinal wall, portal vein, and peritoneal cavity can be detected.

In ileus, bowel distention may be diffuse or it may manifest adjacent to an inflammatory site, producing a sentinel loop, as in appendicitis or pancreatitis. With concurrent peritonitis, the bowel wall may thicken. Colonic gas may be more prominent in ileus, whereas gaseous distention of the small intestine predominates in partial or complete obstruction of the small intestine. Pure colonic dilation, most prominent in the cecum, is the defining feature of acute colonic pseudo-obstruction. Stepladder air-fluid levels may appear in either ileus or obstruction, but with obstruction they are more pronounced and longer. A string-of-beads pattern of the air-fluid interfaces is most suggestive of high-grade obstruction of the small intestine. A diffusely hazy pattern with central localization of bowel loops is characteristic of ascites.

Structural Studies

Contrast radiography should be performed if the differentiation between ileus and obstruction cannot be made or to localize the anatomic site of the obstruction. Barium is the superior contrast agent, but water-soluble medium should be used with suspected perforation because of the intense inflammatory effects of barium on the peritoneum. If there is doubt about the site of obstruction, colonoscopy should be performed before upper gastrointestinal barium radiography to exclude a colonic cause. Upper endoscopy is useful with suspected esophageal, gastric, or duodenal lesions and offers the additional capability of therapeutic dilation of any stricture. Enteroscopy has been recently made available for inspection of the small intestine. A sonde enteroscope is advanced slowly, over several hours, by peristalsis into the distal small intestine. Its drawbacks are a lack of steering control of its tip and the inability to perform therapeutic maneuvers. Push enteroscopy uses a steerable enteroscope that has a central channel for biopsy and therapeutic intervention, but it usually cannot be advanced beyond the jejunum. A computed tomographic scan may establish the diagnosis of an intra-abdominal inflammatory or neoplastic process; ultrasound is generally not useful because of the obscuring effects of intralumenal gas. Angiography is indicated in patients with suspected mesenteric ischemia and infarction.

Functional Studies

In patients with prolonged ileus or suspected chronic intestinal pseudo-obstruction, functional testing of gut motility may be considered. Gastric emptying scintigraphy may document gastroparesis, whereas esophageal or gastroduodenal manometry may show the characteristic hypomotility pattern of visceral myopathy or the random, intense bursts of contractions in visceral neuropathy. Some centers have proposed using gastroduodenal manometry in cases of suspected obstruction of the small intestine in which the radiographic studies are normal. In these instances, manometry shows clusters of contractions separated by periods of quiescence, called the *minute rhythm*.

PRINCIPLES OF MANAGEMENT

Fluid Replacement

Correction of fluid, electrolyte, and acid-base imbalances is guided by laboratory determination of hematocrit, electrolyte, blood urea nitrogen, creatinine, and blood gas levels. With severe hypovolemia, fluid resuscitation should be performed with concurrent monitoring of urine output, central venous pressure, and blood pressure. In patients with superimposed cardiorespiratory or renal disease, a Swan-Ganz catheter may be needed. In mild to moderate hypovolemia, one-half of the deficit should be replaced using crystalloid solutions (e.g., lactated Ringer's solution, normal saline) within 24 hours, and one-half in the second 24 hours. Maintenance fluid requirements average 1500 to 2500 ml per day in an afebrile person with normal renal function. Additional fluids are given with fever or with fluid losses, as from nasogastric suction. With gastric outlet obstruction, potassium chloride is often needed after establishment of normal urine output because renal potassium losses are high in this condition. Sodium bicarbonate is given for profound metabolic acidosis (e.g., pH <7.1). The bicarbonate deficit can be calculated by the formula (24 mEq per liter − $[HCO_3^-]$) × body weight. One-half of the deficit should be given to raise plasma bicarbonate to 16 mEq per liter in the first 12 to 24 hours. Overaggressive correction of acidosis can produce intracellular volume depletion, neurologic dysfunction, and decreased blood oxygen delivery.

Bowel Decompression

Abdominal distention increases gastrointestinal secretion and causes nausea and vomiting, thereby increasing the risk of aspiration. Nasogastric suction is appropriate in ileus and obstruction. The use of longer tubes (e.g., Cantor, Miller-Abbott) is controversial. The patient should be given nothing by mouth, relying on intravenous fluids and nutrients for support. For patients with acute colonic pseudo-obstruction, some clinicians advocate therapeutic colonoscopic decompression, although there are few objective data to support this practice. Placement of a rectal tube or administration of tap water enemas may reduce colonic distention in some patients. Drugs that inhibit motor activity should be withheld.

Surgical Management

As a rule, complete obstruction is surgically relieved as soon as resuscitation is completed and nasogastric suction is achieved, because strangulation cannot be excluded using clinical criteria in this setting. Antibiotics are given preoperatively to reduce the likelihood of wound infections resulting from enterotomy of an unprepared bowel. With strangulation, any necrotic bowel should be resected.

Intraoperative Doppler ultrasound and fluorescein dye injection can be used to assess the viability of the adjacent intestine. In questionable cases, a second-look laparotomy may be needed. In partial obstruction, immediate surgery and antibiotics are of no proven benefit; however, if fever, peritoneal signs, leukocytosis, or hyperamylasemia develop, laparotomy is indicated. With multiple prior operations, immediate surgery usually is not indicated because bowel fixation from intraperitoneal scarring makes strangulation unlikely. Colonic obstruction nearly always requires surgery; nasogastric suction may have little effect in this setting. If bowel cleansing cannot be performed, many surgeons perform a two-stage operation: resection of the obstructed segment and placement of a diverting colostomy followed by anastomosis at a later date to reduce wound infection.

Nonsurgical Management

Nonsurgical therapy can be provided for some disorders. Sigmoid volvulus may be treated by aspiration of colonic gas through a colonoscopically placed tube or by gentle hydrostatic pressure with rectally introduced contrast agents. Endoscopic dilation of adhesions or radiation-induced strictures may be possible. Inoperable colorectal cancer may be palliatively treated by Nd:YAG laser recanalization of the colonic lumen. The use of prokinetic agents in ileus (e.g., cisapride and erythromycin) has been promoted, although studies documenting their efficacy are inconclusive. Prokinetic drugs, including cisapride, metoclopramide, erythromycin, and octreotide are commonly used for chronic intestinal pseudo-obstruction. Unfortunately, in advanced cases, no medical therapy provides impressive relief, and total parenteral nutrition may be required.

COMPLICATIONS

The most serious complication of obstruction or ileus is bowel infarction, with resulting peritonitis and possible death. Other complications include aspiration pneumonia, electrolyte abnormalities, and malnutrition, all of which may have serious consequences in unstable patients who have other concurrent disease. Many of the diseases that produce ileus and obstruction have serious sequelae, in addition to those that result from the involvement of the bowel.

CHAPTER 12

Approach to the Patient with Diarrhea

DIFFERENTIAL DIAGNOSIS

The average daily fecal weight of a person on a Western diet is 100 to 200 g, although a person on a fiber-supplemented diet may pass 500 g per day. In the United States, a daily stool weight of >250 g is considered abnormal. In Western society, 99% of persons note between three bowel movements per week and three per day. Diarrhea is categorized into those disorders that produce stool outputs of >250 g per day and those that produce normal stool output (Table 12-1). High-output diarrheas are further divided according to osmotic, secretory, and mucosal inflammation patterns. Normal-output diarrheas include colonic motility disturbances and disorders of continence. Diarrhea is also classified as acute, which lasts <3 weeks, or chronic, which lasts >3 weeks. Some diseases produce diarrhea by more than a single mechanism. For example, intestinal pseudo-obstruction is a primary motility disorder that leads to secondary bacterial overgrowth and malabsorption. Bacteria in the small intestine deconjugate intralumenal bile acids, which in turn stimulate colonic water and electrolyte secretion.

Osmotic High-Output Diarrhea

Normally, most ingested nutrients are absorbed proximal to the ileocecal junction. However, with osmotic diarrhea, some of the consumed material is not absorbed, and it acts as an osmotic agent to draw free water into the intestinal lumen that is then evacuated as diarrheal stool. The most common cause of osmotic diarrhea is lactase deficiency, in which the lactose in dairy products is not hydrolyzed by brush border disaccharidase activity, thus drawing water into the intestinal lumen. When unhydrolyzed lactose exits the small intestine, colonic bacteria metabolize the sugar molecules to short-chain fatty acids, further increasing the number of osmotically active molecules in the stool. The high-risk groups for lactase deficiency include Asians and Native Americans (90% prevalence), African Americans, Jews, Hispanics, and southern Europeans (60% to 70%), with 10% to 15% prevalence in individuals of northern European descent. Similarly, some persons exhibit incomplete absorption of the sugars

TABLE 12-1
Causes of Diarrhea

High-output osmotic
    Nonabsorbed solutes
        Saline and phosphate laxatives
        Sorbitol, fructose, lactulose
    Disaccharidase deficiency
        Lactase deficiency
        Isomaltase-sucrase deficiency
        Trehalase deficiency
    Small intestinal mucosal disease
        Celiac sprue
        Tropical sprue
        Viral gastroenteritis
        Whipple's disease
        Amyloidosis
        Intestinal ischemia
        Lymphoma
        Giardiasis
    Pancreatic insufficiency
        Chronic pancreatitis
        Pancreatic carcinoma
        Cystic fibrosis
    Reduced intestinal surface area
        Small intestinal resection
        Enteric fistulae
        Jejunoileal bypass
    Bile salt malabsorption
        Bacterial overgrowth
        Ileal resection
        Crohn's disease
    Defective transport
        Congenital chloridorrhea
High-output secretory
    Laxatives
        Bisacodyl
        Phenolphthalein
        Ricinoleic acid
        Dioctyl sodium sulfosuccinate
    Bacterial toxins
        Vibrio cholerae
        Toxigenic *Escherichia coli*
        Clostridium perfringens
    Hormonally induced
        Vasoactive intestinal polypeptide
        Serotonin
        Calcitonin
        Glucagon
        Gastrin
        Substance P
        Prostaglandins

(continued)

TABLE 12-1 *(Continued)*

Defective neural control
    Diabetic diarrhea
Bile acid diarrhea
    Ileal resection
    Crohn's disease
    Bacterial overgrowth
    Postcholecystectomy
Mucosal inflammation
    Collagenous colitis
    Lymphocytic colitis
Villous adenoma
High-output injury
    Inflammatory bowel disease
        Crohn's disease
        Ulcerative colitis
    Acute infections
        Viruses (rotavirus, Norwalk agent)
        Parasites (*Giardia, Cryptosporidium, Cyclospora*)
        E coli
        Shigella
        Salmonella
        Campylobacter
        Yersinia enterocolitica
        Entamoeba histolytica (amebiasis)
    Chronic infections
        *E histolytica (*amebiasis)
        Clostridium difficile
    Ischemia
        Atherosclerosis
        Vasculitis
Normal output
    Motility disorders
        Irritable bowel syndrome
    Endocrinopathies
        Hyperthyroidism
    Proctitis
        Ulcerative proctitis
        Infectious proctitis
    Fecal incontinence
        Surgical and obstetrical trauma
        Hemorrhoids
        Anal fissures
        Perianal fistulae
        Anal neuropathy (diabetes)

fructose and sorbitol, which naturally sweeten fruits (e.g., pears, prunes, peaches, and apples). Commercially, fructose is used in soft drinks and sorbitol is added as an artificial sweetener in gum and candy. Sorbitol is also responsible for diarrhea that occurs after the ingestion of the elixir forms of certain medications (e.g., potassium chloride and theophylline). Congenital defects of carbohydrate absorption include sucrase-isomaltase deficiency, trehalase deficiency, and glucose-galactose malabsorption. Other nonabsorbable solutes may produce diarrhea if consumed to excess (e.g., magnesium-containing antacids and sodium or phosphate laxatives).

Osmotic diarrhea may result from the malabsorption of nutrients other than carbohydrates. Intralumenal maldigestion complicates cirrhosis and bile duct obstruction because of the impaired delivery of bile salt to the small intestine, which then leads to poor micelle formation with ingested fats. Bacterial overgrowth produces steatorrhea from bile salt deconjugation, brush border injury, mucosal inflammation, and hydroxylation of fats, leading to fatty acid diarrhea. Pancreatic exocrine insufficiency caused by chronic pancreatitis, malignancy, cystic fibrosis, or somatostatinomas leads to steatorrhea as a result of the impaired delivery of lipases to the intestine.

Disorders of mucosal function produce malabsorption by various mechanisms. Drugs such as colchicine, neomycin, para-aminosalicylic acid, and the fenamate class of analgesics induce steatorrhea by enterocyte damage, whereas cholestyramine binds intralumenal bile acids. Intestinal infection with *Giardia*, *Cryptosporidium*, *Isospora*, and *Mycobacterium avium* complex organisms produces brush border and intramucosal damage. The immune diseases, systemic mastocytosis, and eosinophilic gastroenteritis grossly distort the intestinal mucosa. Celiac sprue results from hypersensitivity to dietary gluten. Patients with this disease have varied symptoms, including diarrhea and steatorrhea caused by profound villous flattening in the small intestine. Tropical sprue is an infectious disease of unknown origin that is seen in the Indian subcontinent, Asia, the West Indies, northern South America, central and southern Africa, and Central America. It produces diarrhea and malabsorption in persons who have resided in these regions for as few as 1 to 3 months. Villous atrophy may be present; treatment involves a combination of tetracycline and folic acid. Crohn's disease may cause malabsorptive diarrhea with involvement of the small intestine. Whipple's disease, which results from infection with *Trophyerma whippelii*, is diagnosed by mucosal biopsy specimens of the small intestine that show characteristic periodic acid–Schiff (PAS)-positive macrophages. Associated neurologic symptoms (e.g., hypersomnolence and oculo-facial-skeletal myorhythmias), arthralgias, fever, hypotension, and lymphadenopathy characterize the disease. The patient with the congenital defect of chylomicron formation, abetalipoproteinemia, presents in childhood with steatorrhea, red blood cell acanthocytosis, ataxia, and retinitis pigmentosa. Intestinal lymphangiectasia, which is either congenital or acquired (caused by trauma, lymphoma, or carcinoma), causes protein-losing enteropathy with steatorrhea because of the obstruction of lymphatic channels. In this condition, amino acid and carbohydrate absorption are normal because the lymphatic pathways are not involved with these nutrient classes. Adrenal insufficiency causes generalized disturbances in mucosal absorption.

Disorders that manifest as reduced intestinal mucosal surface area and contact time produce malabsorption and diarrhea. Short bowel syndrome and fistulae reduce the villous surface area available for nutrient uptake. Other conditions (e.g., postvagotomy diarrhea and thyrotoxicosis) accelerate intestinal transit, which leaves inadequate time for nutrient assimilation.

Secretory High-Output Diarrhea

Under physiologic conditions, only 1.5 of the 9 liters of fluid that pass the ligament of Treitz each day reach the proximal colon. The colon absorbs all but 100
to 200 ml of this fluid before fecal evacuation. Diarrhea results when this net
absorption is converted to net secretion. The most common causes of secretory
diarrhea result from ingested bacterial enterotoxins produced by enterotoxigenic
Escherichia coli, Staphylococcus aureus, Shigella spp., *Bacillus cereus*, or *Clostridium
perfringens*. Viruses (e.g., rotavirus, Norwalk agent) also likely act through toxins. Prolonged diarrhea may be caused by organisms yet to be identified (e.g.,
Brainerd diarrhea, which was associated with consumption of raw milk). Certain
infections in patients with acquired immunodeficiency syndrome (AIDS) (e.g.,
those caused by *Cryptosporidium* spp. and *M avium* complex) are secretory in
nature. Worldwide, *Vibrio cholerae* is an important infectious cause of secretory
diarrhea. The other prevalent cause of secretory diarrhea is laxative ingestion,
including ricinoleic acid, bisacodyl, senna, cascara, aloe, rhubarb, frangula, danthron, dioctyl sodium sulfosuccinate, and phenolphthalein. Approximately 15%
of patients referred for evaluation of diarrhea and 25% of patients with documented secretory diarrhea are found to be surreptitiously ingesting either laxatives or diuretics.

Rare patients with diarrhea present with symptoms secondary to overproduction of circulating agents that stimulate secretion. Patients with carcinoid
syndrome present with watery diarrhea, flushing, skin changes, bronchospasm,
and cardiac murmurs, which are symptoms caused by the secretion of serotonin, histamine, catecholamines, kinins, and prostaglandins by the tumor
masses. Even without these classic symptoms, carcinoid syndrome should be
considered because one-third of these patients present with diarrhea alone.
Diarrhea is the major clinical manifestation in 10% of patients with gastrinoma;
it has both secretory and osmotic components. Overproduction of vasoactive
intestinal polypeptide (VIP) by vipoma tumors produces the syndrome of
watery diarrhea, hypokalemia, and achlorhydria (WDHA), in which patients
often pass >3 liters of stool daily. Pain and flushing may also be reported in
WDHA syndrome. Medullary carcinoma of the thyroid, which may be sporadic or part of the multiple endocrine neoplasia (MEN type IIA) syndrome,
causes secretory diarrhea because of the release of calcitonin, although these
tumors also produce prostaglandins, VIP, kinins, and serotonin. Glucagonoma
patients have mild diarrhea as well as characteristic rashes (migratory necrolytic
erythema), glossitis, cheilitis, neuropsychiatric manifestations, and thromboembolism. Systemic mastocytosis produces a mixed secretory and osmotic
diarrhea associated with flushing, tachycardia, hypotension, headache, cognitive dysfunction, nausea, ulcer disease, syncope, and urticaria. Histamine and
prostaglandins have been proposed as mediators of this condition. Villous adenomas of >3 cm in diameter produce secretory diarrhea, possibly secondary to
prostaglandin production.

Other disorders also produce secretory diarrhea. Diabetic diarrhea usually
manifests in patients who have long-standing diabetes; it may be profuse,
watery, nocturnal, and associated with severe urgency. This condition is multifactorial; however, the response of this condition to the somatostatin analog
octreotide suggests a secretory component. Furthermore, the response to the
α-adrenoceptor agonist, clonidine, suggests that the complication may result
from an imbalance between absorptive adrenergic and secretory cholinergic
mucosal function. The mucosal inflammatory conditions, collagenous and

microscopic colitis, produce diarrhea by several mechanisms, including increased colonic secretion. Bile salt diarrhea results from stimulation of colonic secretion. Chronic alcoholics may develop severe watery diarrhea, which is multifactorial. Ten percent to 25% of long-distance runners may develop diarrhea, which has been postulated to result from the release of gastrin, motilin, VIP, or prostaglandins. Congenital causes of secretory diarrhea include congenital chloridorrhea, congenital sodium diarrhea, and microvillous inclusion disease. A small subset of patients exhibit chronic idiopathic secretory diarrhea or pseudopancreatic cholera syndrome; it is identified after a thorough exclusion of other causes of gut secretion. Many patients respond to therapy and the disease is often self-limited, disappearing spontaneously in 6 to 24 months.

High-Output Diarrhea Associated with Mucosal Inflammation

Conditions that injure the mucosa of the small intestine or colon result in passive secretion of fluids through the damaged epithelia and altered absorption of electrolytes and water. Most infectious agents that produce mucosal injury diarrhea affect the colon (e.g., *Shigella* and *Salmonella* spp., enteroinvasive or enterohemorrhagic *E coli*, *Campylobacter jejuni*, *Clostridium difficile*, or *Entamoeba histolytica*). Patients present with watery or bloody diarrhea with or without systemic symptoms (e.g., fever, chills, and abdominal pain). In contrast, many infections of the small intestine produce little inflammation, with the exception of yersiniosis, tuberculosis, and histoplasmosis. Inflammatory bowel disease (i.e., Crohn's disease and ulcerative colitis) produces mucosal injury that results in watery or bloody diarrhea. Other inflammatory causes include eosinophilic gastroenteritis, in which eosinophils infiltrate any layer of the gut; milk and soy protein allergy, in which infants present with watery or bloody diarrhea; and radiation enterocolitis, in which inflammation appears after radiation doses of more than 4 to 6 Gy. Other diseases that manifest as miscellaneous inflammatory diarrheas include Behçet's syndrome, Cronkhite-Canada syndrome, graft-versus-host disease, Churg-Strauss syndrome, and mesenteric ischemia.

Normal-Output Diarrhea

Some patients with complaints of diarrhea have daily stool weights of <250 g, but they report frequent, small, well-formed stools in association with rectal urgency, which suggests an underlying motility disorder. The most common cause of chronic diarrhea in the United States is irritable bowel syndrome, which may alternate with constipation and be associated with abdominal pain. Patients with endocrinopathies (e.g., hyperthyroidism) may present with multiple low-volume stools because of altered colonic transit. Anorectal disease may be associated with normal volume diarrhea. Proctitis that involves only a short rectal segment may be sufficient to cause tenesmus and urgency but not active secretion or loss of absorptive capacity. Fecal impaction in institutionalized or hospitalized patients may cause diarrhea that results from flow of fluid around the obstructing bolus. Fecal incontinence secondary to anal disease, instrumentation, surgery, or neuropathy may be misinterpreted as diarrhea by some patients.

WORKUP

History

The duration of diarrhea should be assessed in the history. Acute diarrhea (<3 weeks' duration) usually results from infectious causes, drugs, or ingestion of osmotic substances. The patient should be questioned concerning recent travel; sexual practices; ingestion of well water and poorly cooked food and shellfish; and exposure to high-risk persons in day care centers, hospitals, mental institutions, and nursing homes. The characteristics of the diarrhea provide clues to the causative organism. Watery diarrhea with nausea but little pain is most consistent with toxin-producing bacteria, whereas invasive bacteria may produce more pain and bloody diarrhea. Viruses induce watery diarrhea in association with significant pain and fever with mild to moderate vomiting. Homosexual men, prostitutes, and intravenous drug abusers are prone to diarrhea acquired through oral-fecal transfer. The incidence of acute infectious diarrhea in healthy homosexual men has decreased as a result of "safe sex" practices; however, this has been offset by the high incidence of enteric infections in patients with AIDS. Antibiotic-associated colitis must be suspected if there is a history of recent antibiotic use. Recently initiated medication regimens or inadvertent use of over-the-counter preparations with laxative effects (e.g., antacids containing magnesium) should be determined. Common drugs that produce diarrhea include antiarrhythmics, antihypertensives, diuretics, central nervous system drugs, antiarthritics, cholesterol-lowering medications, and theophylline.

The differential diagnosis of chronic diarrhea (>3 weeks' duration) is more extensive, and a detailed history is mandatory. To gain insight into the cause of diarrhea, the clinician must ascertain what the patient means by "diarrhea." Frequent passage of voluminous stools that do not abate with food avoidance is consistent with a secretory process, whereas passage of low-volume, loose stools at a normal frequency may be secondary to a motor disturbance. Foul-smelling, bulky, greasy stools suggest fat malabsorption. Soft stools that float or disperse in the toilet water and resolve with fasting are reported by some patients with carbohydrate malabsorption, especially if they occur after the ingestion of specific foodstuffs (e.g., dairy products or fruits). However, mild degrees of malabsorption, as with bile duct obstruction or mild chronic pancreatitis, may be asymptomatic and suspected only if complications supervene (e.g., anemia, bleeding, osteopenia, tetany, and amenorrhea). The presence of pain, bloody stools, or weight loss is indicative of one of the inflammatory causes of diarrhea. Incontinence suggests possible structural or functional anal disease.

Coexisting diseases and risk factors may be important in determining the cause of chronic diarrhea. Diabetes and scleroderma may be associated with intestinal dysmotility or bacterial overgrowth. Heat intolerance, palpitations, and weight loss suggest possible hyperthyroidism, and flushing and wheezing are reported by some patients with endocrine neoplasms. A prior history of radiation therapy or known atherosclerotic disease may be relevant. Abdominal surgery (e.g., vagotomy or cholecystectomy) can lead to chronic diarrhea. Lifestyle choices (as listed previously) increase the risk of AIDS-related diarrhea. Chronic ethanol abuse can lead to diarrhea by affecting the function of the small intestine or by producing pancreatic exocrine insufficiency. A family history of diarrhea warrants evaluation for inflammatory bowel disease, celiac sprue, hereditary pancreatitis, or multiple endocrine neoplasia.

Physical Examination

The physical examination results can determine the aggressiveness of the evaluation. Orthostatic hypotension, decreased skin turgor, and dry mucous membranes indicate the need for intravenous hydration and possible hospital admission, especially in individuals at high risk for recurrent dehydration (e.g., the very young or very old, patients with mental impairment, those with high fever or unable to tolerate oral intake, and persons with precarious cardiorespiratory or renal disease who cannot tolerate small changes in intravascular volume).

Clues about the cause of diarrhea may be provided by selected physical findings. Emaciation, cheilosis, and glossitis result from severe malabsorption. The associations of dermatitis herpetiformis with celiac sprue, pyoderma gangrenosum with inflammatory bowel disease, and sclerodactyly with scleroderma indicate the importance of skin inspection. Arthritis may complicate inflammatory bowel disease or Whipple's disease. Resting tachycardia suggests hyperthyroidism, whereas pulmonic stenosis and tricuspid regurgitation are found in carcinoid syndrome. Peripheral or autonomic neuropathy may correlate with visceral neuropathy in diabetes and intestinal pseudo-obstruction. Neuropsychiatric findings may be a manifestation of Whipple's disease. An abdominal mass suggests the presence of malignancy, Crohn's disease, and diverticulitis. Localized abdominal tenderness implicates an inflammatory condition. A digital rectal examination may reveal perianal disease with Crohn's disease; reduced sphincter tone, which could lead to incontinence; and occult or gross fecal blood, which occurs with infectious, inflammatory, and neoplastic conditions.

Additional Testing

Acute Diarrhea

The management of patients with diarrhea depends on the duration and severity of the diarrhea. If a noninfectious cause (e.g., a medication) is found for acute diarrhea, this should be corrected before any further evaluation. If there is no bloody diarrhea, severe dehydration, or host factors that impair the ability to clear the infection, the patient with acute infectious diarrhea should be treated symptomatically with antidiarrheal agents and rehydration if necessary. With complicated or prolonged infection that is unresponsive to supportive care, liquid stools should be sent for culture, especially if there has been recent travel or there is a suspicion of food-borne illness. Stools can be sent for routine culture for the detection of *Salmonella*, *Shigella*, or *Campylobacter* organisms. Special culture techniques are required for the detection of *Yersinia* and *Plesiomonas* organisms and enterohemorrhagic *E coli*. If there is suspicion of parasitic disease, stool samples may be sent for the detection of ova and parasites to find *Giardia*, *Cryptosporidium*, *E histolytica*, or *Strongyloides* organisms. Not infrequently, parasites are difficult to detect in the stool, and aspiration of duodenal juice or biopsy of the small intestine by endoscopy or fluoroscopy is required. The string test also is available for noninvasive diagnosis of giardiasis in the small intestine. In patients with recent antibiotic use, stools should be sent for *C difficile* culture and toxin determination. Twenty percent to 40% of acute infectious diarrheas remain undiagnosed despite laboratory evaluation.

Screening Evaluation of Chronic Diarrhea

Most patients with chronic diarrhea require additional tests to complement the history and physical examination findings (Fig. 12-1). The stools should be evaluated for leukocytes to search for evidence of mucosal injury. Qualitative examination of the stool for fat droplets (Sudan stain) is used to evaluate for malabsorption. Fresh, loose stool samples should be directly examined for parasites, or in rare instances, sent for culture. With antibiotic use, *C difficile* should be excluded as a possible cause. Serum electrolyte values and a complete blood count should be obtained. The erythrocyte sedimentation rate is a crude screening test for systemic inflammatory disease. Serum albumin and globulin may be reduced with malabsorption, malnutrition, or protein-losing enteropathy. Additional blood tests to assess for malnutrition include carotene, iron, folate, vitamin B_{12}, cholesterol, alkaline phosphatase, and prothrombin time. Flexible sigmoidoscopy is performed to exclude proctitis, pseudomembranes, and melanosis coli that is secondary to anthracene laxative abuse. If the rectosigmoid endoscopic appearance is normal, random biopsies can detect microscopic and collagenous colitis in rare cases. In those patients with normal findings on screening studies and relatively low-volume diarrhea, a diagnosis of irritable bowel syndrome is probable.

Directed Evaluation of Chronic Diarrhea

If the screening evaluation is unrevealing, subsequent testing should be directed to the suspected cause. To evaluate for malabsorption, a 72-hour stool specimen can be sent for fecal fat determination, although the values often will be normal in mild cases of disease of the small intestine or pancreatic insufficiency. If malabsorption secondary to disease of the small intestine is suspected, endoscopic biopsy of the small intestine can provide definitive diagnoses of Whipple's disease, *M avium* complex, giardiasis, coccidiosis, strongyloidiasis, Crohn's disease, amyloidosis, eosinophilic gastroenteritis, mastocytosis, lymphangiectasia, lymphoma, and abetalipoproteinemia. The technique further defines abnormal but not diagnostic mucosa in celiac and tropical sprue, bacterial overgrowth, and severe viral enteritis. Duodenal juice can be aspirated for detection of parasites or sent for quantitative culture to diagnose bacterial overgrowth. If bacterial overgrowth is believed to result from dysmotility of the small intestine, manometry may show characteristic myopathic or neuropathic patterns. Barium radiography of the small intestine can demonstrate fistulae, strictures (Crohn's disease, radiation damage, postoperative state), diverticula, and fold thickening (amyloidosis, lymphoma, Whipple's disease). Other tests for malabsorption of the small intestine include the D-xylose test as well as specific breath tests for bile acid malabsorption, fat malabsorption, lactase deficiency, and bacterial overgrowth (see Chapter 10).

Conversely, if pancreatic exocrine insufficiency is a suspected cause of malabsorption, plain abdominal radiographs may reveal calcifications that occur with chronic pancreatitis. Ultrasound and computed tomographic (CT) scanning provide anatomic characterization of the pancreas and may suggest a diagnosis of chronic pancreatitis or malignancy. The most accurate means of identifying the structural changes of chronic pancreatitis or a small pancreatic malignancy is endoscopic retrograde cholangiopancreatography or endoscopic ultrasound. In addition to the quantitation of fecal fat, a functional assessment of pancreatic enzyme output can be obtained with the bentiromide test, which has only moderate sensitivity and

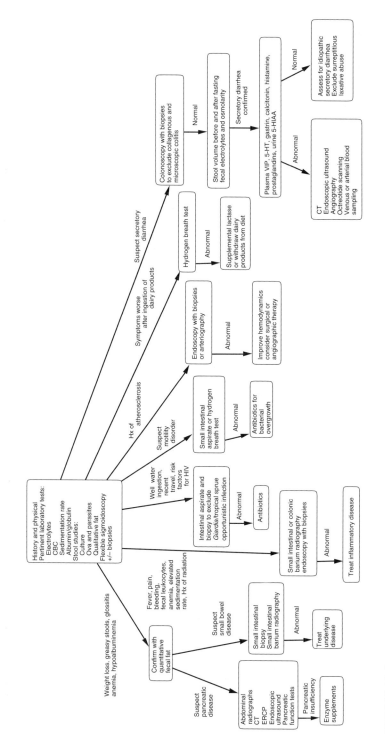

FIGURE 12-1. Workup of a patient with diarrhea. (CBC = complete blood count; CT = computed tomography; ERCP = endoscopic retrograde cholangiopancreatography; HIV = human immunodeficiency virus; Hx = history; 5-HT = serotonin; 5-HIAA = hydroxyindoleacetic acid; VIP = vasoactive intestinal polypeptide.)

specificity, or the pancreatic function tests, in which duodenal juice is assayed for bicarbonate and enzyme content after intravenous secretin and cholecystokinin injection, respectively. Schilling's test can provide suggestive evidence of severe intestinal mucosal disease, bacterial overgrowth, and pancreatic insufficiency.

With suspected secretory diarrhea, barium radiographic structural studies provide limited information, although they may detect carcinoid tumors in rare cases. Colonoscopic biopsies may provide definitive diagnoses of collagenous and microscopic colitis. A secretory process is confirmed by a 24-hour stool quantitation that usually exceeds 1 liter and does not significantly decrease with fasting. Conversely, osmotic diarrheas are lower in volume and decrease with fasting. A secretory diarrhea that abates with nasogastric suction is suggestive of a gastric source (e.g., gastrinoma). Stool pH is usually neutral in secretory diarrhea, but it may be acidic with certain osmotic causes. If prolonged stool collection is not practical, determination of stool electrolytes may provide useful information in some cases. A stool osmolarity of 100 mOsm greater than twice the sum of stool sodium and potassium suggests an osmotic cause, but if the osmolarity approximates twice the sum of the fecal cations, a secretory process is probable. If these investigations suggest secretory diarrhea, blood may be sent for the measurement of gastrin, VIP, glucagon, serotonin, calcitonin, histamine, and prostaglandins. Levels of 5-hydroxyindoleacetic acid in the urine may be measured in selected patients with suspected endocrine neoplasia. If overproduction of one of these mediators is documented, an abdominal CT scan and endoscopic ultrasound are the most sensitive methods for detecting metastatic and primary pancreatic tumor masses, respectively. In cases in which these studies are unrevealing, angiography with or without selective venous sampling, octreotide scanning, and diagnostic laparotomy may be performed.

For diarrhea secondary to suspected inflammatory disease, barium radiography may show diagnostic evidence of inflammatory bowel disease, generalized abnormalities in eosinophilic gastroenteritis, and radiation damage. Upper or lower gastrointestinal endoscopy with biopsy is likely to be the most useful in providing specific diagnoses (e.g., infectious colitis, Crohn's disease, ulcerative colitis, radiation enterocolitis, and ischemia). Rare patients will benefit from ^{111}In-labeled leukocyte tests for inflammatory disease or ^{51}Cr-albumin or α_1-antitrypsin tests that demonstrate protein-losing enteropathy.

Some cases of diarrhea will remain undiagnosed after the appropriate directed evaluation. In these instances, laxative abuse should be considered. Phenolphthalein can be detected by stool alkalinization with NaOH or KOH. A change in color to red or pink is diagnostic of phenolphthalein ingestion. Stool samples may be tested for sulfate, magnesium, and phosphate if these osmotic laxatives are suspected. Bisacodyl, oxyphenisatin, anthraquinones, and castor oil are detectable in urine and stool. In patients who are hospitalized for diarrhea evaluation, a thorough room search can be performed while the patient is away for a test.

PRINCIPLES OF MANAGEMENT

The therapy for diarrhea depends on its severity and its cause. In patients with severe dehydration or electrolyte disturbances, intravenous resuscitation is indicated, possibly as an inpatient treatment. Many patients with severe inflammatory disease need to be admitted to the hospital for intravenous administration of specific medications and to be observed for potential surgical complications (e.g., megacolon and perforation).

Agents for Mild Diarrhea

For diseases that have no specific therapy and for which symptoms are mild, several antidiarrheals are available. Bismuth subsalicylate has anti-inflammatory and bactericidal activity, but it may produce salicylate toxicity and black stools. Over-the-counter opiates (e.g., loperamide) are effective and indicated if there is no sign of significant inflammatory disease. Diphenoxylate with atropine similarly may be prescribed for mild to moderate diarrhea. Other prescription opiates (e.g., codeine and paregoric) are more potent but have the added problems of sedation and drug dependence and should be used judiciously. Kaolin and pectin preparations are extensively promoted but they have limited efficacy. Cholestyramine binds bile acids and some toxins and may be useful in some cases.

Antibiotics for Acute Infectious Diarrhea

Antibiotic therapy of acute infectious diarrhea is controversial. Antibiotics are indicated for persons with shigellosis, cholera, some traveler's diarrhea, antibiotic-associated colitis, parasites, and sexually transmitted infections. Antibiotic treatment is usually recommended for noncholera vibrios; prolonged *Yersinia* infection; early *Campylobacter, Aeromonas,* and *Plesiomonas* infections; and day care outbreaks of enteropathogenic *E coli*. Viral diarrhea and cryptosporidiosis usually are not treated specifically. Regardless of the cause, patients with malignancy, immunosuppression, cardiovascular compromise, vascular prostheses, hemolytic anemia, and refractory infection should receive antibiotics, as should those who are very young or very old. These guidelines were developed for *Salmonella* species but they are also valid for other organisms.

Therapy for Osmotic Diarrhea

The treatment of osmotic diarrhea is tailored to the underlying disease. For carbohydrate malabsorption resulting from lactase deficiency or fructose or sorbitol intolerance, dietary modification may be useful. Lactase supplements are available for those who wish to consume dairy products. Malabsorption in the small intestine usually is specifically treated (e.g., dietary gluten restriction for celiac sprue, antibiotics for tropical sprue and Whipple's disease, and steroids or 5-aminosalicylate for Crohn's disease). Pancreatic exocrine insufficiency is managed with pancreatic enzyme supplements.

Therapy for Secretory Diarrhea

Management of severe secretory diarrhea can be challenging. The somatostatin analog, octreotide, has antisecretory and motor-retarding properties, making it an important agent in treating secretory diarrhea that results from endocrine neoplasia, AIDS, and diabetes. Octreotide may also prevent other clinical manifestations of hormone oversecretion—for example, the flushing and tachycardia that occur with carcinoid tumors. Parenteral calcitonin has shown some utility in controlling diarrhea from vipoma and carcinoid tumors. The α-adrenoceptor agonist clonidine has been used to treat diarrhea associated with opiate withdrawal and diabetic diarrhea; however, its use may be limited by hypotensive side effects. Indomethacin is occasionally effective in patients with neuroendocrine tumors and food allergy, but not in patients with inflammatory bowel disease because it may exacerbate symptoms. Lithium carbonate, bromocriptine, and nicotinic acid are used in rare instances. Phenothiazines, calcium channel antagonists, and serotonin receptor antagonists (e.g., methysergide and cyproheptadine) have antisecretory properties in some cases.

Therapy for Inflammatory Diarrhea

The treatment of inflammatory conditions (e.g., Crohn's disease and ulcerative colitis) involves specific anti-inflammatory drugs (e.g., 5-aminosalicylate and corticosteroid). Refractory cases may require immunosuppressive medications (e.g., azathioprine, 6-mercaptopurine, methotrexate, and cyclosporine).

COMPLICATIONS

Most cases of diarrhea in the United States result only in the inconvenience of frequent defecation, which leads to the loss of productive work and personal time. However, worldwide, diarrhea is a major cause of morbidity and mortality, especially in children and in certain high-risk groups in the United States (e.g., persons with AIDS). Diarrhea causes up to 8 million deaths of children yearly because of severe volume depletion. This group requires aggressive fluid and electrolyte replacement, intravenously with crystalloid formulations, or orally with glucose-electrolyte combinations (e.g., the World Health Organization solution) or commercial formulas (e.g., Pedialyte and Infalyte).

CHAPTER 13

Approach to the Patient with Constipation

DIFFERENTIAL DIAGNOSIS

Constipation, the most prevalent digestive complaint in the United States, has no single definition that can be applied to all cases. Stool frequency lends itself to quantitation; using population-based surveys, constipation may be defined as a frequency of defecation of twice weekly or less. Other patients with constipation may complain instead of straining on defecation, a sensation of incomplete fecal evacuation, or passage of hard, dry stools. The causes of constipation are numerous, including secondary causes and idiopathic disorders, and relate either to impairment of colonic transit or to structural or functional obstruction to fecal evacuation (Table 13-1).

Mechanical Colonic Obstruction

Lesions that obstruct fecal flow to the point of producing constipation must be advanced and distally located. Colorectal neoplasms are an obvious concern in the differential diagnosis of a patient older than 40 to 50 years, but, in general, near-circumferential masses in the left and rectosigmoid colon produce symptomatic constipation, whereas proximal colonic tumors have less effect on bowel movement pattern. Benign causes of colonic obstruction (e.g., strictures from diverticulitis, ischemia, inflammatory bowel disease, or endometriosis) may produce similar symptoms. Anal narrowing and spasm from strictures, neoplasm, foreign bodies, painful fissures, and hemorrhoids may also prevent stool expulsion.

Metabolic and Endocrine Disorders

The most common endocrine causes of constipation are diabetes, pregnancy, and hypothyroidism, with 60% of diabetics reporting the symptom. Although symptoms usually are mild, life-threatening megacolon may develop in myxedema.

TABLE 13-1
Causes of Constipation

Colonic obstruction
    Colorectal neoplasms
    Benign strictures (e.g., diverticulitis, ischemia)
    Inflammatory bowel disease
    Endometriosis
    Anal strictures or neoplasms
    Rectal foreign bodies
    Anal fissures and hemorrhoids
Neuropathic and myopathic disorders
    Peripheral and autonomic neuropathy
    Hirschsprung's disease
    Chagas' disease
    Neurofibromatosis
    Ganglioneuromatosis
    Hypoganglionosis
    Intestinal pseudo-obstruction
    Multiple sclerosis
    Spinal cord lesions
    Parkinson's disease
    Shy-Drager syndrome
    Transection of sacral nerves or cauda equina
    Lumbosacral spinal injury
    Meningomyelocele
    Low spinal anesthesia
    Scleroderma
    Amyloidosis
    Polymyositis/dermatomyositis
    Myotonic dystrophy
Metabolic and endocrine disorders
    Diabetes mellitus
    Pregnancy
    Hypercalcemia
    Hypothyroidism
    Hypokalemia
    Porphyria
    Glucagonoma
    Panhypopituitarism
    Pheochromocytoma
Medications
    Opiates
    Anticholinergics
    Tricyclic antidepressants
    Antipsychotics
    Antiparkinsonian agents
    Antihypertensives
    Ganglionic blockers
    Vinca alkaloids
    Anticonvulsants

    Calcium channel antagonists
    Iron supplements
    Aluminum antacids
    Calcium supplements
    Barium sulfate
    Heavy metals (i.e., lead, arsenic, mercury)
Idiopathic constipation
    Colonic inertia
    Megarectum/megacolon
    Rectosphincteric dyssynergia
    Rectocele/rectal prolapse
    Irritable bowel syndrome

Other endocrine causes of constipation include hypercalcemia, hypokalemia, porphyria, panhypopituitarism, pheochromocytoma, and glucagonoma.

Neuropathic and Myopathic Disorders

Diseases of both the extrinsic and enteric innervation of the colon and anus may produce constipation. Transection of the sacral nerves or cauda equina, lumbosacral spinal injury, meningomyelocele, and low spinal anesthesia induce constipation associated with hypomotility, colonic dilation, decreased rectal tone and sensation, and impaired defecation. Colonic reflexes are preserved in patients with high spinal lesions; thus, digital stimulation can trigger defecation, although these patients can have reduced meal-induced colonic motor activity and impaired rectal sensation and compliance. Constipation is prevalent with multiple sclerosis, cerebrovascular accidents, and disorders of autonomic function (e.g., Parkinson's disease and Shy-Drager syndrome), although in these entities, medication effects must also be considered.

The classic enteric nervous system disorder that produces constipation is Hirschsprung's disease, which most often presents with obstipation and proximal colonic dilation at birth. In contrast to normal function, the internal anal sphincter does not relax with rectal stimulation because of an absence of ganglion cells in the submucosal and myenteric plexuses, which causes a functional blockage to fecal expulsion. Some patients with disease involvement of a very short segment of bowel present in adulthood with either constipation or, in rare instances, incontinence. Other enteric neural diseases include zonal colonic aganglionosis (in which patchy areas of the colon are devoid of neurons either congenitally or secondary to ischemia), intestinal pseudo-obstruction (myopathic and neuropathic), Chagas' disease (resulting from infection with *Trypanosoma cruzi*), neurofibromatosis, long-standing laxative abuse, and diabetes mellitus (which impairs colonic reflex activity).

Rheumatologic disorders produce constipation as a result of impaired colonic transit. Disorders such as dermatomyositis and myotonic dystrophy act through myopathic dysfunction. Amyloidosis and scleroderma may produce either myopathic or neuropathic disease. Constipation in systemic lupus erythematosus has multiple mechanisms including local ischemia secondary to vasculitis.

Medications

Many medications produce mild or severe constipation that may limit their use. Drugs with anticholinergic properties include antispasmodics, tricyclic antidepressants, antipsychotics, and anti-parkinsonian agents. Cation-containing agents include iron, aluminum antacids, calcium, barium, and heavy metals (i.e., arsenic, lead, mercury). Agents that inhibit propulsive neural function are opiates, certain antihypertensives, ganglionic blockers, vinca alkaloids, anticonvulsants, and calcium channel antagonists.

Idiopathic Constipation

Most constipated patients have no demonstrable structural or functional cause for their symptoms and are classified as having idiopathic constipation. Chronic constipation in childhood is multifactorial, involving physiologic and psychological factors. Childhood constipation often manifests as impaction and rectosigmoid dilation, and delayed transit usually of the distal colon or rectum. The cause of childhood constipation is uncertain; impaired rectal sensation and altered anal tone are not reliably demonstrable. Many children exhibit a failure of the puborectalis muscle to relax on attempted defecation, termed *rectosphincteric dyssynergia*, which may be a learned behavior in response to prior painful defecation problems.

Young to middle-aged adults with chronic constipation are predominantly women. Approximately 30% of patients in this group who complain of infrequent defecation actually have normal colonic transit; they exhibit evidence of psychosocial stress, as in irritable bowel syndrome. The other 70% have slow transit, usually of the proximal colon (colonic inertia), which is not associated with psychosocial dysfunction. The physiologic cause of inertia is unknown, although abnormal meal-induced colonic motility has been demonstrated in some patients. Subsets of patients with colonic inertia have a motility disorder of the esophagus or small intestine or a bladder dysfunction suggestive of a diffuse, smooth muscle disorder. Outlet obstruction, in contrast to inertia, is defined by the delay in transit in the rectum. Outlet obstruction is common in nonambulatory patients, patients with megarectum, and those with abnormal pelvic muscle responses to defecation. Normal defecation involves the coordinated relaxation of the puborectalis muscle and anal sphincter. With rectosphincteric dyssynergia, ineffective defecation is associated with impaired relaxation or paradoxical contraction of the puborectalis muscle or anal sphincter. As with children, this condition is probably a learned behavior. The most common cause of constipation in association with abdominal pain in young to middle-aged adults is irritable bowel syndrome.

Constipation in elderly populations is multifactorial, including underlying structural disorders, functional motility disorders, medication effects, and idiopathic dysfunction. The elderly often report constipation as straining with defecation rather than infrequent stool passage, possibly explaining the prevalence of laxative use in this age group. In elderly institutionalized patients, fecal impaction is a common problem because of mental confusion, immobility, or inadequate toilet arrangements.

Idiopathic megacolon is divided into primary and secondary disorders. Primary megacolon is thought to be associated with neuropathic dysfunction. Secondary megacolon and megarectum develop later in life, usually in response to chronic fecal retention. This disorder may be confused with Hirschsprung's disease on anorectal manometry if large enough volumes of rectal distention are not used to elicit anal relaxation on reflex testing.

WORKUP

History

A careful history from the patient with constipation involves delineation of the duration and characteristics of the presenting symptoms. Lifelong constipation usually suggests a congenital condition. A recent change in bowel habits in an adult patient demands exclusion of organic obstructive disease, whereas a history of a period of years is more consistent with functional disease. Associated symptoms (e.g., straining, anal or abdominal pain, bloating, rectal bleeding, or a sense of incomplete evacuation) may be significant. Extracolonic symptoms (e.g., heartburn, nausea, dyspepsia, early satiety, and genitourinary symptoms) are prevalent in functional disorders (e.g., irritable bowel syndrome) as well as generalized dysmotility syndromes. The presence of skin or hair changes, temperature intolerance, or weight gain suggests possible hypothyroidism, whereas weight loss raises concern for malignancy. Underlying systemic illness (e.g., diabetes or a rheumatologic condition) should be determined. A careful history of medication use, including laxative use, is essential. In children, inquiry should be made regarding nightmares, enuresis, school performance, and family tension.

Physical Examination

Physical examination includes a search for gastrointestinal and nongastrointestinal diseases that can cause constipation. Particular attention should be given to the neurologic examination, which may provide evidence of a peripheral or autonomic neuropathy in association with a neuropathic disorder. Abdominal masses, hepatomegaly, or lymphadenopathy suggest possible obstructing malignancy. Anorectal examination can detect tumors, strictures, fissures, hemorrhoids, and rectal prolapse. The neuromuscular function of the anus is evaluated by assessment of resting anal tone and by evidence of prolapse or rectosphincteric dyssynergia on straining. Occult fecal blood warrants a search for underlying structural disease. Pelvic examination in women may demonstrate a rectocele with straining. Abnormalities of perineal sensation and the anal wink (anal contraction elicited by perianal stimulation) suggest neural dysfunction.

Additional Testing

Laboratory Studies

In patients with unexplained constipation, a complete blood count may show microcytic anemia, which might occur with an obstructing colonic lesion

(Fig. 13-1). Other appropriate screening tests include measurement of calcium levels to exclude hyperparathyroidism and measurement of thyroid-stimulating hormone levels to exclude hypothyroidism. Specific serologic tests can detect rheumatologic disease, Chagas' disease, or paraneoplastic pseudo-obstruction, whereas other assays are used for catecholamines, porphyrins, and glucagon.

Structural Studies

Studies of colorectal structure are important to exclude organic disease. In young patients, flexible sigmoidoscopy excludes distal occlusive lesions and can detect melanosis coli, a brown-black mucosal discoloration resulting from chronic anthraquinone laxative use. For patients older than 40 to 45 years, it is important to evaluate the entire colon because of the increased risk of colorectal neoplasm, either with barium enema radiography or with colonoscopy. Barium radiographs can show megarectum and megacolon as well as the denervated segment with Hirschsprung's disease. Deep rectal biopsy specimens may be obtained at least 3 cm above the anal verge to exclude Hirschsprung's disease, when clinically indicated.

Functional Studies

After structural disease has been excluded, most patients are given an empirical trial of medical therapy for constipation. However, patients with severe constipation or symptoms refractory to medication can be considered for functional testing if surgical or biofeedback treatments are under consideration. Colonic transit studies are useful for evaluating patients with infrequent defecation. The patient is placed on a high-fiber diet (20 to 30 g per day) without other laxatives, and radiopaque markers are ingested according to a standard protocol. Serial abdominal radiographs are obtained to determine the times required for marker expulsion. Regional examination can distinguish whether transit is diffusely slowed or if a particular anatomic site provides a functional obstruction to marker passage. Colonic transit testing provides important prognostic and therapeutic information. Those patients with self-reports of infrequent defecation but normal transit have high rates of psychological dysfunction. In contrast, patients with profound colonic inertia have more normal psychological profiles, but unfortunately they often respond poorly to medical laxative therapy. Some centers perform colonic transit scintigraphy; however, this technique has few advantages over radiopaque marker studies and has not achieved widespread use.

Anorectal manometry assesses rectal sensation, compliance, anal tone and maximal squeeze pressure, internal anal sphincter relaxation, and simulated defecation and is most useful in assessing a patient with straining and suspected rectoanal disease. Sensation is quantitated by patient reports of symptoms with progressive rectal balloon inflation, whereas compliance involves simultaneous measurement of rectal volumes and pressures. Some patients with irritable bowel syndrome tolerate balloon distention poorly and have low rectal compliance, whereas patients with megarectum accommodate large balloon volumes with highly compliant rectal walls. Balloon inflation should relax the internal anal sphincter, a phenomenon known as the *rectoanal inhibitory reflex*. This reflex is absent in Hirschsprung's disease, although deep rectal biopsy specimens are needed to confirm the diagnosis. Falsely absent rectoanal inhibitory reflexes may be demonstrated with megarectum if inadequate rectal

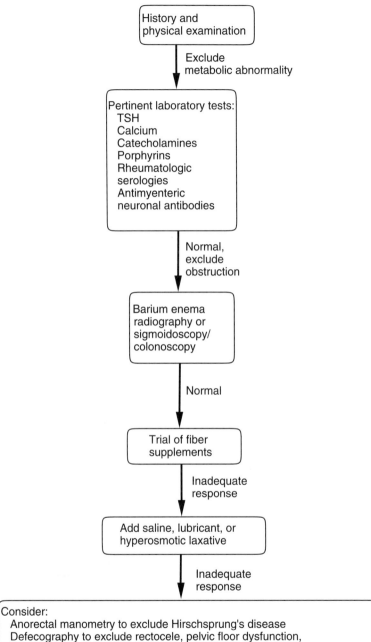

FIGURE 13-1.   Workup of a patient with constipation. (TSH = thyroid-stimulating hormone.)

volumes are given. Attempted defecation should reveal increased rectal pressures concurrent with anal relaxation, although some patients may exhibit paradoxical anal contraction. Manometry may be complemented by electromyography of the anal sphincter.

Defecography is a technique in which thickened barium is introduced into the rectum. Evacuation of the barium bolus is recorded by videofluoroscopy to exclude anatomic abnormalities (e.g., rectoceles and rectal prolapse) and to assess the anorectal angle at rest and with defecation to exclude rectosphincteric dyssynergia in patients with defecatory straining. Rectal expulsion of fluid-filled balloons or solid spheres can assess defecatory function but cannot provide anatomic definition of the defecation process.

PRINCIPLES OF MANAGEMENT

Dietary Approaches

When possible, directed therapy should be given to patients with constipation secondary to a definable disease (e.g., hypothyroidism). For those patients who cannot be managed simply by control of the underlying condition, dietary adjustments are the first line of intervention. Many constipated persons respond to increases in fiber intake to 20 to 30 g per day. Wheat bran with supplemental fluid intake is most effective in increasing stool weight and accelerating colonic transit, followed by fruits and vegetables, oats, corn, cellulose, soya, and pectin. In patients with irritable bowel syndrome, fiber should be gradually increased to minimize bloating.

Behavioral Approaches

Habit training is often effective in the management of constipation. The patient is encouraged to attempt routine defecation after a meal to take advantage of the increase in colonic motility that occurs postprandially. Because exercise may increase colonic motor activity, a daily walking or running routine may be suggested. Selected patients with defined inappropriate contraction of the internal anal sphincter or puborectalis muscle with defecation may benefit from learning biofeedback techniques for retraining of rectosphincteric coordination taught at referral centers.

Pharmacologic Therapy

Bulk-forming laxatives (e.g., psyllium, methylcellulose, and polycarbophil) may be given to patients who do not respond to dietary measures. These agents increase stool volume and diameter, retain fecal water, and increase colonic bacterial mass, resulting in shortened transit time and reduced straining. Mineral oil penetrates and softens the stool but may reduce absorption of vitamins A, D, and K. Docusate salts are anionic surfactants that reduce fecal surface tension, allowing better mixing of aqueous and fatty substances, thus softening the stool.

If bulking and softening agents are ineffective, osmotic laxatives may be useful. Sorbitol and lactulose are nonabsorbable sugars that are degraded by colonic bacteria to short-chain fatty acids that increase stool osmolarity. Cationic laxatives (e.g., saline and magnesium products [milk of magnesia, magnesium citrate]) are relatively nonabsorbable and increase intralumenal water content by osmotic effects. The use of magnesium products should be avoided in cases of renal failure. Saline laxatives may be given rectally.

Stimulant laxatives include castor oil, anthraquinones (e.g., cascara, senna, casanthranol, and danthron), and phenylmethanes (e.g., phenolphthalein and bisacodyl). The use of anthraquinones may produce melanosis coli; danthron has reported hepatotoxic effects. Phenolphthalein may produce skin eruptions and fatal allergic reactions. The use of some stimulant laxatives has been postulated to result in long-term damage of colonic neural integrity.

Other medication classes may be useful in some subsets of patients with constipation. Prokinetic agents (e.g., cisapride) have weak stimulatory effects on colonic transit. The prostaglandin analog misoprostol has had impressive stimulatory effects in small studies of patients who have constipation refractory to other agents. However, this agent has significant gastrointestinal side effects and should be used cautiously by women with reproductive potential because of its abortifacient properties. Small reports suggest that colchicine may also have laxative properties. Preliminary studies suggest that oral naloxone may increase stool volume in constipated elderly patients.

Surgical Treatment

Surgery is the treatment of choice for Hirschsprung's disease. Anal myotomy can be beneficial with short segment involvement, whereas in classic disease, treatment of the aganglionic segment includes resection, bypass, or endorectal pull-through. In selected patients with colonic inertia that is unresponsive to medical management, subtotal colectomy with ileorectal anastomosis may be beneficial. Radiologic and manometric evaluation of the upper gut should be performed to establish that the disease is confined to the colon. Surgical resection or reduction of large rectoceles may be performed; however, this should be considered only if finger pressure on the posterior vaginal wall results in improved fecal evacuation. Rectal prolapse may be surgically treated with suspension or rectopexy procedures, although this often has no effect on the underlying defecation problem. Surgery for rectosphincteric dyssynergia is contraindicated because of a high risk of postoperative incontinence.

COMPLICATIONS

Chronic constipation may lead to rectal prolapse, hemorrhoidal bleeding, or anal fissure development. Fecal impaction may produce colonic obstruction or stercoraceous ulcers, which can bleed or perforate. Large fecalomas may cause extrinsic ureteral compression, resulting in recurrent urinary infections. Fecal incontinence results from anal sphincter damage or perineal nerve dysfunction from straining or prolapse.

CHAPTER 14

Approach to the Patient with Ileostomy or Ileal Pouch

STANDARD END ILEOSTOMY

Technique

Proctocolectomy with end ileostomy (Brooke's ileostomy) is performed for patients who require excision of the entire colon and rectum for ulcerative colitis, familial adenomatous polyposis, or multiple colonic malignancies. The ileostomy is made from the terminal ileum and is positioned in the right lower quadrant of the abdomen (Table 14-1). The fecal effluent is collected in an external appliance that the patient wears continuously. If properly constructed, Brooke's ileostomies are remarkably safe and reliable; however, because of the advent of continence-preserving procedures, the operation is presently reserved for older patients and obese individuals in whom construction of an ileal pouch–anal canal anastomosis would be technically difficult.

Preoperatively, the nutritional and hemodynamic statuses are stabilized. Patients who are taking corticosteroids are given stress doses for the perioperative and early postoperative period. The appropriate site for the stoma is selected preoperatively by positioning a sample appliance on the patient's abdomen. Once constructed, the ileostomy usually begins discharge of effluent by the third postoperative day. The normal ileostomy output averages 600 ml per day. Volumes of >1 liter per day may mandate intravenous fluid replacement. Patients are discharged and encouraged to chew their food carefully or, alternatively, to eat diets low in indigestible fiber, which can obstruct an ileostomy.

Complications

Infection, abscess, and bleeding can occur in the early postoperative period. Stomal obstruction, retraction, and prolapse can occur in the late postoperative period, as can diarrhea and peristomal hernias, but these complications are rare (<5% of patients). Surgical revision may be required to treat these complications. Development of urinary or sexual dysfunction can be minimized if the

TABLE 14-1
Characteristics of Ileostomy and Ileal Pouch Operations

PROCEDURE	CONTINENCE RETAINED	STOMA PRESENT	INTUBATIONS REQUIRED	DISADVANTAGES
End ileostomy (Brooke's ileostomy)	No	Yes	No	Ileostomy bag required
Continent ileostomy (Kock pouch)	Yes	Yes	Yes	Valve malfunction, pouchitis
Ileal pouch–anal canal anastomosis	Yes	No	No	Occasional fecal leakage, pouchitis

excision of the rectum and anus is done in the intersphincteric or submucosal plane away from the nerve bundles. Patients with end ileostomy are susceptible to two long-term metabolic complications—urinary stones and gallstones. Mild chronic dehydration and acidosis develop in many patients, which predispose to precipitation of uric acid stones because of the low output of acidic urine. This complication is prevented by adequate fluid intake, with supplemental alkali in rare cases. Gallstones result from depletion of the bile salt pool in patients who have had significant ileal resection in addition to the colectomy. No adequate prophylaxis has been developed for this complication.

Outcome

After end ileostomy, patients are quickly restored to good health and can expect good stomal function over the long term. The appliances may be unsightly, uncomfortable, and mildly odorous, and noises may emanate from the stoma, all of which may reduce the patient's acceptance of the operation. With ill-fitting appliances, stool or gas leakage can occur, which may lead to possible skin breakdown. Because of these factors, 15% of patients note mild to moderate restriction of daily activities, and 9% report severe restrictions.

CONTINENT ILEOSTOMY

Technique

The continent ileostomy, or Kock pouch, consists of three parts: a pouch made of distal ileum, a valve made of terminal ileum interposed between the pouch and the exterior, and an efferent ileal limb leading from the valve to the stoma. In contrast to the Brooke's ileostomy, the Kock pouch provides continence, which eliminates the need for an ileostomy appliance (see Table 14-1). Because of this, the stoma may be fashioned flush with the skin and placed nearer the pubis to make it less conspicuous. The pouch is emptied at regular intervals through a catheter that is placed into the stoma and drained directly into a toilet. The catheter is removed, washed, and carried by the patient until it is needed again. In general, Kock pouches are indicated in young or middle-aged adults who require total proctocolectomy, whereas the procedure is contraindicated in very young, very old, and obese patients and in those patients with persistent disease of the small intestine (e.g., Crohn's disease).

Postoperatively, the pouch is drained continuously for 1 month to ensure appropriate healing. Subsequently, pouch drainage is performed every 2 hours for an additional month. When matured, Kock pouches require emptying four times daily, with no nightly intubation needed. Dietary advice is similar to that given to patients with end ileostomies. The pouch should be irrigated free of debris once daily with warm water or saline.

Complications

Complications specific to the Kock pouch include slippage of the valve, valve prolapse, stomal stenosis, and pouch-related diarrhea. Valve slippage results from partial loss of the surgically placed intussuscepted segment within the pouch. This leads to difficulty intubating the pouch and pouch leakage and usually requires reoperation. Valve prolapse usually requires surgery to replace and reanchor the valve into the pouch and narrow the opening in the abdominal wall. Stomal stenosis results from local ischemia and is correctable by local construction of a new stoma. Diarrhea occurs in one-third of patients secondary to pouchitis, which is caused by bacterial overgrowth. Symptomatic diarrhea usually responds to antibiotic therapy (e.g., metronidazole). A rarer cause of diarrhea is partial obstruction of the small intestine.

Outcome

In general, patients achieve good control over fecal discharge, although the above complications lead to leakage and other symptoms in significant subsets of patients. Currently, the ileal pouch–anal canal anastomosis has become the procedure of choice for maintenance of continence after a colectomy. At the present time, the Kock pouch is used mainly to provide continence for patients who already have undergone proctocolectomy and placement of a Brooke's ileostomy.

ILEAL POUCH–ANAL CANAL ANASTOMOSIS

Technique

The ileal pouch–anal canal anastomosis, combined with colectomy and rectal mucosal stripping, excises the entire span of colorectal disease in ulcerative colitis, familial adenomatous polyposis, and multiple colorectal malignancies and preserves transanal defecation and fecal continence (see Table 14-1). Because the rectal mucosal stripping is performed endorectally, the nerve supply to the anus, bladder, and genitalia is usually not disturbed; therefore, anal, urinary, and sexual dysfunction postoperatively is rare. Contraindications to ileal pouch–anal canal anastomosis include Crohn's disease (high risk of recurrence in the pouch), distal rectal cancer (cannot ensure adequate tumor-free margins), poor preoperative anal function, and age of older than 65 years (high risk of local complications and incontinence) (Table 14-2). Relative contraindications to the procedure include massive obesity (increases technical difficulty), severe inanition, chronic high-dose steroids, and indeterminate colitis. The operation is usually not performed in an emergency setting (i.e., acute severe colitis, toxic megacolon, colonic perforation with peritonitis, and acute colonic obstruction). In these instances, a temporary Brooke's ileostomy is formed, the rectum is closed at its proximal end, and the ileal pouch–anal canal anastomosis is accomplished at a second operation 6 to 12 months later.

The goal of the operation is to remove all diseased colonic tissue. In most instances, a 3- to 5-cm mucosally stripped region of the rectal muscle serves as the anchor for the ileal pouch and preserves the innervation to the anus. The ileal pouch is then constructed from the distal 30 to 35 cm of ileum; J-shaped pouches are most prevalent, although S-, H-, and W-shaped pouches are also satisfactory. All pouches produce capacities similar to the healthy rectum (300 ml), have similar distensibility, and can evacuate 65% to 85% of their content within 15 seconds. Backwash ileitis is not a contraindication to the construction of a pouch and does not increase the risk of postoperative pouchitis. The most dependent aspect of the pouch is anastomosed at the dentate line, with the surgeon making certain that

---

TABLE 14-2
Indications and Contraindications for Ileal Pouch–Anal Canal Anastomosis

Indications
    Chronic ulcerative colitis
    Familial adenomatous polyposis
    Multiple colorectal malignancies
Contraindications
    Crohn's disease
    Distal rectal or anal malignancy
    Poor anal sphincter function
    Anal sphincter excised
    Age >65 years
Relative contraindications
    Massive obesity
    Emergency operation
    Inanition
    Prolonged steroid use
    Indeterminate colitis

---

there is no tension or compromise of the ileal pouch blood supply. Most patients should undergo a temporary diverting ileostomy to ensure anastomotic healing; the ileostomy is closed 2 months later. Patients younger than 30 years of age, with minimal inflammation, in good health, and who are not taking high-dose steroids may not require this temporary diverting colostomy. Postoperatively, patients are started on low-fiber diets and given loperamide to reduce stool frequency for 1 month. Afterward, the dietary restrictions are gradually lifted as tolerated.

Complications

Early postoperative complications appear in 46% of patients. The most common complication is obstruction (20%), which requires reoperation half of the time. Infection, which occurs in 5% to 10% of patients, can have adverse long-term effects on the use of the pouch. In patients who develop sepsis, pouch removal is necessary in approximately 50% of cases.

Outcome

The overall quality of life after an ileal pouch–anal canal anastomosis is excellent, with 75% to 90% of the patients experiencing improved or satisfactory social, sexual, occupational, and domestic performance. Digestive function, including nutrient absorption, is unimpaired by the ileal pouch–anal canal anastomosis. Vitamin B_{12} malabsorption has not been reported. Enteric output averages 650 ml per day, leading to mild compensatory reductions in urine output. Defecation frequency stabilizes to six small, soft stools during the day and one movement during the night, although older patients may have a higher stool number. Patients with familial adenomatous polyposis have fewer bowel movements than those with colitis. The resting anal pressure is reduced initially by 10% and returns to normal within 1 year; anal squeeze pressures are normal. Episodic decreases in anal tone occur during rapid eye movement sleep, as they do in healthy controls, which may predispose some patients to nocturnal fecal leakage. At 4 years after surgery, 75% of patients are perfectly continent at night, with the remainder reporting some spotting of the undergarments. Anal canal sensation is intact; however, the rectoanal inhibitory reflex is usually lost without apparent effect on defecatory function. Urinary function is unaltered after the second postoperative week. After surgery, 2% of men experience prolonged impotence, and 2% report retrograde ejaculation, while 7% of women note temporary dyspareunia. Pregnancy is a viable option for women patients, with normal vaginal delivery.

Aerobic and anaerobic bacteria proliferate in the ileal pouch and distal ileum, probably secondary to pouch stasis. Nonspecific inflammation of the pouch occurs in 22% of colitis patients and 7% of polyposis patients within the first 4 postoperative years. Pouchitis is heralded by watery diarrhea (occasionally with blood), fever, malaise, pelvic pain, arthralgias, and uveitis. Endoscopy reveals mucosal edema, friability, and punctate erosions. Clinical symptoms usually diminish with antibiotic treatment (e.g., metronidazole), although multiple courses may be needed for recurrent attacks.

CHAPTER 15

Approach to the Patient with Jaundice

Library Resource Center
Renton Technical College
3000 N.E. 4th St.
Renton, WA 98056

DIFFERENTIAL DIAGNOSIS

Jaundice, a yellow discoloration of the sclera, skin, and mucous membranes, results from the accumulation of bilirubin, a by-product of heme metabolism. It must be distinguished from yellow pigmentation caused by the ingestion of foods rich in carotene (carrots) or lycopene (tomatoes) or drugs such as quinacrine (Atabrine) or busulfan. Of the 250 to 300 mg of bilirubin produced daily, 70% results from the reticuloendothelial breakdown of senescent erythrocytes. Bilirubin is cleared by the liver in a three-step process. Bilirubin is first transported into hepatocytes by specific membrane carriers. It is then conjugated to one or two molecules of glucuronide. Finally, the conjugated bilirubin moves to the canalicular membrane, where it is excreted into the bile canaliculus by another carrier protein. Once in the bile, most conjugated bilirubin is excreted in the feces, although a small amount is deconjugated by colonic bacteria and reabsorbed. Colonic bacteria also reduce bilirubin to urobilinogens that are reabsorbed and excreted in the urine.

Normal bilirubin levels are 0.4 ± 0.2 mg per dl, with >95% unconjugated. Hyperbilirubinemia is defined as a total bilirubin level of >1.5 mg per dl, an unconjugated level of >1.0 mg per dl, and a conjugated level of >0.3 mg per dl. Generally, the serum bilirubin level must exceed 2.5 to 3.0 mg per dl for jaundice to be visible. Hyperbilirubinemia is separated into two classes: unconjugated (>80% of total bilirubin) and conjugated (>30% of total bilirubin) (Table 15-1). With prolonged jaundice, circulating bilirubin may bind covalently to albumin, preventing its elimination until the albumin is degraded. Therefore, with certain cholestatic disorders, measurable hyperbilirubinemia persists after resolution of the disease. Conjugated bilirubin is cleared by renal glomeruli; in renal failure, bilirubin levels may increase enormously.

Unconjugated Hyperbilirubinemia

Hemolysis and Ineffective Erythropoiesis

Hemolysis and ineffective erythropoiesis lead to an overproduction of bilirubin that exceeds the conjugative capability of the liver. Hemolysis may result from sickle cell anemia, thalassemia, glucose-6-phosphate deficiency, paroxysmal nocturnal hemoglobinuria, ABO blood group incompatibility, or medications. Severe hemolysis rarely elevates serum bilirubin levels above 5 mg per dl, although hepatocyte dysfunction or Gilbert's syndrome can magnify the hyperbilirubinemia. Iron deficiency, vitamin B_{12} deficiency, lead toxicity, sideroblastic anemia, and dyserythropoietic porphyria produce unconjugated hyperbilirubinemia due to ineffective erythropoiesis. Resorption of large hematomas may also increase production of unconjugated bilirubin.

Neonatal Jaundice

Physiologic neonatal jaundice is noticed in the first 5 days of life in term infants, with unconjugated bilirubin levels peaking near 6 mg per dl by day 3 and then decreasing to normal within 14 days because of the increased activity of uridine diphosphate glucuronosyltransferase (UDPGT), the hepatic enzyme responsible for bilirubin conjugation. Preterm infants may have higher levels of unconjugated bilirubin, which persist for up to 1 month. Nonphysiologic causes in neonates include ABO blood group incompatibility between mother and infant, glucose-6-phosphate dehydrogenase deficiency, pyruvate kinase deficiency, and hypothyroidism. Lucey-Driscoll syndrome is transient unconjugated hyperbilirubinemia resulting from a UDPGT inhibitor in the mother's blood. Breast milk jaundice, which may produce bilirubin levels up to 20 mg per dl, results from an inhibitor of UDPGT activity in the breast milk. Severe unconjugated hyperbilirubinemia produces kernicterus in infants, which manifests as lethargy, hypotonia, and seizures.

TABLE 15-1
Causes of Jaundice

Unconjugated hyperbilirubinemia
    Hemolysis
        Glucose-6-phosphate deficiency
        Pyruvate kinase deficiency
        Medications
    Bilirubin overproduction
        Ineffective erythropoiesis
        Large hematoma
        Pulmonary embolism with infarction
    Neonatal causes
        Physiologic jaundice
        Lucey-Driscoll syndrome
        Breast milk jaundice
    Uridine diphosphate glucuronosyltransferase deficiencies
        Gilbert's syndrome
        Crigler-Najjar syndromes (I and II)
    Miscellaneous causes
        Medications
        Hypothyroidism
        Thyrotoxicosis
        Fasting
Conjugated hyperbilirubinemia
    Congenital causes
        Rotor's syndrome
        Dubin-Johnson syndrome
        Choledochal cysts
    Familial disorders
        Benign recurrent intrahepatic cholestasis
        Cholestasis of pregnancy
    Hepatocellular defects
        Ethanol abuse
        Viral infection
    Cholestatic syndromes
        Primary biliary cirrhosis
        Primary sclerosing cholangitis
        Biliary obstruction
        Pancreatic disease
    Systemic disease
    Infiltrative disorders
    Postoperative complications
    Renal disease
    Sepsis
    Medications

Uridine Diphosphate Glucuronosyltransferase Deficiencies

Gilbert's syndrome, which is inherited in an autosomal-dominant fashion, is the most common cause of unconjugated hyperbilirubinemia, affecting 3% to 8% of the population. One-half of the patients have mild associated hemolysis, and some have splenomegaly. Gilbert's syndrome results from a partial defect of bilirubin conjugation (50% of normal). However, affected patients are asymptomatic, exhibiting jaundice (up to 6 mg per dl) with intercurrent illness, fasting, stress, fatigue, and ethanol use, or in the premenstrual period. Crigler-Najjar type I syndrome is an autosomal-recessive disorder characterized by the absence of UDPGT activity. Untreated patients develop profound unconjugated hyperbilirubinemia and die by 18 months. Treatment consists of phototherapy, plasmapheresis, or liver transplantation. Crigler-Najjar type II syndrome (Arias' disease) is an autosomal-dominant condition with 10% of normal UDPGT activity leading to jaundice by age 1 year in most cases. Crigler-Najjar type II syndrome often needs no treatment unless it affects the very young who are at risk of development of kernicterus.

Other Causes of Unconjugated Hyperbilirubinemia

Probenecid and rifampicin decrease hepatic bilirubin uptake. Sulfonamides, aspirin, contrast dye, and some parenteral nutrition formulations displace bilirubin from albumin, thereby reducing its transport into the hepatocyte. Penicillin, quinine, and α-methyldopa induce hemolysis.

Conjugated Hyperbilirubinemia

Congenital Forms

Rotor's syndrome is a rare, asymptomatic, autosomal recessive disorder manifesting mild conjugated hyperbilirubinemia (2 to 5 mg per dl) in childhood. It is unclear whether the primary defect involves impaired hepatocyte secretion or impaired storage of bilirubin; although oral cholecystograms appear normal, biliary scintigraphy shows absent or delayed secretion. Dubin-Johnson syndrome is an asymptomatic autosomal recessive disorder resulting from the impaired secretion of bilirubin, which produces serum bilirubin levels of 2 to 5 mg per dl. The results of scintigraphy and oral cholecystography are abnormal, whereas histologic examination of the liver reveals darkly pigmented tissue. Patients with Byler's disease present with watery diarrhea, cholestasis, fat-soluble vitamin deficiency, and recurrent infection caused by defective hepatic secretion of bile acids. Choledochal cysts and Caroli's disease manifest as jaundice or cholangitis and can be complicated by the development of cholangiocarcinoma.

Familial Forms

Benign recurrent intrahepatic cholestasis presents with intense pruritus and elevated alkaline phosphatase levels, with mild increases in levels of aminotransferases and serum bilirubin (<10 mg per dl). Attacks, which begin from age 8 to 30 years, can last weeks to months, only to recur every several months to years. Liver biopsy specimens reveal centrilobular cholestasis, which appears to be related to altered bile acid transport and enterohepatic circulation. Cholestasis of pregnancy presents with pruritus in the third trimester and is inherited in an autosomal-dominant fashion. It is mandatory to distinguish this benign condition from acute fatty liver of pregnancy, toxemia, acute cholecystitis, and hepatitis.

Acquired Forms

Acquired disorders constitute the largest group of diseases manifesting with conjugated hyperbilirubinemia. Many of these conditions are associated with cholestasis and present with pruritus, hypercholesterolemia, and steatorrhea. Intrahepatic cholestasis may result from liver disease (fulminant hepatitis, chronic hepatitis with significant hepatocellular dysfunction, the recovery phase of acute hepatitis), infections, and medications. Hyperbilirubinemia occurs in alcoholic patients with acute fatty liver, alcoholic hepatitis, and cirrhosis. Of patients with alcoholic hepatitis, 10% to 20% present with a predominantly cholestatic picture, which may have a poor prognosis if bilirubin levels exceed 10 mg per dl or if encephalopathy, renal failure, or coagulopathy develop. Primary hepatic malignancy, lymphoma, and metastatic carcinoma cause hyperbilirubinemia late in their courses, whereas cholangiocarcinoma and other biliary obstructing lesions produce early jaundice. Bone marrow transplant patients may develop jaundice because of chemotherapy-induced veno-occlusive disease and acute or chronic graft-versus-host disease. Postoperative jaundice may result from anesthesia, intrahepatic cholestasis, transfusions, hypotension, hypoxia, and hemolysis. Rheumatologic disorders (e.g., rheumatoid arthritis, systemic lupus erythematosus, scleroderma) elevate alkaline phosphatase levels but rarely produce jaundice. Sjögren's syndrome has an increased incidence of antimitochondrial antibodies and is associated with primary biliary cirrhosis, which produces jaundice late in its course. Congestive heart failure, shock, and trauma may produce hyperbilirubinemia, whereas renal failure can exacerbate hyperbilirubinemia from any cause. Furthermore, obstructive jaundice increases the risk of renal insufficiency, especially in the postoperative period.

Infections cause jaundice by bile duct obstruction (e.g., ascariasis), cholestasis (e.g., tuberculosis), or by sepsis and endotoxemia. Infections with *Legionella*, *Escherichia coli*, *Klebsiella*, *Pseudomonas*, *Proteus*, *Bacteroides*, and *Streptococcus* organisms produce conjugated hyperbilirubinemia. Two-thirds of patients with acquired immunodeficiency syndrome have elevated levels of aminotransferases or alkaline phosphatase because of hepatitis, infectious sclerosing cholangitis, papillary stenosis, acalculous cholecystitis, malignancy, or medication effects, and all of these disorders may elevate bilirubin levels.

Hepatotoxicity accounts for 3.5% of adverse drug effects. Oral contraceptives produce jaundice in up to 4 of 10,000 patients because of intrahepatic cholestasis. NSAIDs cause hepatitis, cholestasis, granulomatous liver disease, and hypersensitivity reactions. Acetaminophen produces dose-dependent hepatotoxicity, which occurs at lower doses in alcoholics. Isoniazid produces jaundice in 1% of patients. Chemotherapeutic agents delivered into the hepatic arterial circulation may cause a syndrome similar to sclerosing cholangitis. Numerous other medications affect the liver; when identified, the offending medication should be discontinued. Total parenteral nutrition causes hyperbilirubinemia as a result of intrahepatic cholestasis, infection, and the development of gallstones.

The common extrahepatic obstructive causes of jaundice include stones, blood, and malignant and benign strictures. Gallstone disease represents the most common cause of obstructive jaundice in the United States, although biliary parasitic infection is a common problem in certain areas of the world. The most common malignant causes include pancreatic carcinoma, cholangiocarcinoma, and lymphoma. Pancreatitis may produce swelling of the pancreatic head, leading to common bile duct obstruction. Primary sclerosing cholangitis is most commonly associated with inflammatory bowel disease. With obstructive jaundice, alkaline phosphatase levels are elevated concurrently. For hyperbilirubinemia to develop, most of the bile ducts must be obstructed, and ductal dilation may not be detectable on radiographic studies for 72 hours.

WORKUP

History

The primary aim in the evaluation of the jaundiced patient is to determine if the hyperbilirubinemia is unconjugated or conjugated and if the process is acute or chronic. If it is unconjugated, the roles of increased production, decreased uptake, or impaired conjugation must be assessed. For conjugated hyperbilirubinemia, the process must be localized to an intrahepatic or extrahepatic site. Fever, abrupt-onset jaundice, right upper quadrant pain, and tender hepatomegaly suggest acute disease. Shaking chills and high fever point to cholangitis or to a bacterial infection, whereas low-grade fevers and flulike symptoms are more common with viral hepatitis. Pain radiating to the back may be indicative of pancreatic disease. Pruritus is reported with obstructive jaundice of more than 3 to 4 weeks' duration, regardless of the cause. Weight loss, anorexia, nausea, and vomiting are seen nonspecifically in many hyperbilirubinemic disorders.

Related historical features may provide etiologic clues. Recent blood transfusions, intravenous drug abuse, and sexual exposure suggest possible viral hepatitis. Drugs, solvents, ethanol, or oral contraceptives produce jaundice by cholestasis or hepatocellular damage. A history of gallstones, prior biliary surgery, and previous episodes of jaundice suggest bile duct disease. A family history of jaundice raises the possibility of a defect in bilirubin transport or conjugation or a heritable liver disease (e.g., Wilson's disease, hemochromatosis, or α_1-antitrypsin deficiency). Patients younger than 30 years of age are likely to present with acute parenchymal disease, whereas those older than 65 years are at risk for stones or malignancy. Conditions more common in men include alcoholic liver disease, pancreatic or hepatocellular carcinoma, and hemochromatosis. Disorders that are more prevalent in women include primary biliary cirrhosis, gallstones, and chronic active hepatitis.

Physical Examination

The examination can assess the cause, severity, and chronicity of jaundice. Fever may be seen with acute or chronic disease, although high fever warrants a search for a bacterial process. Cachexia, muscle wasting, palmar erythema, Dupuytren's contracture, parotid enlargement, xanthelasma, gynecomastia, and spider angiomas suggest chronic liver disease. A shrunken, nodular liver with splenomegaly signals cirrhosis, whereas masses or lymphadenopathy raise the possibility of malignancy. Liver spans of >15 cm suggest fatty infiltration, congestion, malignancy, or other infiltrative diseases. A friction rub may be found in malignancy. Ascites is found with cirrhosis, malignancy, and severe acute hepatitis. A palpable, distended gallbladder suggests malignant biliary obstruction. Asterixis and changes in mental status are noted with advanced liver disease.

Additional Testing

Laboratory Studies

Laboratory testing can confirm suspicions raised by the history and physical examination results (Fig. 15-1). The reticulocyte count, lactate dehydrogenase and haptoglobin levels, and examination of the peripheral blood smear can provide evidence of hemolysis. If hemolysis is documented, specific testing of the immune mechanisms and tests for vitamin B_{12} deficiency, lead intoxication, thalassemia, and sideroblastic anemia can be performed. In the absence of hemolysis, most patients with pure, unconjugated hyperbilirubinemia are diagnosed with Gilbert's syndrome.

Initial testing of patients with conjugated hyperbilirubinemia to distinguish hepatocellular causes from cholestatic causes includes determination of the levels of aminotransferases, alkaline phosphatase, total protein, and albumin. If the alkaline phosphatase level is normal, then extrahepatic biliary obstruction is unlikely. Although neither aspartate nor alanine aminotransferase levels are specific for liver disease, levels of >300 IU per ml are uncommon in nonhepatobiliary disease. Aminotransferase elevations of <300 IU per ml characterize ethanol and most drug-induced injury, whereas elevations of >1000 IU per ml usually indicate acute hepatitis, certain drug responses (e.g., acetaminophen), or ischemic injury. An aspartate aminotransferase level greater than that of alanine aminotransferase characterizes ethanol injury, whereas in viral hepatitis, the ratio is reversed. Leucine aminopeptidase, 5'-nucleotidase, or γ-glutamyltransferase can help to distinguish alkaline phosphatase elevations caused by hepatobiliary disease from those of bony sources. Specific liver diseases can be evaluated by blood testing (e.g., antimitochondrial antibody with primary biliary cirrhosis, hepatitis serologic findings with viral hepatitis, α_1-antitrypsin levels, iron studies, ceruloplasmin in hereditary liver disease, α-fetoprotein in malignancy, sedimentation rate, immunoglobulins, antinuclear and smooth muscle antibodies with autoimmune disease). Elevated globulin levels with hypoalbuminemia support the diagnosis of cirrhosis, as does failure of the prothrombin time to correct after vitamin K administration. Hypercholesterolemia is found with cholestasis.

Noninvasive Imaging Studies

Ultrasound is the initial test for detection of biliary obstruction, with an accuracy of 77% to 94%. With acute obstruction, it may take 4 hours to 4 days for biliary dilation to be evident. Partial or intermittent obstruction may not produce dilation. Ultrasound is inconsistent in defining the site of obstruction because the distal common bile duct is difficult to visualize. Furthermore, 24% to 40% of patients with choledocholithiasis have bile ducts with normal diameters. Computed tomography (CT) may be performed if ultrasound findings are equivocal or nondiagnostic. CT scans may provide better definition of intra- and extrahepatic mass lesions. Fine needle aspiration of mass lesions is possible with both modalities. Radionuclide imaging with ^{99m}Tc-labeled iminodiacetic acid derivatives is the procedure of choice to detect cystic duct obstruction resulting from acute cholecystitis. The inability to visualize the gallbladder after 6 hours is diagnostic of cystic duct obstruction, whereas common bile duct obstruction is reported if no contrast passes into the intestine within 60 minutes. False-positive test results (i.e., lack of gallbladder or duct filling) can occur with prolonged fasting, parenteral nutrition, and bilirubin levels of >5 mg per dl. Di- and p-isopropyl iminodiacetic acid tracers allow biliary ductal visualization with greater degrees of jaundice.

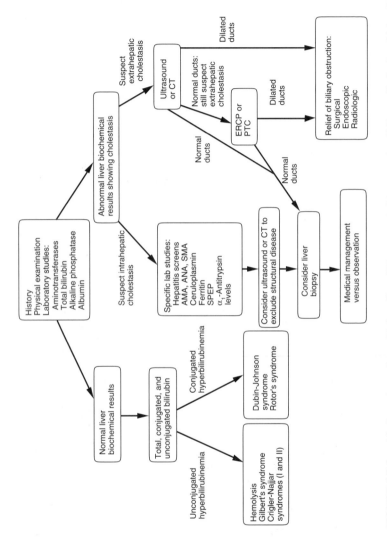

FIGURE 15-1. Workup of a patient with jaundice. (CT = computed tomography; ANA = antinuclear antibody; AMA = antimitochondrial antibody; SMA = anti–smooth muscle antibody; ERCP = endoscopic retrograde cholangiopancreatography; PTC = percutaneous transhepatic cholangiography; SPEP = serum protein electrophoresis.)

Invasive Diagnostic Studies

Endoscopic retrograde cholangiopancreatography (ERCP) and percutaneous transhepatic cholangiography (PTC) use cholecystographic dye and radiography to visualize the biliary tree. ERCP is successful in localizing the site of biliary obstruction in 90% of cases and is of particular utility in patients with choledocholithiasis because of the therapeutic capability of endoscopic sphincterotomy. The complications of ERCP include pancreatitis, cholangitis, bleeding, and perforation. Unsuccessful ERCP may result from the inability to cannulate the ampulla of Vater or to reach the ampulla (e.g., the patient with a Roux-en-Y gastrojejunostomy). PTC localizes the site of biliary obstruction in 90% of patients with dilated ducts, but it is less useful if the ductal diameter is normal. Contraindications to PTC include thrombocytopenia, severe coagulopathy, and ascites. PTC complications include infection, bleeding, pneumothorax, and peritonitis. Both ERCP and PTC afford the capability of biopsy or brushing of suggestive biliary strictures and provide the possibility of stent placement for benign and malignant biliary strictures.

If obstruction has been excluded or hepatocellular disease is suspected, a liver biopsy should be performed. Specific findings on liver biopsy include hepatitis, cirrhosis, granulomas, infection, malignancy, certain autoimmune diseases, venous congestion, infiltrative processes, and hereditary liver disease. For 15% of cases, a liver biopsy is not helpful in determining the cause of hyperbilirubinemia. Dilated ducts are a relative contraindication to liver biopsy. Liver biopsy complications include bleeding, pneumothorax, infection, and puncture of the gallbladder, gut, or kidney.

PRINCIPLES OF MANAGEMENT

Management of a jaundiced patient depends on the underlying cause. In general, a patient with hereditary unconjugated hyperbilirubinemia does not need or does not respond to therapy, although phenobarbital may reduce bilirubin levels in Crigler-Najjar type II syndrome and Gilbert's syndrome. Hemolysis may subside with discontinuation of an offending medication or with corticosteroid treatment of an underlying autoimmune process. Certain hepatocellular diseases may respond to specific therapies—for example, interferon for chronic active hepatitis C infection and phlebotomy programs for hemochromatosis.

The goals of the treatment of a patient with bile duct obstruction are to drain bile from above the blockage to provide relief of pruritus, to decrease the risk of complications, and to remove or bypass the cause of the obstruction. For an otherwise healthy patient with choledocholithiasis, laparoscopic cholecystectomy with common bile duct exploration and removal of the biliary stones is the standard of care, although some clinicians recommend preoperative ERCP in some patients. For elderly or frail patients who cannot undergo surgery, ERCP with endoscopic sphincterotomy may represent the safest alternative. If a stone cannot be removed with standard endoscopic techniques, surgical extraction is indicated; for patients with exceptional surgical risk, endoscopic stenting or percutaneous transkepotic extraction is the alternative. If a malignant biliary obstruction cannot be drained endoscopically or radiographically, a surgical procedure (e.g., cholecystojejunostomy or choledochojejunostomy) may be necessary to bypass the obstructed segment.

COMPLICATIONS

The potential for complications depends on the cause and severity of the jaundice and on patient characteristics. Infants with unconjugated hyperbilirubinemia who have bilirubin levels of >20 mg per dl are at risk of kernicterus, in which bilirubin deposition in the thalamus, hypothalamus, and cerebellum produces irreversible impairment of motor and cortical function. Many hepatic diseases carry the risk of morbidity or death from the underlying disorder. Extrahepatic biliary obstruction may result in secondary biliary cirrhosis, bacterial cholangitis, or hepatic abscess formation, all of which are life-threatening if the obstruction is not relieved.

CHAPTER 16

Approach to the Patient with Abnormal Liver Chemistry Values

DIFFERENTIAL DIAGNOSIS

Evaluation of suspected liver disease requires an understanding of the diverse tests of liver function and serum markers of hepatobiliary disease. Abnormalities in liver chemistry values may result from cholestasis, hepatocellular injury, and infiltrative diseases of the liver (Table 16-1). The approach to the patient with jaundice is discussed in detail in Chapter 15. Hepatocellular disorders produce elevations in liver enzymes that are released by damaged hepatocytes. Infiltration resulting from malignancy, granulomas, amyloid, and other conditions results in elevations of enzymes that are localized to the bile canalicular membrane, usually without development of jaundice.

TABLE 16-1
Causes of Abnormal Liver Chemistry Values

Cholestasis
    Obstructive
        Choledocholithiasis
        Biliary stricture
        Malignancy (bile duct, pancreas, ampullary, duodenal)
        Extrinsic compression
        Sclerosing cholangitis
    Intrahepatic
        Primary biliary cirrhosis
        Medications
        Sepsis
        Rotor's syndrome
        Dubin-Johnson syndrome
        Benign recurrent intrahepatic cholestasis
        Cholestasis of pregnancy
Hepatocellular injury
    Acute viral hepatitis
        Hepatitis A, B, C, D, and E
        Miscellaneous (cytomegalovirus, Epstein-Barr virus, herpes simplex virus, varicella-
            zoster virus)
    Chronic viral liver disease
        Chronic persistent hepatitis B and C
        Chronic active hepatitis B and C
        Cirrhosis
    Alcoholic liver disease
        Steatosis
        Alcoholic hepatitis
        Cirrhosis
    Hereditary liver disease
        Wilson's disease
        Hemochromatosis
        α_1-Antitrypsin deficiency
    Congestive/ischemic disease
        Congestive heart failure
        Constrictive pericarditis
        Hypotension
        Budd-Chiari syndrome
        Inferior vena cava occlusion
        Veno-occlusive disease
    Liver disease in pregnancy
        Acute fatty liver of pregnancy
        Eclampsia
    Medications
Infiltrative disorders
    Malignancy
        Hepatocellular carcinoma
        Lymphoma
        Leukemia
        Metastases
    Granuloma
        Tuberculosis
        Sarcoidosis
        Histoplasmosis
        Medications

Cholestatic Disorders

Cholestasis may result from intrahepatic or extrahepatic processes. Intrahepatic causes of cholestasis include primary biliary cirrhosis (PBC), sepsis, medications, postoperative cholestasis, familial conditions (e.g., benign recurrent intrahepatic cholestasis and cholestasis of pregnancy), and congenital disorders (e.g., Rotor's syndrome, Dubin-Johnson syndrome, and Byler's disease). Extrahepatic biliary obstruction is caused by choledocholithiasis, benign and malignant strictures, extrinsic compression, and sclerosing cholangitis.

Disorders with Hepatocellular Injury

Hepatocellular injury may result from a diverse group of diseases. Acute viral hepatitis in the United States most commonly results from infection with hepatitis A, B, or C viruses. Hepatitis D complicates the course of infection in chronic hepatitis B carriers. Hepatitis E occurs primarily in developing countries and is often fulminant in pregnant women. Other viral causes of hepatitis include cytomegalovirus, herpes simplex virus, Epstein-Barr virus, and varicella-zoster virus. Chronic infection with either hepatitis B or C viruses may also produce chronic hepatitis or cirrhosis. Ethanol consumption produces a broad range of liver disease, including fatty liver, alcoholic hepatitis, and cirrhosis. Hereditary liver diseases that produce hepatocellular injury are Wilson's disease, hemochromatosis, and α_1-antitrypsin deficiency. Congestive and ischemic disease in the liver is caused by congestive heart failure, constrictive pericarditis, hypotension, Budd-Chiari syndrome, inferior vena cava occlusion, and veno-occlusive disease. Pregnancy may be complicated by acute fatty liver of pregnancy and hepatocellular damage secondary to toxemia. Medication- and toxin-induced causes of injury must also be considered.

Infiltrative Diseases

Malignant diseases including primary tumors (e.g., hepatocellular carcinoma), metastases, lymphoma, and leukemia, may produce infiltrative liver disease. Granulomatous liver infiltration may result from infections (e.g., tuberculosis and histoplasmosis), sarcoidosis, and numerous medications.

WORKUP

History

An accurate history is critical in assessing the patient whose laboratory studies provide evidence of liver disease. The presenting symptoms provide important diagnostic clues. Pruritus is a presenting symptom with cholestasis. Although classically associated with PBC and sclerosing cholangitis, pruritus is also reported in extrahepatic biliary obstruction and hepatocellular disease. Many conditions that produce abnormal liver chemistry values are painless, but acute biliary obstruction from stones can produce intense right upper quadrant pain. Concurrent high fever raises concern for cholangitis. Acute hepatitis produces a less well-defined right upper quadrant discomfort with profound fatigue, whereas hepatic tumors may cause subcostal aching.

Numerous factors in the patient's history increase the risk of certain hepatic disorders. Family histories are useful in diagnosing and evaluating hereditary hemolytic states, benign recurrent intrahepatic cholestasis, hemochromatosis, Wilson's disease, and α_1-antitrypsin deficiency. Exposure to hepatotoxic medications, ethanol, and industrial and environmental toxins should be identified. Alcoholic patients should be questioned about acetaminophen use, because hepatotoxicity occurs even with therapeutic dosing in these persons. Intravenous drug abuse, sexual contact, and blood transfusions suggest viral hepatitis, whereas sudden worsening of liver chemistry values in a chronic hepatitis B carrier suggests possible hepatitis D superinfection. Waterborne outbreaks of viral hepatitis have been reported in Southeast Asia and India, underscoring the importance of obtaining a travel history. Risk factors for hepatitis A include recent ingestion of raw or undercooked oysters or clams, male homosexuality, or exposure through day care.

Associated diseases should be ascertained. Right-sided congestive heart failure, hypotension, and shock are recognized causes of abnormal liver chemistry findings. Chronic pancreatitis may produce abnormal liver tests because of the stenosis of the common bile duct. Hepatobiliary manifestations of inflammatory bowel disease may occur in 10% of patients. Hematologic disorders (e.g., polycythemia rubra vera, myeloproliferative disorders, and paroxysmal nocturnal hemoglobinuria) predispose to hepatic vein thrombosis. Hemoglobinopathies (e.g., sickle cell anemia and thalassemia) lead to pigment stone formation. Rashes, arthritis, renal disease, and vasculitis may develop with viral hepatitis. The presence of hypogonadism, heart disease, and diabetes suggests possible hemochromatosis. Concurrent lung disease is found with α_1-antitrypsin deficiency, and central neural findings are associated with Wilson's disease. Patients with leptospirosis present with hepatic and renal abnormalities. Renal cell carcinoma manifests as abnormal liver chemistry values in the absence of metastases. Obesity is a risk factor for fatty liver, as are diabetes and corticosteroid use. Recent surgery should be noted because anesthetic exposure, perioperative hypotension, and blood transfusions all may affect the liver. Recent biliary tract surgery raises concern for bile duct stricture. Cirrhosis is a late complication of jejunoileal bypass surgery for morbid obesity.

Physical Examination

Physical findings are of discriminative value in a patient with abnormal liver chemistry findings. Fever is suggestive of an infectious cause or hepatitis. Jaundice is seen when the serum bilirubin concentration exceeds 2.5 to 3.0 mg per dl. Spider angiomas, palmar erythema, parotid enlargement, gynecomastia, Dupuytren's contracture, and testicular atrophy are stigmata of chronic liver disease. Hyperpigmentation is seen with hemochromatosis and PBC. Ichthyosis and koilonychia are found with hemochromatosis. Lichen planus is associated with autoimmune liver disease and PBC. Xanthomas and xanthelasma appear in chronic cholestasis. Kayser-Fleischer rings and sunflower cataracts suggest Wilson's disease. Conjunctival suffusion raises the possibility of leptospirosis. A liver span of >15 cm is suggestive of passive congestion or liver infiltration. Splenomegaly is found with portal hypertension or infiltrative processes. Abdominal tenderness suggests an inflammatory process (e.g., cholecystitis, cholangitis, pancreatitis, or hepatitis) whereas a palpable, nontender gallbladder raises the possibility of an obstructive malignancy. Murphy's sign (i.e., inspiratory arrest during deep, right upper quadrant palpation) is highly suggestive of acute cholecystitis. A pulsatile liver suggests tricuspid insufficiency, and hepatic bruits or rubs raise the possibility of hepatocellular carcinoma. Occult or gross fecal blood on rectal examination suggests possible inflammatory bowel disease or neoplasm.

Additional Testing

Hepatic Function Tests

Measurements of hepatic function evaluate the liver's ability to excrete substances and assess its synthetic and metabolic capacity.

Bilirubin. Serum bilirubin determination provides a measure of hepatic conjugation and organic anion excretion capabilities. Hyperbilirubinemia can occur from increases in the unconjugated or conjugated bilirubin fractions. Increased production of bilirubin because of hemolysis and defective conjugation produces unconjugated hyperbilirubinemia, whereas hepatocellular disorders and extrahepatic obstruction cause conjugated hyperbilirubinemia. A third form of bilirubin, seen with prolonged cholestasis, is covalently bound to albumin. The presence of this albumin-bound bilirubin explains the slow resolution of jaundice in convalescing patients with resolving liver disease. The urine bilirubin level is elevated in conjugated, not unconjugated, hyperbilirubinemia.

Albumin. Total serum albumin is a useful measure of hepatic synthetic function. With a half-life of 20 days, albumin is a better index of disease severity in chronic rather than acute liver injury. Hypoalbuminemia may result from increased catabolism of albumin, decreased synthesis, dilution with plasma volume expansion, and increased protein loss from the gut or urinary tract. Prealbumin has a shorter half-life (1.9 days) than albumin and therefore has been proposed as a useful measure of hepatic synthetic capacity after acute injury (e.g., acetaminophen overdose).

Clotting Factors. The prothrombin time detects activity of the vitamin K–dependent coagulation factors (II, VII, IX, and X). Synthesis of these factors requires adequate intestinal vitamin K absorption and intact hepatic synthesis. Therefore, prolonged prothrombin times result from hepatocellular disorders that impair synthetic functions and from cholestatic syndromes that interfere with lipid absorption. Parenteral vitamin K administration distinguishes these possibilities. Improvement in the prothrombin time by 30% within 24 hours of vitamin K administration indicates that synthetic function is intact and suggests vitamin K deficiency. A prolonged prothrombin time is a poor prognostic finding; it signifies severe hepatocellular necrosis in acute hepatitis and the loss of functional hepatocytes in chronic liver disease. Individual clotting proteins may be useful clinical guides. Factor VII is the best indicator of liver disease severity and prognosis.

Miscellaneous Tests of Hepatic Function. Serum bile acid determination has been advocated for the assessment of suspected liver disease, although poor diagnostic sensitivity in mild disease has prevented widespread application. However, the finding of normal levels of bile acids in a patient with unconjugated hyperbilirubinemia supports a diagnosis of Gilbert's syndrome in questionable cases. Plasma clearance of sulfobromophthalein, an organic anion, may help distinguish between Dubin-Johnson syndrome and Rotor's syndrome. Serum globulin determinations give useful diagnostic information. Levels in excess of 3 g per dl are primarily observed in autoimmune liver disease, whereas selective increases in levels of immunoglobulin A (IgA) are noted in alcoholic cirrhosis. Elevated serum ammonia levels may be noted with severe acute or chronic liver disease and correlate roughly with hepatic encephalopathy. Acute viral and alcoholic hepatitis produce decreases in the alpha and pre-beta bands on serum protein electrophoresis because of reduced activity of lecithin-cholesterol acyltransferase, whereas the beta band may be broad because of altered triglyceride lipase activity resulting in elevated low-density lipoproteins. Breath tests of antipyrine clearance and aminopyrine demethylation measure impaired hepatic drug metabolism.

Serum Markers of Hepatobiliary Dysfunction

Aminotransferases. Aspartate aminotransferase (AST, SGOT) and alanine aminotransferase (ALT, SGPT) are markers of hepatocellular injury. Because AST is also found in muscle, kidney, heart, and brain, ALT elevations are more specific for liver processes. The highest elevations occur in viral, toxin-induced, and ischemic hepatitis, whereas smaller (<300 IU per ml) elevations are observed in alcoholic hepatitis and other hepatocellular disorders. An AST/ALT ratio of >2 is suggestive of alcoholic liver disease, whereas a ratio of <1 characterizes viral infection and biliary obstruction. When evaluating a patient with liver disease, decreases in AST and ALT levels usually suggest resolving injury, although decreasing aminotransferase levels may also be an ominous indicator of overwhelming hepatocyte death in fulminant liver failure.

Alkaline Phosphatase. Alkaline phosphatase originates in the bile canalicular membranes. Elevations of this enzyme are prominent in cholestasis and infiltrative liver disease; smaller increases are observed in other liver diseases. Alkaline phosphatase activity is also present in bone, placenta, intestine, kidney, and some malignancies. Low levels of alkaline phosphatase may be observed in acute hemolysis complicating Wilson's disease as well as in hypothyroidism, pernicious anemia, and zinc deficiency.

Miscellaneous Markers of Hepatobiliary Dysfunction. Serum levels of γ-glutamyltransferase (GGT), 5'-nucleotidase, and leucine aminopeptidase (LAP) are elevated in cholestatic syndromes and may help distinguish hepatobiliary from bony sources of alkaline phosphatase elevations. Levels of GGT are also elevated with pancreatic disease, myocardial infarction, uremia, lung disease, rheumatoid arthritis, and diabetes. Alcohol, anticonvulsants, and warfarin induce hepatic microsomal enzymes, producing striking GGT level increases. Levels of LAP may be elevated in normal pregnancy. The hepatic mitochondrial enzyme glutamate dehydrogenase is elevated in alcoholic patients and in patients with liver disease secondary to congestive heart failure. The lactate dehydrogenase concentration is frequently obtained as a "liver function test"; however, it has limited specificity for liver processes.

Disease-Specific Markers

Viral Serology. Hepatitis A IgM antibody (anti-HAV IgM) is initially detectable at the onset of clinical illness and persists for 120 days. Anti-HAV IgG is a convalescent marker that may persist for life. Hepatitis B surface antigen (HBsAg) precedes aminotransferase elevations and symptom development and persists for 1 to 2 months in self-limited infections. Antibody to core antigen (anti-HBc) is detected 2 weeks after the appearance of HBsAg, and initially is of the IgM class. Antibody to HBsAg (anti-HBs) appears sometime after the disappearance of HBsAg and may persist for life. During the window period between the disappearance of HBsAg and appearance of anti-HBs, anti-HBc IgM may be the only marker of recent hepatitis B infection. Hepatitis B e antigen and antibody, hepatitis B viral DNA, and DNA polymerase determinations can be used to further characterize the presence of active viral replication in some patients with chronic hepatitis B infection. Enzyme-linked immunosorbent assays (ELISAs) are screening tests for detection of hepatitis C exposure. Recombinant immunoblot assays are used as a supplement to ELISAs in the diagnosis of hepatitis C. These tests may produce negative findings for up to 6 months after acute infection; therefore, if hepatitis C is a diagnostic possibility, repeat testing should be performed at a later date. To determine if hepatitis C viremia is present, a polymerase chain reaction determination of hepatitis C RNA is required. Hepatitis D infection in patients with HBsAg positivity is measured by hepatitis D viral RNA and anti–hepatitis D antibodies. Persistence of anti-HDV IgM predicts progression to chronic hepatitis D infection. A subset of patients who test negative for the above viral markers will exhibit positive serologic findings for cytomegalovirus, herpes simplex, coxsackievirus, or Epstein-Barr virus.

Immunologic Tests.   Markers that may be detected in autoimmune liver disease include antinuclear antibody (ANA, homogeneous pattern in a titer of $\geq$1:160) and the anti–smooth muscle antibodies (SMAs). SMAs are detected in 70% of patients with autoimmune chronic active hepatitis but may also be present in PBC. The presence of anti-liver/kidney microsomal antibodies (anti-LKM$_1$) with reduced titers of anti-actin or ANAs identifies a subset of patients with autoimmune chronic active hepatitis that presents with an aggressive course in young women. Antimitochondrial antibodies (AMAs) are present in 90% of patients with PBC and 25% of patients with chronic active hepatitis or drug-induced liver disease. Antibodies to the Ro antigen and to anticentromere antibodies are observed with PBC, especially in patients with sicca syndrome or scleroderma.

Copper Storage Variables.   Ceruloplasmin is a copper transport protein in the plasma that circulates in low concentrations in Wilson's disease; low levels (<20 mg per dl) are found in 90% of homozygotes and 10% of heterozygotes. Reductions may also be observed with severely depressed synthetic function caused by other end-stage liver diseases. Alternate diagnostic tests for Wilson's disease include urinary copper, which exceeds 100 mg per 24 hours in nearly all patients, and free serum copper, which is markedly elevated.

Iron Storage Variables.   Serum iron level and total iron-binding capacity (transferrin) are useful measures in the diagnosis of hemochromatosis. Transferrin is normally 25% to 40% saturated, but in hemochromatosis, the serum iron concentration approaches the transferrin level. False elevations in transferrin saturation are observed in alcoholic liver disease. Serum ferritin more closely correlates with hepatic and total body iron stores, although ferritin may be elevated in inflammatory disease because it is an acute phase reactant. For a definitive diagnosis of hemochromatosis, liver biopsy is performed for quantitative determination of tissue iron.

α_1-Antitrypsin. α_1-Antitrypsin is a hepatic glycoprotein that migrates in the α_1-globulin fraction on serum protein electrophoresis. Homozygotes for the PiZZ variant of this protein exhibit decreased serum α_1-antitrypsin activity, which predisposes to development of chronic liver and pulmonary disease. Hepatocytes that are unable to excrete the Z protein accumulate periodic acid–Schiff (PAS)-positive, diastase-resistant globules as seen in liver biopsy specimens.

α-**Fetoprotein.** α-Fetoprotein (AFP) is present in the serum of 70% to 90% of patients with hepatocellular carcinoma, although small resectable tumors may not produce AFP. AFP levels are also elevated with germ cell tumors, other gut malignancies, PBC, and acute and chronic hepatitis. To reliably exclude these disorders, a level of >400 mg per ml is said to be specific for hepatocellular carcinoma, although this level excludes nearly one-third of patients with the disorder.

Thyroid Function Tests. Acute hepatocellular injury is associated with elevated levels of serum thyroxine and thyroxine-binding globulin (TBG), the latter caused by TBG release from damaged hepatocytes. Triiodothyronine (T_3) levels are low because of impaired conversion from thyroxine, whereas reverse T_3 levels are elevated. Hypothyroidism may also be a presenting feature of PBC.

Percutaneous Liver Biopsy

As a general rule, direct forms of liver injury tend to cause predominant centrizonal necrosis; immunologically mediated forms of hepatocyte injury are localized to the periportal region; and cholestatic injury is recognized by the accumulation of canalicular bile and feathery degeneration of hepatocytes in the absence of a significant inflammatory infiltrate. Clinical applications of liver biopsy include evaluation of persistently abnormal liver chemistry values and establishment of the diagnosis in unexplained hepatomegaly. Contraindications to liver biopsy are an uncooperative or unstable patient, ascites, right-sided empyema, and suspected hemangioma or echinococcal cyst. Impaired coagulation function is a relative contraindication.

Coordinated Diagnostic Approach

Liver disease is classified into three groups: cholestasis, hepatocellular injury, and hepatic infiltration. Screening the patient by determining levels of AST and ALT activity, serum alkaline phosphatase, serum total and direct bilirubin, serum protein and albumin, and prothrombin time can direct the subsequent evaluation into one of these three groups of liver disease (Fig. 16-1).

  Cholestatic liver disease usually results in increased serum bilirubin and alkaline phosphatase levels with normal to mildly elevated aminotransferase levels, although in early biliary obstruction, transient profound aminotransferase elevations may occur. In extrahepatic cholestasis, the serum bilirubin level increases by 1.5 mg per dl per day, reaching a maximum of 35 mg per dl in the absence of renal failure. In partial biliary obstruction, the bilirubin level may remain normal in the face of an elevated alkaline phosphatase concentration. The most direct approach to the evaluation of suspected cholestasis is to perform ultrasound to assess bile duct size. If malignancy or pancreatic disease is suspected, computed tomography (CT) may provide better anatomic definition of the desired structures. If biliary dilation is detected, endoscopic retrograde cholangiopancreatography (ERCP) or percutaneous transhepatic cholangiography (PTC) can further define and potentially be used to treat the abnormality (see Chapter 15). In some cases of extrahepatic obstruction, bile duct size will be normal; in these cases, ERCP or PTC may still be indicated because of a high

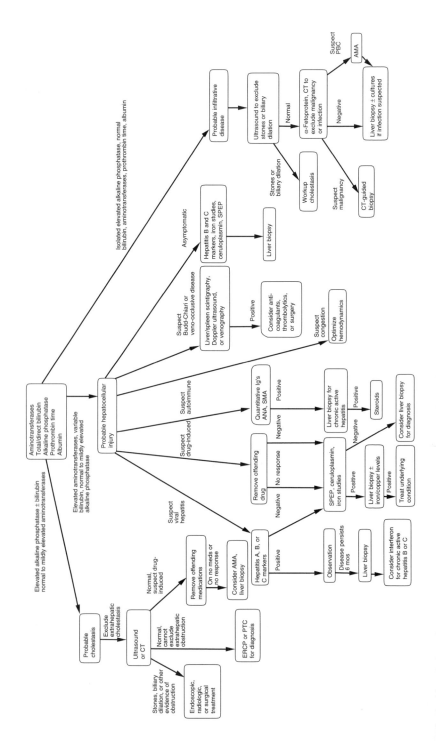

128

clinical suspicion. In questionable cases, percutaneous liver biopsy may provide a definitive diagnosis. However, intrahepatic cholestasis cannot always be distinguished from extrahepatic cholestasis on liver biopsy specimens.

Hepatocellular injury is suggested by aminotransferase levels of >400 IU per ml; levels of >300 IU per ml are nonspecific and are observed with cholestasis as well as with hepatocellular disease. Alkaline phosphatase and bilirubin elevations are variable in hepatocellular disease, depending on the cause and severity of the clinical condition. Prolongation of the prothrombin time and decreases in serum albumin levels indicate significant hepatic synthetic dysfunction. In the setting of acute malaise, anorexia, nausea, jaundice, tender hepatomegaly, and elevated levels of aminotransferases, viral markers should be obtained to exclude hepatitis A, B, or C viruses, depending on the patient risk factors. With disease duration of >6 months, additional studies (e.g., serum protein electrophoresis, ferritin or iron studies, and ceruloplasmin) should be added to the viral serologic studies to exclude hereditary liver disease. Eosinophilia suggests possible drug hypersensitivity. For a patient with prominent systemic symptoms suggestive of autoimmune disease, the clinician should determine the sedimentation rate; serum protein electrophoresis; quantitative immunoglobulins; and the presence of ANA, AMA, and SMA. A hepatocellular pattern is observed with ischemic and congestive liver disease, but measures to improve hepatic blood flow in these conditions can produce brisk reductions in aminotransferases to near normal levels within 72 hours. With congestive liver disease, the prothrombin time may be prolonged out of proportion to other signs of liver disease. Hepatic vein thrombosis (Budd-Chiari syndrome) may be suggested by a liver-spleen scintigraphic pattern showing relatively increased caudate lobe uptake. Doppler ultrasound may suggest the condition; angiography or magnetic resonance imaging can provide a definitive diagnosis. Most acute elevations in aminotransferase levels do not require further evaluation. If aminotransferase levels remain high for >6 months without an identifiable cause, however, a liver biopsy is indicated for diagnosis and to offer prognostic information about possible progression to cirrhosis. Many of these persons are obese or use ethanol, and the usual finding on liver biopsy is fatty liver. However, the unexpected finding of chronic active hepatitis in a subset of these patients provides support for biopsy even in asymptomatic individuals.

Isolated elevation of alkaline phosphatase levels of hepatic origin (confirmed by LAP, 5'-nucleotidase, or GGT) suggests an infiltrative process. These patients should undergo diagnostic imaging as described above, however, to rule out extrahepatic cholestasis. A more than threefold increase in the alkaline phosphatase level in a patient with known cirrhosis raises concern for hepatocellular carcinoma. In these patients, levels of α-fetoprotein should be measured, and an ultrasonographic or CT scan performed to exclude mass lesions. An elevated alkaline phosphatase level, detectable titers of AMA, and an elevated serum IgM level in a middle-aged woman is consistent with PBC. If imaging studies are nondiagnostic, liver biopsy is essential to exclude neoplasm, infection, cholestasis, or granuloma.

FIGURE 16-1. Workup of a patient with abnormal liver chemistry values. (ANA = antinuclear antibody; SMA = anti–smooth muscle antibody; SPEP = serum protein electrophoresis; ERCP = endoscopic retrograde cholangiopancreatography; PTC = percutaneous transhepatic cholangiography; CT = computed tomography; AMA = antimitochondrial antibody; PBC = primary biliary cirrhosis.)

PRINCIPLES OF MANAGEMENT

The management of patients with abnormal liver chemistry values is dependent on obtaining an accurate diagnosis. For extrahepatic obstruction, the goal of treatment is to relieve or bypass the obstruction (see Chapter 15). In drug-induced intrahepatic cholestasis, removal of the offending medication (e.g., antipsychotic medications) is indicated, although this does not always produce prompt normalization of liver chemistry values. Management of PBC depends on the stage of disease. Colchicine, immunosuppressives, and bile acids have been given in the early stages of the disease with questionable success; advanced liver failure in PBC usually warrants liver transplantation. Cholestyramine, rifampicin, phenobarbital, or ondansetron are given for pruritus in the cholestatic disorders.

Specific therapies for many hepatocellular disorders have been well described. Hemochromatosis is managed with phlebotomy, or alternatively, desferrioxamine. Wilson's disease is initially treated with D-penicillamine; maintenance regimens may include oral zinc to reduce intestinal copper absorption. Patients with severe acute hepatitis may require hospitalization for supportive care. An encephalopathic patient may need mechanical ventilation, intracranial pressure monitoring, and possible emergency liver transplantation to avert a fatal outcome. Interferon-α, with or without other antiviral agents, may eliminate the virus or slow disease progression in chronic active hepatitis B and C. Autoimmune chronic active hepatitis is usually responsive to corticosteroids, although some patients require long-term immunosuppressives. Congestive and ischemic hepatopathy improves with control of the underlying hemodynamic state. Anticoagulants or thrombolytic agents may be used in the early stages of Budd-Chiari syndrome or veno-occlusive disease, although these do not prevent clinical deterioration in many patients. Drug-induced hepatocellular injury is managed by medication withdrawal, although some agents have the potential for fatal hepatic necrosis (e.g., acetaminophen). With recent acetaminophen ingestion, administration of *N*-acetylcysteine is indicated.

Many of the causes of infiltrative liver disease have no effective treatment. Hepatic tuberculosis and candidiasis are exceptions; they respond to appropriate antimicrobial therapy. Although hepatocellular carcinoma usually has a poor prognosis, small tumors (<3 cm in diameter) may be resectable for cure. The fibrolamellar variant of hepatocellular carcinoma in young patients has a better prognosis. Multiple metastatic carcinomas are usually unresectable and have dismal prognoses, although prolonged survival has been reported after excision of the primary tumor and three or fewer solitary hepatic metastases.

COMPLICATIONS

Patients with chronic cholestasis or hepatocellular injury may progress to end-stage liver disease, depending on the cause. With hepatocyte loss, coagulopathy and hypoproteinemia develop, increasing the risks of hemorrhage, edema, ascites, and infection. Portal hypertension may lead to ascites, hydrothorax, and hemorrhage from esophageal or gastric varices or portal gastropathy. Other complications of end-stage liver failure include hepatic encephalopathy and hepatorenal syndrome. Infiltrative fungal infections of the liver may progress to abscess formation and death. Infiltrative malignancy usually is fatal.

Hepatitis B and C may be transmitted to contacts of the infected patient, usually by transfer of bodily fluids (e.g., blood), although sexual transmission of hepatitis B (and to a much lesser degree, hepatitis C) is possible. Patients who report body fluid contact with an HBsAg-positive patient should receive hepatitis B immune globulin, and, in most instances, they will benefit from a vaccination against hepatitis B. Immune serum globulin is recommended for individuals potentially exposed to hepatitis A. The role of immune serum globulin in hepatitis C prophylaxis is controversial.

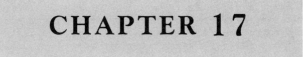

CHAPTER 17

Approach to the Patient with Ascites

DIFFERENTIAL DIAGNOSIS

Ascites refers to the pathologic accumulation of fluid within the peritoneal cavity. It is important to establish a cause for its development and to initiate a rational treatment regimen to avoid some of the complications of ascites. Most cases of ascites in the United States result from liver disease, although disorders involving other organ systems may produce abdominal fluid accumulation in certain situations (Table 17-1).

Hepatic Disease

Portal hypertension is a prerequisite for ascites formation in patients with liver disease. In general, ascites is a complication of chronic liver diseases (e.g., cirrhosis), but some acute diseases (e.g., acute alcoholic hepatitis or fulminant hepatic failure) may result in ascites. In such cases, ascites development signifies a poor prognosis, with 80% mortality in patients with fulminant disease. Ascites may complicate Budd-Chiari syndrome because of venous out-

TABLE 17-1
Causes of Ascites

CAUSE	PERCENTAGE OF TOTAL
Chronic parenchymal liver disease	81.4
Malignancy	10.0
Heart failure	3.0
Tuberculosis	1.7
Nephrogenous (dialysis ascites)	1.0
Pancreatic	0.9
Fulminant hepatic failure	0.7
Biliary	0.5
Lymphatic tear	0.3
Chlamydia infection	0.3
Nephrotic syndrome	0.2

flow obstruction. Three theories have been proposed to explain fluid accumulation. The underfill theory postulates that an imbalance of Starling forces produces intravascular fluid loss into the peritoneum, with resultant hormonally mediated renal sodium retention. The overfill theory proposes that primary renal sodium retention produces intravascular hypervolemia that overflows into the peritoneum. The peripheral arterial vasodilation theory proposes that portal hypertension leads to vasodilation and reduced effective arterial blood volume, which increases renal sodium retention and promotes fluid accumulation. With the vasodilation theory, the underfill mechanism is operative in early compensated cirrhosis, whereas the overflow mechanism operates in advanced disease.

Renal Disease

Nephrotic syndrome is a rare cause of ascites in adults. It results from protein loss in the urine, leading to decreased intravascular volume and increased renal sodium retention. Nephrogenous ascites is a poorly understood condition that develops with hemodialysis; its optimal treatment is undefined and its prognosis is poor. Continuous ambulatory peritoneal dialysis is an iatrogenic form of ascites that takes advantage of the rich vascularity of the parietal peritoneum to effect elimination of endogenous toxins. Urine may accumulate in the peritoneum in newborns or as a result of trauma or renal transplantation in adults.

Cardiac Disease

Ascites is an uncommon complication of both high- and low-output heart failure. High-output failure is associated with decreased peripheral resistance; low-output disease is defined by reduced cardiac output. Both lead to renal sodium retention. Pericardial disease is a rare cardiac cause of ascites.

Pancreatic Disease

Pancreatic ascites develops as a complication of severe acute pancreatitis, pancreatic duct rupture in acute or chronic pancreatitis, or leakage from a pancreatic pseudocyst. Underlying cirrhosis is present in many patients with pancreatic ascites. Pancreatic ascites may be complicated by infection or left-sided pleural effusion.

Biliary Disease

Most cases of biliary ascites result from gallbladder rupture, which usually is a complication of gangrene of the gallbladder in elderly men. Bile also can accumulate in the peritoneal cavity after biliary surgery or biliary or intestinal perforation.

Malignancy

Malignancy-related ascites signifies advanced disease in most cases and is associated with a dismal prognosis. Exceptions are ovarian carcinoma and lymphoma, which may respond to debulking surgery and chemotherapy, respectively. The mechanism of ascites formation depends on the location of the tumor. Peritoneal carcinomatosis produces exudation of proteinaceous fluid into the peritoneal cavity, whereas liver metastases or primary hepatic malignancy induces ascites likely by producing portal hypertension, either from vascular occlusion by the tumor or arteriovenous fistulae within the tumor.

Infectious Disease

In the United States, tuberculous peritonitis is a disease of Asian, Mexican, and Central American immigrants, and it is also a complication of the acquired immunodeficiency syndrome (AIDS). One-half of patients with tuberculous peritonitis in the absence of AIDS have underlying cirrhosis, usually secondary to ethanol abuse. Patients with liver disease tolerate antituberculous drug toxicity less well than patients with normal hepatic function. Exudation of proteinaceous fluid from the tubercles lining the peritoneum induces ascites formation. *Coccidioides* organisms cause infectious ascites formation by similar mechanisms. For sexually active women who have a fever and inflammatory ascites, chlamydia-induced Fitz-Hugh–Curtis syndrome should be considered. Gonococcus may also produce this condition.

Chylous Ascites

Chylous ascites results from the obstruction of or damage to chyle-containing lymphatic channels. The most common causes are lymphatic malignancies (e.g., lymphomas, other malignancies, surgical tears, and infectious causes). Patients with chylous ascites exhibit more of a hypovolemic response to paracentesis than those with other forms of ascites.

Other Causes of Ascites Formation

Serositis with ascites formation may complicate systemic lupus erythematosus. Meigs' syndrome, which is characterized by the development of ascites and pleural effusion, is caused by benign ovarian neoplasms. Ascites with myxedema appears to be secondary to disease-related cardiac disease. Mixed ascites occurs when the patient has two or more separate causes of ascites formation.

WORKUP

History

The history can help to elucidate the cause of ascites formation. Increasing abdominal girth as a result of ascites may be part of the initial presentation of patients with alcoholic liver disease; however, the laxity of the abdominal wall and the severity of underlying liver disease suggest that the condition can be present for some time before it is recognized. Patients who consume ethanol only intermittently may report cyclic ascites, whereas patients with nonalcoholic disease usually have persistent ascites. Other risk factors for viral liver disease should be ascertained (i.e., drug abuse, sexual exposure, blood transfusions, and tattoos). A positive family history of liver disease raises the possibility of a heritable condition (e.g., Wilson's disease, hemochromatosis, or α_1-antitrypsin deficiency) that might also present with symptoms referable to other organ systems (diabetes, cardiac disease, joint problems, and hyperpigmentation with hemochromatosis; neurologic disease with Wilson's disease; pulmonary complaints with α_1-antitrypsin deficiency). Patients with cirrhotic ascites may report other complications of liver disease including jaundice, pedal edema, gastrointestinal hemorrhage, or encephalopathy. The patient with long-standing stable cirrhosis who abruptly develops ascites should be evaluated for possible hepatocellular carcinoma.

Information concerning possible nonhepatic disease should be obtained. Weight loss or a prior history of cancer suggests possible malignant ascites, which may be painful and produce rapid increases in abdominal girth. A history of heart disease raises the possibility of cardiac causes of ascites. Some alcoholics with ascites have alcoholic cardiomyopathy rather than liver dysfunction. Tuberculous peritonitis usually presents with fever and abdominal discomfort. Patients with nephrotic syndrome usually have anasarca. Patients with rheumatologic disease may have serositis. Patients with ascites associated with lethargy, cold intolerance, and voice and skin changes should be evaluated for hypothyroidism.

Physical Examination

Ascites should be distinguished from panniculus, massive hepatomegaly, gaseous overdistention, intra-abdominal masses, and pregnancy. Percussion of the flanks can be used to rapidly determine if the patient has ascites. The absence of flank dullness excludes ascites with a 90% accuracy. If dullness is found, the patient should be rolled into a partial decubitus position to test if the air-fluid interface shifts (shifting dullness). The fluid wave has less value in the detection of ascites. The puddle sign detects as little as 120 ml of ascitic fluid, but mandates that the patient assume a hands-knees position for several minutes.

The physical examination can help in determining the cause of ascites. Palmar erythema, abdominal wall collateral veins, spider angiomas, splenomegaly, and jaundice are consistent with liver disease. Large veins on the flanks and back indicate blockage of the inferior vena cava that is caused by webs or malignancy. Masses or lymphadenopathy suggest underlying malignancy. Distended neck veins, cardiomegaly, and auscultation of an S_3 or pericardial rub suggest cardiac causes of ascites, whereas anasarca may be observed with nephrotic syndrome.

Additional Testing

Blood and Urine Studies

Laboratory blood studies can provide clues to the cause of ascites (Fig. 17-1). Abnormal levels of aminotransferases, alkaline phosphatase, and bilirubin are seen with liver disease. Prothrombin time prolongation or hypoalbuminemia is also observed with hepatic synthetic dysfunction, although low albumin levels are noted with renal disease, protein-losing enteropathy, and malnutrition. Hematologic abnormalities, especially thrombocytopenia, suggest liver disease. Renal disease may be suggested by electrolyte abnormalities or elevations in blood urea nitrogen and creatinine. Urinalysis may reveal protein loss with nephrotic syndrome or bilirubinuria with jaundice. Specific tests (e.g., α-fetoprotein) or serologic tests (e.g., antinuclear antibody) may be ordered for suspected hepatocellular carcinoma or immune-mediated disease, respectively.

Ascitic Fluid Analysis

Abdominal paracentesis is the most important means of diagnosing the cause of ascites formation. It is appropriate to sample ascitic fluid in all patients with new-onset ascites as well as in all those admitted to the hospital with ascites, as there is a 10% to 27% prevalence of ascitic fluid infection in the latter group. Paracentesis is performed in an area of dullness either in the midline between the umbilicus and symphysis pubis, as this area is avascular, or in one of the lower quadrants. Needles should not be inserted close to abdominal wall scars with either approach because of the high risk of bowel perforation; puncture sites too near the liver or spleen should be avoided as well. In 3% of cases, ultrasound guidance may be needed. The needle is inserted using a Z-track insertion technique to minimize postprocedure leakage, and 25 ml or more of ascitic fluid is removed for analysis.

Analysis of ascitic fluid should begin with gross inspection. Most ascitic fluid resulting from portal hypertension is yellow and clear. Cloudiness raises the possibility of infectious processes, whereas a milky appearance is seen with chylous ascites. A minimum density of 10,000 erythrocytes per μl is required to provide a red tint to the fluid, which raises the possibility of malignancy if the paracentesis is atraumatic. Pancreatic ascitic fluid is tea colored or black. The ascitic fluid cell count is the most useful test. The upper limit of the neutrophil cell count is 250 cells per μl, even in patients who have undergone diuresis. If

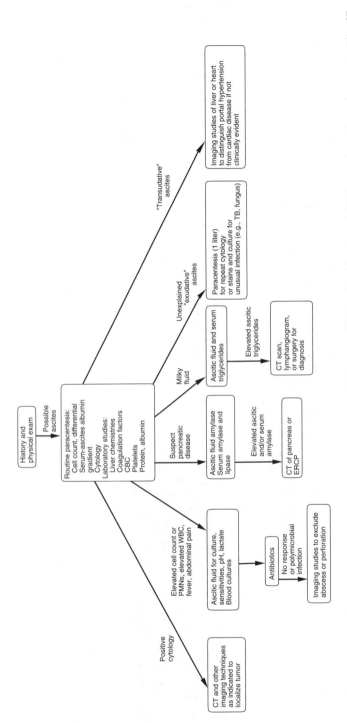

FIGURE 17-1. Workup of a patient with ascites. (CBC = complete blood count; WBC = white blood count; PMNs = polymorphonuclear neutrophils; CT = computed tomography; ERCP = endoscopic retrograde cholangiopancreatography; TB = tuberculosis.)

paracentesis is traumatic, only 1 neutrophil per 250 erythrocytes and 1 lymphocyte per 750 erythrocytes can be attributed to blood contamination. With spontaneous bacterial peritonitis (SBP), the neutrophil count exceeds 250 cells per µl and represents >50% of the total white cell count in the ascitic fluid. Chylous ascites may produce increases in ascitic lymphocyte counts. If infection is suspected, ascitic fluid should be inoculated into blood culture bottles at the bedside and sent for bacterial culture. Gram's stain is insensitive for the detection of bacterial infection, and results should not be considered reliable if negative, as 10,000 organisms per milliliter are needed for Gram's stain positivity, whereas spontaneous peritonitis may occur with only 1 organism per milliliter. Similarly, the direct smear has only a 0% to 2% sensitivity for the detection of tuberculosis. If 1 liter of fluid is cultured for tuberculosis, the sensitivity is 62% to 83%. If tuberculosis is strongly suspected, peritoneal biopsy is indicated using direct visualization of the peritoneal surface with a laparoscope, rather than blind biopsy. Certain infections can reduce ascitic fluid glucose levels, but because glucose concentrations usually are normal with SBP, this measure has limited utility. Similarly, testing of ascitic fluid pH and lactate levels has been proposed to evaluate for infected fluid; however, their sensitivities are low.

The serum-ascites albumin gradient provides important information about the cause of the ascites. Calculating the gradient involves subtracting the albumin concentration in the ascitic fluid from the serum value. If the serum albumin minus ascitic albumin concentration is 1.1 g per dl or higher, the patient can be diagnosed with portal hypertension with 97% accuracy. Causes of high-gradient ascites include cirrhosis, alcoholic hepatitis, cardiac ascites, massive liver metastases, Budd-Chiari syndrome, portal vein thrombosis, veno-occlusive disease, acute fatty liver of pregnancy, myxedema, and some mixed ascites. Conversely, a gradient of <1.1 g per dl signifies ascites that is not caused by portal hypertension. Low albumin gradient ascites may result from peritoneal carcinomatosis, tuberculosis, pancreatic or biliary disease, nephrotic syndrome, or connective tissue disease. Previous means of assessing the cause included measurement of total ascitic fluid protein and ascitic fluid-to-serum lactate dehydrogenase ratios. Although sometimes still used to distinguish "exudative" from "transudative," the accuracy of these measures is only 55% to 60%.

The detection of malignancy in ascitic fluid can be a diagnostic challenge. Although nearly 100% of patients with peritoneal carcinomatosis have positive results on cytologic analysis of the peritoneal fluid, patients with liver metastases, lymphoma, and hepatocellular carcinoma usually give negative cytology results. Peritoneal biopsy is rarely needed for peritoneal carcinomatosis. The value of ascitic fluid levels of carcinoembryonic antigen and humoral tests of malignancy in detection of malignant ascites is undefined.

Other ascitic fluid tests may be ordered depending on the clinical scenario. In uncomplicated cirrhotic ascites, the ascitic fluid amylase level is low with an ascitic fluid-to-serum ratio of 0.4. With pancreatic ascites, the levels may exceed 2000 IU per liter and amylase ratios may increase to 6. With milky ascitic fluid, a triglyceride level is obtained. Chylous ascites triglyceride levels exceed 200 mg per dl versus 20 mg per dl in cirrhotic ascites. For patients with brown ascitic fluid, an ascitic level of triglycerides greater than the serum level suggests biliary or bowel perforation.

Structural Testing

Radiographic, endoscopic, and scintigraphic means can be used to assess the cause of ascites. Barium radiography or upper or lower endoscopy may detect a primary tumor that is responsible for malignant ascites. Computed tomography or ultrasound may define mass lesions of the liver, pancreas, or ovaries or show findings suggestive of cirrhosis. Upper endoscopy may show varices or portal gastropathy, indicative of portal hypertension. Liver-spleen scintigraphy may show colloid shifting in cirrhosis. Doppler ultrasound or angiography may detect Budd-Chiari syndrome. Chest radiography may show apical disease consistent with tuberculosis. Abdominal radiography also is useful in assessing complications of ascites. Plain abdominal radiographs can be assessed for free subdiaphragmatic air in patients with peritonitis to exclude bowel perforation as a cause. Kidney biopsy may be necessary to evaluate renal causes of ascites.

PRINCIPLES OF MANAGEMENT

Ascites Unrelated to Portal Hypertension

In patients with peritoneal carcinomatosis, the peripheral edema responds to diuretic administration but the ascites does not. The mainstay of management of these patients is periodic therapeutic paracentesis. Peritoneovenous shunts may be performed in selected cases; however, in most instances, the short life expectancy does not warrant this aggressive intervention. Nephrotic ascites will respond to sodium restriction and diuretics. Tuberculous peritonitis requires specific antituberculosis agents. Pancreatic ascites may resolve spontaneously, respond to octreotide therapy, or require endoscopic stenting or surgery if a ductal leak is present. Postoperative lymphatic leaks may require surgical intervention or peritoneovenous shunting. Nephrogenous ascites may respond to vigorous dialysis.

Portal Hypertension–Related Ascites

For patients with ascites secondary to portal hypertension, dietary sodium restriction to a daily level of 2 g is essential. Fluids do not need to be restricted unless the serum sodium is <120 mEq per liter. If single-agent diuretic therapy is planned, spironolactone at a daily dose of 100 mg is the best choice. For patients who experience spironolactone side effects (e.g., painful gynecomastia), amiloride may be given at 10 mg per day. The physician should expect a slow response to spironolactone because of its long half-life; weight loss may not be evident for 2 weeks. It is often reasonable to add a loop diuretic (e.g., furosemide) at 40 mg per day to maximize natriuresis. Doses may slowly be increased to maximums of 400 mg per day of spironolactone and 160 mg per day of furosemide. If diuresis is still suboptimal, metolazone or hydrochlorothiazide may be added, although the hyponatremic and hypovolemic effects of such triple drug regimens mandate close physician follow-up, often on an inpatient basis. There should be no limit to the amount of weight that can be diuresed daily if pedal edema is present. Once the dependent edema has resolved, diuretics should be adjusted to achieve a daily weight loss of 0.5 kg. Urine sodium levels may be used to direct diuretic therapy. Patients with urine sodium excretion of <5 mEq every 24 hours may need very high diuretic doses for effective natriuresis. Similarly, the inability of diuretic treatment to increase urine sodium output of >10 mEq every 24 hours predicts probable treatment failure. Development of encephalopathy, a serum sodium level of <120 mEq per liter, or serum creatinine of >2 mg per dl are relative indicators for discontinuation of diuretic therapy. Because concurrent use of NSAIDs promotes renal failure, inhibits the efficacy of diuretics, and may cause gastrointestinal hemorrhage, their use is discouraged.

Various nonmedical means to treat refractory ascites are available. Large-volume paracentesis, with removal of 5 liters of fluid, can be performed in as little as 20 minutes. Total paracentesis, with withdrawal of 20 liters or more of fluid, is now known to be safe. The issue of concurrent administration of intravenous albumin is controversial. Some clinicians advocate albumin infusion as a means to prevent paracentesis-induced changes in electrolytes and creatinine. Other physicians avoid albumin infusion in view of its cost, particularly because differences in long-term survival have not been demonstrated with such measures. Transjugular intrahepatic portosystemic shunts (TIPSs) are effective in some patients with diuretic-resistant ascites. Peritoneovenous shunts (e.g., Denver and LeVeen) drain ascitic fluid into the central venous circulation; however, they have not achieved widespread use because of a lack of efficacy, shunt occlusion, and side effects (e.g., pulmonary edema, variceal hemorrhage, diffuse intravascular coagulation, and thromboembolism). Surgical portocaval shunt procedures were used in the past, but frequent postoperative complications (e.g., encephalopathy) have tempered enthusiasm for the techniques. Liver transplantation may be indicated in some patients.

COMPLICATIONS

Infection

SBP is defined as ascitic fluid infection with pure growth of a single organism and an ascitic fluid neutrophil count of >250 cells per μl without evidence of a surgically remediable intra-abdominal cause. SBP occurs only in the setting of liver disease, for all practical purposes, although it has been reported with nephrotic syndrome. Ascites is a prerequisite for SBP; however, it may not be detectable on physical examination. Infection usually occurs with maximal fluid accumulation. *Escherichia coli*, *Klebsiella pneumoniae*, and *Pneumococcus* organisms are the most common isolates in SBP, with anaerobes being the causative organism in 1% of cases. Eighty-seven percent of SBP patients present with symptoms, most commonly fever, abdominal pain, and changes in mental status, although the clinical manifestations may be quite subtle. Antibiotics should be initiated when an ascitic fluid neutrophil count of >250 cells per μl is documented before obtaining formal culture results. The most well-accepted antibiotic for SBP is the third-generation cephalosporin cefotaxime, to which 98% of offending bacteria are sensitive. When susceptibility testing is available, a drug with a more narrow spectrum may be substituted. Most infectious disease experts recommend 10 to 14 days of therapy, although a randomized trial comparing 5 to 10 days of therapy showed no difference, supporting a shorter antibiotic course. A repeat paracentesis that demonstrates a reduction in neutrophil counts 48 hours after initiating antibiotic treatment indicates that the antibiotic choice was appropriate. If the correct antibiotics are given in a timely manner, the mortality rate of SBP should not exceed 5%; however, many patients succumb to other complications of the underlying liver disease. Oral quinolones are given as prophylactic agents after an initial episode of SBP because of a reported 1-year recurrence rate of 69% in unprophylaxed patients.

SBP is not the only infectious complication of ascites. *Monomicrobial bacterascites* is defined as the presence of a positive result on ascitic fluid culture for a single organism with a concurrent fluid neutrophil count of <250 cells per µl. One series of patients with bacterascites demonstrated a predominance of gram-positive organisms, whereas another showed flora similar to SBP. Because of the high mortality rate of untreated bacterascites (22% to 43%), antibiotic treatment is warranted for many patients. Alternatively, paracentesis may be repeated for cell count and culture. *Culture-negative neutrocytic ascites* (CNNA) is defined as ascitic fluid with a neutrophil count of >250 cells per µl with negative fluid culture results in patients who have received no prior antibiotics. Patients with CNNA usually have spontaneously resolving SBP, but empirical antibiotics usually are given. A decline in ascitic neutrophil counts on repeat paracentesis indicates an appropriate response to therapy. If there is no response to antibiotics, cytologic analysis and culture of the ascitic fluid for tuberculosis may be indicated. *Secondary bacterial peritonitis* manifests as a polymicrobial infection with a very high ascitic fluid neutrophil count with an identified intra-abdominal source such as appendicitis, diverticulitis, or intra-abdominal abscess. In contrast to SBP, secondary peritonitis usually requires surgical intervention. Gut perforation is suspected with two of the following three criteria: ascitic protein concentration of >3 g per dl, glucose level of <50 mg per dl, and lactate dehydrogenase level of >225 mU per ml. Water-soluble contrast enemas are used in older patients to exclude a perforated colonic diverticulum, whereas young patients should have an upper gastrointestinal study using water-soluble dye because of the probability of a perforated ulcer. In patients with secondary peritonitis but no perforation, repeat paracentesis 48 hours after initiating antibiotic treatment will usually demonstrate increasing neutrophil counts. *Polymicrobial bacterascites* with an ascitic neutrophil count of >250 cells per µl is diagnostic of inadvertent gut perforation by the paracentesis needle. It is usually treated with broad-spectrum antibiotics that include coverage for anaerobes. Alternatively, the decision to treat may be deferred until the results of a repeat paracentesis are obtained.

Tense Ascites

Some patients develop tense ascites with abdominal discomfort or dyspnea with as little as 2 liters of ascitic fluid, whereas others may accumulate 20 liters or more before becoming tense. Therapy for tense ascites relies on large-volume paracentesis, which may have the added benefit of increasing the venous return to the heart with resultant improvement in cardiac output and stroke volume.

Abdominal Wall Hernias

Umbilical and inguinal hernias are common in patients with ascites. These hernias may produce skin ulceration or rupture (Flood's syndrome), or they may become incarcerated. More than one-half of these patients will need surgery, which is performed after preoperative paracentesis. More aggressive surgery is needed for ulceration, rupture, or incarceration because of the risks of systemic infection. The mortality of rupture is significant (11% to 43%), and it increases in patients with jaundice or coagulopathy.

Hepatic Hydrothorax

Pleural effusions (usually right-sided) are prevalent in cirrhotic ascites. Left-sided effusions are more common with tuberculosis or pancreatic disease. Hepatic hydrothorax is postulated to result from a defect in the diaphragm, which preferentially permits fluid passage into the thorax during the negative pressures generated by normal inspiration. Infection of this fluid is unusual, except in a patient with concurrent SBP. Therapy of hepatic hydrothorax is often challenging because it often does not respond to diuretics. Pleurodesis has been tried, but complications (e.g., leaks) are very common. TIPSs and peritoneovenous shunts have also been used for hepatic hydrothorax.

Meralgia Paresthetica

Large-volume ascites causes pressure-induced injury to the lateral femoral cutaneous nerve, producing paresthesias along the lateral thigh. This condition, termed *meralgia paresthetica*, is treated by reducing the ascitic volume.

CHAPTER 18

Skin Lesions Associated with Gastrointestinal Disease

CUTANEOUS MANIFESTATIONS OF INFLAMMATORY BOWEL DISEASE

Chronic ulcerative colitis and Crohn's disease are associated with numerous immunologically mediated cutaneous disorders (Table 18-1). Generalized erythema may be morbilliform (macules and papules) or scarlatiniform (confluent) and often results from a medication or transfusion reaction. Multiple annular areas of erythema may also be seen with inflammatory bowel disease (IBD). Urticaria is characterized by dermal edema and erythema that resolve within 24 hours. In patients with IBD, urticaria usually results from medications or from causes independent of the underlying gastrointestinal illness. Therapy for urticaria relies on removal of the offending agent and use of antihistamines.

Erythema multiforme is a self-limited mucocutaneous syndrome with target-like skin lesions and serum sickness symptoms (e.g., fever and arthralgias), which may result from IBD or the drugs used in its treatment. The minor form of erythema multiforme is limited to the skin, whereas the major form is more severe, with significant mucosal involvement, a condition known as Stevens-Johnson syndrome. Toxic epidermal necrolysis, which overlaps with Stevens-Johnson syndrome, manifests as a burnlike appearance and usually results from medications. Gastrointestinal complications of toxic epidermal necrolysis include esophagitis and esophageal stricture. Corticosteroids are used for these conditions; ophthalmologic consultation is required for eye involvement.

Erythema nodosum is characterized by tender subcutaneous nodules, usually on the legs; results from immune complex-mediated involvement of subcutaneous fat vessels; and may occur in association with fever, malaise, arthralgias, and arthritis. The incidence of erythema nodosum is 7% with ulcerative colitis but is lower with Crohn's disease. Erythema nodosum generally resolves with control of the underlying disease, although NSAIDs or acetaminophen may be used to reduce systemic symptoms.

TABLE 18-1
Cutaneous Conditions Associated with Inflammatory Bowel Disease

Erythemas (including annular erythemas)
Urticaria
Erythema nodosum
Necrotizing vasculitis
Large vessel necrotizing vasculitis
Pustular vasculitis
Pyoderma gangrenosum
Oral lesions
    Specific granulomas (Crohn's disease only)
    Aphthosis
    Angular cheilitis
    Pyostomatitis vegetans
Metastatic Crohn's disease
Finger clubbing
Acquired acrodermatitis enteropathica (zinc deficiency)
Striae
Epidermolysis bullosa acquisita
Psoriasis
Exfoliative erythroderma
Vitiligo
Lichen planus
Lichen nitidus

Leukocytoclastic vasculitis produces immune complex–mediated endothelial swelling of postcapillary venules with neutrophilic invasion and fibrinoid necrosis. Patients present with palpable purpura. Similar vascular lesions may occur in the central and peripheral nervous system, synovium, pleura, pericardium, gastrointestinal tract, and kidneys. This condition, which is found rarely in ulcerative colitis and Crohn's disease, is managed by controlling the underlying disease. Severe cases may require corticosteroids, immunosuppressives, or plasmapheresis.

Pyoderma gangrenosum appears as a cutaneous ulcer with a purple undermined border that may heal with cribriform scarring or worsen with local trauma. Underlying IBD should be excluded in any patient with pyoderma gangrenosum, although chronic hepatitis, rheumatoid arthritis, and myeloproliferative disorders may produce similar cutaneous findings. Pyoderma gangrenosum is treated aggressively with corticosteroids, immunosuppressives, or sulfones because of the risk of local infection or sepsis.

Thirty percent of patients with ulcerative colitis have oral lesions (e.g., aphthous ulcers or angular stomatitis). Patients with Crohn's disease may have these also, as well as granulomas of the lips and mouth. Patients with numerous oral aphthous ulcers should be evaluated to exclude ulcerative colitis, Crohn's disease, and Behçet's disease. Pyostomatitis vegetans is an oral papular eruption with a cobblestone appearance and is associated with IBD.

Other cutaneous manifestations of IBD include "metastatic" Crohn's disease (i.e., noncaseating cutaneous granulomas), pustular vasculitis, and other skin disorders that relate to specific nutritional deficiencies.

CUTANEOUS MANIFESTATIONS
OF RHEUMATOLOGIC DISEASES

Many rheumatologic diseases—for example, systemic lupus erythematosus and rheumatoid arthritis—have a broad range of cutaneous manifestations. The cutaneous findings in dermatomyositis include periungual telangiectasia, cuticular dystrophy, and violaceous poikiloderma (hypo- or hyperpigmentation, telangiectasia, epidermal atrophy), which may present over the eyes (heliotrope rash), knuckles (Gottron's sign), and extensor surfaces. There may be a photosensitivity component to violaceous poikiloderma. Because dermatomyositis may develop as a paraneoplastic phenomenon, a search for an underlying neoplasm should be performed in adult patients with recent onset of the disease.

Primary amyloidosis manifests as macroglossia as well as cutaneous papules, plaques, and nodules with pinch purpura, whereas patients with secondary amyloidosis do not exhibit visible cutaneous involvement.

Scleroderma may occur in several forms: a localized cutaneous form (morphea); a relatively mild, systemic CREST variant (calcinosis, Raynaud's phenomenon, esophageal dysmotility, sclerodactyly, telangiectasia); or the more severe, progressive systemic sclerosis. Sclerosis occurs acrally and periorally and may affect the trunk. A salt-and-pepper pigment change may be noted over sclerotic areas in darker skinned patients. Telangiectases are boxlike or matlike on the face, hands, oral mucosa, and other sites.

Behçet's disease is defined by the presence of oral aphthous ulcers in the absence of IBD or collagen vascular disease plus two or more of the following symptoms: genital aphthous ulcers, synovitis, posterior uveitis, cutaneous pustular vasculitis, and meningoencephalitis. Aphthous ulcers may occur at any gastrointestinal site with Behçet's disease. The oral lesions of Behçet's are distinguished from the psoriasiform oral lesions of Reiter's disease. Recurrent herpes simplex must be excluded as a cause of the oral and genital lesions. The synovitis produces an asymmetric, migratory, nonerosive oligoarthritis.

Twenty percent of patients who have undergone jejunoileal bypass for morbid obesity develop pustular cutaneous vasculitis, arthritis, and a serum sickness-like illness. Similar syndromes occur with IBD or with creation of a blind loop during ulcer surgery (e.g., Billroth II). The skin lesions appear in crops that last 1 to 2 weeks and occur at intervals from one to several months. The syndrome may resolve with systemic antibiotics (e.g., metronidazole, tetracycline, or erythromycin) or with restoration of normal intestinal anatomy.

SKIN DISEASE AND
GASTROINTESTINAL HEMORRHAGE

Various diseases manifest as skin findings and gastrointestinal hemorrhage. Patients with hereditary hemorrhagic telangiectasia (i.e., Osler-Weber-Rendu disease), which is an autosomal dominant disorder, present with numerous 1- to 3-mm telangiectases on the lips, tongue, face, hands, chest, and feet. Blue rubber bleb nevus syndrome is an autosomal dominant disorder characterized by cutaneous, blue-colored, rubbery, compressible, and sometimes painful nodular vascular malformations up to 10 cm in diameter. Bleeding and intussusception may result from gastrointestinal lesions. Patients with Kaposi's sarcoma, which occurs in acquired immunodeficiency syndrome (AIDS) and in endemic form in elderly individuals of Mediterranean descent, present cutaneously with red-purple macules to large vascular tumors. In older men, the lesions begin on the lower extremities, extending proximally in association with peripheral edema. Gastrointestinal lesions, most commonly of the small intestine, may produce hemorrhage or partial obstruction. The endemic form of Kaposi's sarcoma carries a good prognosis. Malignant atrophic papulosis (Degos' disease) is an idiopathic disorder with discrete, painless papules with umbilicated porcelain-white centers surrounded by telangiectatic rims. Patients who have gastrointestinal involvement with this condition may present with fatal gastrointestinal hemorrhage.

Gastrointestinal bleeding may complicate the course of many connective tissue diseases. Pseudoxanthoma elasticum is a genetic disorder characterized by elastic fiber alterations that produce cutaneous, visceral, ocular, and cardiovascular manifestations. Cutaneous yellow papules and plaques that resemble chicken skin may affect the buccal mucosa as well as the neck, axilla, and other flexures. The characteristic yellow, cobblestone-appearing mucosa may be associated with hemorrhage. Ehlers-Danlos syndrome, a heterogeneous group of genetic disorders with defective collagen production, produces hyperextensible and fragile skin with impaired wound healing, purpura from easy bruising, cigarette paper-thin scars, fishmouth scars, and pseudotumors over joints. Gastrointestinal complications of this condition include hemorrhage and perforation. Cutis laxa, a group of autosomal and X-linked disorders characterized primarily by abnormalities of elastic fibers, gives the appearance that the skin is too large for the patient's body, with areas of sagging and wrinkling. In the gut, diverticula and hernias may develop. Neurofibromatosis (von Recklinghausen's disease) is an autosomal dominant disorder presenting with café au lait macules, axillary freckles, and cutaneous neurofibromas. Gastrointestinal ulceration, bleeding, volvulus, obstruction, perforation, and intussusception may occur.

CUTANEOUS FINDINGS IN GASTROINTESTINAL POLYPOSIS SYNDROMES

Hereditary and sporadic gastrointestinal polyposis syndromes have characteristic cutaneous findings that may suggest or confirm a specific diagnosis. Gardner's syndrome is an autosomal dominant inherited condition related to familial polyposis coli that manifests in adolescence with multiple colorectal polyps; osteomas; and epidermoid cysts of the scalp, face, and extremities. Desmoid tumors are locally aggressive fibrous tumors that may affect the abdominal wall. Peutz-Jeghers syndrome is also an autosomal dominant disease. Patients present in infancy with multiple gastrointestinal hamartomatous polyps and melanotic macules involving the lips, palms, soles, digits, periorbital skin, anus, and buccal mucosa. Cronkhite-Canada syndrome is a sporadic disorder characterized by alopecia, onychodystrophy, intestinal polyps, and hyperpigmented macules that coalesce to form plaques primarily on the upper extremities, occasionally with development of vitiligo. The cutaneous findings in Cowden disease, an autosomal dominant disorder with multiple gastrointestinal hamartomas, include facial and oral mucosal papules (tricholemmomas), oral cobblestoning, acral keratoses, lipomas, hemangiomas, neuromas, and café au lait macules as well as a scrotal appearance to the tongue. Muir-Torre syndrome is an autosomal dominant condition with multiple visceral carcinomas in association with cutaneous sebaceous neoplasms (i.e., hyperplasia, adenoma, epithelioma, carcinoma), basal cell carcinomas, and keratoacanthomas. The association of gastrointestinal polyps with acrochordons (skin tags) is controversial and unproved.

CUTANEOUS SIGNS OF GASTROINTESTINAL MALIGNANCY

When detected on physical examination, certain characteristic skin lesions should raise concern for gastrointestinal malignancy. Extramammary Paget's disease exhibits an erythematous scaling or lichenified patch with surface erosion and crusting and is considered to represent a cutaneous adenocarcinoma. Its development in a perianal site is associated with gastrointestinal malignancy (usually rectal or cloacogenic carcinoma) in at least 25% of cases. Therapy includes surgery or radiation therapy. Acanthosis nigricans is a condition characterized by smooth, thickened, hyperpigmented skin in body fold areas (e.g., the axilla, neck, palms, soles, and oral regions) that occurs in association with gastric adenocarcinoma as well as other tumors. Acanthosis nigricans may precede the diagnosable tumor by several years or may signal the development of metastatic disease in patients with known malignancy; remission of the skin disease parallels cure of the underlying neoplasm. Tylosis, keratoderma of the palms and soles, presents with diffuse or punctate yellow keratosis of the palmar or plantar surfaces in patients with gastrointestinal malignancy, especially esophageal squamous cell carcinoma. The Howel-Evans syndrome is an autosomal disorder in which 95% of those affected develop esophageal carcinoma and tylosis by 65 years of age. Generalized erythroderma is observed in some patients with gastrointestinal lymphoma, esophageal, or occult carcinoma. Hypertrichosis lanuginosa acquisita refers to the sudden appearance of fine, downy hair in association with gastrointestinal malignancy, including the involvement of the gallbladder and pancreas. Patients with Plummer-Vinson (Paterson-Kelly) syndrome present with koilonychia (brittle, spoon-shaped nails), atrophic tongue, and angular stomatitis in association with iron deficiency anemia and postcricoid esophageal carcinoma.

Endocrine neoplasms may produce characteristic dermatologic findings, including flushing with carcinoid syndrome and necrolytic migratory erythema in glucagonoma syndrome, which usually affects perioral, lower abdominal, and perineal sites with erythema, erosions, superficial necrosis, and scaling.

The skin examination also can provide evidence of a direct extension of malignancy and metastatic disease. Skin metastases from gastrointestinal malignancy are firm, pink, dermal to subcutaneous masses in the abdomen or pelvis. The Sister Mary Joseph nodule is an indurated nodule of the umbilicus and is found in some patients with malignancy, especially gastric or colonic adenocarcinoma. Rarely, extensive dermal infiltration may result from tumor involvement of lymphatics in the abdomen or thigh.

BULLOUS SKIN DISEASES THAT AFFECT THE GASTROINTESTINAL TRACT

Bullous skin diseases may produce characteristic lesions of the gastrointestinal tract. *Epidermolysis bullosa* refers to a spectrum of diseases, both dominant and recessive, in which blisters occur spontaneously, often at sites of friction soon after birth. Rarely, pyloric atresia is the presenting manifestation in infants, apparently the results of mucosal blistering and scarring in utero. The major gastrointestinal sites of involvement are the mouth, esophagus, and anus. Esophageal lesions present with dysphagia, often caused by bullae or weblike scarring near the cricopharyngeal area. Anal involvement may produce constipation. Epidermolysis bullosa acquisita is a late-onset disorder occurring in association with IBD.

Pemphigus vulgaris manifests oral erosions and cutaneous lesions that are characterized by acantholytic blistering and the presence of IgG in the intraepidermal space on biopsy. Symptomatic esophageal involvement is unusual, but lower gastrointestinal involvement may produce hemorrhage.

Bullous pemphigoid occurs in older patients and exhibits tense cutaneous bullae, with oral involvement in one-third of cases and less often in the esophagus or anus. Bullous pemphigoid has been associated with gastrointestinal malignancy, especially colonic carcinoma. Skin biopsy specimens show subepidermal blistering with linear IgG deposition in the basement membrane zone.

SKIN CONDITIONS ASSOCIATED WITH ABDOMINAL PAIN

Several disorders with prominent abdominal pain have associated cutaneous findings. Patients with variegate porphyria, the most common porphyria with pain and skin lesions, present with uninflamed blisters and erosions in sun-exposed sites, which may progress to milia formation, hyperpigmentation, facial hypertrichosis, and sclerosis. The skin findings in the lysosomal storage condition, Fabry's disease, are punctate, small (1 mm), nonblanching, red-blue angiokeratomas appearing in the region of the midabdomen to the knees. Reduced sweat production may occur with this disease. Mastocytosis is a disorder of mast cell proliferation with red-brown macules (urticaria pigmentosa) that are pruritic and develop a wheal or vesicle when stroked (Darier's sign). Angioedema, characterized by edema in a deep dermal or subcutaneous location, may present as part of a hereditary or acquired C1 esterase deficiency syndrome or after ingestion of certain medications. The condition may result in gastrointestinal mucosal edema and abdominal pain. Varicella zoster reactivation in the T7 through L1 dermatomes may produce abdominal pain in association with clustered vesicles.

Pancreatic disease can produce characteristic cutaneous findings. Periumbilical purpura (Cullen's sign) and left flank purpura (Grey-Turner's sign) result from retroperitoneal dissection of blood along fascial planes from acute hemorrhagic pancreatitis. Panniculitis caused by pancreatitis exhibits tender, red, subcutaneous nodules, occurring most commonly on the lower extremities. Fluctuant areas of fat necrosis may be part of the initial presentation in patients with pancreatitis and pancreatic carcinoma. The eruption of yellow-red papules over extensor surfaces and the buttocks in a patient with pancreatitis suggests eruptive xanthomatosis secondary to hypertriglyceridemia or type IV or V hyperlipoproteinemia.

SKIN CONDITIONS ASSOCIATED WITH MALNUTRITION AND MALABSORPTION

There is considerable overlap in the cutaneous manifestations of the specific nutrient deficiency syndromes. Marasmus (total starvation) is characterized by dry, loose skin, prominent facial lanugo hair, hyperkeratosis around hair follicles, and an absence of edema. In kwashiorkor (carbohydrate excess with protein deficiency), there are hypo- or hyperpigmented scaling patches and purpura with epidermal peeling over edematous sites, joints, or flexural areas (flaky paint sign). Hair pigment may show alternating dark and light bands (flag sign). Cutaneous lesions in essential fatty acid deficiency, especially linoleic acid, include diffuse, erythematous scales with alopecia and traumatic purpura.

Vitamin and mineral deficiencies produce characteristic syndromes. Patients with vitamin A deficiency present with multiple keratotic papules on the extremities (phrynoderma) with mucosal keratinizing metaplasia. Conversely, vitamin A excess causes alopecia, a sunburn appearance, cheilosis, skin fragility, and brittle nails. Deficiencies of the B vitamins (riboflavin, pyridoxine, niacin) produce seborrheic dermatitis of the face and a smooth tongue. With niacin deficiency (pellagra), painful, erosive, pigmented scaling patches may occur in sun-exposed sites. Occurrence on the upper chest is known as a *Casal's necklace*. Cutaneous manifestations of vitamin B_{12} deficiency include generalized hyperpigmentation of the palms, soles, and nails, whereas white hair, alopecia areata, or vitiligo may occur in pernicious anemia. Folate deficiency may cause a lemon-yellow skin discoloration. Purpura, petechiae, perifollicular hemorrhages, corkscrew hairs, and gingival erosions are prominent features of vitamin C deficiency. Zinc deficiency (acrodermatitis enteropathica) produces erythematous, scaling, vesiculopustular or eroded, acrally distributed plaques, with associated alopecia, impaired wound healing, and stomatitis.

Certain malabsorptive conditions manifest characteristic skin diseases—for example, dermatitis herpetiformis with celiac sprue. Dermatitis herpetiformis is characterized by intense pruritus and multiple, grouped vesicles distributed symmetrically, especially on the scalp and extensor surfaces. Skin biopsy specimens show subepidermal blistering with neutrophilic infiltration of the dermal papillae and IgA deposition at the dermal-epidermal junction or within the dermal papillae. Even if gastrointestinal symptoms are not present, nearly all patients with dermatitis herpetiformis have some degree of villous atrophy of the small intestine and inflammatory infiltration secondary to gluten sensitivity. The skin disease may be treated with dietary gluten restriction or, if necessary, with dapsone or sulfapyridine.

PERINEAL SKIN LESIONS

Physical examination may reveal distinct cutaneous findings in the perianal or perineal areas (Table 18-2). Vesicles or erosions on an erythematous base suggest possible herpes simplex, whereas varicella zoster produces dermatomal clustering of vesicles. Perianal erosions and ulcers also occur in Crohn's disease, amebiasis, primary and secondary syphilis, or in nontreponemal venereal disease. Flesh-colored, pedunculated papules may be condyloma acuminata (venereal warts). Erythema with scaling or maceration in the gluteal fold raises concern for candidal infection, psoriasis, seborrheic dermatitis, contact dermatitis from fecal soiling, or bacterial impetigo. These lesions should be scraped and treated accordingly; biopsy is indicated to exclude extramammary Paget's disease for lesions that do not respond to treatment. Idiopathic pruritus ani presents commonly in middle-aged men with superimposed psychological factors and responds to removal of any triggering factors, careful cleaning techniques, topical or locally injected corticosteroids, or cryosurgery.

TABLE 18-2
Perineal Skin Lesions

Erythema with scale or maceration
    Contact dermatitis
    Seborrheic dermatitis
    Psoriasis
    Candidiasis
    Dermatophytosis
    Secondary syphilis
    Extramammary Paget's disease
    Nutritional deficiencies
    Bowen's disease
Vesicles, erosions, ulcers
    Herpes simplex
    Varicella zoster
    Impetigo (streptococcal, staphylococcal)
    Syphilis (primary or secondary)
    Chancroid
    Deep fungal, acid-fast bacilli, protozoal
    Bullous pemphigoid
    Pemphigus
    Ecthyma
Nodules, tumors, ulceration
    Condyloma acuminata
    Hidradenitis suppurativa
    Squamous or basal cell carcinoma
    Crohn's disease
    Carcinoma
    Kaposi's sarcoma
    Granulomatous herpes simplex

CHAPTER 19

Approach to Gastrointestinal Problems in the Elderly

ALTERATIONS IN PHYSIOLOGY AND PHARMACOLOGY IN ELDERLY PATIENTS

In elderly patients, age-related physiologic events must be distinguished from problems that result from disease. A common mistake is to ascribe a constellation of symptoms and signs to the aging process when a correctable condition is present. A number of pathologic disorders primarily affect older individuals and should be given more serious consideration than in younger patients. Vascular diseases (e.g., mesenteric ischemia) affect older persons who have well-documented atherosclerosis. Atrophic gastritis and its consequences rarely appear in young persons. Aging leads to a decline in helper and killer T-cell function, with little deterioration in B-cell, plasma cell, or antigen-presenting cell function, indicative of selected defects in immune responses in the elderly. Intraepithelial lymphocytes are reduced in advanced age, impairing gut-associated immunity.

Changes in drug pharmacodynamics and pharmacokinetics occur with aging. Benzodiazepines have greater pharmacodynamic effects in elderly persons, whereas α-adrenoceptor agonists and antagonists are less effective. Distribution and clearance of drugs may be altered by changes in body weight and composition. Fat represents approximately 40% of total body weight in an elderly patient, compared with 25% in a young patient, thereby changing the distribution of lipid- and water-soluble medications. Renal creatinine clearance falls progressively after age 60 years, reaching at age 80 years levels one-third those of a young person. Hepatic blood flow also is reduced with age. Therefore, drugs that are cleared by the kidney or liver may exhibit delayed excretion in an older patient. More drug side effects may occur in patients whose bodies have undergone age-related changes in physiology. For example, corticosteroids may produce dangerous bone demineralization in an elderly patient with osteoporosis, or they may accelerate cataract development.

Clinical disorders may differ in the elderly for several reasons. Presenting symptoms and signs may be altered because of central nervous system disease, depression, or a fear of complex medical care. Acute abdominal pain in some conditions (e.g., appendicitis) is muted by age, providing inappropriate reassurance to the clinician that the patient does not have a serious problem. Chemical peritonitis from ulcer perforation may be absent if the patient is achlorhydric. The differential diagnosis of acute pain is different in the elderly, with an increased incidence of cholecystitis and malignancy. Pain localization may be atypical in persons older than 60 years. Laboratory data should not be considered differently in an older patient than in a younger person, as most test results do not change as a result of aging. Diagnostic endoscopic or radiographic studies should not be avoided in the elderly. These procedures usually are well tolerated unless there is severe cardiorespiratory disease, although the sedative requirements may be reduced. The site of gastrointestinal hemorrhage does not differ greatly with age and should be managed aggressively in elderly patients. Abdominal surgery should not be avoided merely on the basis of age; it is now recognized that surgical risk more closely correlates with associated diseases than with the age of the patient.

DISORDERS OF SWALLOWING AND FOOD INGESTION

Differential Diagnosis

Disorders of swallowing and food intake are prevalent in the elderly and result from anorexia, forgetfulness, depression, physical inability to prepare food or to eat, dental problems, ill-fitting dentures, diseases that impair bolus transfer to the esophagus, and diseases of esophageal transfer. The muscles of the mouth and pharynx may weaken, altering mastication. Pharyngeal muscle dyscoordination may result from neuromuscular diseases (e.g., Parkinson's disease, cerebrovascular accidents, polymyositis, dermatomyositis, myasthenia gravis). Altered pharyngeal sensation and proprioception can change taste acuity and altered discrimination of bolus size and consistency. Lip closure may be impaired with advanced age. The cumulative effects of these age-related changes are slowed tongue function, food spills, prolonged swallowing, and drooling. Although the number and sensitivity of taste buds decrease with age, taste disturbances most commonly result from medication effects, inadequate oral hygiene, or denture problems. Certain pharyngeal disorders (e.g., Zenker's diverticulum and cricopharyngeal achalasia) occur primarily in elderly individuals.

A number of physiologic changes in esophageal function occur in the elderly population. Dyssynchrony of deglutition and respiration occurs, the duration of swallowing is prolonged, the upper esophageal sphincter pressure is less, and upper esophageal sphincter relaxation is altered. Radiographically demonstrated corkscrew esophagus or presbyesophagus and manometrically documented tertiary contractions are more prevalent in the elderly but have little or no pathophysiologic consequence. The resting lower esophageal sphincter pressure has not been convincingly shown to decrease with age; however, acid reflux episodes are more frequent. True disorders of esophageal motility usually occur in the setting of other systemic disorders (e.g., diabetes and rheumatologic disease), although studies using crude technetium-99m–labeled fluid test meals have shown delays in esophageal transit in older persons. Esophageal disorders in the elderly to which the clinician should give special consideration include pill-induced esophagitis, achalasia, and esophageal carcinoma. Older patients who take medications at bedtime are at risk of pill-induced esophageal injury because salivation and swallowing are reduced during sleep (Table 19-1). Secondary achalasia must be more carefully considered in older patients than in younger persons.

TABLE 19-1
Medications Associated with Esophageal Injury

Doxycycline hydrate
Tetracycline hydrochloride
Clindamycin
Emepronium bromide
Potassium chloride
Ferrous sulfate or succinate
Alprenolol hydrochloride
Quinidine
Aspirin
Sustained release theophylline
Alendronate

Principles of Management

The examination and treatment of an elderly patient with a swallowing dysfunction are not significantly different from the treatment of a younger patient. Barium
swallow and upper gastrointestinal radiography are used to exclude esophageal and
gastric structural lesions. Upper endoscopy can diagnose neoplasms, esophagitis,
pill-induced injury, and ulcer disease. Manometry may demonstrate esophageal
dysmotility, whereas 24-hour pH testing may document gastroesophageal reflux
disease. Drug therapy is similar for elderly and young patients, but there may be a
greater need for instruction in swallowing techniques from a qualified speech
pathologist or other therapist for the patient with oropharyngeal dyscoordination.

PEPTIC DISEASE AND GASTRIC DISORDERS

Differential Diagnosis

The incidence of peptic ulcer disease is greater in the elderly than in the young
because of the increased use of NSAIDs, smoking, poor nutrition, and other factors.
Gastric acid secretion does not decrease in the majority of older persons; only 25% to
30% show acid hyposecretion. Duodenal bicarbonate secretion may fall in the elderly,
whereas gastric emptying, intrinsic factor secretion, and other physiologic functions
of the stomach usually do not change with age. Gastric ulcers manifest in a more
proximal location in older patients, often near the cardia. Intrathoracic ulcers located
within hiatal hernias may produce atypical chest pain. Giant gastric ulcers (>2.5 cm
in diameter) occur more frequently in the elderly and may be difficult to distinguish
from malignancy. Infection with *Helicobacter pylori* is more prevalent in the elderly
and is probably responsible, in part, for the increased incidence of ulcer disease and
gastric malignancies in these patients.

Hypochlorhydria, caused by chronic atrophic gastritis, is a disorder of the
elderly. Gastric polyps develop with atrophic gastritis, but the long-term risk of gastric cancer development is increased only three- to fourfold. Gastric hypochlorhydria increases the proximal duodenal pH, predisposing the patient to infection with
Salmonella species, *Vibrio cholera*, *Giardia* species, and perhaps *Clostridium diffi-*

cile, and also increasing the risk of bacterial overgrowth in the small intestine. Hypochlorhydria may also cause malabsorption of iron, calcium, and vitamin B_{12}.

Principles of Management

The symptoms of ulcer disease are more variable and subtle in older patients, often only reported as anorexia and vague discomfort that does not radiate. Substernal chest pain may mimic angina. One-third of patients report no pain at all. Complications from ulcer hemorrhage are common in older patients, including more frequent rebleeding after initial control of hemorrhage, more severe hypotension as a result of blood loss, and significant cardiorespiratory compromise with fluid resuscitation. The mortality rate for ulcer perforation is high in the elderly.

Examination of an older patient with suspected ulcer disease must be thorough and aggressive, with early upper endoscopy. If an uncomplicated ulcer is found, appropriate management with acid-suppressive drugs (i.e., histamine H_2-receptor antagonists or proton-pump inhibitors) is initiated. There is no evidence that standard doses of these drugs have significant age-related side effects. Prolonged use of the proton-pump inhibitor omeprazole may impair iron and vitamin B_{12} absorption. Drug-drug interactions, especially with medications such as theophylline and warfarin, may occur, and monitoring of blood levels may need to be intensified. If *H pylori* infection is found, it should be treated; if NSAIDs are causative, they should be withdrawn if possible. If NSAIDs are not restarted, maintenance acid-suppressive therapy is not required. If continued NSAID use is necessary, full-dose H_2-receptor antagonist or proton-pump inhibitor therapy may have efficacy, especially for patients with duodenal lesions. Misoprostol, the prostaglandin E_1 analog, may provide protection against NSAID-induced ulcer disease and may have some role in treating acute ulcer disease as well, although a frequent dosing schedule and side effects (e.g., diarrhea and abdominal pain) may limit its use.

If surgery is required, its performance on an elective basis is indicated whenever possible because of the hazards of emergency surgery in the elderly. Surgical mortality and morbidity are directly related to the number and severity of other diseases present in an older patient. Long-term postgastrectomy problems (e.g., diarrhea) are difficult to manage in the elderly.

In general, a patient with hypochlorhydria needs no special intervention, although complications such as nutrient malabsorption and bacterial overgrowth may be dealt with specifically. The role of endoscopic surveillance of an elderly patient with hypochlorhydria or pernicious anemia is controversial. For most older patients, follow-up endoscopic biopsies to exclude the new development of dysplasia need not be performed more frequently than every 5 years, if at all.

MALABSORPTION DISORDERS

Differential Diagnosis

In general, intestinal absorption and proximal intestinal epithelial histology do not change with advanced age. Fecal fat excretion is not increased in the elderly, nor is xylose absorption altered. Pancreatic size diminishes in some older patients; this has little functional consequence, with no alterations in pancreatic enzyme output compared with that of younger persons. Calcium absorption falls in some elderly patients because of reduced renal production of 1,25-dihydroxycholecalciferol, lowered serum concentrations, or impaired intestinal responsiveness to 1,25-dihydroxycholecalciferol. Age-related lactase deficiency may lead to reduced milk intake and to lower total body calcium. Malabsorption of nutrients may occur with gastric hypochlorhydria, as detailed above.

Among elderly patients with malabsorption who are referred to a specialist, 44% have pancreatic disease and 25% have celiac sprue. Other causes of malabsorption prevalent in nursing home populations include multiple intestinal diverticula, post-gastrectomy syndromes, and bacterial overgrowth secondary to intestinal strictures or dysmotility. The true prevalence of pancreatic insufficiency in older individuals is unknown because of the extensive exocrine reserve of the normal pancreas. However, a specific idiopathic syndrome of elderly women is characterized by mild pain, hypergammaglobulinemia, weight loss, pancreatic calcifications, and fever. Up to one-third of patients with newly diagnosed celiac sprue are older than age 60 years. These patients may present with vague dyspepsia and malaise rather than with diarrhea and weight loss. Complications of celiac sprue (e.g., osteomalacia, hypoprothrombinemia, ulcerations, intestinal pseudo-obstruction, and lymphoma) are more common in the elderly. Mesenteric vascular disease rarely produces malabsorption with pain in older patients. The prevalence of covert ethanol abuse is high in elderly populations; therefore, the effects of alcohol on mucosal function of the small intestine must be considered. Bacterial overgrowth may result from strictures (e.g., Crohn's disease, radiation therapy, postoperative, malignancy) and diverticula of the small intestine, intestinal pseudo-obstruction, or coloenteric fistulae. Gastric achlorhydria and reduced intestinal lysozyme and IgA production may also contribute to development of bacterial overgrowth in the small intestine.

Principles of Management

The examination of an elderly patient with suspected malabsorption is based on known risk factors. Prior surgery or established Crohn's disease should suggest possible bacterial overgrowth from intestinal strictures or the presence of fistulae. A long history of ethanol abuse raises the possibility of chronic pancreatitis or absorptive dysfunction in the small intestine. If there is no obvious cause, screening laboratory studies and radiographic evaluation may detect anemia, mineral and vitamin deficiencies, and pancreatic calcifications. Further evaluation with breath testing and barium radiography and small bowel biopsy may detect intestinal causes of malabsorption. Conversely, structural and functional testing of the pancreas may detect pancreatic exocrine dysfunction. Therapy should be based on a defined pathologic state but should also include appropriate replacement of minerals and vitamins as needed.

CONSTIPATION

Differential Diagnosis

Constipation is often described by elderly persons as painful, difficult, or incomplete stool evacuation rather than infrequent defecation. The problem of constipation is especially prevalent in older, less mobile patients in nursing homes or other chronic care facilities. Although colonic transit usually is normal, delayed rectal evacuation is found in elderly patients with constipation because of reduced rectal wall elasticity, decreased sensitivity to rectal wall distention, and abnormalities in colonic ganglia cells.

TABLE 19-2
Constipation in the Elderly: Causes and Contributing Factors

Obstruction (e.g., malignancy)
Neuromuscular disease (e.g., parkinsonism, laxative colon)
Endocrine disease (e.g., hypothyroidism, hyperparathyroidism, diabetes)
Psychiatric disease (e.g., depression)
Dietary alterations (e.g., decreased food or fluid intake, inadequate bulk in diet)
Decreased defecatory sensation
Medications (e.g., laxative abuse, sedatives, tranquilizers, antihypertensives, ganglionic
  blockers, opiates, calcium-containing antacids)

Several specific causes of constipation and predisposing factors should be considered in the examination of a constipated older person (Table 19-2). Megacolon is caused by long-standing fecal retention and predominates in patients who are institutionalized, who are taking psychotropic medications, and who have Parkinson's disease or organic mental syndromes. Acute pseudo-obstruction may also occur in patients with electrolyte disturbances, infection, or hemodynamic instability. Endocrine disorders (e.g., hypothyroidism) should be considered in patients with appropriate clinical manifestations. Medications such as antihypertensives, antidepressants, antispasmodics, or narcotics should be considered. Volvulus of the cecum or sigmoid colon is most prevalent in elderly individuals, especially in institutionalized patients who have underlying mental syndromes. Structural obstruction from malignancy is the most worrisome cause of constipation in elderly patients and should be excluded if surgical intervention is feasible.

Principles of Management

An elderly patient with new-onset constipation should be carefully examined to exclude systemic disorders and colonic obstruction. If indicated, serum calcium and thyroid stimulating hormone levels can be used to screen for hyperparathyroidism and hypothyroidism. Colonoscopy or flexible sigmoidoscopy plus contrast radiography are helpful in excluding obstructing colonic malignancy or occlusion secondary to postoperative strictures or Crohn's disease. Therapy should begin by increasing fiber intake along with fluid supplementation. Osmotic agents such as laxatives that contain magnesium or poorly absorbable sugars (e.g., lactulose, sorbitol) may be slowly introduced with observation for increased bloating. If simple measures are ineffective, pelvic floor testing with retraining of rectosphincteric dyssynergia should be considered.

DIARRHEA

Differential Diagnosis

In contrast to constipation, diarrhea is not a common gastrointestinal problem in the elderly. New-onset diarrhea may result from medication side effects, as a paradoxical response to fecal impaction, abuse of laxatives, diabetic neuropathy, and rarely, as a result of infection with *Escherichia coli*, *C difficile*, *Campylobacter jejuni*, or other organisms. Fecal incontinence, a common complaint of older patients, is frequently misreported as diarrhea. Causes of incontinence include rectal prolapse, obstetrical trauma in the remote past, fecal impaction, neuropathy, prior surgery, and radiation therapy.

Inflammatory bowel disease (IBD) is more common in elderly patients than generally is recognized. Two-thirds of older patients with Crohn's disease are women who show predominantly colonic involvement, often in a left-sided distribution similar to that found in diverticular disease. Ulcerative colitis restricted to the rectum and sigmoid colon occurs more commonly in older patients. Surgery is necessary less often in elderly than in young patients, and disease recurrences are less frequent. Extraintestinal complications of IBD occur less frequently in the elderly. The mortality rate of IBD in the elderly is two to three times that of younger persons. Specifically, mortality from the first attack of IBD is significantly higher in the elderly primarily because of delays in diagnosis resulting in the need to perform risky emergency surgery. Other conditions may produce clinical presentations similar to IBD, including colonic ischemia, postradiation colitis, and diverticulitis.

Principles of Management

The management of diarrhea in the elderly depends on its cause. Offending medications should be withdrawn. Relief of fecal impaction may provide improvement in some patients. Stool samples should be obtained for *C difficile* toxin assay if there is a history of recent antibiotic use. In a patient with suspected infection, stool samples for culture and for examination for ova and parasites are obtained as indicated. In a patient with unexplained diarrhea, evaluation for surreptitious laxative abuse should be performed.

For elderly patients with fecal incontinence, treatment must be individualized. Patients with rectal prolapse or fecal impaction may respond best to treatment of underlying constipation. Rare patients may respond to surgical reconstruction of the anorectal angle. Anal repair surgery usually has limited success in patients with anal sphincter dysfunction. Conversely, biofeedback retraining of the external anal sphincter may be successful in some elderly patients, although bed-bound patients are unlikely to benefit from this technique.

A patient with suspected IBD should undergo evaluation to exclude conditions that produce similar symptoms. Abdominal radiography may show thumbprinting with mesenteric ischemia, whereas barium enema radiography may demonstrate segmental involvement with ulceration or stricture formation. Flexible sigmoidoscopy or colonoscopy may show similar endoscopic appearances in ulcerative colitis, Crohn's disease, ischemia, and radiation colitis. Biopsy specimens may help in distinguishing the conditions, but often the diagnosis is clinical, depending on the presence of other concurrent diseases and the distribution of colitis. Endoscopy is relatively contraindicated in a patient with suspected megacolon. Angiography may play a role in some patients, but those with colonic ischemia caused by a low-flow state may have normal mesenteric vessels. Diverticulitis may mimic the presentation of Crohn's disease. Fecal blood and perianal disease are more consistent with Crohn's disease. Computed tomography may show sigmoid thickening and fluid collection with both conditions. Although barium radiography and endoscopy are usually discouraged in suspected diverticulitis, gentle flexible sigmoidoscopy without air insufflation may demonstrate proctitis with IBD.

The medical treatment of IBD in elderly patients should be approached with care. Response to treatment may be less complete than in younger individuals. Opiates and anticholinergics should be used only sparingly because of sedating side effects, cardiac complications, and the potential for inducing megacolon. In general, sulfasalazine and 5-aminosalicylates, as well as immunosuppressives, such as azathioprine and 6-mercaptopurine, are well tolerated. Metronidazole can prolong prothrombin times in patients taking warfarin. Osteopenia, hyperglycemia, cataracts, glaucoma, and behavioral changes induced by corticosteroids are increased in elderly populations. In an elderly IBD patient, corticosteroids should be withdrawn as quickly as possible, with early institution of long-term immunosuppressive therapy if needed. For older patients who require surgery for ulcerative colitis, construction of an ileal pouch–anal canal anastomosis may not be practical because of increased defecation frequency and problems with fecal incontinence. For these individuals, placement of a Brooke ileostomy may provide superior overall bowel function.

HEPATOBILIARY DISORDERS

Differential Diagnosis

Liver structure and function change little with age, and liver chemistry abnormalities strictly referable to advanced age are not reported. Elevations in alkaline phosphatase levels occur in 27% of elderly patients; these are caused by bone disease in 50% and liver disease in 25%. Unsuspected hyperbilirubinemia usually indicates congestive heart failure, whereas transaminase elevations suggest hepatocellular injury. Hepatitis in elderly patients may be milder, but often produces more severe complications. Drug-induced hepatotoxicity should be considered in elderly patients with new liver chemistry abnormalities.

The prevalence of gallstones increases with age, reaching 35% by age 80 years. Juxtapapillary duodenal diverticula are most common in elderly patients and are associated with gallstones in 65% to 85% of patients. Postcholecystectomy bile duct stones may occur. The common clinical presentations of this disorder include biliary colic, cholecystitis, cholangitis, and pancreatitis. Cholecystitis may present as a vague discomfort or altered mental status, whereas cholangitis may produce hypotension. Gallbladder empyema has a high mortality but also may produce only mild symptoms. Gallstone pancreatitis is potentially fatal. The clinical scoring systems to predict disease severity are less accurate in patients older than 75 years, and computed tomographic (CT) scans may provide better prognostic information. Acalculous cholecystitis is difficult to diagnose and carries a high mortality rate. Obstructive jaundice from choledocholithiasis is common in the elderly and may mimic the presentation of pancreatic carcinoma.

Principles of Management

The management of an elderly patient with suspected hepatic disease differs little from that for younger patients. Isolated alkaline phosphatase elevations should be evaluated for bony or hepatic causes. Potentially hepatotoxic drugs should be withdrawn if possible. Infectious, immune, or heritable causes of liver dysfunction should be evaluated with specific tests if clinically suspected. Liver biopsy should be considered if the information obtained will modify therapy for the older patient.

Elderly patients with suspected biliary disease should be aggressively managed because of the potentially high morbidity and mortality. If infection is suspected, blood samples should be obtained for culture, and antibiotics should be instituted early in the course of infection. Ultrasound may detect bile duct dilation, pericholecystic fluid, or gallbladder wall thickening. Demonstration of gallstones is of limited value, as asymptomatic gallstones are prevalent in older patients. CT may also define infection or pancreatitis. The diagnosis of bile duct disease in the elderly is best made with endoscopic retrograde cholangiopancreatography (ERCP), which also offers the capabilities of sphincterotomy and stone extraction in patients with gallstone pancreatitis, cholangitis, or obstructive jaundice. In an unstable patient with symptomatic common bile duct and gallbladder stones, ERCP with sphincterotomy represents a safe alternative to cholecystectomy in the prevention of further serious complications. Percutaneous transhepatic cholangiography provides an alternative approach to the biliary tree. When possible, elective cholecystectomy by the laparoscopic approach should be performed because of the 10% to 20% mortality of emergency biliary surgery. Asymptomatic gallstones do not warrant surgical intervention. Patients who do not respond to endoscopic or radiologic approaches and who are not surgical candidates may be treated with lithotripsy or direct gallbladder instillation of methyl-ter-butyl ether for gallstone dissolution.

CHAPTER 20

Approach to the Female Patient with Gastrointestinal Disease

GASTROINTESTINAL DISEASES AND PREGNANCY

Alterations in Physiology and Pharmacology in Normal Pregnancy

Profound physiologic changes occur during pregnancy, many of which are advantageous for the mother and fetus. The increases in blood volume and red cell mass in pregnancy facilitate oxygen delivery to the fetus and protect the mother from excess blood loss during delivery. Many of the pregnancy-related changes stem from hormonal and anatomic factors. Hydronephrosis and hydroureter result from the relaxant effects of progesterone on the ureters and from partial obstruction at the pelvic brim by the enlarging uterus. Levels of human chorionic gonadotropin (hCG), which is derived initially from the trophoblast, then later from the placenta, peak in the first trimester and appear to maintain the corpus luteum until the placenta produces sufficient progesterone. hCG also regulates fetal and placental steroid production and has immune-modulating and thyroid-stimulating effects. Although peak levels of serum hCG correlate temporally with the nausea of pregnancy, direct evidence supporting a pathogenic role for the hormone is lacking. Progesterone, which is synthesized initially by the ovary and then by the placenta, maintains the myometrium in a relaxed state, has inhibitory effects on contractile function in other smooth muscle structures, and modulates immune maintenance of fetal tissue. Estrogens (e.g., estradiol, estrone, estriol), which are synthesized by the placenta, increase uteroplacental blood flow and may have weak relaxant effects on smooth muscle. Levels of progesterone and estrogens increase with advancing gestation.

Pregnancy induces changes in the absorption, distribution, and elimination of drugs. Slowed gastric emptying delays peak drug levels, whereas prolonged intestinal transit increases drug absorption or metabolism. Decreased acid secretion may alter drug solubility. Increases in the maternal and fetal plasma volumes increase the volume of drug distribution, whereas the decrease in albumin increases unbound plasma drug levels. A 50% increase in glomerular filtration rate accelerates drug elimination.

Placental and fetal factors determine the effect of medications on the developing fetus. Drugs enter the fetal circulation by diffusion and by facilitated or active transport. The placenta contains enzymes for drug oxidation, reduction, hydrolysis, and conjugation. Fetal albumin levels initially are very low, causing blood levels of drugs that are normally bound to albumin to be high. Serum albumin rises progressively with increasing gestation. Drugs are responsible for 1% to 5% of fetal malformations, usually through unknown mechanisms. Major malformations occur in the first trimester during the period of critical organogenesis, whereas exposure to teratogens in the second and third trimesters produces growth and mental retardation.

Nausea and Vomiting and Hyperemesis Gravidarum

Pathophysiology

Nausea and vomiting occur in 50% to 90% of pregnancies, usually in the first trimester, but do not have deleterious effects on pregnancy outcome, birth weight, or the number of congenital malformations. Intractable vomiting, which produces dehydration, electrolyte disturbances, and nutritional deficiencies, is termed *hyperemesis gravidarum*. It is a complication of 3.5 of every 1000 deliveries. In general, hyperemesis gravidarum has few adverse effects on pregnancy, although increases in fetal central nervous system and skeletal abnormalities have been reported, and the condition may be a risk factor for future testicular cancer in male children.

Estrogen and progesterone have been proposed as mediators of nausea in the first trimester of pregnancy because of the strong correlation between nausea and oral contraceptive use. Also, nausea of pregnancy occurs more often in nulliparous, nonsmoking, and obese women, all of whom exhibit high circulating estrogen levels. The nausea of pregnancy is associated with rhythm disturbances of gastric electrical activity, effects mimicked by exogenous estrogen and progesterone in nonpregnant women, raising the possibility that gastric pacemaker disruption induces symptoms. However, the hormone that exhibits the greatest temporal association with the nausea of pregnancy is hCG, although the pathogenic role of this mediator is unproved. Serum levels of thyroxine increase during the first trimester, probably because of the thyroid-stimulating effects of hCG. However, the role of thyroxine in producing nausea is unknown.

Principles of Management

Nausea and vomiting typically begin in the sixth week of gestation and subside in the second trimester, although 60% of patients with hyperemesis gravidarum may experience symptoms beyond 20 weeks. Management of mild nausea in pregnancy involves ingestion of multiple small meals and avoidance of situations known to aggravate symptoms; medications are rarely necessary. With a failure to gain weight or symptom onset in the second or third trimester, the clinician should consider hyperemesis gravidarum, pre-eclampsia, urinary infection, appendicitis, and intrahepatic cholestasis. In addition to fluid, electrolyte, and nutrient deficits, hyperemesis gravidarum may produce Mallory-Weiss tears, pulmonary aspiration, retinal hemorrhage, and neurologic abnormalities. Hospitalization for fluid and electrolyte replacement often is necessary for hyperemesis gravidarum. Intravenous hyperalimentation is used in extreme cases. Phenothiazines and anti-histamines are used with some success, although their safety in pregnancy has not been confirmed.

Gastroesophageal Reflux Disease

Pathophysiology

Decreases in lower esophageal sphincter (LES) pressure and mechanical effects of the gravid uterus have been proposed as contributing to gastroesophageal reflux in pregnancy. In late pregnancy, LES pressure is reduced in patients with heartburn. However, even in early pregnancy, LES responses to contractile agents are blunted, which indicates impairment of LES competence before symptoms develop. The LES pressure response is probably mediated by circulating hormones, as both estrogen and progesterone relax LES smooth muscle. Theories about mechanical factors are based on the positive correlation between reflux symptoms and the size of the gravid uterus. The effects of pregnancy on other mechanisms of gastro-esophageal reflux (e.g., transient LES relaxations) are unknown.

Principles of Management

A compatible history given by a pregnant patient usually is sufficient to diagnose gastroesophageal reflux, and further diagnostic testing is not indicated. Endoscopy is safe during pregnancy, but should be performed only for complications such as stricture or hemorrhage. Treatment regimens must consider medication side effects and fetal well-being. Antireflux programs suggest small meals; no food before bed-time; elevation of the head of the bed; and avoidance of caffeine, ethanol, and tobacco. Antacids and sucralfate are safe in the second and third trimesters. The safety of H_2-receptor antagonists in pregnancy is undefined, although cimetidine has been used for peptic ulcer without apparent adverse effects. Similarly, prokinetic agents (e.g., metoclopramide and cisapride) are used to treat severe gastro-esophageal reflux, but their safe use in pregnancy has not been confirmed.

Peptic Ulcer Disease

Pathophysiology

Peptic ulcer disease is rare during pregnancy; its prevalence may not be different from that in age-matched, nonpregnant controls. In fact, symptoms in pregnant patients with known peptic ulcer disease may improve because of reduced gas-tric acid production, although this remains controversial because many studies show no change in acid secretion. Complications of peptic ulcer disease are exceedingly rare in pregnancy but may occur late in the third trimester or in the postpartum period when serum gastrin levels increase.

Principles of Management

The diagnosis of peptic ulcer disease during pregnancy is based on typical symp-tomatology and nonspecific tenderness on abdominal examination. Because invasive tests are usually avoided, the true incidence of this condition in pregnant women is unknown. More aggressive evaluation should be reserved for patients with hemorrhage or suspected obstruction. Endoscopy is preferred to upper gastrointestinal barium radiography to avoid radiation exposure. Suspected perforation should be aggressively diagnosed and treated. As with gastroesophageal reflux, antacids are the safest choice, although H_2-receptor antagonists are often used. In a pregnant patient with *Helicobacter pylori*–induced ulcer disease, the choice of antibiotics should be made carefully to avoid harming the fetus (e.g., metronidazole has teratogenic effects).

Gallstone Disease

Pathophysiology

Because of multiple factors, cholesterol cholelithiasis is more prevalent in women than in men, especially in women with prior pregnancies. Gallbladder size increases during pregnancy and ejection efficiency declines. During the second and third trimesters, there is a decrease in the total bile salt pool, which increases the fractional concentration of cholesterol. It is unknown whether complications of cholelithiasis occur more frequently in pregnant than in nonpregnant women.

Principles of Management

The signs and symptoms of acute cholecystitis are similar to those in nonpregnant women. The diagnosis is based on typical symptoms, laboratory findings, and ultrasound demonstration of gallstones with or without gallbladder wall thickening or pericholecystic fluid. Ultrasound results may be difficult to interpret in late pregnancy because of gallbladder displacement. Oral cholecystography and biliary scintigraphy should be avoided. Many patients with acute cholecystitis are managed medically with analgesics, fluid resuscitation, and antibiotics. Because of the increased risk of fetal loss associated with surgery in the first trimester, cholecystectomy should be deferred to the second trimester whenever possible. Gallstone pancreatitis has a high morbidity and mortality in pregnancy; therefore, early cholecystectomy and common bile duct exploration is recommended. Endoscopic retrograde cholangiopancreatography has been used in pregnancy, but few data are available concerning its safety.

Inflammatory Bowel Disease

Pathophysiology

Pregnancy has variable effects on the activity of inflammatory bowel disease (IBD). Patients with quiescent ulcerative colitis at the onset of pregnancy are likely to remain quiescent, whereas those with active disease are apt to experience a worsening of symptoms. The course of ulcerative colitis during a single pregnancy does not predict disease patterns with future pregnancies. Exacerbations, when they occur, usually present in the first trimester. Crohn's disease behaves in a similar fashion during pregnancy. Ulcerative colitis has little effect on the rates of congenital abnormalities and fetal loss, although severe colitis may increase the risks of spontaneous abortion and stillbirth. Active Crohn's disease confers a twofold-increased risk of spontaneous abortion, stillbirth, and premature delivery, although quiescent disease has little effect. Ulcerative colitis has little or no effect on fertility. Women with Crohn's disease have a slightly increased rate of infertility related to disease activity and nutritional status; however, some cases of apparent reduced fertility in Crohn's disease result from the patient's choice not to have children.

Principles of Management

Medical therapy of IBD during pregnancy can be accomplished without harm to the fetus. Sulfasalazine has not been associated with an increase in prematurity, low birth weight, or spontaneous abortion. The experience with 5-aminosalicylates in pregnancy is limited, although no complications have been reported. Patients taking sulfasalazine should receive supplemental folate because of sulfasalazine-induced inhibition of transport and metabolism of folate. Corticosteroids do not increase the risk of low birth weight, spontaneous abortion, or fetal abnormalities. Metronidazole and immunosuppressive agents have teratogenic effects in animals; therefore, their use in pregnancy is not advisable. Discontinuation of immunosuppressives is recommended at least 6 months before considering pregnancy.

Constipation

Pathophysiology

Constipation is prevalent in pregnancy and usually results from colonic hypomotility. Increases in colonic transit times correlate with increases in progesterone levels. Animal studies document reduced contractile efficiency of colonic smooth muscle after exposure to progesterone. Other factors include rectosigmoid compression by the gravid uterus, increased colonic water and electrolyte absorption, and prenatal vitamin supplements.

Principles of Management

Constipation during pregnancy rarely mandates extensive evaluation. Increases in dietary fiber and fluid intake are often effective. If constipation persists, a fiber supplement (e.g., psyllium) can safely be recommended. Bisacodyl and docusate stool softeners have been used without apparent adverse effects.

Acute Abdominal Pain

Differential Diagnosis

The differential diagnosis of acute abdominal pain in pregnancy includes the same nonobstetric causes that are seen in nonpregnant patients (Table 20-1). Appendicitis is the most common gastrointestinal condition requiring surgery during pregnancy. The enlarging uterus may displace the location of the appendix cephalad. Guarding, rigidity, and fever are less common with pregnancy, and the physiologic leukocytosis of pregnancy reduces the diagnostic utility of a complete blood count. Pyuria and hematuria may result from local compression and irritation of the ureter. Abscess formation may stimulate premature uterine contractions and delivery. Most cases of acute pancreatitis are associated with cholelithiasis or

---

TABLE 20-1
Causes of Acute Abdomen in Pregnancy

Nonobstetric causes
    Acute appendicitis
    Acute cholecystitis
    Acute pancreatitis
    Hepatic rupture
    Intestinal obstruction
    Adnexal torsion
    Sickle cell crisis
Obstetric causes
    Ectopic pregnancy
    Abruptio placentae
    Red degeneration of a uterine myoma
    Uterine rupture

---

with an underlying lipoprotein disorder. Other causes include hyperparathyroidism and ethanol abuse. Acute pancreatitis in pregnancy carries a high risk of maternal and fetal mortality as well as of complications such as pseudocyst formation. Hepatic rupture may occur in the setting of pre-eclampsia with associated disseminated intravascular coagulation, usually near term or immediately postpartum. Spontaneous splenic rupture and rupture of splenic arterial aneurysms are rare causes of acute abdominal pain and are usually associated with significant intraperitoneal hemorrhage. Intestinal obstruction usually results from adhesions from prior surgery and is most common in the third trimester, presumably because of pressure on pre-existing adhesions from the expanding uterus. An ovarian cyst in a twisted adnexa can produce an acute abdomen during pregnancy. Its presentation may mimic that of acute appendicitis. Sickle cell anemia in crisis may produce acute abdominal pain and is associated with high maternal and fetal mortality rates.

The differential diagnosis of acute abdominal pain also includes causes specific to pregnant women. The most common cause of acute abdomen in the first trimester is ectopic pregnancy. Abruptio placentae is an important cause of acute pain in late pregnancy. Classically, patients present with pain, uterine tenderness, and vaginal bleeding, which are caused by separation of the placenta from its uterine attachment. Abruptio placentae may be self-limited, or it may cause fetal demise or severe maternal complications, including blood loss, disseminated intravascular coagulation, and renal cortical necrosis. Red degeneration of a uterine myoma is caused by hemorrhagic infarction of a uterine fibroid and is characterized by focal acute pain. Uterine rupture generally occurs late in pregnancy—spontaneously or during labor—in patients who have undergone prior cesarean section. It usually results in fetal demise and intra-abdominal hemorrhage. Acute granulomatous peritonitis may result from premature rupture of fetal membranes or meconium spillage into the peritoneal cavity during cesarean section.

Principles of Management

Acute abdominal pain during pregnancy should be aggressively evaluated and treated according to the underlying cause, because many of the causative conditions have potentially fatal outcomes for both the fetus and mother. Early surgery is indicated in appendicitis because mortality rates increase with development of peritonitis. Emergency surgery is nearly always required for ectopic pregnancy, hepatic rupture, splenic or splenic artery rupture, uterine rupture, and adnexal torsion, whereas elective surgery is usually performed for intestinal obstruction. Medical therapy is appropriate for acute pancreatitis and sickle cell anemia. Treatment of abruptio placentae consists of blood replacement and expeditious delivery.

GYNECOLOGIC DISEASE AS A CAUSE OF LOWER ABDOMINAL PAIN

Acute and chronic abdominal and pelvic pain in women may result from various gynecologic causes (Table 20-2).

Acute Presentations

Differential Diagnosis

Pelvic Inflammatory Disease. Acute pelvic inflammatory disease (PID) results from the ascent of bacteria into the uterus and fallopian tubes. Salpingitis (i.e., tubal infection) is the most characteristic manifestation, although peritonitis, intra-abdominal abscess formation, or sepsis may result. Risk factors for developing PID include sexual activity with multiple partners, the presence of an intrauterine device, and prior pelvic instrumentation. Oral contraceptives decrease the risk because of increased cervical mucus viscosity. Cervicitis resulting from sexually transmitted *Chlamydia trachomatis* or *Neisseria gonorrhoeae* commonly precedes PID development, whereas PID associated with an intrauterine device is caused by normal vaginal flora. Patients classically present with the triad of fever, lower abdominal pain, and vaginal discharge, although there is a wide spectrum of presentations.

TABLE 20-2
Gynecologic Causes of Abdominal and Pelvic Pain in Reproductive-Age Women

Acute presentation
    Pelvic inflammatory disease
    Ectopic pregnancy
    Mittelschmerz
    Ruptured ovarian cyst
        Corpus luteum
        Ovarian endometrioma
    Adnexal torsion
Chronic presentation
    Endometriosis
    Ovarian carcinoma
    Dysmenorrhea

Ectopic Pregnancy. Ectopic pregnancy is the leading cause of maternal mortality and should especially be considered in a patient with acute lower abdominal pain with a history of prior PID, previous pelvic surgery, progestin-only oral contraceptive, intrauterine device use, previous ectopic pregnancies, and use of advanced reproductive technologies. Tubal ectopic pregnancies are most common, but extrauterine implantation may also occur in the ovaries, cervix, and abdominal cavity. Patients typically present with abdominal pain, abnormal or absent uterine bleeding, breast tenderness, and nausea. A ruptured ectopic pregnancy may produce hypotension or pain referral to the left shoulder.

Midcycle Ovulatory Pain. Pain from intraperitoneal bleeding associated with physiologic rupture of an ovarian follicle can range from mild discomfort to severe pain prompting emergency evaluation. Ovulatory pain (i.e., mittelschmerz) is sudden, sharp, and unilaterally localized, lasting several hours.

Ruptured Ovarian Cysts. Acute abdominal pain may result from hemorrhage into a corpus luteum cyst with subsequent rupture, or rupture of an ovarian endometrioma. Hemorrhage into the cystic cavity usually occurs late in the menstrual period, often immediately before menstruation. Clinical presentations typically include lower quadrant pain, delayed menses, abnormal uterine bleeding, and an enlarged, tender adnexal mass. Leakage from an ovarian endometrioma may evoke intense chemical peritonitis, resulting in development of low-grade fever and rectal irritation.

Ovarian Torsion. Ovarian or adnexal torsion is most commonly associated with ovarian neoplasms (e.g., benign cystic teratomas and fibromas), fallopian tube tumors, or paratubal structures (e.g., paramesonephric cysts). Patients typically present with sharp pain that is brief, irregular, and repetitive if torsion is intermittent. Symptoms may occur when patients rise out of a chair or stoop over. With ovarian necrosis, pain may become dull and less precise, and over 4 to 6 hours, generalized peritonitis may develop. Rarely, the process may wall off with omentum or bowel and produce low-grade chronic pain.

Principles of Management

All female patients with acute lower quadrant abdominal pain should be examined for possible gynecologic causes. Therefore, careful pelvic examination is required. Patients with salpingitis have marked tenderness on bimanual examination, although unilateral tenderness is rare. A Gram's stain of cervical secretions may suggest gonococcal cervicitis. However, secretions should be rigorously tested for *N gonorrhoeae* and *C trachomatis* by culture, fluorescent antibody smear, or enzyme-linked immunoassay techniques. Virtually all patients with ectopic pregnancy have abdominal or adnexal tenderness, although an adnexal mass is palpable in only 50% of cases. Some patients will exhibit blue coloration of the cervix.

Blood testing should include pregnancy testing, a white blood cell count, hemoglobin concentration, and in some cases, a sedimentation rate. However, only 45% of patients with salpingitis exhibit leukocyte counts in excess of 8000 cells per µl and only 75% have a sedimentation rate of >15 mm per hour. Pregnancy testing is performed in all women to assess for possible ectopic pregnancy.

Other diagnostic studies may be of use. Pelvic and vaginal ultrasound studies have limited use in PID unless a palpable adnexal mass is noted, although they may show evidence of ectopic pregnancy, ovarian cysts, or ovarian torsion. Culdocentesis may recover purulent fluid in PID or blood in ectopic pregnancy or with ovarian cyst rupture. Diagnostic laparoscopy may distinguish PID, ectopic pregnancy, ovarian lesions, and appendicitis.

The management of acute pain secondary to gynecologic disease depends on its cause. Most patients with PID respond to parenteral cefoxitin plus oral doxycycline or intravenous clindamycin plus gentamicin. If an intrauterine device is present, it should be removed. Surgery is indicated in PID for patients with sepsis or a ruptured abscess. Transvaginal or transabdominal drainage may be needed in rare cases that are unresponsive to antibiotics. Surgery is the mainstay of therapy for suspected or documented ectopic pregnancy. In stable patients, laparoscopic salpingectomy or salpingostomy may be possible, but emergency laparotomy is needed if hemodynamic compromise is present. Patients should be followed postoperatively with determination of hCG levels to exclude the possibility of residual trophoblastic tissue. Medical or direct injection techniques for ectopic pregnancy are being tested. Midcycle ovulatory pain usually resolves, but patients may need oral contraceptives for ovarian suppression. Patients with ovarian cysts and torsions may require surgical intervention.

Chronic Presentations

Differential Diagnosis

Dysmenorrhea. Dysmenorrhea is defined as pelvic pain in association with menstruation and may range from mild discomfort to severe, debilitating symptoms. Primary dysmenorrhea may result from elevated uterine prostaglandin production, which can enhance uterine contractility and sensitize intrauterine pain fibers to mechanical and chemical stimuli. Secondary dysmenorrhea may result from endometrial polyps, submucous myomas, intrauterine devices, endometriosis, adenomyosis, and cervical stenosis. Dysmenorrhea is described as sharp, crampy, lower midabdominal pain that may radiate to the back or thigh. The pain usually starts before the onset of vaginal bleeding and peaks on the first day of menstruation.

Endometriosis. Endometriosis is characterized by the ectopic growth of hormonally responsive endometrium outside the uterus, usually in close proximity to the fallopian tubes, ovaries, cul-de-sac, and uterosacral ligament. Endometriosis involving the gastrointestinal tract is localized most frequently to the rectosigmoid colon, with less likely attachment to the rectovaginal septum, small intestine, cecum, appendix, and other sites. Hemoperitoneum may be present during menstruation. Extra-abdominal sites of implantation include the central and peripheral nervous systems and the lungs. Patients typically present with pain and cramping with or slightly before the onset of menstruation. Gastrointestinal involvement may produce rectal pain, pain on defecation, constipation, or colonic obstruction with severe disease. Rare symptoms include intussusception, obstruction of the small intestine, hemorrhagic ascites, protein-losing enteropathy, and bowel perforation.

Ovarian Malignancies. Ovarian cancer is most prevalent in peri- and postmenopausal women and most commonly occurs in patients with histories of late childbearing, late marriage, and infertility. Oral contraceptives appear to reduce the risk of ovarian cancer. Ovarian cancer spreads by contiguous invasion and intraperitoneal seeding and is confined to the ovary at the time of diagnosis in <30% of patients. Sites of metastasis include the fallopian tubes, uterus, bladder, and rectum. Diffuse involvement of the intestinal serosa may produce severe gastrointestinal dysfunction. Bowel encasement may further produce intestinal obstruction. Malignant ascites is present in 35% of women at the time of diagnosis. Rarely, the disease may metastasize to lymph nodes, lung, or liver.

Principles of Management

Physical examination can provide clues to the cause of chronic lower abdominal pain of gynecologic etiology. Patients with primary dysmenorrhea usually have a normal examination, whereas those with secondary dysmenorrhea may exhibit uterine masses, cervical stenosis, or endometriosis. Patients with endometriosis may have nodular thickening and tenderness along the uterosacral ligaments, on the posterior uterus, and in the cul-de-sac that are most prominent at the time of menstruation. Physical findings in ovarian cancer include ascites, abdominal or pelvic masses, signs of intestinal obstruction, and pleural rubs or effusions. In a postmenopausal woman, the presence of a palpable ovary, even in the absence of symptoms or other findings, should raise concern about ovarian malignancy.

Diagnostic testing usually is not necessary for primary dysmenorrhea, although ultrasound may occasionally be useful for some patients with secondary dysmenorrhea. Ultrasound may also detect ovarian endometriomas. Laparoscopy allows confirmation of endometriosis with the appropriate clinical presentation, whereas endoscopy or barium radiography may define gastrointestinal manifestations. Ultrasound is useful in differentiating ovarian neoplasms from ovarian cysts and may document ascites, liver metastasis, lymphadenopathy, and ureteral dilation. Computed tomography may provide further definition of the spread of malignant disease. The tumor marker CA-125 is 80% to 90% accurate in differentiating malignant ovarian tumors from benign disease when levels exceed 65 U per ml. α-Fetoprotein elevations may suggest ovarian endodermal sinus tumors, whereas hCG levels may rise with choriocarcinoma and embryonal carcinoma. Surgical staging and peritoneal fluid sampling are required before determining appropriate treatment for a patient with ovarian cancer.

Management of chronic abdominal pain in women depends on the cause. Patients with primary dysmenorrhea may respond to NSAIDs or, in severe cases, oral contraceptives. Surgical resection may be necessary for some causes of secondary dysmenorrhea. Endometriosis may be pharmacologically treated with oral contraceptives, progestational agents, danazol, or gonadotropin-releasing hormone analogs (e.g., leuprolide). Laparoscopic laser treatments may be beneficial in patients with severe pain caused by endometriosis, whereas total hysterectomy with bilateral salpingo-oophorectomy may be recommended in severely affected patients who do not desire further pregnancy or when pregnancy is not possible because of disease involvement. With ovarian malignancies confined to a single ovary, primary treatment is unilateral salpingo-oophorectomy. Surgical debulking and chemotherapy are used as palliative therapy for extensive disease.

CHAPTER 21

Approach to the Patient Requiring Nutritional Support

DIFFERENTIAL DIAGNOSIS

Causes of Nutrient Deficiency

Most people are able to ingest the necessary fluids, nutrients, vitamins, and minerals to maintain health. However, certain patients, because of disease or surgical procedures, cannot satisfy their nutritional requirements with oral intake alone. In general, the recommended daily allowances of nutrients provide a large margin of safety. In a stable patient, 20 ml of fluid and 20 to 25 kcal per kg are required for fluid and weight maintenance, although in severely malnourished individuals, the calorie requirement may be as high as 35 kcal per kg.

Many conditions produce nutrient deficiencies, which in turn produce various clinical findings (Table 21-1). Inadequate intake is the most common cause of nutrient deficiency worldwide. Decreased intake is most likely to affect nutrients that have small body stores, such as folate, water-soluble vitamins, and protein. Malabsorptive conditions, especially those that impair the effective mucosal absorptive surface area of the small intestine (e.g., celiac sprue, short bowel syndrome, Whipple's disease), may produce profound nutrient deficiency. In addition to malabsorption of oral intake, patients with these conditions lose endogenous stores of minerals, vitamins, and proteins that are not reabsorbed from gastric, pancreaticobiliary, and small intestinal secretions. When steatorrhea is present, divalent cations (calcium, magnesium, zinc) are especially prone to malabsorption because they combine with unabsorbed fatty acids to form nonabsorbable soaps. Drugs may induce malabsorption. Cholestyramine binds fats and fat-soluble vitamins, whereas neomycin precipitates bile salts. Sulfasalazine inhibits folate absorption, and colchicine inhibits enterocyte release of fat-soluble vitamins. Antacids decrease phosphorus absorption. Increased losses of fluid and electrolytes may occur in the absence of malabsorption as a result of diarrhea, vomiting, enterocutaneous fistulae, gastric suctioning, and renal wasting. Finally,

---

TABLE 21-1
Physical Signs of Deficiencies of Specific Nutrients

Hair
  Thin, sparse (protein, zinc, biotin)
  Flag's sign (transverse pigmentation) (protein, copper)
  Easy pluckability (protein)
Nails
  Spoon-shaped (i.e., koilonychia) (iron)
  No luster, transverse ridging (protein, energy)
Skin
  Dry, scaling (i.e., xerosis) (vitamin A, zinc)
  Seborrheic dermatitis (essential fatty acids, zinc, pyridoxine, biotin)
  Flaky paint dermatosis (protein)
  Follicular hyperkeratosis (vitamin A, vitamin C, essential fatty acids)
  Nasolabial seborrhea (niacin, pyridoxine, riboflavin)
  Petechiae, purpura (vitamin C, vitamin K, vitamin A)
  Pigmentation, desquamation (niacin)
  Pallor (folate, iron, cobalamin, copper, biotin)
Eyes
  Angular palpebritis (riboflavin)
  Blepharitis (B vitamins)
  Corneal vascularization (riboflavin)
  Dull, dry conjunctiva (vitamin A)
  Bitot's spot (vitamin A)
  Keratomalacia (vitamin A)
  Fundal capillary microaneurysms (vitamin C)
  Ophthalmoplegia (Wernicke's encephalopathy) (thiamine)
Other
  Delayed wound healing (vitamin C, protein, zinc, essential fatty acids)
  Hypogonadism, delayed puberty (zinc)
  Glucose intolerance (chromium)
Mouth
  Angular stomatitis (B vitamins, iron, protein)
  Cheilosis (riboflavin, niacin, pyridoxine, protein)
  Atrophic lingual papillae (niacin, iron, riboflavin, folate, cobalamin)
  Glossitis (niacin, pyridoxine, riboflavin, folate, cobalamin)
  Decreased taste and smell (vitamin A, zinc)
  Swollen, bleeding gums (vitamin C)
Glands
  Parotid enlargement (protein)
  Sicca syndrome (vitamin C)
  Thyroid enlargement (iodine)
Heart
  Enlargement, tachycardia, high-output failure (i.e., beriberi) (thiamine)
  Small heart, decreased output (protein, energy)
  Cardiomyopathy (selenium)
  Cardiac arrhythmias (magnesium, potassium)
Extremities
  Edema (protein, thiamine)
  Muscle weakness (protein, energy, selenium)
  Bone and joint tenderness (vitamin C, vitamin A)
  Osteopenia, bone pain (vitamin D, calcium, phosphorus, vitamin C)
Neurologic
  Confabulation, disorientation (i.e., Korsakoff's psychosis) (thiamine)
  Decreased position and vibration sense, ataxia (cobalamin, thiamine)
  Decreased tendon reflexes (thiamine)
  Weakness, paresthesias (cobalamin, pyridoxine, thiamine)
  Mental disorders (cobalamin, niacin, thiamine, magnesium)

increased caloric and fluid needs are noted in many conditions such as pregnancy, lactation, sepsis, trauma, and burns.

Certain clinical conditions are associated with nutrient deficiencies. Ethanol abuse depresses appetite and causes nausea and vomiting, diarrhea, pancreatitis, and cirrhosis. Ethanol is toxic to the enterocytes in the small intestine, causing decreased transport of glucose, amino acids, folate, and thiamine. Protein and calorie malnutrition resulting from anorexia, nausea, dietary restriction, and increased utilization from inflammation or corticosteroid use may complicate Crohn's disease. Specific deficiencies that are common in Crohn's disease include those of calcium, vitamin D, iron, vitamin B_{12}, zinc, and potassium. Nutrient deficiencies in short bowel syndrome result from profound malabsorption of exogenous and endogenous nutrients. Other causes of intestinal failure that result in malabsorption include radiation enteritis, intestinal pseudo-obstruction with bacterial overgrowth, chronic adhesive peritonitis, and mucosal diseases without effective treatment (collagenous sprue). Advanced liver disease may alter the plasma amino acid profile.

Mineral Deficiency States

Major Minerals

Sodium. Sodium deficiency results from increased losses caused by vomiting, diarrhea, diuresis, salt-wasting renal disease, fistulae, or adrenal insufficiency. Severe sodium depletion in association with dehydration produces nausea and vomiting, exhaustion, cramps, seizures, and cardiorespiratory collapse. Pseudohyponatremia may result from excess lipid, glucose, blood urea nitrogen, mannitol, or glycerin in the serum. Among hospitalized patients, hyponatremia commonly results from free water excess caused by cardiac, renal, or hepatic insufficiency.

Potassium. Total body potassium depletion usually results from gastrointestinal or urinary losses. (Causes of urinary loss include diuretics, alkalosis, mineralocorticoid excess, antibiotics, cisplatin, renal tubular acidosis, hypomagnesemia, and hypothermia.) Hypokalemia also results from potassium shifts from the extracellular to the intracellular compartments, as may occur with alkalosis, administration of insulin or glucose, treatment with β_2-adrenoceptor agonists or α_1-antagonists, treatment of megaloblastic anemia, or periodic paralysis. Symptoms of potassium depletion include confusion, lethargy, weakness, cramps, myalgias, cardiac arrhythmias, glucose intolerance, nausea, vomiting, diarrhea, ileus, and gastroparesis.

Calcium. Calcium is the most abundant cation in the body. Conditions that cause hypocalcemia include vitamin D deficiency, failure of vitamin D synthesis or action, hypoparathyroidism, hypomagnesemia, acute pancreatitis, osteoblastic malignancies, malabsorption, and medications (e.g., aminoglycosides, cisplatin, calcitonin, furosemide, mithramycin, citrated blood, phosphates, and anticonvulsants). Manifestations of hypocalcemia include a positive Chvostek or Trousseau sign, tetany, hyperreflexia, paresthesias, seizures, mental status changes, increased intracranial pressure, bradycardia, heart block, and choreoathetotic movements. Chronic calcium deficiency causes rickets in children and osteomalacia in adults.

Phosphorus. Phosphorus is the major intracellular anion, and 80% to 85% of body stores are in bone. Hypophosphatemia occurs in 2% to 3% of hospitalized patients as a result of decreased intestinal absorption (antacids, malabsorption, vitamin D deficiency, hypoparathyroidism), increased renal excretion (proximal tubule disease, alkalosis, diuretics, hyperparathyroidism, burns, corticosteroids), and intracellular shifts (respiratory alkalosis, carbohydrate administration). Severe hypophosphatemia produces hemolysis, encephalopathy, seizures, paresthesias, muscle weakness, rhabdomyolysis, decreased glucose utilization, and reduced oxygen delivery.

Magnesium.   Magnesium is the second most abundant intracellular cation, with 70% of total body stores contained in bone. Intestinal absorption is decreased in malabsorption syndromes. Excessive urinary loss results from hypercalcemia, volume expansion, tubular dysfunction, alcoholism, diabetes, hyperparathyroidism, hypophosphatemia, and medications (e.g., diuretics, aminoglycosides, cyclosporin, amphotericin, cisplatin, digoxin). Shifts into the intracellular space may result from refeeding, treatment of diabetic ketoacidosis, pancreatitis, and correction of acidosis in renal failure. Patients with hypomagnesemia present with tremors, myoclonic jerks, ataxia, tetany, psychiatric disturbances, coma, ventricular arrhythmias, hypotension, or cardiac arrest.

Trace Minerals

Iron.   Ten percent of ingested iron is absorbed in the duodenum and upper jejunum, although this may increase to 30% in deficiency states. Absorption is enhanced by gastric acid and decreased when insoluble iron complexes form (e.g., iron with phytates, phosphates, or antacids). Iron deficiency results from gastrointestinal bleeding, excessive menstrual blood loss, multiple pregnancies, and malabsorption (celiac sprue, achlorhydria). Clinical manifestations of iron deficiency stem from the resulting anemia and include weakness, lightheadedness, decreased exercise tolerance, and tachycardia.

Zinc.   Twenty percent of ingested zinc is absorbed in the small intestine, and the major route of excretion is in the bile. Zinc deficiency results from malabsorption, cirrhosis, alcoholism, nephrotic syndrome, sickle cell anemia, pregnancy, pica, pancreatic insufficiency, penicillamine use, and chronic diarrhea of any cause. Clinical manifestations of zinc deficiency include growth retardation, scaling skin, alopecia, diarrhea, apathy, night blindness, poor wound healing, and dysgeusia.

Copper.   Copper is absorbed with 40% efficiency in the stomach and small intestine, although its absorption may be inhibited by iron and zinc. Copper deficiency in adults is rare, occurring with parenteral nutrition without copper supplements and during penicillamine therapy. Clinical manifestations of copper deficiency include microcytic anemia, leukopenia, neutropenia, and skeletal abnormalities.

Selenium.   Selenium is absorbed in the small intestine and excreted in the urine and stool. Selenium deficiency occurs with malabsorptive conditions in the small intestine, fistulae, alcoholism, cirrhosis, acquired immunodeficiency syndrome, cancer, and with administration of parenteral nutrition formulas without supplemental selenium. In the United States, symptoms of selenium deficiency are rare but may include myositis, weakness, and cardiomyopathy.

Chromium.   Only 2% of dietary chromium is absorbed. Chromium deficiency occurs with short bowel syndrome and in patients receiving poorly supplemented parenteral nutrition formulas. Clinical manifestations include hyperglycemia, insulin insensitivity, encephalopathy, peripheral neuropathy, and weight loss.

Iodine.   Thirty percent of iodine absorbed by the gastrointestinal tract is excreted by the thyroid. Iodine deficiency usually is caused by inadequate intake, and it results in hypothyroidism and thyroid hyperplasia and hypertrophy. Iodine supplements are rarely needed in parenteral nutrition solutions, presumably because sufficient iodine is present as a contaminant or it is absorbed from the skin.

Other Minerals.   Several minerals are considered essential, but human deficiency syndromes have not been reported for these elements. Fluoride is almost completely absorbed from the gut and it is avidly retained by bone. It is essential for growth, reproduction, and iron absorption. Molybdenum is needed for metabolism of purines and sulfur-containing compounds. Manganese is a cofactor for pyruvate carboxylase and manganese superoxide dismutase. Vanadium, nickel, cobalt, tin, and silicon are considered essential in mammals, but no human deficiency has been reported. Cadmium, lead, boron, aluminum, arsenic, mercury, strontium, and lithium eventually may prove to be essential, but no replacement is currently needed.

Vitamin Deficiency States

Fat-Soluble Vitamins

In general, deficiencies of the fat-soluble vitamins (A, D, E, and K) take years to develop because large stores are present in adipose tissue. Vitamin D is made endogenously in sun-exposed skin. Vitamins that undergo enterohepatic circulation (e.g., A and D) may be vulnerable to loss in malabsorptive conditions. Blood values for fat-soluble vitamins are difficult to interpret because of adipose stores and plasma-binding proteins.

Vitamin A.   Vitamin A or its carotenoid precursors are present in animal products (e.g., liver, kidney, dairy products, eggs) and in green and yellow vegetables. Vitamin A deficiency usually results from decreased intake and fat malabsorption, although impaired carotenoid conversion in mucosal disease, inability to store the vitamin in liver disease, and increased urinary losses (e.g., as from tuberculosis, cancer, pneumonia, urinary tract infection) may be contributing factors. Symptoms of deficiency are night blindness, xerophthalmia, follicular hyperkeratosis, altered taste and smell, increased cerebrospinal fluid pressure, and increased infections.

Vitamin D.   Vitamin D occurs naturally in fish liver oils, eggs, liver, and dairy products and is absorbed by the small intestine. Cholecalciferol (vitamin D_3) is also synthesized on ultraviolet exposure of the skin. Vitamin D deficiency may result from inadequate sun exposure, steatorrhea, severe liver or kidney disease, Crohn's disease, or resection of the small intestine. Clinical manifestations of deficiency include hypocalcemia, hypophosphatemia, bone demineralization, osteomalacia in adults, rickets in children, and bony fractures.

Vitamin E.   Vitamin E is a fat-soluble antioxidant and free radical scavenger found in plants and vegetable oils. Gastrointestinal absorption requires bile salts and pancreatic enzymes. Deficiency is rare in humans, but may occur in abetalipoproteinemia, cystic fibrosis, cirrhosis, malabsorption, biliary obstruction, and as a result of excess mineral oil ingestion. It may produce histologic changes in the spinal cord and medulla, hemolysis, and a progressive neurologic syndrome (areflexia, gait disturbance, decreased vibratory and proprioceptive sensation, and gaze paresis).

Vitamin K.   Vitamin K is abundant in the diet and is synthesized by intestinal bacteria. Deficiency results very rarely from poor intake. When it occurs, it is usually caused by fat malabsorption, diminished liver function or bile secretion, or antibiotic inhibition of bacterial production. The most significant clinical manifestation of vitamin K deficiency is prolongation of the prothrombin time with increased risk of hemorrhage.

Water-Soluble Vitamins

In contrast to fat-soluble vitamins, water-soluble vitamins are not stored in large quantities in the body. Vitamins such as folate or vitamin B_{12}, which undergo enterohepatic circulation, may be deficient in patients who have diseases that impair this function. Blood levels of water-soluble vitamins usually reflect body stores and fall before clinical manifestations of vitamin deficiency develop.

Thiamine.   Thiamine (vitamin B_1) is readily available in the diet in the United States, and deficiency generally presents only in alcoholics or in patients with malabsorption, severe malnutrition, prolonged fever, or on chronic hemodialysis. Worldwide, thiamine deficiency causes beriberi, which exhibits easy fatigability, weakness, paresthesias, and high-output congestive heart failure. Other clinical manifestations of deficiency include peripheral neuropathy, cerebellar dysfunction, subacute necrotizing encephalomyelopathy, and Wernicke's encephalopathy (characterized by mental changes, ataxia, nystagmus, paresis of upward gaze). Thiamine deficiency may also play a role in Korsakoff's syndrome.

Riboflavin.   Riboflavin (vitamin B_2) is prevalent in milk, eggs, and leafy green vegetables. Deficiency occurs in conjunction with other B-vitamin deficiencies in alcoholism and malabsorption. Riboflavin deficiency produces angular stomatitis, cheilosis, glossitis, seborrhea-like dermatitis, pruritus, photophobia, and visual impairment.

Niacin.   Niacin (vitamin B_3) and its amino acid precursor, tryptophan, are found in animal proteins, beans, nuts, whole grains, and enriched breads and cereals. Niacin deficiency occurs rarely as a complication of alcoholism or malabsorption. It can also occur in patients with carcinoid syndrome or Hartnup disease. The clinical result of niacin deficiency is pellagra. Patients with this condition present with a scaly, hyperpigmented dermatitis localized to sun-exposed surfaces; diarrhea; and central nervous system dysfunction, including irritability and headache progressing to psychosis, hallucinations, and seizures.

Pyridoxine.   Pyridoxine (vitamin B_6) is provided by ingestion of animal protein and whole grain cereals. Pyridoxine deficiency most commonly occurs secondary to treatment with pyridoxine antagonists such as isoniazid, hydralazine, and penicillamine, but it may also occur in alcoholics or patients with malabsorption. Clinical findings in pyridoxine deficiency include peripheral neuropathy, seborrheic dermatitis, glossitis, angular stomatitis, cheilosis, seizures, and sideroblastic anemia.

Folate. Folate is abundant in vegetables, legumes, kidney, liver, and nuts. In developed countries, folate deficiency is most commonly caused by poor intake as a result of alcoholism or by poor absorption as a result of malabsorptive syndromes, sulfasalazine therapy, anticonvulsant use, or the effects of ethanol on mucosal function in the small intestine. Folate deficiency produces macrocytic anemia, thrombocytopenia, leukopenia, glossitis, diarrhea, fatigue, and possibly neurologic findings.

Cobalamin. Cobalamin (vitamin B_{12}) is found in animal tissues. A dietary deficiency may occur in vegetarians who do not consume any foods of animal origin. Cobalamin deficiency is also caused by pernicious anemia, gastrectomy, ileal disease or resection, or bacterial overgrowth, in which bacteria bind dietary cobalamin so that it cannot be absorbed. Clinical findings of deficiency include macrocytic anemia, anorexia, loss of taste, glossitis, diarrhea, dyspepsia, hair loss, impotence, and neurologic disease (i.e., peripheral neuropathy, loss of vibratory sensation, incoordination, muscle weakness and atrophy, irritability, and memory loss).

Ascorbic Acid. Ascorbic acid (vitamin C) is present in fruits (especially citrus) and vegetables. Scurvy develops after 2 to 3 months of a diet deficient in ascorbic acid. Other causes of deficiency include alcoholism, malabsorption, and Crohn's disease. Vitamin C deficiency produces weakness, irritability, aching joints and muscles, and weight loss, which progress to perifollicular hyperkeratotic papules, petechiae, and swollen, hemorrhagic gums.

Biotin. Biotin is abundant in food. Deficiency may occur in persons whose diet is high in egg whites, which contain a biotin-binding glycoprotein, and in patients taking hyperalimentation solutions without a biotin supplement. The effects of deficiency include anorexia, nausea, dermatitis, alopecia, mental depression, and organic aciduria.

Essential Fatty Acid Deficiency

Essential fatty acids are long-chain fatty acids that cannot be synthesized by mammals (i.e., linoleic, linolenic, and arachidonic acids). Because humans can synthesize arachidonic acid from exogenous linoleic acid, only linoleic acid (and to a lesser degree, linolenic) is required in the diet. Vegetable oils are rich in dietary sources. Parenteral nutrition lipid emulsions consist of soybean or safflower oil, which are predominantly linoleic acid. Clinical manifestations of essential fatty acid deficiency, usually caused by fat-free hyperalimentation, appear within 3 to 6 weeks as scaly dermatitis, alopecia, coarse hair, hepatomegaly, thrombocytopenia, diarrhea, and growth retardation.

Protein-Calorie Malnutrition

Although there are few clinically useful measures for quantitating protein-calorie malnutrition, some studies suggest that 20% to 60% of inpatients are undernourished. Healthy adults can die of starvation after 60 to 90 days if no proteins or calories are provided. In hypermetabolic conditions, this period may decrease to as few as 14 days. Malnutrition is associated with weakness, impaired immune responses, skin breakdown, infection, apathy, and irritability. If malnutrition is severe, full recovery of cardiac and skeletal muscle function may not occur.

TABLE 21-2
When to Begin Nutritional Support in Patients Who Are Not Eating

PATIENT GROUP	BEGIN TUBE FEEDINGS IF POSSIBLE	BEGIN TOTAL PARENTERAL NUTRITION
Neither hypercatabolic nor malnourished	7–10 days	14–21 days
Either hypercatabolic or malnourished	1–5 days	1–10 days
Both hypercatabolic and malnourished	1–3 days	1–7 days

PRINCIPLES OF MANAGEMENT

Implementation of Nutritional Support

The ultimate goal of nutritional support is to decrease morbidity and mortality by providing nutrients or modifying nutrient metabolism. Deciding when to institute nutritional support is a matter of informed clinical judgment. A calorie count by the dietary staff may provide an assessment of nutrient intake. Allowance must be made for fecal wastage in a patient with malabsorption. Next, nutrient expenditure must be determined. The resting energy expenditure for a healthy adult is 20 kcal per kg, but this may double in highly catabolic conditions (e.g., burns). Finally, the degree of protein and calorie malnutrition is estimated. Several variables have been proposed to quantitate this last measure, including serum albumin, creatinine-height index, serum transferrin, skin testing, serum transthyretin, and skinfold thickness, but none of these is reliable by itself. The Subjective Global Assessment of nutrition status suggested by Detsky and colleagues correlates well with predicting clinical outcome after surgery. This scale rates patients as well nourished, moderately malnourished, or severely malnourished based on weight loss, dietary intake, gastrointestinal symptoms, functional capacity, and physical examination findings. In patients who are not eating, enteral feeding is provided within 7 to 10 days in well-nourished, non-catabolic patients, in 1 to 5 days in catabolic or malnourished patients, and in 1 to 3 days in catabolic and malnourished patients (Table 21-2). If parenteral nutrition is required, this should be initiated in 14 to 21 days, 1 to 10 days, and 1 to 7 days for each category of patients, respectively.

When initiating a nutritional program, energy and protein goals must be set. The energy goals for most inpatients range from 25 to 35 kcal per kg per day with protein contents of 1 to 2 g per kg per day. It is recommended that most critically ill patients receive no more than 5 to 7 g per kg per day of glucose. Intravenous lipid emulsions provided in excess of 1 g per kg per day are associated with hypoxemia, bacteremia, and impaired immune function. For patients who are not critically ill, optimal calorie support is obtained if they receive energy equal to 100% to 120% of their total daily energy expenditure, which is composed of the basal energy expenditure and factors contributed by stress hypermetabolism; nonshivering thermogenesis; diet-induced thermogenesis; energy expenditure of activity; energy expenditure for weight gain; and abnormal fecal, urinary, and wound energy losses. A crude calculation of the energy goal for a given patient is to estimate the basal energy expenditure (20 kcal per kg per day) and multiply by a stress factor for the severity of illness, which ranges from 1.0 for mild disease to 2.0 for severe burns. An additional 0% to 20% of the basal energy expenditure is added for activity level, and if weight gain is desired, an additional 500 to 1000 kcal per day is included. The protein goal is set to 0.8 to 2.0 g per kg per day if energy intake is adequate. Occasionally, patients with severe renal or liver failure may require <0.8 g per kg per day, whereas highly catabolic patients, such as those with burns, may require 2.0 g per kg per day of protein.

Enteral Nutrition

The delivery of nutrients into the gastrointestinal tract using a tube is the preferred method of feeding patients who cannot ingest by mouth calories adequate for their needs but who have normal digestion and absorption. Nasogastric feeding is the most appropriate route for short-term feeding of cooperative patients. To reduce the risk of pulmonary aspiration in individuals with delayed gastric emptying and regurgitation, feedings may be delivered to the distal duodenum or jejunum. If long-term feedings (i.e., >1 month) are anticipated, endoscopic, surgical, or radiologic placement of a gastrostomy tube is a safe and relatively easy option. Similarly, jejunal feedings may be given through a surgically placed jejunostomy. Some clinicians have had success with jejunostomy extensions through a pre-existing gastrostomy tube, but these extended tubes may be propelled back into the stomach over time.

Tube feeding solutions must be individualized for each patient. For stable patients with normal gastric function, bolus feedings through a gastrostomy are safe, providing efficient nutrient support that requires little of the caregiver's time. For patients who have gastroesophageal reflux with pulmonary aspiration, tube feedings through a gastrostomy should be continuous with the patient in a partially upright position, and residual gastric volumes should be determined periodically to prevent gastric retention. All small intestinal nutrient perfusions are performed on a continuous basis to avoid inducing a dumping syndrome. Most tube feeding products have a caloric density of 1 kcal per ml, although more concentrated formulas are available if fluid restriction is necessary. Formulas more concentrated than 1 kcal per ml are not suitable for patients who cannot drink water in response to thirst. The protein content of commercial products ranges from 20 to 75 g per liter. Most preparations contain whole protein, which is suitable for most patients. The value of formulas with free amino acids or peptides for patients with severe intestinal disease or severe diarrhea remains to be determined. Essential amino acid-predominant preparations are useful for treating patients with renal failure to delay the initiation of dialysis, whereas solutions with a higher concentration of branched-chain amino acids and a lower concentration of aromatic amino acids may be useful for some patients with hepatic failure. For patients with glucose intolerance, a 50% to 60% fat-containing formula may be used, whereas a low-fat, elemental preparation is best for patients with fat malabsorption, pancreatitis, or delayed gastric emptying. Low-electrolyte formulas may be chosen for patients with cardiac, renal, or hepatic failure. Most enteral feeding formulas provide the necessary trace elements and vitamins.

Parenteral Nutrition

Intravenous alimentation or total parenteral nutrition (TPN) is indicated for patients who are unable to meet their nutritional needs through gastrointestinal feedings. Parenteral nutrition may be administered through a peripheral vein or through a central venous catheter. Peripheral parenteral nutrition is reserved for patients of near normal nutritional status who need to maintain lean body mass over a relatively short time, such as patients undergoing elective surgery who will not receive enteral nutrition for 3 to 7 days or for patients who need supplementation of suboptimal oral or enteral intake. In contrast, central TPN is considered for hospitalized patients with protein-calorie malnutrition or for patients who cannot meet their nutritional needs with enteral intake lasting >10 days.

The advent of safe intravenous lipid emulsions has made peripheral parenteral nutrition practical because the emulsions are calorically dense (3 kcal per ml), yet isotonic. Peripheral parenteral nutrition solutions contain 5% to 10% glucose, 2% to 5% amino acids, and electrolytes. Lipid emulsions of 10%, 20%, or 30% are mixed into the solution or administered separately. To provide adequate daily calories in an acceptable volume, lipid emulsions must be used. They will thus provide 50% to 70% of nonprotein calories. This is acceptable in relatively well patients, but it raises concern about immunosuppression in severely ill patients. Peripheral parenteral nutrition is hyperosmotic (500 to 1000 mOsm per kg) and is given at a rate of 2 to 3 liters per day. The risk of phlebitis is minimized by using fine-bore silicon catheters that are rotated frequently.

With central TPN, the problem of hypertonicity-induced phlebitis is avoided by delivering the nutrients into a vessel with high-volume flow, usually the superior vena cava. Catheters are aseptically placed into the subclavian or internal jugular veins and advanced into the middle to lower part of the superior vena cava. Use of the inferior vena cava route is discouraged except as a last resort because of the risk of infection. When possible, central TPN should be administered through single-lumen catheters. For patients who need TPN beyond their inpatient stay, permanent catheters (e.g., Hickman or Broviac) are surgically placed for home TPN administration.

As with other nutritional regimens, central TPN programs must be individualized. Crystalloid amino acids are the only available nitrogen source for central TPN, of which 45% are essential, 20% are branched-chain, and 12% are aromatic amino acids plus methionine. Special mixtures with increased essential or branched-chain amino acids are available for patients with renal and hepatic failure, respectively. TPN formulations with 20% to 30% of nonprotein calories as fat are associated with few complications. Increased-lipid, decreased-glucose mixtures are used for patients with diabetes or pulmonary failure to provide less glucose and less carbon dioxide production, respectively. If fluid restriction is important, concentrated intravenous nutrients are available—70% dextrose in water, 30% lipid emulsion, and 15% amino acid solution. Standard TPN electrolyte formulations are suitable for 50% to 80% of patients. Fifteen millimoles of phosphorus and 30 to 40 mEq potassium should be provided per 800 glucose kcal. Most formulas contain 30 to 50 mEq sodium, 5 to 10 mEq magnesium, and 5 to 10 mEq calcium per liter. Chloride and acetate are added to TPN to prevent acidosis. Heparin, insulin, and H_2-receptor antagonists are added as needed. Trace elements and vitamins are routinely added to central TPN formulations to prevent deficiencies. Iron is not routinely included. Therefore, if iron deficiency occurs, supplemental iron may be added. Vitamin K preparations should be included at least weekly.

Central TPN has been shown to be of benefit in several clinical settings. The most unequivocal indication for home TPN is intestinal failure from any cause. TPN is also the primary therapeutic modality that leads to closure of enterocutaneous fistulae in 30% to 50% of patients. However, if spontaneous closure does not occur after 30 to 60 days of TPN, continuation of this therapy is unlikely to be successful. Central TPN is used in the management of inflammatory bowel disease, although bowel rest with central TPN is not useful as primary therapy, nor does it decrease the need for surgery in ulcerative colitis or Crohn's colitis. In contrast, central TPN has a more important role in treating Crohn's disease involving the small intestine, correcting disease-induced vitamin, mineral, and nutrient deficiencies. For patients with complicated acute pancreatitis, central TPN is indicated if enteral feeding exacerbates abdominal pain or if ascites, fistulae, or pseudocysts are present. Lipid emulsions are given cautiously and should be reduced if serum triglyceride levels exceed 400 mg per dl.

COMPLICATIONS

Enteral Nutrition

The major complications of enteral tube feedings are pulmonary aspiration, diarrhea, metabolic abnormalities, and infection. The risk of aspiration is reduced by tube placement distal to the ligament of Treitz. With gastric feedings, the upper body should be elevated at least 30 degrees above horizontal. Residual volumes of 200 ml with nasogastric feedings and 100 ml with gastrostomy feedings indicate an increased risk of aspiration. Diarrhea may result from a too rapid infusion rate, concurrent use of antibiotics and antacids, sorbitol-containing elixir, inadequate fiber supplementation, too much lipid with fat malabsorption, hypertonic formulation, vitamin or mineral deficiency, or hypoalbuminemia. If no remediable cause of diarrhea is found, loperamide elixir, diphenoxylate with atropine, or tincture of opium may be given. Infectious complications are pneumonia as well as recolonization of the gut, gastroenteritis, and sepsis from contaminated formulas.

Parenteral Nutrition

The potential complications of central TPN include mechanical, septic, and metabolic problems. The risks of catheter insertion include pneumothorax, hemorrhage, brachial plexus injury, air or guidewire embolism, cardiac tamponade, and death. Catheters can become occluded by blood, fibrin, intravenous lipid, or precipitated drugs. Vascular catheters are responsible for one-third of nosocomial bacteremias and one-half of candidemias. The most commonly observed organisms include *Staphylococcus epidermidis*, other staphylococcal species, *Candida* organisms, other yeasts, and gram-negative rods. The risk of septicemia with central TPN is 3 to 5 infections per 100 catheters. The most common metabolic complications are hyperglycemia, hypophosphatemia, and hypokalemia. Undetected hyperglycemia may produce osmotic diuresis, hyperosmolar dehydration, coma, and death. Patients who are alcoholic, severely malnourished, or receiving antacids are at increased risk of hypophosphatemia because of shifts from the extracellular to the intracellular compartment. Similarly, hypokalemia results from shifts into the intracellular spaces. Other metabolic complications of central TPN include hypomagnesemia, hyponatremia, fluid overload or dehydration, fat intolerance, hypoglycemia, and hypercalcemia. Abnormalities of the liver occur frequently with central TPN, including calculous and acalculous cholecystitis and hepatic steatosis. TPN-induced liver abnormalities may be minimized by not exceeding caloric needs of the patient, especially the glucose component. Daily cholecystokinin injections may reduce biliary complications of central TPN.

CHAPTER 22

Approach to the Patient with Alcohol or Drug Dependency

Alcohol and drug dependency is prevalent in the United States. There are approximately 18 million alcohol abusers, 700,000 heroin addicts, and tens of millions who have tried cocaine or marijuana. Three percent to 16% of pre-employment drug screening tests produce positive results. Furthermore, patients with chronic pain syndromes are at risk for addiction to narcotics. Most drugs produce tolerance with continued use, causing the abuser to increase the dose. Tolerance is often but not invariably accompanied by physical dependence, which is an adaptive state that manifests itself by intense physical disturbances when drug use is suspended, or by psychic dependence, a condition in which the agent produces satisfaction or a psychic drive that requires periodic drug use for its maintenance. If drug discontinuation affects neural systems, the withdrawal syndrome will be physiologically violent (e.g., seizures), whereas withdrawal from psychic dependence may produce depression and drug craving. Many classes of agents with different physiologic and psychological effects produce drug dependency.

ETHANOL

Clinical Features and Diagnosis

The risk of alcoholism involves a genetic component that is highly sensitive to environmental factors, with a lifetime risk of 20% to 25% for men and 5% for women. Symptoms of intoxication include somnolence, dysarthria, ataxia, nystagmus, and impaired judgment. The alcohol dependence syndrome has several features: narrowing of the drinking pattern such that there is little variability from day to day; an awareness of the compulsion to drink; tolerance to the intoxicating effects of ethanol; physical dependence; early drinking to relieve "morning after" symptoms; the inability of negative consequences (e.g., family, social, professional, health) to deter drinking; and rapid reinstatement of the syndrome with recurrent drinking. These issues should be raised with the patient and the family members. The CAGE test is a simple, nonthreatening series of four questions (Table 22-1) that has a 93%

TABLE 22-1
The CAGE Test for Alcohol Dependency

Questions
Have you felt the need to **Cut** down on drinking?
Are you **Annoyed** by questions about your drinking behavior?
Do you feel **Guilty** about your drinking and its effects?
Do you need an **Eye-opener** (early morning drink) to feel better?

sensitivity and 76% specificity with two or more positive responses. There is no biochemical test to quantitate drinking behavior; however, elevations in mean corpuscular volume, uric acid, triglycerides, and γ-glutamyl transpeptidase may support the suspicions of the family or clinician. Within 6 to 12 hours of ingestion, alcohol can be detected by analysis of breath, blood, or urine. In general, ethanol is cleared at a rate of 100 mg per kg per hour, but this may vary up to threefold according to individual metabolism.

Principles of Management

Ethanol detoxification, with intensive counseling, behavior modification, and support group enrollment, may be undertaken on an outpatient basis in the absence of major medical illness or withdrawal symptoms; otherwise, hospitalization should be considered. In the 1 to 2 days of abstinence, tremor and tachycardia occur, which may progress to hallucinations in 10% to 20% of cases. Seizures and delirium tremens, which is characterized by hallucinations and severe sympathetic overactivity (e.g., tachycardia, fever, dilated pupils, hypertension, diaphoresis), develop later in a minority of patients. Benzodiazepines and barbiturates are effective in preventing ethanol withdrawal symptoms, and calcium channel antagonists and clonidine have shown efficacy in preventing withdrawal or seizures in animal models. The response to detoxification programs depends on the underlying support system. Those with stable support have abstinence rates of 60% for up to 18 months, compared with 30% for unemployed individuals in lower socioeconomic strata. The use of medications to maintain sobriety has provided mixed results. Serotonin-reuptake inhibitors (e.g., fluoxetine, zimeldine) have been somewhat effective, as have opiate antagonists (e.g., naltrexone). Alcohol-sensitizing drugs (e.g., disulfiram) inhibit aldehyde dehydrogenase, leading to nausea, tachycardia, flushing, and hypotension as a result of acetaldehyde accumulation. However, the largest controlled trial showed no difference in abstinence rates with disulfiram and placebo.

SEDATIVE-HYPNOTICS

Clinical Features and Diagnosis

Barbiturates and benzodiazepines are used for sedation, muscle relaxation, seizure control, anxiety, and panic disorders. High doses produce emotional lability, dysarthria, ataxia, and rarely, delirium, disorientation, and altered perception, all of which may be increased by concurrent ethanol use. Dependence on barbiturates occurs in 1 month, whereas benzodiazepine dependence requires about 20

TABLE 22-2
Guidelines for Screening Tests for Drug Abuse

Duration of positive urine screening tests
    Ethanol: 6–12 hours
    Barbiturates and benzodiazepines: several days
    Opiates: 2–5 days
    Cocaine: 2–4 days
    Amphetamines: 2–4 days
    Marijuana: 30 days
    Phencyclidine: 8 days
Sources of false-positive urine screening tests
    Barbiturates and benzodiazepines: ibuprofen
    Opiates: poppy seeds (morphine), dextromethorphan
    Amphetamines: ephedrine, phenylpropanolamine, pseudoephedrine, other sympa-
      thomimetics
    Marijuana: ibuprofen, naproxen, fenoprofen, passive smoke inhalation
Sources of false-negative urine screening tests
    Adulteration of sample with acids, bases, benzalkonium chloride (e.g., Visine), soap
    Dilution of urine (including with diuretics)
    Short time elapsed after use
    Ibuprofen may interfere with confirmation testing (gas chromatography-mass spec-
      trometry) for marijuana
Drugs for which screening tests not available
    Lysergic acid diethylamide (LSD)
    Mescaline
    Psilocybin
    Designer drugs

---

weeks of use. Users of benzodiazepines develop tolerance to the sedative effects of the drugs but not to their anxiolytic effects. Barbiturates and benzodiazepines are reliably detected with urine drug screening tests for several days after the last use (Table 22-2).

Principles of Management

Abrupt withdrawal from barbiturates and benzodiazepines produces tremor, dysphoria, insomnia, hyperreflexia, anxiety, and, rarely, seizures. Barbiturate withdrawal may be as dangerous as delirium tremens. Seizures may occur in patients who are dependent on benzodiazepines if they are administered flumazenil, a benzodiazepine antagonist. Safe withdrawal is accomplished by gradual dose reductions of 10% per day.

OPIATES

Clinical Features and Diagnosis

Heroin is the choice of most narcotic addicts, but prescription drugs such as codeine, methadone, meperidine, and oxycodone are also widely abused. Fentanyl may be abused by medical personnel. Methylphenyltetrahydropyridine is a synthetic derivative of meperidine that caused an outbreak of toxic parkinsonism in the 1970s by destroying substantia nigra neurons in victims. No tolerance to the miotic or constipating effects of opiates develops, so these manifestations may provide clues to narcotic abuse. Urine tests for opiates may produce positive results for 2 to 5 days after the last use. Although ingestion of poppy seeds can give a false-positive result, the cough suppressant dextromethorphan usually does not give a positive test result. Fentanyl is difficult to detect in the blood of users because it is highly potent at very low doses.

Principles of Management

Fully developed symptoms of opiate withdrawal result from overactivity of the sympathetic nervous system and include lacrimation, rhinorrhea, dilated pupils, piloerection, diaphoresis, yawning, hypertension, tachycardia, and fever. In contrast, hallucinations, tremor, and delirium are not typical of opiate withdrawal and suggest other drug use. Withdrawal symptoms can be blocked by clonidine, which inhibits the activity of neurons in the locus caeruleus that are hyperactive secondary to the suspension of opiates. Methadone may be used to wean the patient from shorter-acting opiates. Relapse may be prevented by chronic use of oral naltrexone, but this drug is potentially hepatotoxic.

COCAINE AND OTHER STIMULANTS

Clinical Features and Diagnosis

Cocaine may be taken nasally, intravenously, or by freebasing (i.e., smoking of heated vapors). It induces tolerance, but only relatively mild withdrawal. Nonetheless, it has the highest abuse potential of drugs in current use. Amphetamines are active orally or intravenously. The sympathetic effects of cocaine and amphetamines include pupillary dilation, tachycardia, hypertension, cardiac arrhythmias, myocardial infarction, aortic dissection, myocarditis, intestinal ischemia, disseminated intravascular coagulation, rhabdomyolysis, ulcer perforation, and seizures. Use during pregnancy causes microcephaly, growth retardation, intrauterine cerebral infarction, and cerebral hemorrhage in the fetus. Amphetamines can produce hallucinations and delirium. If taken intravenously, they can cause necrotizing angiitis. Cocaine metabolites can be detected on drug screening for up to 48 hours after use. The detection of amphetamines is complicated by cross-reactions with over-the-counter sympathomimetics (e.g., ephedrine, pseudoephedrine, phenylpropanolamine, phentermine, fenfluramine).

Principles of Management

Withdrawal from stimulants produces depression, fatigue, disturbed sleep with increased dreaming, and intense drug craving. Treatment is usually performed on an outpatient basis and consists of complete abstinence, which is documented by mandatory urine testing. Cocaine craving is treated by intensive counseling. Desipramine may reduce dysphoria and improve sobriety. Extinction therapy, in which the user watches videotapes of cocaine use or handles drug paraphernalia without using the drug, has been used for some patients.

CANNABIS

The active ingredient of marijuana, 9-tetrahydrocannabinol, causes euphoria, relaxation, subjective intensification of perception, altered sense of time, and impaired psychomotor function, as well as vasodilation (tachycardia, conjunctival injection) and appetite stimulation. Five percent of episodes of cannabis use result in anxiety attacks or paranoia. Prolonged use may cause an "amotivational" syndrome of passivity, preoccupation with drug use, decreased drive, and memory loss. Cannabis withdrawal produces restlessness, insomnia, and nausea. Urine tests may produce positive results for up to 30 days after the last use of the drug.

PHENCYCLIDINE

Phencyclidine (PCP) may be taken by any route, including smoking. It produces euphoria at low doses and sympathetic activation, hyperactivity, and hallucinations at higher doses. The hallucinations are frequently auditory, thus producing behavior that mimics paranoid schizophrenia. Physical findings of drug use include vertical and horizontal nystagmus, sympathetic overactivity, numbness, increased pain thresholds, ataxia, and dysarthria. PCP may be detected on urine testing for up to 8 days after use; however, false-positive results occur with over-the-counter decongestants.

HALLUCINOGENS

Lysergic acid diethylamide (LSD) and hallucinogenic amphetamines are sympathomimetics and produce hypertension, pupillary dilation, tachycardia, hyperreflexia, and disordered perception. Users may experience loss of control, flashbacks (i.e., re-experiencing of drug-induced perceptions), and "bad trips" (i.e., terrifying hallucinations). Tolerance develops after three to four doses, but there is little physical dependence or craving. Screening urine tests are not widely available for detection of LSD.

TOBACCO

Clinical Features

Tobacco is highly addictive because the nicotine is absorbed through the oral mucosa and lungs. Nicotine produces manifestations of increased sympathetic activity (e.g., tachycardia, mental arousal) and muscle relaxation. Tolerance to nicotine occurs rapidly (within hours) and a withdrawal syndrome that consists of restlessness, irritability, anxiety, impatience, and impaired concentration is common. Tobacco may also increase metabolism of imipramine, lidocaine, oxazepam, propranolol, and theophylline.

Principles of Management

To reduce the severity of tobacco withdrawal, several nicotine delivery systems have been developed, including the use of nicotine polacrilex in nicotine gum and a number of transdermal nicotine patches. When used in conjunction with counseling, these agents demonstrate efficacy superior to that seen with placebos. Nicotine preparations should be used cautiously in patients with angina, cardiac arrhythmias, or a recent myocardial infarction.

ANABOLIC STEROIDS

Clinical Features and Diagnosis

Anabolic steroids are used in 4- to 12-week cycles by athletes to augment training, especially in power sports such as weightlifting and football. Several drugs are often used together in a practice referred to as stacking. Hepatic complications of anabolic steroid abuse include reversible elevations in liver chemistry values, jaundice, liver cell hyperplasia, hepatic adenoma, hepatocellular carcinoma, angiosarcoma, and fatal peliosis hepatis. Other adverse effects include increases in low-density lipoproteins, with concurrent decreases in high-density lipoproteins, prostate hypertrophy, prostate carcinoma, testicular atrophy, decreased sperm counts, gynecomastia, premature epiphyseal closure in adolescents, irreversible masculinization in women, mood changes, psychosis, and aggressive behavior.

Principles of Management

Anabolic steroid abuse may be suspected by prominent muscular development in a patient as well as by development of adverse side effects. Needle tracks may be visible on the thighs or buttocks. Anabolic steroid use may be detected by gas chromatography-mass spectrometry and by measurement of serum gonadotropins. Testosterone is found by detecting increased ratios of testosterone to epitestosterone in urine. Treatment of a patient who abuses steroids involves strict suspension of drug use. No significant withdrawal syndrome occurs after discontinuation of anabolic steroids.

CHAPTER 23

Advice to Travelers

TRAVEL-RELATED ISSUES

Pretravel Preparations

Before travelers embark on a trip to an area where infectious disease acquisition is possible, a complete travel itinerary should be prepared at least 6 weeks in advance to identify specific locations to be visited and to determine the length of stay at each locale, so that the need for prophylaxis can be determined. Although not required by the United States, some governments require evidence of yellow fever vaccination in persons who have recently traveled to areas where the disease is endemic. No countries officially require cholera vaccination as a condition of entry, although some customs officials may still make this demand. Some diseases, such as traveler's diarrhea, present soon after arrival, whereas the risk of contracting other diseases, such as hepatitis, increases with length of stay. Other conditions are seasonal. Risk of illness may be increased by choosing adventure trips instead of the usual tourist routes, by camping or staying in primitive housing, or by animal exposure. Medical risk factors for disease acquisition include allergies to drugs or to indigenous flora, impaired immune function, chronic obstructive pulmonary disease, diabetes, glucose-6-phosphate deficiency, malabsorption, achlorhydria secondary to gastric surgery or possibly medications, and extremes of age.

Modes of Travel

Air travel may be associated with disruption of the sleep-wakeful cycle known as "jet lag." It is useful to gradually shift the sleep cycle before departing. Use of a short-duration benzodiazepine (e.g., triazolam) during a long air flight or immediately after arrival may assist in sleep cycle adjustment, although this agent may produce retrograde amnesia when taken with ethanol. Reduced pressures in aircraft cabins produce dehydration, which, when coupled with immobility, increase the risk of thromboembolic disease. In high-risk persons, low-dose aspirin may be advisable to prevent this complication. The reduced oxygen tension in an aircraft at high altitude may exacerbate symptoms in patients with obstructive lung disease.

Sea travel is often complicated by motion sickness. Over-the-counter diphenhydramine or dimenhydrinate may be used to prevent motion sickness. Severe cases may require promethazine or prochlorperazine in suppository form.

TABLE 23-1
Halogen Treatment of Unpurified Water

TREATMENT	AMOUNT PER QUART	DESIRED CONCENTRATION
Iodine tablet (tetraglycine hydroperiodide)	1 tablet for warm, clear water	7 ppm
	2 tablets for cool or cloudy water	14 ppm
Tincture of iodine	5 drops for warm, clear water	
	10 drops for cool or cloudy water	
Chlorine tablets (calcium hypochlorite)	Variable	5–10 ppm as determined by portable colorimetric kit

Water Supplies

Unpurified water may contain bacterial, viral, or parasitic pathogens. Carbonated beverages are usually safe, but bottled water cannot be relied on. Water should be boiled or disinfected by halogen treatment or filtration. Effective halogen regimens per quart of water include the following: one iodine tablet (tetraglycine hydroperiodide) for warm, clear water to achieve a level of 7 parts per million (ppm) or 2 iodine tablets for cool or cloudy water to achieve a level of 14 ppm; 5 drops of tincture of iodine for warm, clear water or 10 drops of tincture of iodine for cool or cloudy water; or sufficient chlorine tablets to achieve levels of 5 to 10 ppm (Table 23-1).

Medical Care Overseas

If necessary, the U.S. embassy or consulate may provide recommendations for local physicians, hospitals, or emergency services. When possible, all medications for prophylaxis and treatment should be carried by the traveler, as overseas medications may have different names and strengths. Overseas, over-the-counter medications may have dangerous constituents; thus, they should be avoided.

DISEASES FOR WHICH IMMUNIZATION IS AVAILABLE

The vaccination schedule should take into consideration interactions of vaccines with each other and with immune serum globulin (ISG). If possible, live-virus vaccines should be separated by 30 days or given simultaneously at separate sites. Yellow fever and cholera vaccines should be given at least 3 weeks apart. Some live vaccines should not be given sooner than 6 weeks after receiving ISG to maximize the immune response, whereas ISG should not be given for 2 weeks after measles, mumps, and rubella vaccination to avoid impairing the immune response. Malaria prophylaxis with chloroquine may depress immune function; therefore, vaccination should be performed 2 weeks before initiating the drug.

Vaccines That May Be Required

Yellow Fever

Yellow fever is limited to tropical Africa, northern South America, and Panama. It is prevalent especially in forested areas and is transmitted by mosquitoes. Fatality rates approach 40%, so vaccination is mandatory. The live-virus vaccine is highly effective (>90%) beginning 10 days after vaccination. Boosting is recommended at 10-year intervals. Vaccination is not recommended in immunocompromised patients, in infants younger than 6 months, or in pregnant women.

Cholera

The risk of cholera is extremely low (1 in 500,000) for travelers to Asia and Africa, and, with good hygiene and dietary discretion, it is not a significant problem in regions with periodic pandemics (e.g., Central and South America). Given the availability of antibiotics (e.g., tetracycline), the low incidence of disease, the high incidence of adverse reactions to the vaccine, and the limited efficacy of the vaccine, cholera vaccination is rarely recommended. Vaccination should be limited to travelers working under high-risk unsanitary conditions. The killed whole-cell bacterial vaccine has 50% efficacy for 3 to 6 months and induces local reactions in 1% to 2% of recipients. Newer vaccines are being tested.

Recommended Immunizations for Travelers

Hepatitis A

Hepatitis A virus (HAV) is prevalent in Africa, Asia, and Central and South America, especially in rural or unsanitary urban areas. Transmission is by contaminated food, beverages, ice, or person-to-person contact. ISG is given as passive immunization at a dose of 0.02 ml per kg for trips of <3 months and 0.06 ml per kg for longer trips up to 5 months. Because 20% to 35% of adults in the United States are immune to HAV, determination of anti-HAV antibody titers may obviate the need for ISG. Frequent or long-term travelers should consider receiving the hepatitis A vaccine (1 dose at least 4 weeks before departure and one booster dose 6 to 12 months later. Protection has been estimated to last for 10 years.

Hepatitis B

Risk for hepatitis B virus (HBV) infection is increased in Asia, the South Pacific, and sub-Saharan Africa. Risk factors include drug abuse, sexual activity, blood transfusions, and medical exposures, although casual transmission may occur in highly endemic areas. HBV vaccines are administered in three doses over 6 months to health care workers, long-term (>6 months) residents, persons who are sexually active with the local populace, persons who receive local medical care, and frequent travelers.

Typhoid Fever

Typhoid is prevalent in Africa, Asia, and South and Central America. Vaccination is recommended for those who travel to these areas, especially if exposure to potentially contaminated food and water is possible. Vaccination is especially recommended for persons traveling for >2 weeks. Four doses of the live oral attenuated *Salmonella typhi* strain Ty21a are ingested over 1 week and are 70% to 90% effective for prophylaxis. Children younger than 5 years of age, immunosuppressed individuals, and patients with febrile or gastrointestinal illness should not be vaccinated with the live strain. Booster doses are recommended every 5 years. The parenteral killed *S typhi* vaccine is also effective (70% to 90%); however, local reactions, fever, malaise, and risks for pregnant women make this vaccine less desirable.

Rabies

Canine rabies is widespread in urban and rural areas of Asia, Africa, and Latin America, whereas mongooses in the Caribbean and vampire bats in Latin America may also transmit the disease. The human diploid cell rabies vaccine (HDCV) or rabies vaccine absorbed is recommended for those planning visits of 30 days or longer. Three doses of HDCV are given over 21 to 28 days, with boosters required every 2 years. HDCV does not eliminate the need for postexposure immunization in persons who have sustained a bite, but it reduces the number of postexposure HDCV injections from five to two and eliminates the need for rabies immune globulin.

Meningococcal Disease

Epidemics of meningococcal disease are common in sub-Saharan Africa during the dry season (December to June) and may also occur in New Delhi, Nepal, and Saudi Arabia. A tetravalent capsular polysaccharide vaccine is 75% to 100% effective for serogroups A and C, but it is much less effective in children, especially those younger than 2 years.

Plague

Although plague is endemic in rodents, it occurs very rarely in humans in the western United States, South America, Africa, the Middle East, and Central and Southeast Asia. Although vaccine reactions are common, the parenteral-killed plague bacillus vaccine should be considered by travelers to plague-endemic areas where it is difficult to avoid rodents and fleas.

Viral Encephalitis

Japanese encephalitis is a mosquito-borne illness endemic to Central and Southeast Asia, especially where rice culture and pig farming are common. An inactivated vaccine is available. Tick-borne encephalitis occurs in Russia and Central and Eastern Europe, where risks are increased in forested areas and by ingesting unpasteurized dairy products from infected animals. Although effective vaccines are available, vaccination is not necessary for most travelers.

Recommended Vaccines for Both Travelers and Nontravelers

Polio is prevalent in the developing world. Thus, previously immunized adult travelers should receive a booster dose of the oral live or parenteral enhanced inactivated polio vaccine. Measles, mumps, and rubella are also common in the developing world. For those born after 1956 without measles immunity, a dose of the live, attenuated measles vaccine is recommended before travel. The schedule for tetanus and diphtheria boosters should be accelerated to 5-year intervals for travelers who will be at risk of dirty wounds. All of these vaccines should also be part of a routine immunization schedule in nontravelers.

DISEASES FOR WHICH CHEMOPROPHYLAXIS IS RECOMMENDED

Malaria

Most cases of severe malaria are caused by the parasite *Plasmodium falciparum*. Travelers should understand that no antimalarial is 100% effective. Therefore, they should minimize the risk of mosquito bites by wearing long-sleeved clothing and using insect repellents containing DEET (*N,N*-diethyl-meta-toluamide) on the skin. Mosquito nets should be used while sleeping. In those areas in which the organisms are sensitive, the drug of choice remains chloroquine at 300 mg per week from 2 weeks before until 4 weeks after travel. Chloroquine resistance is increasing in Africa, Southeast Asia, India, South America, and Oceania, with multidrug-resistant strains appearing in some areas. Mefloquine is available for chloroquine-resistant malaria and is the drug of choice for most regions of the world except for certain Caribbean areas, parts of Central America, and the Middle East. Mefloquine is given at 250 mg weekly, from 2 weeks before entry until 4 weeks after departure from the malarious region. Drug side effects include gastrointestinal upset, dizziness, and, rarely, seizures and convulsions. Mefloquine should not be used in children who weigh <15 kg, in travelers taking β-blockers or drugs that alter cardiac conduction, and in travelers with epilepsy or psychiatric disease. Doxycycline at 100 mg per day for 1 to 2 days before and 4 weeks after travel is an alternative drug for chloroquine-resistant malaria. For mefloquine- and doxycycline-intolerant travelers, chloroquine may be used, and the individual is instructed to start taking pyrimethamine-sulfadoxine if malaria symptoms arise, although this agent may cause fatal reactions in 1 in 20,000 users. Resistance to pyrimethamine-sulfadoxine is now reported in Southeast Asia, in the Amazon basin, and in sub-Saharan Africa. Primaquine at 45 mg per week for 8 weeks is indicated to eradicate the asymptomatic extraerythrocytic stage of *Plasmodium vivax* and *Plasmodium ovale* after the traveler leaves the endemic area, although testing for glucose-6-phosphate dehydrogenase should be performed to prevent drug-induced hemolysis.

Leptospirosis

Leptospirosis is transmitted by water contaminated by the urine of infected animals. In rare instances (e.g., military jungle maneuvers), doxycycline at 200 mg per week may have prophylactic efficacy.

DISEASES REQUIRING TREATMENT DURING TRAVEL

Traveler's Diarrhea

Traveler's diarrhea attack rates in travelers to Latin America, Africa, the Middle East, or Asia are 30% to 70%, with the usual onset of symptoms occurring within 2 to 3 days of arrival. Diarrhea usually persists for 3 to 4 days and rarely longer than 1 week. Causes of traveler's diarrhea include enterotoxigenic *Escherichia coli*, shigellae, salmonellae, *Campylobacter jejuni*, *Yersinia enterocolitica*, *Giardia lamblia*, *Entamoeba histolytica*, *Cryptosporidium* species, and *Cyclospora* species. Vaccines are still under development. Therefore, current prophylaxis rests on dietary discretion (e.g., avoiding tap water, ice, fresh vegetables, and salads). Bismuth subsalicylate taken four times daily in liquid (60 ml) or solid (two 300-mg tablets) form decreases the incidence of traveler's diarrhea by 50%. Routine use of prophylactic antibiotics is not recommended for most travelers because of the concerns about possible side effects and the existence of antibiotic-resistant organisms. However, certain high-risk travelers who cannot tolerate dehydration or travelers on brief trips who cannot miss scheduled appointments may be given prophylactic doxycycline, trimethoprim-sulfamethoxazole, or norfloxacin, which can reduce the incidence of traveler's diarrhea by 90%.

Patients affected with traveler's diarrhea should begin treatment at the onset of symptoms. Maintenance of hydration with glucose and salt solutions is essential. Packets of oral rehydration salts containing glucose, sodium chloride, potassium chloride, and sodium citrate have been developed by the World Health Organization. Opiates (e.g., loperamide and diphenoxylate with atropine) may be used for mild to moderate traveler's diarrhea for up to 3 days, although they should be avoided in patients with bloody diarrhea or high fever. Bismuth subsalicylate taken every 30 minutes can reduce diarrhea, but it is not as effective as the opiate agents. Prompt initiation of a 3-day course of twice-daily antibiotics (e.g., ciprofloxacin, 500 mg; trimethoprim, 160 mg/sulfamethoxazole, 800 mg; trimethoprim, 200 mg alone; doxycycline, 100 mg; norfloxacin, 400 mg) can shorten the duration of symptoms of severe traveler's diarrhea. Synergistic therapeutic effects may be obtained by combining an antibiotic course with an antidiarrheal agent.

Altitude Sickness

Rapid ascent to altitudes above 8000 feet can produce insomnia, headache, nausea, vomiting, and pulmonary or cerebral edema, which are related to the degree of exertion and the altitude attained. Sleep may increase the symptoms as a result of decreased vascular integrity associated with hypoventilation-induced hypoxia. Prevention of altitude sickness is best accomplished by slowing the ascent. Acetazolamide, which induces metabolic acidosis with compensatory respiratory alkalosis, and dexamethasone decrease the incidence of altitude sickness. For pulmonary or cerebral edema, oxygen is administered at 6 to 12 liters per minute and descent is immediate. Dexamethasone, acetazolamide, or nifedipine may reduce symptoms but should not be used to delay descent.

Typhus

Treatment of the rare condition typhus with tetracycline or chloramphenicol is curative.

DISEASES WITHOUT IMMUNOPROPHYLAXIS OR TREATMENT

Hepatitis E

Hepatitis E is endemic and epidemic in India, Pakistan, China, Mongolia, Hong Kong, North Africa, and Mexico. It has an incubation period of 45 days. Hepatitis E infection has a 15% to 20% mortality in pregnant women. ISG from sources in the United States is not protective against infection.

Human Immunodeficiency Virus

Human immunodeficiency virus (HIV) infection rates are high in Africa, India, and Southeast Asia. Risk factors for HIV infection include intravenous drug abuse, use of infected blood products, and sexual contact. Live viral vaccines should not be given to HIV-infected patients who have symptoms or CD4 counts of <200 cells per μl.

DISEASES IN THE RETURNING TRAVELER

Asymptomatic Illness

Travelers who experienced a febrile or diarrheal illness overseas may require a screening evaluation on their return, including complete blood count, liver chemistry determinations, tuberculin testing, fecal ova and parasites examination, and specific serologic tests for indigenous diseases, even if they are asymptomatic. The presence of eosinophilia suggests possible filariasis, liver flukes, or intestinal helminth infection.

Symptomatic Illness

Travelers who return with a febrile illness should be evaluated for possible malaria, amebic liver abscess, enteric fever, hepatitis, and tuberculosis. Persistent diarrhea is the most common symptom evaluated by gastroenterologists in returning travelers. If diarrhea lasts longer than 2 weeks, *Salmonella, Shigella,* or *Campylobacter* organisms should be considered; northern travel raises the possibility of *Y enterocolitica;* and antibiotic use suggests possible *Clostridium difficile* infection. Persistent *E coli* infections are not detectable by standard cultures. If no agent can be identified, an empiric course of therapy with trimethoprim-sulfamethoxazole or ciprofloxacin should be considered. In more prolonged diarrhea, evaluation for ova and parasites should be initiated by obtaining three fresh stool samples. Some cases of giardiasis may require duodenal aspiration or biopsy or use of the string test to detect small intestinal organisms. Therapy for proven or suspected *Giardia* infection includes quinacrine or metronidazole. *E histolytica* presents with bloody diarrhea, mucus, and hematophagous trophozoites in the stool. Chronic nondysenteric diarrhea may be associated with *E histolytica* cyst passage, but use of antiamebic therapy in this setting is controversial. *Isospora belli* is a rare cause of chronic diarrhea and is treated with trimethoprim-sulfamethoxazole. *Cryptosporidium* infection usually produces self-limited diarrhea in immunocompetent individuals. *Cyclospora* species produce chronic diarrhea, fatigue, and weight loss in travelers from Nepal, but no specific treatment is available. Intestinal helminths (e.g., *Ascaris*, hookworm, *Trichuris*) and *Strongyloides* organisms should be treated specifically. *Schistosoma mansoni* is diagnosed by serologic testing and rectal biopsy. Tropical sprue is considered in a traveler with diarrhea and malabsorption. The D-xylose test result is abnormal and jejunal fluid is culture-positive for several aerobic organisms including *Klebsiella*, *Enterobacter*, and *E coli*. After being confirmed by a biopsy of the small intestine, tropical sprue is treated with tetracycline and folate. Some patients report persistent diarrhea and malabsorption and exhibit flattened intestinal villi. Although this post-travel syndrome may be prolonged, the prognosis is good for ultimate recovery.

CHAPTER 24

Nosocomial Infections and Risks to Health Care Providers

HOSPITAL EPIDEMIOLOGY

Acquisition of Nosocomial Infections

Bacteria are the most common causes of nosocomial infections, but viruses, fungi, mycobacteria, and parasites also are transmitted in the health care setting. Most nosocomial infections arise from endogenous sources within the patients, and the likelihood of transmission is determined by organism pathogenicity, virulence, invasiveness, and the inoculating dose. Certain infections, such as those caused by *Legionella pneumophila*, may arise from exogenous reservoirs such as cooling towers or shower heads. Organisms may be spread by contact (e.g., methicillin-resistant staphylococci from the hands), droplets (e.g., rubella), or common vehicle (e.g., contaminated catheters or endoscopes), or be airborne (e.g., aspergillosis). Increasingly, nosocomial pathogens are identified as resistant bacteria and fungi.

Nosocomial infections occur in 3% to 5% of hospitalized patients; nosocomial pneumonias are most common. The mortality rate of nosocomial infections is 20% to 50%. Risk factors for hospital-acquired pneumonias include age older than 70 years, chronic lung disease, decreased mental status, chest surgery, acid suppression, frequent change of ventilator circuits, and the fall and winter seasons. Nosocomial pneumonia is usually caused by more than one organism, with gram-negative rods involved in >60% of cases. Surgical wound infections are the second most common nosocomial infection and usually are caused by *Staphylococcus aureus*. Increases in postoperative antibiotic-resistant gram-positive bacteria, gram-negative bacteria, coagulase-negative staphylococci, and yeasts have been noted. Risk factors for surgical wound infections include length of preoperative stay, length of operation, use of drains, remote infections, age, timing of antibiotics, and illness severity. Other nosocomial infections include primary bloodstream infections relating to catheters and invasive procedures, and urinary infections that most commonly occur in women or in patients with urinary catheters.

Infection Control

The most basic component of all isolation programs is hand washing before and after every patient contact, although compliance with this recommendation has been poor. Beyond this, there are six isolation categories for which implementation depends on the severity and cause of patient illness. Strict isolation is recommended for highly contagious diseases spread by air and contact (e.g., varicella, pneumonic plague, and viral hemorrhagic fever) and requires a private room with negative-pressure ventilation and masks, gowns, and gloves for health care workers. Contact isolation is recommended for diseases spread by contact (e.g., staphylococcal, herpes simplex, and group A streptococcal skin infections) and requires masks, gowns, and gloves. Respiratory isolation is needed for airborne pathogens (e.g., measles and meningococcus), and a private room and masks are required. Tuberculosis (TB) isolation requires a private room, negative-pressure ventilation, and disposable particulate respirator masks. Enteric precautions are needed for diseases transmitted by pathogens in feces (e.g., hepatitis A [HAV], *Salmonella* species, or *Shigella* species), whereas drainage and secretion precautions prevent transmission of pathogens from purulent secretions. Recommendations for these two categories include gloves and gowns. Universal precautions dictate that all blood and body fluid samples should be handled by gloved personnel. Protective eye or face shields and gowns should be worn if splashing or spraying of fluids is possible. Health care workers with weeping skin lesions should refrain from patient or equipment contact. Often, a patient's diagnosis will not be known. In these cases, the Body Substance Isolation protocol recommends barrier precautions, gloves, gowns, masks, and eyewear to prevent contact between health care workers and all moist body substances.

Health care workers should be immunized against measles, mumps, rubella, diphtheria, pertussis, tetanus, and hepatitis B (HBV) and should receive influenza vaccine annually. If a health care worker is exposed to a potential pathogen, first aid should be performed, including washing of the wound. The exposure should be categorized as high- or low-risk for human immunodeficiency virus (HIV) and HBV transmission. High-risk exposures include needle stick or scalpel injuries with patient blood contact; low-risk exposures include needle sticks from subcutaneous or piggyback injections. For high-risk exposure, HBV and HIV

TABLE 24-1
Indications for Isoniazid Prophylaxis

Any age
    A positive tuberculin skin test and any one of the following:
        Human immunodeficiency virus seropositivity
        Recent conversion of the tuberculin skin test (<2 yrs)
        Abnormal findings on a chest radiograph compatible with old or healed
            tuberculosis
        Presence of a medical risk factor increasing the chance of developing active
            tuberculosis (e.g., diabetes, renal failure, immunosuppression, malignancy,
            silicosis, weight loss, intravenous drug abuse)
        Close contact with someone with active tuberculosis
<35 years of age
    A positive tuberculin skin test, regardless of duration of skin-test positivity

serologic testing of the patient and health care worker is performed at the time of exposure. Additional HIV testing of the health care worker is performed at 6 weeks, 12 weeks, 6 months, and 12 months.

TUBERCULOSIS

Nosocomial transmission of TB has occurred from patients with draining ulcers, those with osteomyelitis, and those undergoing bronchoscopy for unexplained pulmonary infiltrates. In addition, outbreaks of multidrug-resistant TB have been reported on HIV wards. Measures to prevent the spread of TB have been widely implemented by hospitals, but many nosocomial TB outbreaks result from breaches in standard infection control procedures and from improperly functioning isolation rooms. Health care workers should be screened annually for TB exposure through a tuberculin skin test, with workers in high-risk situations undergoing screening every 3 to 6 months. Workers with positive skin test results should be evaluated regularly for active TB with chest radiography. In patients without active TB who are younger than 35 years, isoniazid prophylaxis (300 mg daily) is given for 6 to 12 months (Table 24-1). This regimen is also recommended for workers of any age who are HIV-positive, who have had TB skin test conversion within the past 2 years, who have findings on chest radiographs consistent with old TB, who have a medical risk factor for acquiring TB, or who associate with a TB-infected individual.

BLOOD-BORNE PATHOGENS

Human Immunodeficiency Virus

Percutaneous injuries (84%) are the predominant mode for transmission of HIV to health care workers, followed by mucocutaneous exposure to blood containing HIV (13%), and combined mucocutaneous and percutaneous blood exposure (3%). Percutaneous injuries occur in 7% of operating room cases and occur most commonly from suture needles, from manually holding the tissue, or from instruments held by coworkers. Medical students and house staff are exposed to HIV-positive blood at a rate of 9.5% per person per year. In this group, universal precautions are practiced less than half of the time. Despite the prevalence of blood product contact, the risk of HIV transmission to a health care worker is small. In a survey of 3,400 orthopedists, 3.2% reported previous injury with sharp objects from HIV-positive patients, yet none developed HIV seropositivity.

Several interventions are recommended to reduce HIV transmission including refraining from recapping needles, use of puncture-resistant containers for disposal of sharp objects, and increased glove use (or even double gloving). For workers who sustain percutaneous exposure to known HIV-positive blood, HIV tests should be performed immediately and at 6 weeks, 12 weeks, 6 months, and 12 months. The effectiveness of chemoprophylaxis with zidovudine is unproved, but offering the drug to exposed health care workers has evolved into standard practice. When given, zidovudine is administered in a dose of 200 mg every 4 hours, for 6 weeks, beginning within 4 to 6 hours of exposure. Zidovudine may also be given for 24 to 48 hours to the exposed worker while awaiting HIV serology test results on the patient. Zidovudine is not indicated after exposure to blood splashes, exposure to nonbloody fluid, or penetrating injuries from nonbloody instruments.

Hepatotropic Viruses

Hepatitis A

HAV is an enteric RNA virus that produces a brief viremic period followed by viral replication and fecal shedding. The process lasts about 28 days, with fecal shedding over the final 10 to 14 days. HAV is primarily spread through contaminated food or water, although parenteral transmission rarely is reported. Acute HAV infection is documented by the detection of IgM antibodies to HAV (anti-HAV IgM), whereas the detection of IgG antibodies to HAV (anti-HAV IgG) indicates prior exposure with recovery. Risk factors for HAV infection include homosexuality, drug abuse, contact with others with hepatitis or with children in day care, or foreign travel. If universal precautions are followed, the risks to health care workers are small. In the rare instance of needle exposure, immune serum globulin (ISG) is given at 0.02 ml per kg within 10 days of exposure. HAV vaccine (1 injection with a booster at 6 to 12 months) should be offered to health care providers at high risk.

Hepatitis B

HBV is a DNA virus that is spread horizontally by parenteral and sexual exposure, vertically by perinatal exposure, and in settings of close personal contact such as households and institutions. The diagnosis of acute HBV infection is made by the detection of IgM antibodies to hepatitis B core antigen (anti-HBc IgM), whereas chronic HBV infection is defined by the persistence of hepatitis B surface antigen (HBsAg) positivity. Furthermore, active replication is indicated by high serum levels of hepatitis B e antigen (HBeAg) and HBV DNA. Antibodies to HBeAg (anti-HBe) should not be considered protective against infection as long as HBsAg is present. Anti-HBc IgM is a specific marker of acute infection, although rare cases of chronic hepatitis with high levels of viral replication exhibit this antibody. Persons who have received HBV vaccine are positive for antibodies to HBsAg (anti-HBs) only and are protected against new HBV infection in 95% of cases.

Risk factors for the acquisition of HBV include drug abuse, sexual contact with multiple partners, household contacts and sexual contact with HBV carriers, infants of HBV-infected mothers, exposure in institutions for the developmentally disabled, transfusion of certain plasma products, hemodialysis, exposure to blood products through one's employment, and residence in areas of high HIV endemicity. The risk of needle-stick transmission after exposure to HBsAg-positive blood is 7% to 30%. High HBV replicative status (HBeAg positive, high levels of HBV DNA) confers an increased risk of transmission. In the exposed worker who has not been vaccinated or who has inadequate titers of anti-HBs, prophylaxis with hepatitis B immune globulin (HBIG), 0.06 ml per kg, and revaccination is appropriate (Table 24-2). Booster injections are not currently recommended for HBV. However, in immunocompromised patients, a booster dose is indicated if anti-HBs titers are <10 mIU per ml. In the health care setting, HBV-infected health care workers should not perform procedures that put the patient at risk of contact with that worker's blood.

Hepatitis D virus (HDV, delta virus) is an RNA virus that infects and replicates only in the presence of HBsAg positivity. During acute infection, HDV antigen (Ag) and IgM antibodies to HDV (anti-HDV IgM) are present, whereas chronic infection is marked by the presence of HDV Ag and the absence of anti-HDV IgM. The primary recommendation for avoidance of HDV infection is adequate HBV vaccination. In exposed workers, HBIG therapy and HBV vaccination decreases the risk of HDV infection.

Hepatitis C

Hepatitis C virus (HCV) is an RNA virus transmitted by parenteral and other routes. HCV acquisition can occur via sexual transmission, but the risk is low. The presence of HIV infection may act as a cofactor for transmission of both HIV and HCV. Similarly, vertical maternal-to-fetal HCV transmission is rare unless the mother is also HIV positive. Both of these phenomena probably result from higher rates of HCV replication in HIV-positive women compared with those who are seronegative for HIV. HCV RNA is not present in saliva, urine, sweat, or semen. Current testing for HCV infection involves enzyme-linked immunosorbent assay (ELISA) or radioimmunoblot assay for HCV antibodies, but these tests measure only exposure and not necessarily active infection. Furthermore, anti-HCV positivity may not develop for up to 12 months after infection. Polymerase chain reaction (PCR) testing for HCV RNA is available in research institutions to document active viral replication.

Risk factors for HCV infection include drug abuse, blood transfusions, employment in a health care environment, and tattoos. Health care workers are at risk from needle sticks, with approximately a 10% transmission rate, and from body fluid exposures. ISG (0.06 ml per kg) should be given to persons with percutaneous exposure as soon as possible after exposure, although its efficacy in prevention of HCV infection is unknown. Future use of tests for active HCV replication (PCR for HCV RNA) may better define individuals who should receive ISG. Infected health care workers should observe universal precautions to prevent transmission to patients.

TABLE 24-2
Prophylaxis for Hepatitis B After Parenteral Exposure

EXPOSED PERSON	HBsAg-POSITIVE SOURCE	HBsAg-NEGATIVE SOURCE	SOURCE HBsAg UNKNOWN
Unvaccinated	HBIG × 1[a] and initiate HB vaccine[b]	Initiate HB vaccine[b]	Initiate HB vaccine[b]
Previously vaccinated, known responder	Test exposed person for anti-HBs: (1) if adequate,[c] no treatment; (2) if inadequate, HB vaccine booster dose	No treatment	No treatment
Previously vaccinated, known nonresponder	HBIG × 2 or HBIG × 1 + 1 dose of HB vaccine	No treatment	If known high-risk source, treat as if source HBsAg-positive
Previously vaccinated, response unknown	Test exposed person for anti-HBs: (1) if adequate,[c] no treatment; (2) if inadequate, HBIG × 1 + HB vaccine booster dose	No treatment	Test exposed person for anti-HBs: (1) if adequate,[c] no treatment; (2) if inadequate, HB vaccine booster dose

HBsAg = hepatitis B surface antigen; HBIG = hepatitis B immunoglobulin; HB = hepatitis B.
[a]HBIG; 0.06 ml/kg intramuscular given immediately after exposure.
[b]HB vaccine; first dose within 1 wk, second dose in 1 mo, third dose in 6 mos.
[c]Adequate anti-HBs is >10 mIU by radioimmunoassay or positive by enzyme immunoassay.

Non-A, Non-B, Non-C Hepatitis

The diagnosis of non-A, non-B, non-C hepatitis is reserved for persons with presumed viral hepatitis and negative serologic tests. Precautions and work restrictions for this entity are similar to those for HCV.

Cytomegalovirus

Cytomegalovirus (CMV) is a ubiquitous DNA virus to which many adults in the United States (30% to 100%) have evidence of prior exposure. Health care providers generally are not at high risk for CMV infection unless they are immunocompromised. In previously unexposed pregnant women, new CMV infection is teratogenic. Serologic tests (CMV IgM) are available, but diagnosis usually requires clinical evidence of invasive infection such as viral isolation from tissue or cytologic specimens. Universal precautions and good hand washing should be protective for health care workers. No work restrictions have been issued for infected care providers.

GASTROINTESTINAL PATHOGENS

Enteric Viruses

Rotavirus is an RNA virus that produces 30% to 50% of the cases of pediatric gastroenteritis as well as rare cases of diarrhea in adults. Infection most commonly occurs during the winter in children younger than 3 years of age and is associated with shedding of large amounts of virus in the stool for up to 3 weeks. Adherence to universal precautions, good hand washing, and meticulous housekeeping of the infected patient's room and linens help to prevent transmission.

Enteric Bacteria

Clostridium difficile

Clostridium difficile is responsible for 70% to 90% of antibiotic-associated colitis and 15% to 25% of antibiotic-associated diarrhea. This pathogen also may be transmitted by person-to-person contact, and carriage by and infection of hospital personnel has been documented. Adherence to universal precautions, hand washing, and use of gloves can prevent transmission.

Escherichia coli

Several groups of pathogenic *Escherichia coli* are known: enteropathogenic, enterotoxigenic, enteroinvasive, enteroadherent, and enterohemorrhagic. Transmission is by the fecal-oral route in areas of poor sanitation and commonly occurs in the summer. The diagnosis depends on a high index of suspicion; however, many laboratories now routinely culture specimens for this organism if the diarrhea is bloody. Observance of universal precautions and hand washing should prevent most transmission.

Salmonella Species

Salmonellae are gram-negative bacilli that cause gastroenteritis, most commonly in the summer and fall, in persons younger than 20 years and older than 70 years, often coincident with outbreaks of food poisoning. The major routes of transmission include person-to-person, via contaminated food (e.g., eggs), and via contaminated common sources (e.g., medications). Infections with *Salmonella* species are prevalent in health care facilities, with an attack rate tenfold higher than for other epidemics and a 7% to 9% mortality. The incubation period is typically 1 to 2 weeks but may be as long as 2 months. Diagnosis of infection is based on culture of organisms from the blood or stool. The presence of *Salmonella* organisms in the stool for longer than 1 year defines the chronic carrier state. Health care workers are at risk for person-to-person transmission, which can be minimized by adherence to universal precautions and good hand washing. Chronic carriers should be given 4 to 6 weeks of antibiotics to eradicate the infection. Chronic carriers with biliary tract disease should receive a 10- to 14-day course of antibiotics plus a cholecystectomy. Health care workers should not have patient contact during the period of fecal shedding.

Shigella Species

Shigellae are gram-negative bacilli that produce gastroenteritis, especially in children between 1 and 4 years of age, most often during the summer and fall. Transmission occurs by the fecal-oral route, and outbreaks may be foodborne or may occur in day care facilities. The diagnosis of shigellosis is made by stool culture. Prevention of transmission is by observance of universal precautions. Health care workers who are infected may have temporary limitations in their patient interactions, but fecal shedding is almost always complete within 1 month. Although usually self-limited, treatment of shigellosis with a quinolone or trimethoprim-sulfamethoxazole is recommended to prevent transmission.

Campylobacter Species

Campylobacter jejuni is responsible for 5% to 7% of cases of gastroenteritis in the United States and can occur in all age groups during the summer and fall. Transmission is by the fecal-oral route, sexual contact, raw milk, poultry, and contaminated water. Special stool culture techniques are necessary to detect *C jejuni*. Universal precautions should be observed. Occasionally, the infection may persist for 3 weeks. It is prudent to treat infected health care workers with erythromycin or a quinolone to reduce fecal excretion of the organism.

Vibrio Species

Vibrio cholerae is an enterotoxigenic pathogen that causes cholera, which is rare in the United States. Infection results from inadequately cooked or raw shellfish and usually occurs in the summer. In contrast, *Vibrio parahaemolyticus* is an enteroinvasive pathogen. These infections are rare in health care providers and can be prevented by universal precautions. Infected workers may be considered for antimicrobial therapy with tetracycline or trimethoprim-sulfamethoxazole.

Aeromonas Species

Clinical illness from *Aeromonas* organisms is more severe in children than in adults and is acquired from water, farm animals, or vegetables. Hand washing and universal precautions can prevent most transmission. Infected health care providers can be considered for tetracycline or trimethoprim-sulfamethoxazole treatment, although most individuals experience self-limited disease.

Yersinia enterocolitica

Transmission of *Yersinia enterocolitica* occurs by contaminated food or by person-to-person spread, with an incubation period of 2 to 11 days. Health care providers may acquire this infection and should observe universal precautions and hand washing. Food handlers should not work when ill.

CHAPTER 25

Structural Anomalies and Miscellaneous Disorders of the Esophagus

ESOPHAGEAL EMBRYOLOGY AND ANATOMY

A small diverticulum on the ventral surface of the foregut is first recognizable in the fourth week of gestation. It eventually separates into the esophagus and trachea. The esophageal circular muscle and myenteric plexus form in the sixth week, and the submucosal blood vessels develop by the seventh week. Epithelial tissue occludes the lumen in the seventh and eighth weeks. Esophageal recanalization occurs by the tenth week, and from the fourth through the ninth month, stratified squamous epithelial tissue develops.

The adult esophagus is 18 to 26 cm in length, with a diameter of 2 to 3 cm. The cervical esophagus extends from the pharyngoesophageal junction to the suprasternal notch (4 to 5 cm) and is bounded anteriorly by the trachea, posteriorly by the spine, and laterally by the carotids and the thyroid. The thoracic esophagus is posterior to the trachea from T4 to T8; crosses anterior to the aorta from T8 to T10; and passes at T10 through the diaphragmatic hiatus, which consists of the muscular crura, the median arcuate ligament, and collagen and elastic fibers of the phrenoesophageal membrane. The abdominal esophagus is short (0.5 to 2.5 cm). The squamocolumnar mucosal junction is visibly located where the pink-gray lining with the linearly oriented vessels of the esophagus changes to the red-orange granular appearance of the gastric cardia. The cervical esophagus is supplied with blood by the inferior thyroid artery with smaller contributions from other sources; the thoracic esophagus is supplied by the aorta, right intercostal, and bronchial arteries; the abdominal esophagus is supplied by the left gastric, short gastric, and left inferior phrenic arteries. Fine intraepithelial channels drain into a subepithelial superficial venous plexus, which then drain into deep intrinsic submucosal veins that communicate with their gastric counterparts. In the thoracic esophagus, venous blood passes into the azygos, hemiazygos, and intercostal veins. There is a high-pressure watershed zone between the portal and azygos systems at the gastroesophageal junction that is prone to the formation of varices in portal hypertension. These dilated veins or varices serve as collateral channels to return portal blood to the systemic circulation. Thus, varices from portal hypertension extend only to the level of the aortic arch, where the azygos circulation drains centrally. The parasympathetic innervation of the esophagus is by the left and right vagus that intertwine with sympathetic fibers to form the esophageal plexus. Sympathetic innervation is provided by the superior cervical ganglion, sympathetic chain, major splanchnic nerve, thoracic aortic plexus, and celiac ganglion. Lymphatics drain to the deep cervical, internal jugular, tracheal, tracheobronchial, posterior mediastinal, and pericardial lymph nodes.

The esophageal wall is composed of the mucosa, submucosa, muscularis externa, and adventitia. The absence of a serosal layer allows easy spread of esophageal malignancies. The mucosa consists of nonkeratinized squamous epithelium, the lamina propria, and the muscularis mucosae. The inner epithelial border is irregular because of projections of the lamina propria called *dermal papillae*. Foci of hyperplastic epithelial cells with intranuclear glycogen (glycogen acanthosis) are seen as focal white elevations in some persons. Epithelial cytotoxic T cells and macrophages, and lamina propria helper T cells and B lymphocytes represent the gut-associated lymphoid tissue of the esophagus. Striated muscle tissue makes up the inferior pharyngeal constrictor, cricopharyngeus, and proximal 6 to 8 cm of the esophagus, and is arranged into an inner circular and outer longitudinal layer. The distal esophagus is composed of circular and longitudinal smooth muscle layers. The physiologic lower esophageal sphincter is immediately cephalad to the diaphragmatic hiatus. Below the diaphragm, the inner circular muscle thickens and oblique fibers from the greater curvature of the stomach are found. The myenteric plexus lies between the circular and longitudinal muscle layers. A submucosal plexus is seen as an irregular network of nerve bundles near the inner coat of the muscularis externa. In the lower esophageal sphincter, nerve endings with varicosities are observed to interact with differentiated cells (i.e., interstitial cells of Cajal) that initiate and coordinate contraction.

DEVELOPMENTAL ANOMALIES

Tracheoesophageal Fistulae and Atresias

Etiology and Pathogenesis

During embryogenesis, disruption in the elongation and separation of the esophagus from the trachea may occur. Tracheoesophageal fistulae (TEFs) result from incomplete fusion of the tracheoesophageal septum, whereas esophageal atresia occurs when esophageal elongation outstrips the foregut proliferative capacity. Five types of TEFs are described, with the most common being a lower esophageal pouch fistula with proximal esophageal atresia. These disorders are commonly associated with prematurity and hydramnios as well as with other congenital abnormalities (e.g., imperforate anus, malrotation, duodenal atresia, and annular pancreas).

Clinical Features, Diagnosis, and Course

Symptoms present in infancy and include regurgitation, respiratory distress during feedings, pneumonia, and abdominal distention. Atresia may be suspected if it is impossible to pass an esophageal catheter. A TEF is suggested by radiographic demonstration of a gasless abdomen or increased distention, depending on the anomaly. The diagnosis of TEF may be based on findings of air insufflation of the esophagus or cautious contrast radiography. The recommended treatment of TEF or atresia is early surgical repair. Long atretic segments may require colonic interposition. Long-term sequelae after surgical repair of TEFs and atresias include esophageal dysmotility, gastroesophageal reflux, and respiratory complications.

Congenital Esophageal Stenoses and Duplications

Etiology and Pathogenesis

Congenital stenosis results from failure of the normal embryonic separation of the trachea and esophagus and may not be diagnosed until late in childhood or adulthood. Duplications arise because of failed coalescence of embryonic lumenal vacuoles during the recanalization phase, with formation of cysts or parallel tubular channels within the esophageal wall that communicate with the lumen at one or both ends. Cystic duplications are the second most common benign esophageal tumor and occur within the esophageal wall, most commonly in the distal esophagus (60%). Gastric, bronchogenic, and neuroenteric cysts as well as cysts with squamous or respiratory epithelia may be found in the esophagus. Many patients with duplication present early in life. Foregut duplication cysts are associated with cervical and thoracic vertebral anomalies.

Clinical Features, Diagnosis, and Management

Symptoms of esophageal stenosis include regurgitation, slow eating, and dysphagia to solids. Barium swallow radiographs show segmental stenosis with ring-like folds, which are also observed on endoscopic examination. Tubular duplications present with symptoms of obstruction or gastroesophageal reflux and are diagnosed from barium swallow radiographs or endoscopic findings. Proximal duplication cysts present in infancy with potentially fatal tracheobronchial compression. Distal esophageal cysts produce dysphagia, epigastric discomfort, chest pain, cough, dyspnea, or regurgitation. Chest radiography may demonstrate the duplication cyst as a mediastinal mass, which can be further defined by barium swallow radiography, ultrasound, or computed tomography. On endoscopic examination, a duplication cyst appears as a soft, compressible extrinsic mass and exhibits a cystic structure on endoscopic ultrasound studies. Resective surgery is recommended for many patients with stenosis or duplication; however, selected patients with stenosis will respond to bougienage. Large duplication cysts may require marsupialization rather than resection. Malignant degeneration within tubular or cystic duplications has been reported.

Esophageal Rings and Webs

Etiology and Pathogenesis

Lower esophageal mucosal rings (i.e., Schatzki's rings) are located at the squamocolumnar junction and consist of mucosa (squamous on the proximal side, columnar or squamous on the distal side) and submucosa. True mucosal rings are circumferential, symmetrical, and >3 mm thick and are associated with a hiatal hernia. In contrast, lower esophageal muscular rings occur 1.5 cm proximal to the squamocolumnar junction and consist of an annular ring of hypertrophied or hypertonic muscle with overlying squamous mucosa. Muscular rings are broader (4 to 5 mm) and are associated with esophageal dysmotility, gastroesophageal reflux, and hiatal hernias. Esophageal webs are thin, transverse squamous mucosal membranes that occur in the upper and middle esophagus with advancing age. Classically, webs that involve the postcricoid esophagus (usually the anterior wall) may be associated with iron deficiency anemia (Plummer-Vinson or Paterson-Kelly syndrome) and have a propensity for development of pharyngeal and esophageal carcinoma. Single or multiple midesophageal webs are believed to be congenital.

Clinical Features, Diagnosis, and Management

Most esophageal mucosal rings are asymptomatic, but if <20 mm in diameter, they may produce intermittent dysphagia in patients older than 40 years. Rings <13 mm in diameter regularly cause solid food dysphagia. Barium swallow radiography is the diagnostic test of choice for esophageal rings. Their detection is enhanced by a Valsalva's maneuver during the swallow or with use of a barium tablet or marshmallow. Endoscopy also may define a Schatzki's ring. Muscular rings occasionally produce dysphagia. Barium swallow radiography in these patients demonstrates a broader, smooth, symmetrical narrowing that may vary in caliber. In some cases, esophageal manometry shows lower esophageal sphincter hypertension that correlates with the level of the ring. The majority of symptomatic patients with mucosal or muscular rings are treated with sequential bougienage to a lumenal diameter of 16.5 to 20.0 mm, although some mucosal rings may require endoscopic cautery incision. Patients with both upper and midesophageal webs present with infrequent intermittent dysphagia that may be treated with bougienage, transendoscopic incision, or rarely, surgery.

Miscellaneous Developmental Esophageal Anomalies

Bronchopulmonary Foregut Malformations

Bronchopulmonary foregut malformations develop when respiratory cell rests or a portion of the lung bud arises from the esophagus. With incomplete involution of the abnormal respiratory tissue, a communication with the gastrointestinal tract can result. Infants may present with respiratory distress or congestive heart failure, whereas older children and adults develop pneumonia, bronchiectasis, hemoptysis, gastrointestinal bleeding, and dysphagia. Associated congenital defects are present in 40% of children. Barium swallow radiography, angiography, and bronchography are useful for diagnosis; the treatment of this condition is surgical resection.

Vascular Compression of the Esophagus

Aortic arch vessel abnormalities are common and result from disruption of the normal developmental formation of the great vessels. Dysphagia lusoria is the symptomatic compression of the esophagus by an aortic arch anomaly, usually an aberrant right subclavian artery. Patients present in infancy, childhood, or adulthood. The physical examination may reveal a reduced right radial pulse. Barium swallow radiography shows an oblique filling defect above the aortic arch. The condition is corrected surgically, although adults with mild dysphagia can be treated with dietary modification. Other vascular anomalies include esophageal compression by an anomalous vertebral artery and right aortic arch, double aortic arch, right aortic arch with patent ductus arteriosus, cervical aortic arch, and aberrant left pulmonary artery.

Heterotopic Gastric Mucosa

Heterotopic gastric mucosa appears at endoscopy as patches of red-orange mucosa typically in the proximal esophagus below the cricopharyngeus (inlet patch), although the condition may present at any esophageal site. Most cases are asymptomatic, although the acid-secretory capabilities of these patches may produce esophagitis. Other complications include cervical webs or rings, TEF, and adenocarcinoma.

DIVERTICULA

Etiology and Pathogenesis

Pharyngoesophageal, or Zenker's, diverticula form by protrusion of posterior hypopharyngeal mucosa between the inferior pharyngeal constrictor and the cricopharyngeus proximal to the esophagus. Development of Zenker's diverticula may stem from high hypopharyngeal pressures during swallowing that are caused by a poorly compliant cricopharyngeus. Diverticula also develop in the middle or distal esophagus and usually are secondary to esophageal dysmotility, whereas distal diverticula occur in patients who have long-standing esophageal strictures. In children, esophageal diverticula may develop proximal to a stricture induced by the ingestion of a foreign body. Esophageal intramural pseudodiverticulosis is a rare condition in which multiple small pseudodiverticula in the esophageal wall form from dilation of the submucosal glands secondary to stasis and inflammation. Esophageal strictures are seen in 70% to 90% of these patients; esophageal candidiasis and prior corrosive injury have been reported as risk factors.

Clinical Features, Diagnosis, and Management

Patients with Zenker's diverticula present after age 50 years with dysphagia for solids and liquids, regurgitation of undigested food, cough, halitosis, gurgling, a neck mass, weight loss, and aspiration pneumonia. Barium swallow radiography with lateral views helps to confirm the diagnosis. Surgery is the recommended treatment. Successful operative procedures include diverticulectomy with or without cricopharyngeal myotomy, diverticular inversion with myotomy, and myotomy alone, as well as endoscopic division of the septum between the diverticulum and proximal esophagus. Complications of Zenker's diverticula include development of squamous cell carcinoma, spindle cell carcinoma, and benign tumors.

Esophageal diverticula and pseudodiverticula are seen on barium swallow radiographs or upper endoscopic studies. Symptoms from these conditions include dysphagia, regurgitation, and substernal chest pain. They often result from the primary stricture rather than the diverticula; thus, surgical diverticulectomy is rarely needed. Dilation of strictures, antireflux therapy, and calcium channel antagonists may be useful in selected cases.

ESOPHAGEAL HIATAL HERNIAS

Etiology and Pathogenesis

A hiatal hernia is defined as the cephalad displacement of the esophagogastric junction into the thorax by a distance of 2 cm or more. They usually appear in later life, more often in women. They are believed to be secondary to esophageal contraction from reflux-induced injury, increased intra-abdominal pressure, and atrophy or weakening of the hiatal region. The phrenoesophageal membrane inserts 2 to 3 cm above the diaphragmatic hiatus and anchors the esophagogastric junction. It is this attachment that has been postulated to stretch with hiatal hernia formation. Straining during defecation while on a low-fiber diet may predispose to hiatal hernia development. The condition is more common in persons with peptic ulcer disease, scleroderma, kyphosis, and ankylosing spondylitis. The precise relationships among hiatal hernia, lower esophageal sphincter function, and gastroesophageal reflux are uncertain; however, it is known that most patients with hiatal hernias are asymptomatic, whereas most patients with symptomatic gastroesophageal reflux have hiatal hernias.

Clinical Features, Diagnosis, and Management

Asymptomatic hiatal hernias need no evaluation. A minority of patients with hiatal hernias present with gastroesophageal reflux, stricture formation, occult or gross hemorrhage, and, rarely, incarceration with pain. Barium swallow radiography will define the hernia, but endoscopy is indicated in potentially complicated cases for control of hemorrhage, stricture dilation, or diagnosis of Barrett's esophagus. Proper medical therapy with acid-suppressing agents or prokinetic drugs controls reflux-induced symptoms so well that surgery is needed in <5% of cases.

CAUSTIC ESOPHAGEAL INJURY

Etiology and Pathogenesis

The ingestion of caustic substances, either accidental or as a result of a suicide gesture, may produce esophageal damage within seconds. First-degree burns produce mucosal hyperemia and edema but no scars. Second-degree burns extend into the muscle layers and produce exudation, mucosal loss, and ulcerations that may progress to scarring over weeks to months. Third-degree burns are transmural, with erosion into the mediastinum, pleural, or peritoneal cavity. Fistula formation and death are possible.

Alkaline agents such as lye, Clinitest tablets (containing copper sulfate, sodium hydroxide, and sodium carbonate), and disc batteries (containing potassium or sodium hydroxide) produce liquefaction necrosis of the esophagus depending on the concentration and duration of contact. Blood vessel thrombosis, edema, cell necrosis, and neutrophilic infiltration are followed by bacterial colonization. Ammonia and bleach generally do not cause severe esophageal damage. Acids in toilet bowl cleaners (e.g., sulfuric, hydrochloric, or phosphoric acid), swimming pool additives, antirust compounds, and soldering fluxes produce coagulation necrosis of the mucosa that may limit penetration of acid into the esophageal wall. In contrast to alkali ingestion, the stomach usually bears the brunt of injury with acid ingestion.

Clinical Features, Diagnosis, and Management

Symptoms of caustic ingestion include burning of the lips, tongue, or pharynx; dysphagia; odynophagia; drooling; vomiting; and dyspnea. Hematemesis and abdominal pain suggest possible gastric injury, whereas hoarseness, wheezing, and stridor are suggestive of airway involvement. Patients with third-degree burns may present with shock, mediastinitis, or peritoneal findings. Initial diagnostic studies should include chest and abdominal radiography, which may detect pneumonitis, pleural effusions, mediastinal and subdiaphragmatic air, and in selected cases, the ingested battery. After intravenous sedation, upper endoscopy is gently performed to assess the extent of damage. Barium swallow radiography should not be performed because of the irritating effects of barium in the setting of perforation and because of the inability to subsequently visualize the mucosa with endoscopy. Computed tomography may further define the extent of damage or detect the development of an abscess.

The first step in the management of patients who have ingested caustic substances is to stabilize the airway. If respiratory distress is present, endotracheal intubation is indicated. Induced emesis is contraindicated and oral intake is prohibited. Intravenous fluids are provided as necessary. The use of antibiotics is reasonable in patients with second- and third-degree burns. The role of corticosteroids is controversial, although most recent studies show no benefit. If they are used, corticosteroids (e.g., prednisone, 60 mg daily for 3 weeks) should be reserved for patients with circumferential burns with a high likelihood of stricture formation. Sucralfate has been shown to be of benefit in one uncontrolled trial. Gentle esophageal dilation is recommended 2 to 4 weeks after caustic ingestion if dysphagia is present. Patients with impending or frank perforation require surgery, which may include esophagectomy and colonic interposition. For disc battery ingestion, immediate endoscopic removal is indicated, if the battery remains in the esophagus, to minimize the burn area and decrease the risk of perforation.

Complications of caustic ingestion include esophageal stricture, carcinoma, and gastric damage. Esophageal stenosis may develop as early as 2 weeks postingestion, and most commonly occurs after full-thickness circumferential burns. After lye ingestion, the risk of squamous cell esophageal carcinoma increases 1000-fold, with a latent period of several decades; therefore, surveillance endoscopy may be indicated in this patient subset. Gastric outlet obstruction may develop 2 to 6 weeks after the ingestion of acid substances. Squamous metaplasia and gastric carcinoma have been reported, but the causative role of ingested caustics is uncertain.

MEDICATION-INDUCED ESOPHAGEAL INJURY

Etiology and Pathogenesis

Whether medications cause esophageal damage depends on several factors. Round tablets take longer to pass through the esophagus than oval pills. Large volumes of water assist transit of gelatin-coated pills or capsules. Taking medications while supine increases the risk of delayed transit across the lower esophageal sphincter. In young patients, antibiotics are the most common cause of pill-induced damage, whereas medications commonly ingested, such as potassium, NSAIDs, and vitamin C, are more likely causes in the elderly. Most cases occur in patients without prior esophageal disease. There is a predilection for pills to lodge at the level of the aortic arch.

Clinical Features, Diagnosis, and Management

Odynophagia and dysphagia are the typical symptoms of pill-induced esophageal damage, usually occurring within hours of ingestion but occasionally days or weeks later. Substernal pain and hematemesis are sometimes reported. The diagnosis is confirmed by upper endoscopy, which often shows a discrete ulcer or ulcers with exudation in the middle esophagus. Biopsy specimens show inflammation and reactive hyperplasia. Barium swallow radiography may show ulceration or stricturing. Therapy focuses on removing the offending medication. Viscous lidocaine, antacids, and analgesics may be used to relieve discomfort. Esophageal dilation may be necessary for chronic stricture formation.

ESOPHAGEAL FOREIGN BODIES

Etiology and Pathogenesis

Populations at risk for foreign body ingestion include adults with dentures, patients with psychiatric illness, prisoners, and young children. Coins are most commonly ingested by children, whereas the most common esophageal foreign bodies in adults are chicken or fish bones. These items tend to lodge in the cervical esophagus, at the level of the aortic arch, above the lower esophageal sphincter, or proximal to a pre-existing stricture. Food impactions often occur in the setting of a Schatzki's ring.

Clinical Features, Diagnosis, and Management

Dysphagia is the most common symptom, followed by odynophagia, choking, drooling, coughing, dyspnea, and wheezing. Chest radiography may detect a radiopaque object or suggest soft-tissue swelling with a radiolucent foreign body. Upper endoscopy usually provides the diagnosis. Most foreign bodies pass through the gut uneventfully, but some objects require endoscopic, fluoroscopic, or surgical extraction. Blunt objects may be removed using a Foley catheter with fluoroscopic control. Endoscopy can be used to remove a broader range of objects; in many cases, an overtube should be used to prevent tracheal aspiration. If the foreign body has been present for a long period of time, surgery may be required for extraction, repair of perforation, drainage of an abscess, or closure of a fistula. Food impactions usually are associated with underlying esophageal disease. Esophageal relaxation with nitroglycerin or glucagon may allow spontaneous passage of the food bolus into the stomach. Upper endoscopy can remove impacted food or gently push it into the stomach if lumenal visualization is adequate. After the esophagus is cleared, acid suppression is begun; esophageal dilation is deferred until a later date. Rarely, surgery is necessary to clear a food impaction.

SYSTEMIC DISEASES THAT AFFECT THE ESOPHAGUS

There are a number of systemic diseases that affect the esophagus. The diseases and esophageal findings are listed in Table 25-1.

Sarcoidosis

Sarcoidosis rarely manifests as granulomatous esophagitis. Patients with sarcoidosis may exhibit dysphagia as a result of long strictures or esophageal dysmotility. More commonly, dysphagia in these patients results from gastroesophageal reflux, esophageal infection, or extrinsic compression by enlarged lymph nodes.

Crohn's Disease

Crohn's disease of the esophagus is extremely rare. Inflammation usually parallels the activity of the disease in other regions of the gastrointestinal tract. Dysphagia occasionally has been the presenting symptom of Crohn's disease; rarely, Crohn's esophagitis has been reported to be the sole manifestation of the disease. Symptoms of esophageal involvement include odynophagia, dysphagia, pyrosis, substernal chest pain, and fistulous tracts to the bronchi, mediastinum, or stomach. The diagnosis of esophageal Crohn's disease is difficult to establish. The esophagus may have a cobblestone appearance on barium radiography. Upper endoscopy is more useful in excluding other disorders, as diagnostic granulomas are rare. Corticosteroids usually are helpful, but sur-

TABLE 25-1
Effects of Systemic Diseases on the Esophagus

DISEASE	ESOPHAGEAL FINDINGS
Sarcoidosis	Long strictures
Crohn's disease	Aphthous ulcers, linear ulcers, impaired motility, strictures, sinus tracts
Behçet's disease	Superficial ulcers, diffuse esophagitis, perforated ulcers, severe stenosis
Graft-versus-host disease	Esophageal mucosal desquamation, webs, strictures, gastroesophageal reflux
Pemphigus vulgaris	Erythema, hemorrhagic bullae, esophageal mucosal desquamation
Bullous pemphigoid	Intraepidermal bullae, esophagitis dissecans superficialis
Benign mucous membrane pemphigoid	Bullae, webs, long strictures
Epidermolysis bullosa dystrophica	Bullae, blebs, ulceration with deep scarring, long strictures, spontaneous dissection

gical resection and esophagogastrostomy may be necessary if medications and bougienage are not successful.

Behçet's Disease

Manifestations of Behçet's disease include oral and genital aphthous ulcerations and ocular inflammation. Esophageal involvement may produce odynophagia, dysphagia, chest and epigastric pain, and hematemesis caused by erosions, diffuse esophagitis, perforated ulcers with mediastinal abscess, and severe esophageal stenosis, usually in the middle to distal esophagus. Endoscopic biopsy specimens show ulceration with nonspecific inflammation and neutrophilic infiltration. Some success in treating Behçet's disease has been reported with whole blood and plasma transfusions, transfer factor, corticosteroids, and cyclosporine.

Graft-Versus-Host Disease

Up to 40% of bone marrow transplant survivors develop chronic graft-versus-host disease (GVHD). GVHD esophagitis presents with odynophagia, dysphagia, pyrosis, and substernal chest pain. Infectious esophagitis complicating chronic immunosuppression is important in the differential diagnosis. Upper endoscopy in a GVHD patient typically reveals erythematous, friable, and peeling mucosa (i.e., desquamative esophagitis). Strictures and webs may be seen and are also detectable by barium swallow radiography. Manometry may show esophageal aperistalsis. Esophageal histologic examination in acute GVHD reveals increases in the number of lamina propria lymphocytes, whereas chronic

GVHD is characterized by a bandlike lymphocytic infiltrate and destruction of the basal layer. Treatment is directed at increasing immunosuppression and providing adequate acid suppression to prevent secondary damage from gastroesophageal reflux. Esophageal strictures usually respond to bougienage. In rare cases, parenteral nutrition or gastrostomy feedings are necessary.

Pemphigus Vulgaris

Pemphigus vulgaris is a chronic disease that usually presents in the fourth to sixth decade of life with flaccid bullae of the skin and oral mucous membranes and occasionally of the esophagus. The disease is more common in women and among people of Jewish and Mediterranean descent. Pemphigus autoantibody against a cell surface cadherin causes loss of cell-cell adhesion and leads to a marked susceptibility to the separation of the superficial epithelium from the basal layer after only minimal trauma. Esophageal complaints include dysphagia, odynophagia, epigastric pain, and pyrosis. Upper endoscopic examination may show esophageal erosions, white plaques, flaccid hemorrhagic bullae, and sheets of peeling mucosa. Biopsy specimens show acantholysis with IgG and complement (C3) deposits in the intracellular spaces. Esophageal pemphigus vulgaris may require high-dose corticosteroids. Alternate therapies include cyclosporin and plasmapheresis.

Bullous Pemphigoid

Bullous pemphigoid is a benign vesiculobullous disease of older patients that infrequently has symptomatic esophageal manifestations. Bullae form as a result of antibodies directed against the squamous epithelial basement membrane, with deposition of IgG and C3 above the basement membrane. Although usually asymptomatic, patients with esophageal bullous pemphigoid may develop cicatrix formation and present with odynophagia, dysphagia, or even emesis of an esophageal cast (i.e., esophagitis dissecans superficialis). The presence of serum anti-basement membrane antibody is diagnostic, but the test is insensitive (only 70% are positive) and thus biopsy and immunohistochemistry may be required to confirm the diagnosis. Prednisone with or without cyclophosphamide is the most effective therapy, although sulfapyridine is occasionally helpful.

Library Resource Center
Renton Technical College
3000 N.E. 4th St.
Renton, WA 98056

Benign Mucous Membrane Pemphigoid

Benign mucous membrane pemphigoid is a chronic blistering disease of the conjunctiva and mouth, usually beginning in the fourth decade of life. It may also involve the esophagus, manifesting as dysphagia, odynophagia, cough, and aspiration pneumonia. Barium swallow radiography may show bullae, webs, or strictures. Bullae are rarely seen endoscopically; biopsy specimens show chronic subepithelial inflammation with a lack of acanthosis. Immunofluorescence reveals IgG and C3 deposits intracellularly and on the basement membrane. Long strictures may temporarily respond to esophageal dilation; however, endoscopy may be hazardous, producing esophageal sloughing. Administration of corticosteroids and dapsone has been beneficial. Colonic interposition may be needed to treat severe esophageal strictures.

Epidermolysis Bullosa Dystrophica

Epidermolysis bullosa dystrophica is a hereditary vesiculobullous or mechano-bullous disease of squamous epithelium. Esophageal involvement is important in the autosomal recessive form of the disease but rarely is significant in the dominant forms. Histopathologically, there is separation of the basal lamina from the underlying dermis resulting from a loss of anchoring fibrils between the two layers. The underlying cause appears to be the defective assembly or transport of type VII collagen. There is also an increase in collagenase activity in the skin from the bullae. Cutaneous bullae present early in life, leading to a recurrent scarring-healing pattern known as mummification. Esophageal bullae ulcerate, bleed, then heal, with scarring and stricture formation. Upper esophageal webs may contribute to dysphagia. Spontaneous dissection of the esophageal wall may occur, creating a double-barrel deformity, whereas esophageal rupture may occur spontaneously or with attempted dilation. Barium swallow radiography is the diagnostic procedure of choice. Upper endoscopy may induce further bulla formation; however, careful endoscopic dilation can be performed in selected cases. Patients should avoid hot or coarse foods, and if necessary, switch to a nutritionally complete liquid diet. Corticosteroids can be effective treatment, but esophagectomy with colonic interposition may be necessary. The condition has an increased risk of esophageal cancer.

TRAUMATIC ESOPHAGEAL INJURY

Etiology and Pathogenesis

Mallory-Weiss tears are linear, nonpenetrating lacerations in the gastric or esophageal mucosa near the esophagogastric junction. They are often induced by retching and vomiting. Tears may be multiple, and they occur in men more frequently than in women. Hiatal hernias are found in 42% to 80% of cases and may be a risk factor for development of Mallory-Weiss tears. Esophageal intramural hematomas occur spontaneously in patients with coagulopathies or with retching or vomiting and are thought to result from sudden changes in intramural pressure. Other causes of hematoma include foreign body ingestion, pill-induced injury, and esophageal variceal sclerotherapy. Esophageal rupture is a life-threatening injury that may result from severe retching (i.e., Boerhaave's syndrome), with a perforated Barrett's ulcer, after thoracic or abdominal trauma, or after esophageal instrumentation. Boerhaave's syndrome is characterized by a spontaneous esophageal rupture, usually in a region of anatomic weakness in the left posterolateral aspect of the esophagus just above the diaphragm. Iatrogenic causes of rupture include endoscopy, bougienage, passage of a nasogastric tube, sclerotherapy, and balloon tamponade for variceal hemorrhage. Blunt thoracoabdominal trauma from motor vehicle crashes or even from the Heimlich maneuver occasionally may produce upper esophageal rupture because of the rapid change in esophageal transmural pressure.

Clinical Features, Diagnosis, and Management

Patients with Mallory-Weiss tears present with upper gastrointestinal hemorrhage, usually with a history of retching or vomiting. Upper endoscopy is most useful for diagnosis and offers the capability of therapeutic intervention (e.g., injection therapy and cautery) if bleeding does not stop spontaneously. Other diagnostic modalities such as angiography are not useful. Surgery is rarely necessary for refractory hemorrhage. Patients with intramural hematomas most often present with chest discomfort or hematemesis. Upper gastrointestinal endoscopy reveals a mass with bluish discoloration protruding into the esophageal lumen. Computed tomography, magnetic resonance imaging, or endoscopic ultrasound rarely may be necessary to distinguish hematomas from benign or malignant esophageal masses. Intramural hematomas usually resolve spontaneously over 2 to 10 days. Coagulopathies should be corrected. Rarely, esophageal perforation may be a complication.

Cervical and upper esophageal perforations present with neck and chest pain, subcutaneous emphysema, dysphagia, odynophagia, nausea, vomiting, hematemesis, hoarseness, or aphonia, whereas distal perforations may produce additional abdominal pain, pneumothorax, or pneumomediastinum. Hamman's crunch, a crackle in cadence with cardiac activity, may be noted on auscultation. Symptoms manifest abruptly with shock, or they may not be reported for the first 8 hours after iatrogenic injury. Chest and abdominal radiographs may demonstrate subcutaneous emphysema, pneumothorax, pneumomediastinum, pleural effusion, and pneumoperitoneum. Contrast esophagography with water-soluble agents may be diagnostic. If no perforation is found, barium swallow radiography or upper endoscopy may provide better definition of the esophageal anatomy. Both of these techniques are potentially hazardous for patients with possible rupture, and they should be used cautiously. Cervical penetrating injuries are a special case requiring preoperative or intraoperative endoscopy. Thoracentesis may reveal pleural fluid with an acidic pH because of the gastric contents and with increased amylase owing to the salivary secretions. With small ruptures, medical management may be adequate; however, most patients require surgical intervention. If diagnosis is delayed, drainage of the infected areas may be needed. The course of treatment is likely to be prolonged in complicated cases, and usually requires parenteral nutrition.

CHAPTER 26

Motility Disorders of the Esophagus

DISORDERS OF THE HYPOPHARYNX, UPPER ESOPHAGEAL SPHINCTER, AND CERVICAL ESOPHAGUS

Incidence and Epidemiology

Dysphagia may result from neurologic and muscle disorders of the hypopharynx, upper esophageal sphincter (UES), and cervical esophagus. Most patients with cervical dysphagia are older; studies show that 30% to 40% of nursing home patients have eating or swallowing abnormalities. Autopsy series show high incidences of aspiration pneumonia secondary to swallowing dysfunction. Certain neurologic and myopathic conditions may appear in younger patients, however, and these may be more amenable to therapy.

Etiology and Pathogenesis

Upper Esophageal Sphincter Disorders

Cricopharyngeal hypertension refers to elevations in UES pressure that contribute to globus sensation in some patients, or alternatively, to dysphagia in Plummer-Vinson syndrome, gastroesophageal reflux disease, and postlaryngectomy patients. Studies suggest that esophageal distention is the major stimulus responsible for UES contraction. In many cases, gastroesophageal reflux of acid is the common denominator that leads to distention, irritation, and subsequent UES hypertension. However, these patients have increased levels of psychosocial dysfunction, which may increase UES pressure and reduce pain tolerance. Abnormally low UES pressure (usually with generalized weakness of the pharyngeal muscles) is observed with amyotrophic lateral sclerosis, myasthenia gravis, and myotonic dystrophy. Primary failure of UES relaxation with swallowing is extremely rare, being found only with central nervous system lymphoma or oculopharyngeal muscular dystrophy, whereas secondary UES relaxation dysfunction may occur after neck surgery. Most reported cases of cricopharyngeal achalasia actually result from weak pharyngeal forces, poor hyoid elevation, or noncompliant UES musculature that may be particularly significant in patients with cricopharyngeal bars. Delayed UES relaxation may be a manifestation of familial dysautonomia (i.e., Riley-Day syndrome), which is an autosomal recessive disease with autonomic dysfunction and altered swallowing and sucking. UES motor abnormalities have been reported with Zenker's diverticulum, including premature closure, altered pharyngeal-UES coordination, and incomplete UES relaxation; however, reduced UES compliance appears to be the primary defect in the development of these diverticula.

Neurologic Disorders

The most common causes of acute cervical dysphagia are cerebrovascular accidents. Symptoms usually appear abruptly and are associated with other neurologic deficits. Multiple brain stem infarctions may be the cause. Alternatively, hemispheric strokes may produce dysphagia as a result of brain stem distortion from adjacent cerebral edema. Degenerative neuronal changes with progressive bulbar palsy and pseudobulbar palsy produce tongue and pharyngeal paralysis. Polio and the postpolio syndrome alter pharyngeal function, as does amyotrophic lateral sclerosis. Hypopharyngeal stasis, aspiration, and UES dysfunction are prevalent in Parkinson's disease. Swallowing abnormalities, including difficult initiation, UES abnormalities, and incoordination, occur in more than one-half of patients with multiple sclerosis. Rare neurologic causes of cervical dysphagia include brain stem tumors, syringobulbia, tetanus, botulism, lead poisoning, alcoholic neuropathy, carcinoma, chemotherapy, and radiation therapy.

Primary Muscle Disorders

Polymyositis and dermatomyositis are characterized by proximal muscle weakness and atrophy, which involves the esophagus in 60% to 70% of cases and produces poor pharyngeal and proximal esophageal contraction, barium pooling in the valleculae, and decreased UES tone. Myotonic and oculopharyngeal dystrophy are the two forms of muscular dystrophy that affect the swallowing mechanism. Myotonic dystrophy presents with myopathic facies, swan neck, myotonia, muscle wasting, frontal baldness, testicular atrophy, and cataracts. Radiographic studies demonstrate impaired pharyngeal emptying and abnormal esophageal body peristalsis. Oculopharyngeal dystrophy presents with ptosis and dysphagia but does not have other gastrointestinal manifestations. Myasthenia gravis affects striated esophageal musculature, producing dysphagia in two-thirds of patients, which worsens as the patient eats a meal. Hyperthyroidism and hypothyroidism affect swallowing, as do sarcoidosis, systemic lupus erythematosus, and the stiff man syndrome.

Clinical Features

Neuromuscular diseases of the hypopharynx and upper esophagus produce a form of dysphagia in which the patient cannot initiate swallowing or propel the food bolus from the hypopharynx into the esophageal body. The patient can usually localize symptoms to the cervical region. Patients may also describe nasal regurgitation, tracheal aspiration, drooling, or the need to manually dislodge impacted food. Gurgling, halitosis, and a neck mass suggest a Zenker's diverticulum, whereas hoarseness may reflect nerve dysfunction or intrinsic vocal cord muscular disease. Dysarthria and nasal speech suggest muscle weakness of the soft palate and pharyngeal constrictors. The examination may show the following symptoms: focal deficits with cerebrovascular accidents, ptosis and end-of-day weakness with myasthenia gravis, and paucity of movement with Parkinson's disease.

Findings on Diagnostic Testing

Cineradiography

Cineradiography records the complex and rapid sequence of events occurring in the mouth, pharynx, and upper esophagus during a swallow. Preliminary soft tissue lateral neck radiographs detect structural problems of the cervical spine, tongue, hyoid, mandible, pharynx, and larynx. Dynamic recordings of the barium swallow include lateral and posteroanterior views after ingestion of thin and thick liquid barium and barium cookies. Motility disturbances manifest as delayed initiation and a prolonged duration of swallowing or a disturbance in the sequence of muscle movements. Barium retention in the pharyngeal recesses is caused by altered mucosal sensitivity, decreased muscle tone, or alterations in recess shape or size. Pharyngeal stasis is another sign of altered motility. Misdirected swallows with laryngeal penetration or aspiration are striking abnormalities. Delayed UES opening may be noted, as in familial dysautonomia. Cricopharyngeal bars have been proposed to represent pharyngoesophageal incoordination or muscular hypertrophy, although most patients with this radiographic finding are asymptomatic.

Manometry

Because of technical limitations, manometry is less helpful in evaluating patients with cervical dysphagia than those with more distal conditions. The primary measurements obtained include resting UES pressure, an approximation of the onset and offset of pharyngeal peristalsis, and the degree of relaxation and coordination between the UES and pharyngeal contractions.

Other Modalities

Upper gastrointestinal endoscopy assists in excluding lumenal lesions at the pharyngeal level, in the proximal esophagus, and in the distal esophagus, which may be the source of referred symptoms. Direct laryngoscopy also visualizes this region, as well as the upper airways, and is helpful in assessing for diffuse neuromuscular disease. Scintigraphic studies can demonstrate hypopharyngeal stasis, regurgitation, and tracheal aspiration. Brain imaging can be obtained with computed tomographic or magnetic resonance imaging studies. Testing with the anticholinesterase agent edrophonium is useful in the diagnosis of myasthenia gravis.

Management and Course

The first step in managing a patient with cervical dysphagia is to recognize and correct reversible causes of symptoms, including Parkinson's disease, myasthenia gravis, hyperthyroidism or hypothyroidism, and polymyositis. Cineradiography can be used to direct the planning of meals based on consistency and swallowing techniques. Some patients with oropharyngeal dysphagia are candidates for cricopharyngeal myotomy to weaken the UES high-pressure zone. Patients with good responses to surgery are those with intact oropharyngeal sensation, including some individuals with neuropathic disease, myopathic disease (oculopharyngeal muscular dystrophy), and UES dysfunction (Zenker's diverticulum). Contraindications to myotomy include gastroesophageal reflux with regurgitation. In patients with cervical dysphagia who cannot safely obtain adequate nutrition, enteral feedings through a nasoenteric tube or gastrostomy may be necessary.

ACHALASIA

Incidence and Epidemiology

Achalasia usually presents in persons between 25 and 60 years of age. Childhood onset should raise concern of a congenital or systemic disease, whereas onset in an elderly person may indicate achalasia secondary to malignancy. The disorder shows no sex preference and shows an annual incidence of 1.1 per 100,000 in the United States.

Etiology and Pathogenesis

Major neuroanatomic changes have been described in primary achalasia, including loss of myenteric ganglion cells in the esophageal body and lower esophageal sphincter (LES), reductions in esophageal body nerve fibers, degeneration of the vagus nerve, and changes in the dorsal motor nucleus of the vagus. The esophageal ganglion cells that remain are surrounded by mononuclear inflammatory cells. Damaged ganglion cells may contain intracytoplasmic hyaline or spherical eosinophilic inclusions (Lewy bodies). Immunohistochemical studies demonstrate reductions in vasoactive intestinal polypeptide (VIP) staining in neurons in the lower esophagus. Because VIP is a potent smooth muscle relaxant, the selective loss of VIPergic innervation could explain the incomplete LES relaxation and increased LES pressure in achalasia. Esophageal muscle tissue from achalasia patients contracts and relaxes in response to direct stimulants or inhibitors but does not respond to ganglionic agents, confirming local denervation of the involved tissues. In vivo, cholecystokinin may produce a paradoxical LES contraction in a patient with achalasia, which is in contrast to the relaxation observed in healthy individuals. The role of changes in the vagus nerve and dorsal motor nucleus in the pathogenesis of achalasia is undefined, although impaired gastric acid secretion and pancreatic polypeptide release in response to sham feeding in some patients are consistent with defective vagal activity. The lower esophageal smooth muscle is thickened in achalasia; however, this may be an adaptive phenomenon rather than a significant factor in the pathologic picture. The roles of genetic factors and infection in the genesis of achalasia are undefined.

Conditions that produce secondary achalasia may exhibit the same characteristics as primary achalasia. Malignancy may produce secondary or pseudoachalasia. Most commonly, these tumors are adenocarcinomas of the gastroesophageal junction, but pancreatic carcinoma, small cell and squamous cell lung carcinoma, prostate carcinoma, and lymphoma may also cause the syndrome either by direct compression of the distal esophagus or by malignant cell infiltration of the esophageal myenteric plexus. Other tumors (e.g., Hodgkin's disease, lung carcinoma, and hepatocellular carcinoma) produce achalasia by a paraneoplastic mechanism. Although most patients with pseudoachalasia are older, have a short duration of symptoms, and report weight loss, these criteria do not have significant predictive value in determining the cause of the disease. Chagas' disease is caused by the protozoan *Trypanosoma cruzi*, which is transmitted by the reduviid (kissing) bug, endemic in Brazil, Venezuela, and Argentina. After an acute septic phase, a chronic destruction of ganglion cells in the gut, urinary tract, heart, and respiratory tract develops over years. The presence of megaureter, megaduodenum, megacolon, or megarectum is helpful in distinguishing Chagas' disease from achalasia. Complement fixation tests are available to confirm the diagnosis. Other causes of secondary achalasia include infiltrative diseases (with amyloid, sphingolipids, eosinophils, or sarcoid), diabetes, intestinal pseudo-obstruction, pancreatic pseudocysts, von Recklinghausen's disease, multiple endocrine neoplasia type IIB, juvenile Sjögren's syndrome, and familial adrenal insufficiency with alacrima.

Clinical Features

All patients with achalasia report solid food dysphagia, and most also report liquid dysphagia. Symptoms may be intermittent and insidious in onset. The duration of symptoms at the time of diagnosis averages 2 years. The patient may have learned special maneuvers such as throwing the shoulders back, lifting the neck, performing a Valsalva maneuver, and drinking carbonated beverages, to promote passage of the esophageal bolus into the stomach. Other manifestations of achalasia include fullness or gurgling in the chest, regurgitation of undigested food eaten hours before, nocturnal regurgitation of food and saliva, choking, coughing, bronchitis, pneumonia, tracheal compression, and lung abscess. Postprandial or nocturnal chest pain is reported by up to one-third of patients. It may be so severe as to cause decreased food intake and weight loss, but it tends to improve as the disease progresses. Heartburn may result from bacterial production of lactic acid in the esophagus.

Findings on Diagnostic Testing

Radiographic Studies

Chest radiography may reveal mediastinal widening with an outline of the esophagus, loss of the gastric air bubble, an esophageal air-fluid level, and chronic pulmonary aspiration changes. Barium swallow radiography is the initial screening test for achalasia and may show impaired contrast transit within a dilated lumen, a loss of peristalsis, impaired LES relaxation, a characteristic tapering of the distal esophagus ("bird's beak"), and, rarely, an esophageal diverticulum proximal to the LES. The presence of mucosal irregularities warrants a search for malignancy.

Upper Gastrointestinal Endoscopy

Upper gastrointestinal endoscopy is always necessary to exclude malignancy. Typically, endoscopy reveals esophageal dilation, atony, and erythema, friability, and ulcerations from chronic stasis. Esophagitis caused by an infection with *Candida* organisms is a common finding and should be treated before therapeutic intervention. The LES may be puckered, but passage of the endoscope

---

TABLE 26-1
Manometric Findings in Achalasia

Absence of peristalsis in esophageal body (required for diagnosis)
Incomplete lower esophageal sphincter relaxation (usually present, not required)
Complete relaxation of short duration may be seen in early achalasia
Elevated resting lower esophageal sphincter pressure (common, not required)
Elevated intraesophageal pressure relative to gastric pressures (common, not required)

---

into the stomach should not be difficult in the absence of malignancy. Careful retroflexion of the endoscope in the gastric fundus is mandatory, and biopsy specimens should be obtained from any suggestive areas.

Esophageal Manometry

The diagnosis of achalasia should always be confirmed by esophageal manometry (Table 26-1). The absence of esophageal body peristalsis is a requirement for diagnosis, although low-amplitude simultaneous contractions are often seen. Vigorous achalasia is a variant of achalasia with high-amplitude (>60 mm Hg) nonperistaltic contractions. Incomplete LES relaxation with swallowing is usually (>80% of cases) but not always present in patients with achalasia because early in the course of disease, some patients exhibit complete LES relaxations of very short duration. Sixty percent of patients have elevated LES pressure (>35 mm Hg). Elevated intraesophageal pressures often are noted but are not required for diagnosis.

Scintigraphic Studies

Esophageal scintigraphic emptying studies may show retention of a semi-solid meal but are rarely useful in the initial diagnosis of achalasia. Scintigraphy is sometimes performed after therapy to assess reductions in esophageal retention.

Management and Course

Achalasia is not curable, and no treatment can restore normal esophageal body peristalsis or complete LES relaxation. Treatment therefore rests with measures to reduce LES pressure sufficiently to enhance gravity-assisted esophageal emptying. The most feared complication of achalasia is squamous cell carcinoma, which results from chronic stasis and occurs in 2% to 7% of patients, usually those who have had unsatisfactory or no treatment.

Medication Therapy

Nitrates and calcium channel antagonists are the most common medical therapies of achalasia. Sublingual isosorbide dinitrate reduces LES pressures by 66% for 90 minutes; however, no placebo-controlled trials have assessed the efficacy of this agent. Sublingual nifedipine lowers LES pressure by 30% to 40%, and a placebo-controlled study showed good to excellent clinical responses in 70% of patients in one study but lower responses in other studies. Medication therapy has significant limitations, such as duration of action and tachyphylaxis. However, elderly patients, patients who refuse more invasive therapy, patients who cannot give consent, and patients with very mild symptoms may benefit from these relaxant drugs.

Injection Therapy

Botulinum toxin, a potent inhibitor of neural acetylcholine release, reduces LES pressure and relieves symptoms for up to 6 months in patients with achalasia. Some ongoing studies suggest that botulinum toxin injections may provide a viable alternative to mechanical dilation or surgery.

Mechanical Dilation

Standard bougienage with a maximum dilator (20 mm) usually produces only transient symptomatic relief. In contrast, pneumatic dilation to >3 cm, which forcefully tears the LES circular muscle, produces long-lasting reductions in LES pressure. Most clinicians use preprocedure sedation despite the concerns about medication-induced LES relaxation minimizing the efficacy of dilation. Balloons are inflated for several seconds to 5 minutes at pressures ranging from 360 to 775 mm Hg, which produce responses in 32% to 98% of cases. A postdilation LES pressure of <10 mm Hg predicts a 100% remission rate at 2 years. Approximately 20% to 40% of patients require further dilation several years later. The most common complication of pneumatic dilation is perforation (1% to 13% of cases). Some clinicians perform a water-soluble radiographic swallow film followed by barium swallow radiography (if no perforation is detected) before sending the patient home. Postprocedure gastroesophageal reflux is rare. Epiphrenic diverticula and large hiatal hernias are considered to be relative contraindications to pneumatic dilation. Patients younger than 18 years usually respond better to surgery than to dilation.

Surgery

Surgical therapy of achalasia usually involves a longitudinal incision of the muscle layers from several centimeters above the LES to 1 cm below (i.e., Heller myotomy). Patients with vigorous achalasia may require more extended myotomy. Thoracoscopic procedures are being developed to replace thoracotomy approaches. Good to excellent responses to myotomy occur in 65% to 92% of patients. Symptomatic gastroesophageal reflux may occur in up to 10% of cases, which may be further complicated by strictures, Barrett's esophagus, and adenocarcinoma.

SPASTIC MOTILITY DISORDERS
OF THE DISTAL ESOPHAGUS

Incidence and Epidemiology

Several disorders of spastic esophageal motor activity have been characterized in patients with noncardiac chest pain. Patients with spastic disorders present at any age; the mean age of onset is 40 years. A predominance of female patients is characteristic of most studies.

Etiology and Pathogenesis

Spastic motor disorders of the esophagus rarely require surgery, so very little tissue is available for pathologic evaluation. Most striking is thickening of the lower esophageal muscle (≤ 2 cm) that is seen in some patients with diffuse esophageal spasm (DES). In contrast to achalasia, loss of ganglion cells has not been demonstrated in the spastic disorders, although changes in vagus nerve integrity have been found in DES. Patients exhibit enhanced esophageal motor responses to cholinergic agonists, edrophonium, and ergonovine, which suggests neural dysfunction. Electromyographic studies show increased spike-independent contractions and increased excitability of spontaneous spike activity, possibly reflecting impaired inhibitory innervation. A role for central nervous system dysfunction has been suggested by the demonstration of simultaneous, repetitive esophageal contractions with stress. In addition to these motor events, patients with noncardiac chest pain of esophageal origin often exhibit hypersensitivity to esophageal distention or acid perfusion, which is suggestive of a pathogenic afferent neural defect. A number of specific spastic disorders of the esophagus have been characterized based on manometric criteria.

Diffuse Esophageal Spasm

The characteristic manometric feature of DES is the simultaneous onset of esophageal body contractions at two or more adjacent recording sites representing >10% of contractile activity, which is usually intermixed with normal peristaltic activity. Other conditions that produce similar findings include diabetic neuropathy, rheumatologic disease, alcoholism, and pseudo-obstruction. Other manometric abnormalities include multiple contractions, high-amplitude contractions, long-duration contractions, and LES abnormalities (e.g., incomplete relaxation and hypertension). Some cases of DES have shown progression to achalasia, suggesting that these manometrically defined abnormalities represent a spectrum of a single encompassing disease in some patients.

Nutcracker Esophagus

Nutcracker esophagus is found in 27% to 48% of patients with noncardiac chest pain. It is characterized by peristaltic esophageal contractions of high amplitude (>180 mm Hg) as well as prolonged duration (>6 seconds) in one-third of patients. The relation between these contractile abnormalities and symptoms is unknown, especially as medical correction of the high-amplitude motor activity does not reliably correlate with reduced chest pain.

Hypertensive Lower Esophageal Sphincter

Hypertensive LES is defined by an LES pressure of >45 mm Hg with normal relaxation and esophageal body peristalsis, although overlap syndromes with DES and nutcracker esophagus are observed. Radiographic and scintigraphic evaluations usually show no delay in bolus passage into the stomach in patients with this condition.

Nonspecific Esophageal Motility Disorders

The nonspecific esophageal motility disorders do fit into well-characterized manometric patterns. The abnormalities include frequent simultaneous contractions, retrograde contractions, low-amplitude contractions, prolonged contractions, and isolated incomplete LES relaxation. The clinical significance of these disorders is unknown.

Clinical Features

Intermittent dysphagia for solids and liquids is present in 30% to 60% of patients with spastic esophageal motor disorders and may be exacerbated by large boluses of food, medications, or foods of extreme temperatures. Dysphagia is usually not severe enough to produce weight loss. Intermittent substernal chest discomfort with radiation to the back, neck, jaw, or arms lasting minutes to hours is reported by 80% to 90% of patients. Features suggesting an esophageal rather than a cardiac cause include pain that is nonexertional, continues for hours, interrupts sleep, is meal related, and is relieved by antacids. Associated heartburn (20% of cases), dysphagia, or regurgitation may favor an esophageal cause; however, no symptom complex applies exclusively to esophageal pain. Heartburn may not be pathologic, but rather may result from hypersensitivity to acid in the esophagus, as suggested by the observation that antireflux therapy is often ineffective. Other disturbances such as urinary and sexual dysfunction, irritable bowel syndrome, anxiety disorders, and depression are common.

Findings on Diagnostic Testing

Radiographic and Endoscopic Studies

Barium swallow radiography should be performed on any patient with dysphagia and should be considered for a patient with noncardiac chest pain. Motor disorders may be suggested by isolated and uncoordinated (tertiary) contractions in the distal two-thirds of the esophagus that entrap and delay barium transit. In general, these abnormalities are transient and are intermixed with normal swallows. "Bird's beak" deformities are not observed, although patients with spastic disorders may have an increased incidence of hiatal hernia formation. Upper endoscopy may be performed to exclude structural lesions or esophagitis as a cause of symptoms.

Manometry and Provocative Testing

The manometric characteristics of each of the spastic disorders is described above. Esophageal dysmotility is more common in patients with dysphagia (53%) than in patients with chest pain (25%) (Table 26-2). Nutcracker esophagus is the most common finding in patients with chest pain, whereas achalasia is the most prevalent cause of dysphagia. Provocative testing is performed to increase the sensitivity of functional testing. Intravenous edrophonium is the most common provocative test and may increase esophageal contractions and produce chest pain in up to 40% of patients. However, the false-positive rate is high. Intravenous ergonovine produces increased contractile activity and chest pain in some patients but has significant cardiac toxicity. Atypical chest pain is frequently reproduced by bethanechol injection, but troubling side effects are common. Esophageal balloon distention produced chest pain in 60% of patients, but in only 20% of controls. This technique may also induce dysphagia.

TABLE 26-2
Incidences of Esophageal Motility Disorders in Patients with Noncardiac Chest Pain and Dysphagia

DYSMOTILITY PATTERN	CHEST PAIN (255 OF 910 PATIENTS)	DYSPHAGIA (132 OF 251 PATIENTS)
Nutcracker esophagus	48%	10%
Nonspecific esophageal dysmotility	36%	39%
Diffuse esophageal spasm	10%	13%
Achalasia	2%	36%
Hypertensive lower esophageal sphincter	4%	2%

Source: Data from PO Katz, CB Dalton, JE Richter, et al. Esophageal testing of patients with noncardiac chest pain or dysphagia. Ann Intern Med 1987;106:593.

Scintigraphic Studies

Abnormal peristalsis and delayed transit may be detected by scintigraphic evaluation, especially in DES, although similar findings are noted on radiographic evaluation. False-negative results on studies are obtained with intermittent spastic disorders or disorders with preserved peristalsis (e.g., nutcracker esophagus).

Ambulatory pH and Motility Recording

Twenty-four-hour esophageal pH monitoring is the best test for identifying abnormal acid reflux and its relation to symptoms. Twenty-four-hour esophageal manometry is presently available only in selected referral centers. It has shown abnormal motor patterns in 16% of chest pain episodes.

Management and Course

Spastic motor disorders of the esophagus are not progressive or life threatening. Treatment should attempt to reduce symptoms without exposing the patient to potential therapeutic complications. Gastroesophageal reflux may produce esophageal dysmotility, similar to DES, independent of visible esophagitis. Patients with esophagitis may also exhibit reduced peristaltic amplitude and LES pressure. If gastroesophageal reflux is suggested by symptoms, structural testing, or 24-hour pH monitoring, aggressive antireflux treatment should be used for 1 to 2 months. If reflux is not a consideration, the most important step is to reassure the patient that there is no serious heart condition or other disease. When reassurance fails, medical, mechanical, and surgical treatment options are available.

Medications

Some DES patients experience relief with nitrates; however, no placebo-controlled studies have been performed. An uncontrolled study of hydralazine has shown some symptomatic improvement in patients with spastic esophageal disorders. Calcium channel antagonists (e.g., nifedipine, diltiazem) reduce esophageal body contractile pressures and LES pressures, but placebo-controlled studies have shown no symptomatic benefit from these drugs. A double-blind, placebo-controlled trial of the antidepressant trazodone produced global improvement and reduced distress from esophageal symptoms in one study; it has been postulated that antidepressants alter visceral pain perception. Similarly, behavioral modification and biofeedback have shown some efficacy in these disorders.

Mechanical Dilation

Bougienage probably does not produce symptomatic benefits greater than placebo dilation. However, pneumatic dilation has reduced symptoms in DES and hypertensive LES, especially if dysphagia is prominent.

Surgery

For patients with dysphagia or intractable pain caused by spastic motor esophageal dysfunction, a Heller myotomy to include the LES and the spastic portions of the esophageal body may produce symptom reductions in >50% of cases. However, the risk of the procedure coupled with the uncertain therapeutic response mandates a cautious approach to surgery.

ESOPHAGEAL MOTILITY DISORDERS ASSOCIATED WITH SYSTEMIC DISEASES

Rheumatologic Disease

Scleroderma

The esophagus is involved in 75% to 85% of patients with scleroderma, regardless of whether the diffuse or CREST (calcinosis, Raynaud's phenomenon, esophageal dysfunction, sclerodactyly, telangiectasia) variants are present. Scleroderma produces smooth muscle atrophy and fibrosis leading to absent distal esophageal contractions and LES incompetence. Clinically, patients present with dysphagia and heartburn. Symptomatic patients usually have Raynaud's phenomenon. The prevalence of erosive or ulcerative esophagitis is up to 60%, with some patients developing Barrett's esophagus and adenocarcinoma. Dysphagia may result from dysmotility, peptic stricture, or *Candida* esophagitis. Barium swallow radiography shows a dilated, aperistaltic esophagus with free gastroesophageal reflux and delayed emptying if the patient is supine. Wide-mouth esophageal diverticula may also be present. Manometry shows low to absent LES pressure, weak or absent distal peristalsis, and normal proximal esophageal peristalsis. Gastroesophageal reflux is aggressively treated with H_2-receptor antagonists or proton pump inhibitors. Frequent bougienage may be necessary for peptic strictures. If antireflux surgery is contemplated for intractable esophagitis, loose 270-degree fundoplications are necessary to minimize postoperative dysphagia.

Mixed Connective Tissue Disease

Mixed connective tissue disease combines features of scleroderma, polymyositis, and systemic lupus erythematosus and is suggested by high titers of antibodies to nuclear ribonucleoprotein antigen. More than 60% of patients have esophageal involvement, including aperistalsis and reduced pressures of both the UES and LES. The efficacy of corticosteroids in these patients is unproved.

Other Diseases

Up to 35% of patients with systemic lupus erythematosus have esophageal manometric abnormalities (DES, reduced peristalsis, and LES pressure), although symptoms are rare. Thirty percent of patients with rheumatoid arthritis exhibit minimal decreases in peristaltic amplitude. One-half of patients with Sjögren's syndrome report dysphagia, but this usually results from diminished lacrimal and salivary secretions.

Endocrine and Metabolic Disorders

Diabetes

More than 60% of diabetics with neuropathy exhibit disordered esophageal motility resulting from autonomic degeneration, but most patients are asymptomatic. Manometric findings in diabetes include decreased peristaltic amplitude, reduced LES pressure with incomplete relaxation, double-peaked waves, and simultaneous and repetitive contractions.

Thyroid Disease

Graves' disease produces acceleration of esophageal peristalsis. DES has been reported with thyrotoxic myopathy. Dysphagia in patients with myxedema may result from decreased peristaltic amplitude and velocity and incomplete LES relaxation.

Amyloidosis

Amyloidosis produces decreased LES pressure, decreased peristaltic amplitude, simultaneous contractions, or an achalasia-like pattern in 60% of patients, which may produce dysphagia.

ETHANOL AND THE ESOPHAGUS

Acute ethanol ingestion reduces the amplitude of peristaltic contractions and LES tone and induces simultaneous contractions. Chronic alcoholics with neuropathy exhibit increased simultaneous contractions and reductions in primary and secondary peristaltic activity. Ethanol withdrawal produces LES hypertension and increases peristaltic amplitude.

AGING AND THE ESOPHAGUS

One study has shown that patients older than 90 years may have reduced peristalsis, incomplete LES relaxation, and increased simultaneous contractions; however, symptomatic manifestations are rare. A subsequent investigation of patients older than 80 years showed only reduced peristaltic amplitude.

CHAPTER 27

Reflux Esophagitis and Esophageal Infections

GASTROINTESTINAL REFLUX DISEASE

Incidence and Epidemiology

Gastroesophageal reflux disease (GERD) refers to the pathologic consequences of the effortless movement of gastric contents to the esophagus, including symptoms or signs referable to the esophagus, pharynx, larynx, and respiratory tract. Some clinicians reserve the term *reflux esophagitis* to describe only those persons with mucosal damage and inflammation. GERD is extremely common, being reported at least once monthly by approximately 40% of adult Americans. Furthermore, 7% report daily heartburn, and nearly 1% have erosive esophagitis. The incidence of severe GERD increases dramatically after age 40 years, and the condition is more common in men than women. Of the patients with GERD, 5% will develop ulceration, 4% to 20% will develop strictures, and 8% to 20% will develop Barrett's esophagus.

Etiology and Pathogenesis

Potency of the Refluxate

Gastric contents that contribute to the potency of the refluxate include hydrochloric acid, pepsin, bile salts, and pancreatic enzymes. The pH of the gastric contents determines which substances are noxious. At a neutral pH, deconjugated bile salts and pancreatic enzymes produce significant tissue damage, whereas these compounds are insoluble and inactivated, respectively, at an acidic pH. With acid reflux, the degree of mucosal damage is accelerated at pH values of <2 or if pepsin or conjugated bile salts are present. Most patients with GERD secrete normal amounts of gastric acid. However, acid seems to be the injurious factor in these patients because minimal bile salts are detected and because pepsin is innocuous at neutral pH. In patients with Zollinger-Ellison syndrome, increased acid production contributes to the development of esophagitis.

Antireflux Barriers

Barriers to reflux of gastric contents include the lower esophageal sphincter (LES), the intra-abdominal segment of the esophagus, the diaphragmatic crura, the phrenoesophageal ligament, the mucosal rosette, and the angle of His. The high-pressure zone is generated mainly by the LES; however, the crura are important during coughing, sneezing, and bending. In healthy individuals, a certain amount of physiologic gastroesophageal reflux occurs by means of transient LES relaxations (TLESRs), which increase after a meal to permit gas to be vented from the stomach. In patients with GERD, there may be spontaneous reflux associated with increased TLESRs, reductions in LES pressure that permit retrograde reflux during increases in intra-abdominal pressure, or free reflux with an incompetent LES. The mechanisms of increased TLESRs in GERD patients are unknown, although a small subset exhibits delayed gastric emptying with gastric distention. Increases in gastric distention with hypersecretory conditions (Zollinger-Ellison syndrome) may increase TLESRs and exacerbate acid-induced esophageal damage. LES pressures may be reduced in pregnancy, diabetes, and scleroderma. The role of hiatal hernias is controversial. Most patients with GERD have hiatal hernias, but only a small minority of patients with hiatal hernias have significant GERD. A nonreducing hernia prolongs the time required for acid clearance from the esophagus from 5 minutes in healthy persons to 10 minutes in affected patients.

Lumenal Acid Clearance

Factors contributing to esophageal lumenal clearance include gravity, peristalsis, and salivary and esophageal bicarbonate secretion. After reflux occurs, most of the bolus is returned to the stomach with one to two swallow-induced peristaltic contractions. The remaining esophageal contents are then neutralized by bicarbonate secreted by the salivary and esophageal glands. The duration, not the frequency, of esophageal acidification correlates best with esophagitis, which indicates the importance of acid clearance mechanisms. However, many patients with GERD do not have delayed esophageal transit or abnormal salivary bicarbonate, and the defects they have in contractile activity are minimal. Nocturnal reflux has the greatest potential for esophageal damage, as most lumenal acid clearance factors are inactive during sleep.

Tissue Resistance

In healthy individuals, the daily acid contact time with esophageal mucosa is estimated at 1 to 2 hours. Therefore, a major factor in symptomatic gastroesophageal reflux is defective tissue resistance to damage. In contrast to the stomach and duodenum, the esophagus does not secrete a protective mucous layer and maintains only a minimal lumen-to-cell H^+ gradient. Protective structural components include cell membranes and intercellular junctions that limit H^+ diffusion into the esophageal tissue. Esophageal cells have the ability to buffer and extrude H^+ by the actions of intracellular phosphate and proteins, bicarbonate production by carbonic anhydrase, and ionic transporters that exchange intracellular H^+ and Cl^- for extracellular Na^+ and bicarbonate. Esophageal blood flow delivers oxygen, nutrients, and bicarbonate and removes H^+ and carbon dioxide in a dynamic fashion. Replication rates of esophageal epithelial cells increase in patients with GERD. The strongest evidence for defective tissue resistance factors comes from studies in which large subsets of patients with esophagitis showed no increase in acid contact time. Nicotine inhibits sodium transport across esophageal epithelium, whereas ethanol and aspirin increase permeability to H^+. Smoking and alcohol also impair LES function and acid clearance.

Clinical Features

The most common symptom of GERD is heartburn, which is described as substernal burning that moves orad from the xiphoid. Heartburn most often occurs after meals and may be relieved by acid-neutralizing agents. The frequency and severity of heartburn correlate poorly with endoscopically defined esophagitis. Patients with GERD may also present with substernal chest discomfort that mimics cardiac-related angina pectoris. Regurgitation of bitter or acid-tasting liquid is common. Water brash is the spontaneous appearance of salty fluid in the mouth resulting from reflex salivary secretion in response to esophageal acid. Solid food dysphagia in a patient with GERD raises the possibility of peptic strictures or adenocarcinoma arising from Barrett's metaplasia. Odynophagia rarely results from severe esophageal ulceration.

Acid damage to the oropharynx may produce sore throat, earache, gingivitis, poor dentition, and globus, whereas reflux damage to the larynx and respiratory tract causes hoarseness, wheezing, bronchitis, asthma, and pneumonia. The association of GERD and pulmonary disease is partly because of shared risk factors (e.g., tobacco smoking). Moreover, pulmonary disease may predispose to the development of GERD because of anatomic changes in the gastroesophageal high-pressure zone and because of medications that lower LES pressure (e.g., theophylline). Bronchospasm may be initiated by acidification of the esophagus alone; thus, tracheal penetration by the refluxate is not a requirement for development of asthma with GERD.

Findings on Diagnostic Testing

A history of heartburn alone is sufficient for the diagnosis of GERD and provides adequate rationale to initiate therapy. Diagnostic studies should be considered for patients with atypical symptoms, symptoms unresponsive to therapy, and symptoms and signs indicative of tissue injury (e.g., dysphagia, odynophagia, hematemesis, guaiac-positive stool, and anemia) (Table 27-1).

Radiographic Studies

Barium swallow or upper gastrointestinal radiography can identify ulcers, strictures, hiatal hernias, or a reticulated mucosal pattern suggestive of Barrett's esophagus, if careful double-contrast techniques are used. Barium radiography may rarely show free gastroesophageal reflux of the contrast agent, a finding that has high specificity but a low sensitivity for the diagnosis of GERD.

Upper Gastrointestinal Endoscopy

Upper gastrointestinal endoscopy with biopsy is the gold standard for documenting reflux-induced injury. Endoscopic findings in patients with GERD include normal mucosa, erythema, edema, friability, exudate, erosions, ulcers, strictures, and Barrett's metaplasia. Histologic hallmarks of esophagitis are

TABLE 27-1
Tests for Assessing Gastroesophageal Reflux

Tests for the presence of reflux
    Barium swallow radiography
    Acid reflux testing
    Esophageal pH monitoring
    Radionuclide ^{99m}Tc scintigraphy
Tests for assessing symptoms
    Bernstein's acid perfusion test
    Esophageal pH monitoring
    Empiric trial of acid-suppressive medications
Tests for assessing esophageal damage
    Barium swallow radiography
    Upper gastrointestinal endoscopy with or without biopsy
    Esophageal potential difference measurement
Tests for assessing disease pathogenesis
    Acid clearance test
    Radionuclide ^{99m}Tc scintigraphy
    Esophageal manometry
    Gastric acid secretory studies

increased height of the esophageal papillae and basal cell hyperplasia. Acute injury to the vascular bed, edema, and neutrophilic (and sometimes eosinophilic) infiltration signify esophageal damage. Chronic inflammation is characterized by the presence of macrophages and granulation tissue. With severe injury, fibroblasts may deposit enough collagen to form a stricture. Long-standing acid damage also promotes aberrant repair of the mucosa by columnar epithelium (i.e., Barrett's metaplasia).

Scintigraphic Studies

Scintigraphy with ^{99m}Tc–sulfur colloid may provide complementary information in the evaluation of a patient with GERD. Gastroesophageal reflux may be detected by scanning the esophagus after instillation of a tracer in the stomach; this procedure has a specificity of 90% and a sensitivity of 14% to 90%. Clearance of a swallowed tracer can estimate esophageal clearance of acid.

Esophageal Manometry

Esophageal manometry is most useful in the management of a patient being considered for surgery. A low LES pressure is associated with a high failure rate of medication therapy; therefore, this technique may be useful in determining which patients may benefit from antireflux surgery. However, 30% to 50% of GERD patients have normal LES pressures (10 to 30 mm Hg), whereas 10% of normal persons have LES pressures of <10 mm Hg. Manometric assessment of esophageal body peristalsis also is important preoperatively, because documentation of abnormal peristalsis may influence the type of antireflux surgery chosen.

Provocative Tests

Provocative tests are sometimes requested as part of a manometric examination to clarify the diagnosis of GERD. The acid reflux test involves measuring esophageal pH 5 cm above the LES in the basal state after straight leg raising, during a Valsalva and Muller maneuver, and during abdominal compression. If these maneuvers do not produce a pH of <4, testing is repeated after perfusion of 300 ml of 0.1 N hydrochloric acid in the stomach. Acid reflux testing has a sensitivity of 54% to 100% and a specificity of 70% to 95%. The Bernstein test can determine if chest discomfort is secondary to esophageal acidification with a sensitivity of 7% to 27% and a specificity of 83% to 94%. Initially, normal saline is infused into the middle esophagus for 5 to 15 minutes followed by infusion of 0.1 N hydrochloric acid. If symptoms are reproduced within 30 minutes of acid infusion, saline is reinfused to relieve symptoms and symptoms are again provoked by acid delivery. The appearance of symptoms with acid infusion in a patient who is blinded to the infusion sequence constitutes a positive test result. Complete symptom relief by saline infusion is not essential.

Ambulatory Esophageal pH Monitoring

Continuous 24-hour pH monitoring is performed with a nasally inserted pH probe positioned 5 cm above the LES. The patient is given an event marker to use with a recording device that is triggered to correlate symptoms with changes in esophageal pH. Maximal sensitivity (93%) and specificity (93%) are obtained by quantitating the percentage of time the pH is <4 using threshold values of 10.5% in the upright position and 6% in the supine position. Esophageal pH monitoring can also be used to correlate atypical symptoms, such as chest pain with acid reflux.

Miscellaneous Tests

The electrical potential difference of squamous epithelium differs from that of columnar epithelium; this transition is used to detect Barrett's metaplasia in research settings. Gastric acid secretory analysis may be performed in a patient who fails to respond to acid-suppressive drugs to exclude acid hypersecretion resulting from conditions such as Zollinger-Ellison syndrome.

Management and Course

The course of GERD is highly variable; 58% of symptomatic patients with abnormal pH monitoring but normal findings on endoscopic examination require medications for >6 months. Despite medical therapy, 15% of cases progress from nonerosive to erosive esophagitis. In patients with documented healing of erosive esophagitis over a 6.5-year follow-up period, 7.7% progressed to Barrett's esophagus, 2.5% developed strictures, and 2.2% developed ulcers.

Lifestyle Modification

Lifestyle modifications should be part of the initial management of the GERD patient (Table 27-2). The head of the bed should be elevated to enhance nocturnal esophageal acid clearance. Smoking and ethanol use, which have deleterious effects on LES pressure, acid clearance, and epithelial function, should be avoided. Reducing meal size and the intake of fat, carminatives, and chocolate

TABLE 27-2
Lifestyle Modifications for Patients with Gastroesophageal Reflux

Elevate the head of the bed 6 in.
Stop smoking
Stop excessive ethanol consumption
Reduce dietary fat
Reduce meal size
Avoid bedtime snacks
Weight reduction (if overweight)
Avoid specific foods
    Chocolate
    Carminatives (e.g., spearmint, peppermint)
    Coffee (caffeinated, decaffeinated)
    Tea
    Cola beverages
    Tomato juice
    Citrus fruit juices
Avoid specific medications (if possible)
    Anticholinergics
    Theophylline
    Benzodiazepines
    Opiates
    Calcium channel antagonists
    β-Adrenergic agonists
    Progesterone (some contraceptives)
    α-Adrenergic antagonists

limits gastric distention, lowers TLESR incidence, and prevents LES pressure reductions. Caffeinated and decaffeinated coffee, tea, and carbonated beverages should be avoided because they stimulate acid production. Tomato juice and citrus products may exacerbate symptoms because of their osmotic effects. Medications that reduce LES pressure should be limited whenever possible (e.g., anticholinergics, theophylline, diazepam, opiates, calcium channel antagonists, β-adrenergic agonists, α-adrenergic antagonists, and progesterone).

Medication Therapy

Acid-suppressive drugs are the mainstay for continuous therapy of GERD. H_2-receptor antagonists (e.g., cimetidine, ranitidine, famotidine, and nizatidine) are safe and effective for treating mild to moderate disease, but they must often be given in doses double those used for the treatment of duodenal ulcer. Mild GERD can be treated with over-the-counter H_2-receptor antagonists. For gross erosive esophagitis, H_2 antagonists are only marginally better than placebo, and when dose reduction is attempted, relapse is common. Proton pump inhibitors (e.g., omeprazole and lansoprazole) are the drugs of choice for endoscopically proven erosive esophagitis and symptomatic GERD refractory to H_2-receptor antagonists. These agents, which are irreversible H^+,K^+-adenosine triphosphatase antagonists, produce superior acid suppression; however, cessation is associated with high rates of recurrence. This has led to concern about the long-term safety of proton pump inhibitors, as they produce twofold to fourfold increases in serum gastrin, which in experimental animals leads to development of enterochromaffin tumors (i.e., carcinoids). Other concerns include the promotion of colonization of the upper gut with a bacterial generation of carcinogenic nitrosamines and the induction of certain hepatic and small intestine cytochrome P-450 enzymes. However, long-term studies have not demonstrated significant adverse sequelae after several years of use.

Prokinetic agents are used as primary therapy or as adjunctive agents for patients with GERD. Cisapride, an agent that acts on serotonin 5-HT$_4$ receptors to facilitate myenteric acetylcholine release, promotes gastric emptying and increases LES pressure. Cisapride is superior to placebo in reducing symptoms and healing erosions, but relapse is common on attempted dose reduction. In patients healed by acid-suppressive therapy, cisapride (20 mg twice daily) often prevents relapse. Metoclopramide and bethanechol have limited efficacy for patients with GERD.

Liquid antacids are indicated for rapid, safe, and effective acute symptom control. They may also heal erosive disease if given at very high doses. However, at high doses, significant side effects (e.g., diarrhea with magnesium antacids and constipation with aluminum antacids) make compliance difficult. Low-sodium antacids (e.g., magaldrate [Riopan]) are preferable for patients on salt-restricted diets. Gaviscon (aluminum hydroxide and magnesium carbonate), an antacid-alginate combination, decreases reflux by producing a viscous mechanical barrier, but it may also adversely affect bowel function. Sucralfate, the basic salt of aluminum hydroxide and sucrose octasulfate, acts topically to increase tissue resistance, buffer acid, and bind pepsin and bile salts, but its efficacy in treating patients with GERD is limited.

Treatment Strategy

For most patients with heartburn, empirical treatment with antacids or H$_2$-receptor antagonists for 4 weeks is reasonable. Those who do not respond to therapy should undergo endoscopy to define any mucosal abnormalities. If erosive esophagitis is not found, therapy should be directed at symptom control with higher doses of H$_2$-receptor antagonists, cisapride, or proton pump inhibitors; follow-up endoscopy is not indicated. For patients with erosive or ulcerative esophagitis, therapy is directed at mucosal healing to prevent complications; follow-up endoscopy may be needed at 2- to 3-month intervals, depending on the clinical setting. Because of the theoretical risks of long-term proton pump inhibitors, attempts should be made to convert patients to maintenance H$_2$-receptor antagonist therapy, either in high doses alone or in combination with cisapride. For patients who require continuous proton pump inhibitor therapy, consideration should be given to surgical management.

Surgical Treatment

The indications for antireflux surgery are the failure of medical therapy to heal or to prevent relapse of erosive esophagitis, the failure of medications to prevent stricture formation, and the development of pneumonia or airway compromise. The Nissen (360-degree wrap) and Belsey (270-degree wrap) fundoplications and the Hill gastropexy produce 85% success rates in relieving symptoms and healing lesions, although symptoms recur in 10% of patients. Two percent to 8% develop postoperative dysphagia or gas-bloat syndrome (i.e., the inability to belch or vomit). The operative mortality for these procedures is 1%. Fundoplications reduce hiatal hernias and enhance LES competency, whereas a gastropexy anchors the gastroesophageal junction to the median arcuate ligament. The Belsey procedure is chosen for patients with impaired esophageal peristalsis to reduce the likelihood of postoperative dysphagia. The Hill operation is used for patients with prior gastric resection.

Management of Complications

Strictures are characterized by progressive dysphagia over months to years and may be associated with reduced heartburn. Stricture development may be accelerated by NSAID use. Although strictures may be defined radiographically, endoscopy is required in all cases to exclude malignancy. Esophageal dilation may be performed without (Maloney, Hurst) or with (Savary) endoscopic guidance. Tight strictures may require pneumatic dilation.

Barrett's esophagus is an acquired condition in which squamous epithelium is replaced by columnar epithelium in response to chronic acid exposure. Development of Barrett's metaplasia initially is protective because the columnar epithelium is relatively acid resistant. However, up to 10% of patients with this condition develop esophageal adenocarcinoma. Some patients may have abnormal mucosa extending <3 cm above the LES; the relative malignant risk of this short-segment Barrett's metaplasia is believed to be lower but still higher than the risk in the general population. Barrett's metaplasia occurs in 10% to 15% of patients with erosive esophagitis and in 40% of patients with strictures. Diagnosis of Barrett's esophagus requires endoscopic biopsy directed at mucosa that is more red-orange than the normal squamous mucosa. If the color distinction is not clear, Lugol's solution will preferentially stain the squamous mucosa blue-black. Barrett's metaplasia may be divided into three histologic types: atrophic gastric-fundic, junctional, and specialized intestinal columnar. The intestinal metaplastic subtype appears to have the greatest risk of malignant degeneration. Endoscopic surveillance is currently recommended for patients with Barrett's esophagus, with esophageal resection performed for development of high-grade dysplasia or adenocarcinoma.

Hemorrhage may occasionally develop from esophageal erosions and ulcers. It may be chronic, with production of iron-deficiency anemia, or acute. Perforation of an esophageal ulcer is a serious complication that may cause life-threatening mediastinitis.

Gastroesophageal Reflux Disease in Infants and Children

Symptoms of GERD in infants and children include regurgitation, irritability, difficulty feeding, rumination, failure to thrive, apnea, asthma, pneumonia, and near sudden infant death syndrome. Many children with GERD outgrow their disease as a result of LES maturation. In children, Barrett's metaplasia has the same color as squamous mucosa, indicating the importance of biopsies in this age group. Infants should be fed small volumes of thickened formula and given acid-suppressive agents in size-adjusted doses. With intractable symptoms or reflux that has produced severe airway disease, a Nissen fundoplication may be considered.

ALKALINE REFLUX ESOPHAGITIS

Alkaline reflux esophagitis develops from prolonged contact of esophageal epithelium with nonacidic gastric or intestinal contents, usually in patients who have undergone ulcer surgery with vagotomy or, less commonly, in patients with achlorhydria who have not undergone surgery. Factors responsible for mucosal damage include deconjugated bile salts and pancreatic enzymes. Medications that may be effective therapy include bile salt–binding agents (e.g., cholestyramine, colestipol, sucralfate) and mucosal coating agents (e.g., antacids). When medications fail, a Roux-en-Y gastrojejunostomy may divert intestinal contents away from the esophagus. Alternatively, fundoplication may be performed in patients with intact stomachs or adequate gastric remnants.

FUNGAL INFECTIONS OF THE ESOPHAGUS

Etiology and Pathogenesis

Esophageal infections are rare in immunocompetent persons, but they are becoming more common because of the increasing numbers of patients with acquired immunodeficiency syndrome (AIDS) and the increasing numbers undergoing organ transplantation (Table 27-3). Immunocompetent patients who develop esophageal infections have impaired esophageal defenses: reduced peristalsis, as in diabetes, scleroderma, and achalasia; altered flora, as occurs with antibiotic use; and local infection that spreads to the esophagus, as in mediastinal tuberculosis. The most prevalent esophageal infections are caused by fungal agents.

The most common esophageal fungal infection is caused by *Candida albicans*, but other *Candida* species (*C tropicalis*, *C parapsilosis*, and *Torulopsis glabrata*) may also cause infection. These organisms are normal components of the oral flora, but they may become pathogenic if their numbers increase (e.g., as with antibiotic use) or if the patient is immunosuppressed (e.g., by therapy with corticosteroids or cyclosporin or by the development of hematologic malignancy or AIDS). Grossly, *Candida* organisms may produce esophageal involvement ranging from scattered white plaques to a dense pseudomembrane that consists of fungi, mucosal cells, and fibrin overlying friable, ulcerated mucosa. In severe cases, lumenal narrowing, pseudodiverticula, and fistulae may develop.

Esophageal aspergillosis, histoplasmosis, and blastomycosis are rare. Histoplasmosis and blastomycosis usually spread to the esophagus from paraesophageal lymph nodes. Infection with *Aspergillus* species causes large, deep ulcers, whereas esophageal histoplasmosis and blastomycosis are characterized by focal lesions and abscesses that may produce odynophagia if muscle layers are involved. Complications of these fungal infections include stricture and tracheoesophageal fistula formation.

Clinical Features

The main symptoms of esophageal fungal infections are dysphagia and odynophagia, which usually are worse with solid foods and may be severe enough to limit oral intake. Oral candidiasis may be associated with esophageal infection in AIDS, whereas chronic mucocutaneous candidiasis may have associated involvement of other mucous membranes, hair, nails, and skin as well as associated adrenal or parathyroid dysfunction. Infections with *Candida* organisms can produce mild blood loss, but life-threatening hemorrhage is rare. Fistulization may lead to pulmonary infection.

TABLE 27-3
Organisms Associated with Infectious Esophagitis

Fungi
    Candida species (especially *C albicans*)
    Aspergillus species
    Histoplasma capsulatum
    Blastomyces dermatitides
Viruses
    Herpes simplex virus type 1
    Cytomegalovirus
    Varicella-zoster virus
Bacteria
    Mycobacterium tuberculosis
    Actinomyces israelii
    Streptococcus viridans
    Lactobacillus acidophilus
    Treponema pallidum

Findings on Diagnostic Testing

Radiographic or endoscopic studies are commonly used to confirm suspected fungal esophageal infection. Barium swallow radiography may reveal a shaggy mucosal appearance, as well as plaques, pseudomembranes, cobblestoning, nodules, strictures, fistulae, and mucosal bridges. However, false-negative rates of 25% and 10% have been reported for single- and double-contrast examinations, respectively. Upper gastrointestinal endoscopy is the most sensitive and specific means of diagnosing fungal esophageal infection. Brushings of mucosal lesions are examined immediately after 10% potassium hydroxide is added or after they are fixed in 95% ethanol before permanent staining. Biopsy specimens are obtained for histologic examination. Brushings are more sensitive for detection of *Candida* organisms than biopsy specimens; however, some patients with positive findings on brushings but negative findings on histologic examination may have fungal colonization rather than infection. The microscopic appearances of *Candida* and *Aspergillus* species are distinctive. In rare cases, culture of the fungus may be necessary to characterize the organism and to determine sensitivity to antifungal agents, especially in patients who have been refractory to prior therapy. Because *Histoplasma* organisms usually do not invade the esophageal mucosa, brushings and biopsy specimens may be nondiagnostic. Therefore, bronchoscopy, mediastinoscopy, or surgery may be necessary to characterize this infection.

Management and Course

Most patients with fungal esophageal infections will have a definitive endoscopic diagnosis before treatment is initiated. For patients with AIDS who have oral candidiasis and symptoms of esophagitis, empiric antifungal therapy may be initiated without embarking on a diagnostic evaluation. Fluconazole and ketoconazole are effective oral imidazole antifungals that alter fungal cell membrane permeability.

Other imidazoles (e.g., clotrimazole and miconazole) are less effective in treating active esophageal infection. In addition to its efficacy in treating infections caused by *Candida* organisms, ketoconazole is also effective against histoplasmosis and blastomycosis. Doses of ketoconazole may need to be increased to treat infection in patients with reduced gastric acid production, such as occurs with AIDS, acid-suppressive medication use, post-gastric surgery, or atrophic gastritis. In contrast, fluconazole absorption is not pH dependent. Adverse effects of these agents include nausea, hepatotoxicity, adrenal insufficiency, decreased gonadal steroid production, and inhibition of cyclosporin metabolism. Intravenous miconazole is occasionally used, but it may produce anemia, thrombocytopenia, hyponatremia, hyperlipidemia, anaphylaxis, cardiac arrest, and acute psychosis.

Polyene antibiotics (e.g., nystatin and amphotericin) bind to fungal membrane sterols, causing cell death. Nystatin is useful for oral thrush, but it is less effective than the imidazoles for esophageal involvement. Intravenous amphotericin B is an agent of last resort for treatment of fungal esophageal infections because of its potential to cause severe side effects (e.g., fever, hypotension, mental status changes, wheezing, renal toxicity, nausea, hypokalemia, hypomagnesemia, and bone marrow suppression). Cessation of therapy or dose reduction is recommended if serum creatinine levels exceed 3 mg per dl. Amphotericin is the drug of choice for treating systemic aspergillosis, and it is also used to treat ketoconazole-resistant histoplasmosis and blastomycosis. Flucytosine is a fluorinated pyrimidine that interferes with fungal RNA translation and may be given in combination with amphotericin; its side effects include rash, hepatitis, diarrhea, and bone marrow suppression. Flucytosine should not be given alone because fungi develop resistance to this drug.

VIRAL INFECTIONS OF THE ESOPHAGUS

Etiology and Pathogenesis

Herpes simplex virus 1 (HSV-1), cytomegalovirus (CMV), and varicella-zoster virus (VZV) are the major viral causes of infectious esophagitis. HSV-1 occurs most often in patients with immunosuppression, although esophageal involvement in healthy individuals may develop. HSV-1 esophageal infection begins as discrete vesicles, which may combine to form larger hemorrhagic ulcerations. Squamous cells at the edge of the ulcers exhibit multinucleation, ground-glass nuclei, and eosinophilic Cowdry's type A inclusions surrounded by halos, with enveloped virions observable on electron microscopy. Cytomegalovirus esophageal infection most commonly complicates the course of AIDS and produces prominent esophageal ulcers, which may be numerous, round or serpiginous, and deep, in some cases reaching the muscularis. Inclusion bodies are seen in the cytoplasm of infected cells. The frequency of esophageal involvement in primary chicken pox is unknown. However, cases of esophageal ulcerations that appear similar to HSV-1 lesions in association with thoracic dermatomal zoster reactivations have been reported. These esophageal ulcerations resolve with resolution of the skin lesions.

Clinical Features

HSV-1 esophageal infection occurs concurrently or after the skin infection. It commonly produces severe odynophagia. In immunodeficient patients, this esophageal infection can produce hemorrhage, cause perforation with tracheoesophageal fistula formation, or disseminate. In contrast, immunocompetent persons usually experience only self-limited infection. CMV esophagitis produces either dysphagia or odynophagia and may be associated with involvement of other organ systems.

Findings on Diagnostic Testing

Radiography and endoscopy have utility in the diagnosis of viral esophageal infections. On barium swallow radiography, HSV-1 infection usually appears as focal ulcerations on a background of normal mucosa. However, a shaggy appearance is common and indistinguishable from that observed in infections with *Candida* organisms. Barium studies of CMV esophagitis show vertical linear ulcers with central umbilication, and, rarely, diffuse thickening of mucosal folds. Confirming the diagnosis of viral esophageal infection requires upper gastrointestinal endoscopy with biopsy. Infection with HSV-1 appears as discrete, punched-out ulcers (0.3 to 2.0 cm diameter) with raised yellow rims (i.e., volcano ulcer), but it may also be characterized by bullae or diffusely hemorrhagic mucosa. Biopsy specimens and brushings taken from the edges of ulcers may reveal multinucleate squamous cells with the characteristic Cowdry's type A inclusions. Esophageal infection with CMV appears as small (0.3 to 0.5 cm diameter), longitudinal, or giant ulcers (1.0 to 3.5 cm diameter) in the distal esophagus or as polypoid masses. Examination of brushings or biopsy specimens, respectively, may reveal epithelial or endothelial CMV inclusions. Viral cultures of esophageal tissue for HSV-1 and CMV may be performed in cases in which the diagnosis is unclear.

Management and Course

In immunocompetent persons, oral viscous lidocaine may be sufficient therapy for HSV-1 esophageal infection, whereas intravenous acyclovir for 7 to 10 days appears to reduce symptoms, shorten viral shedding, and hasten healing in immunocompromised patients. VZV is susceptible to acyclovir, but there is little experience with this agent in treating esophageal infection with VZV. An acyclovir derivative, ganciclovir, appears to be effective in treating CMV esophageal infection, although this agent may cause rash and neutropenia. Foscarnet, a pyrophosphate analog that inhibits viral DNA polymerase and reverse transcriptase, may also be useful in treating CMV infections, but this drug can cause renal failure, anemia, and heart failure.

MYCOBACTERIAL, BACTERIAL, AND TREPONEMAL INFECTIONS OF THE ESOPHAGUS

Etiology and Pathogenesis

Esophageal tuberculosis (TB) involvement has increased since the onset of the AIDS epidemic and usually affects the middle third of the esophagus because spread of infection is from the mediastinal lymph nodes by way of a draining fistula or obstructed lymphatics. Less commonly, TB pharyngitis or laryngitis may spread to the upper esophagus. Swallowed mycobacteria may colonize strictures or malignancies. Multiple esophageal miliary mucosal granulomas may result from the hematogenous spread of infection. Primary esophageal TB is exceedingly rare.

Bacterial esophageal infection is caused by gram-positive organisms such as *Streptococcus viridans*, staphylococci, and bacilli. It usually occurs after esophageal injury from nasogastric tubes, chemotherapy, radiation, or GERD. Rare causes include *Actinomyces israelii*, *Corynebacterium diphtheria*, and *Lactobacillus acidophilus*. The esophagus may appear normal or exhibit erythema, plaques, pseudomembranes, blood vessel infiltration, and hemorrhage. Actinomycosis produces granulomatous esophagitis with drainage of sulfur granules from abscess cavities.

Tertiary syphilis of the esophagus is characterized by a submucosal gumma, mucosal ulcers, or diffuse inflammation with fibrosis in the upper esophagus. Syphilitic periarteritis is evident on histologic examination.

Clinical Features

TB patients with esophageal ulcers may complain of odynophagia, whereas those with strictures will note dysphagia. The presence of meal-induced choking or coughing should suggest possible esophageal fistula formation. Hemorrhage from TB esophageal infection is rare. In neutropenic patients undergoing chemotherapy, bacterial esophagitis appears as odynophagia or dysphagia and may be associated with fever. Patients with syphilitic esophageal involvement present with dysphagia or with complications of fistulous disease; odynophagia is rare.

Findings on Diagnostic Testing

Barium radiographic findings (e.g., ulceration, strictures, masses, and fistulae) are nonspecific findings in patients with esophageal TB infection. Upper gastrointestinal endoscopy with biopsy is essential for the diagnosis of bacterial esophagitis because radiography is nonspecific. Endoscopic biopsy specimens obtained from around the edges of lesions may show granulomas or acid-fast bacilli on microscopic examination and may be cultured for confirmation and determination of antimycobacterial sensitivities. With syphilitic involvement, barium swallow radiography may show a long, ulcerated stricture in the upper esophagus, which is stiff on endoscopic examination. Biopsy may not be helpful in this disorder. Therefore, the diagnosis will rest on clinical judgment or on other disease manifestations.

Management and Course

Multidrug therapy for esophageal TB infection is indicated. If fistulae do not close with medical treatment, surgery may be necessary, including possible colonic interposition. Bougienage may be performed for strictures, whereas emergency surgery may be needed to control hemorrhage from an arterio-esophageal fistula. Bacterial esophagitis should be treated with appropriate antibiotics if the sensitivities of the infecting organisms are known or with empirical high-dose penicillin. However, mortality is more closely related to the underlying immunosuppressive disease. Penicillin is curative of esophageal syphilis infection; however, bougienage or surgery may be necessary to treat complicated disease.

IDIOPATHIC ULCERATIVE ESOPHAGITIS IN ACQUIRED IMMUNODEFICIENCY SYNDROME

Some patients with AIDS present with odynophagia secondary to ulcerative esophagitis of unknown cause, although an infection is likely, as viruslike particles have been identified on biopsy specimens. Radiographic and endoscopic examinations reveal ulcers that are large and longitudinal; some also may exhibit papillomatous overhanging edges. Clinicians should exclude zidovudine-induced ulcers as a possible cause. The most effective therapy is prednisone for several weeks, although recent reports suggest some efficacy with thalidomide.

CHAPTER 28

Esophageal Tumors

SQUAMOUS CELL CARCINOMA

Incidence and Epidemiology

Worldwide, squamous cell carcinoma is the most common malignant tumor of the esophagus, although an increase in the incidence of adenocarcinoma has essentially equalized the incidences of these two tumors in the United States. Large regional variations in the rate of squamous cell cancer occur between and within countries. Portions of Iran, China, and the former Soviet Union have exceptionally high rates, as much as 500-fold greater than in regions of low risk, emphasizing the importance of environmental factors in the pathogenesis of squamous cell cancers.

In the United States, blacks have a fivefold increased risk relative to whites. The risk is threefold higher in men than in women. The annual rates for black males and females are 15 per 100,000 and 7 per 100,000, respectively. The corresponding figures for white males and females are 3 per 100,000 and 1 per 100,000, respectively. The higher incidence in some ethnic groups may be closely related to environmental factors. Also, lower socioeconomic groups have a higher incidence of squamous cell cancer than higher socioeconomic groups.

Etiology and Pathogenesis

Although the events responsible for the pathogenesis of squamous cell tumors remain poorly characterized, the majority of these cancers are attributable to environmental factors. In Western countries, most patients use alcohol or tobacco. The risk of squamous cell cancer increases in a dose-dependent manner for both alcohol and tobacco consumption. This effect appears to be additive, as the risk for patients who smoke and drink excessively is much higher than the risk for patients who use either substance alone. For unknown reasons, alcohol and tobacco do not appear to increase the risk of squamous cell tumors in other areas of the world. Dietary excess of nitrosamines and deficiencies in fruits and vegetables have also been associated with an increased risk of squamous cell cancer. Squamous cell carcinoma of the esophagus occurs in approximately 1% to 6% of patients with squamous cell cancer of the head and neck. The association is consistent with the cancer-promoting effects of ethanol and tobacco for both tumors.

Other risk factors for esophageal squamous cell carcinoma have been elucidated. Lye ingestion that causes an esophageal stricture has been associated with development of squamous cell tumors several decades after the exposure. Although lye ingestion accounts for only a small percentage of all esophageal cancers, it underscores the importance of environmental exposures in this disease. Achalasia also is associated with an increased incidence of esophageal cancer. Whether or not achalasia represents a premalignant condition is controversial, but several series have documented a 10- to 30-fold increase in the rate of squamous cell cancer, which develops 17 to 20 years after the initial symptoms of achalasia. The disease that has the strongest association with squamous cell cancers is tylosis. This rare autosomal dominant condition is characterized by hyperkeratosis of the palms and soles. Although the genetic alteration responsible for this syndrome remains unknown, the development of esophageal cancer is essentially inevitable in affected individuals.

Clinical Features

By the time patients develop symptoms of esophageal cancer, the disease usually is far advanced. Most symptoms are attributable to the mechanical effects of the tumor mass, and dysphagia is the most common presentation. Initially, patients experience difficulty only when swallowing solids. As the dysphagia caused by the malignancy becomes more severe over weeks to months, patients may also have difficulty swallowing liquids. Patients often note a vague retrosternal discomfort, and approximately 50% of patients report odynophagia. Impaired food intake and anorexia may lead to profound weight loss. Involvement of adjacent mediastinal strictures may be indicated by a chronic cough caused by a tracheoesophageal fistula, hoarseness caused by recurrent laryngeal nerve involvement, and, rarely, exsanguination caused by invasion of the cancer into the aorta.

The most striking physical finding often is a generalized loss of muscle mass and subcutaneous fat. In patients with early disease, the physical examination findings may be normal, but patients with metastatic disease may exhibit hepatomegaly, bony pain, and supraclavicular adenopathy.

Findings on Diagnostic Testing

Radiographic Studies

Because the clinical pattern of dysphagia is imprecise in distinguishing between benign and malignant disorders of the esophagus, all patients with dysphagia should undergo esophageal imaging. Barium swallow radiography is very sensitive in detecting cancers large enough to produce dysphagia, but its sensitivity for detecting early lesions is only 75%, limiting its usefulness as a screening test for patients at high risk. This study is particularly useful in evaluating dysphagia because fluoroscopic examination can often detect motility abnormalities or proximal diverticula that may not be appreciated on endoscopic studies. Early esophageal cancers may appear as a tiny ulceration or plaquelike elevation. Advanced cancers assume one of three patterns: a polypoid intralumenal protrusion, a stricture or loss of distensibility as a result of infiltration, or a discrete ulceration, often with protruding edges. Because some malignancies may produce a smooth symmetric stricture, these tumors cannot be distinguished reliably from benign peptic strictures on barium-enhanced radiographs.

Endoscopic Studies

Upper gastrointestinal (GI) endoscopy with biopsy and brushings is the procedure of choice for diagnosing esophageal cancer. Early cancers can be detected as elevated plaques or small erythematous erosions. If the tumor mass precludes passage of the endoscope, gentle, fluoroscopically guided dilation may permit completion of the examination. All mucosal abnormalities should undergo brushing and biopsy for cytologic and histologic examination, respectively. The sensitivity of biopsy alone is 70% to 90%, and with the addition of cytologic examination, nearly all cancers are detected. Because a sampling error occasionally leads to false-negative biopsy and cytology results, any lesion that is highly suggestive of malignancy should be rebiopsied.

Management and Course

All patients with esophageal cancer should have the tumor staged on the basis of the depth of invasion (T stage), the nodal status (N stage), and the presence of distant metastatic disease (M stage) (Table 28-1). Although current techniques have a limited accuracy compared with pathologic staging, establishing the TNM stage assists the clinician in determining an appropriate treatment strategy and provides the single best indicator of prognosis. Computed tomographic (CT) scanning is the most commonly used staging procedure. Although it is a sensitive means of documenting aortic invasion, CT scanning may overstage tumors, and it has low accuracy in determining nodal involvement. CT scanning is the procedure of choice for detecting hepatic metastases. Magnetic resonance imaging has also been used to stage esophageal tumors, but it does not appear to provide an advantage over CT scanning. The most accurate means of determining the T and N stages in all types of esophageal

---

TABLE 28-1
TNM Staging System for Esophageal Cancer

Primary tumor (T)
- TX   Primary tumor cannot be assessed
- T0   No evidence of primary tumor
- Tis   Carcinoma in situ
- T1   Tumor invades the lamina propria or submucosa
- T2   Tumor invades the muscularis propria
- T3   Tumor invades the adventitia
- T4   Tumor invades adjacent structures

Lymph node (N)
- NX   Regional lymph nodes cannot be assessed
- N0   No regional lymph node metastasis
- N1   Regional lymph node metastasis

Distant metastases (M)
- MX   Presence of distant metastasis cannot be assessed
- M0   No distant metastasis
- M1   Distant metastasis

---

tumors is endoscopic ultrasound (EUS) examination. EUS has an accuracy of about 90% and 85% for establishing the T and N stages of a tumor, respectively. Although EUS can detect celiac lymph nodes, it has only a limited capacity for determining the M stage of a tumor. In addition, tight esophageal strictures may preclude a complete examination, reducing the overall accuracy of EUS.

Surgical resection is the primary therapy for all patients with tumors that are confined to the esophagus. Although curative resection is unlikely for T3 or N1 lesions, palliative resection can provide 1 to 2 years of symptom-free survival. Locally advanced (T4) or metastatic (M1) disease is not amenable to curative resection, and the poor long-term survival of these patients makes surgical palliation an unfavorable option.

The most common surgical procedure is a transthoracic esophagectomy with esophagogastric anastomosis. An alternate procedure for lesions in the upper one-third of the esophagus involves a subtotal esophagectomy with a gastric pull-up into the neck and requires a combined abdominal and cervical approach. Both procedures provide the adequate exposure and tissue resection margins necessary for a cancer operation. An innovative procedure for lower esophageal tumors involves transhiatal resection and primary anastomosis, but there are concerns whether the exposure and margins are adequate in this approach. In the past, operative mortality rates have ranged from 20% to 30%, rendering esophagectomy among the most morbid gastrointestinal operations performed. More recent series suggest a mortality rate of 5% to 10%. The high incidence of comorbid conditions in these patients increases the risk of cardiopulmonary complications, and a high rate of anastomotic leaks leads to numerous septic complications.

Despite improvements in surgical technique, the overall 5-year survival of patients undergoing resection is 6%. If only the patients with an apparently curative resection are analyzed, the 5-year survival still is only 25%. High rates of recurrence have prompted trials of perioperative chemotherapy and radiation therapy to improve systemic and regional control of the tumor. Several trials have investigated the role of radiation alone, chemotherapy alone, and the combination of radiation with chemotherapy before and after surgical resection, but there is no definitive evidence that these interventions improve survival. However, postoperative radiation therapy does decrease local recurrence in patients who receive a palliative resection. Large ongoing trials may clarify the role of perioperative cytoreductive therapy.

If surgical resection is not performed because of excessive surgical risk or unresectable disease, radiation therapy is an effective means of palliation. Most patients experience improvement in dysphagia, but <15% have relief that lasts more than 12 months. The overall 5-year survival rate is 6%, which is equivalent to surgical series. Patients with tumors of <5 cm have better survival rates. Clinical trials have found that the combination of radiation therapy with chemotherapy regimens using 5-fluorouracil and cisplatin improves survival relative to radiation therapy alone. Whether this regimen is superior to surgery remains unknown.

Several endoscopic interventions may palliate the symptoms of esophageal cancer. Esophageal stents can be placed across stenotic mass lesions to restore swallowing function. The recent introduction of expandable metallic stents represents an advance over the rigid plastic stents that are technically difficult to place. Metallic stents with a silicone coating can be placed across tracheoesophageal fistulae, permitting the patient to swallow saliva and food without aspirating. Metallic stents do have a high rate of complications, including intractable chest pain, stent migration, perforation, and bleeding. Laser photocoagulation and bipolar electrocoagulation may also be used to reduce tumor bulk. Percutaneous endoscopic gastrostomies can be placed to maintain nutritional intake in the setting of severe dysphagia.

ADENOCARCINOMA

Incidence and Epidemiology

For unclear reasons, the incidence of adenocarcinoma of the esophagus and gastroesophageal junction in the United States is increasing faster than any other tumor. The disease primarily affects white males older than 40 years; the incidence of adenocarcinoma in this group now exceeds the rate of squamous cell cancers.

Etiology and Pathogenesis

Essentially all esophageal adenocarcinomas arise in areas of Barrett's metaplasia. Similarly, adenocarcinoma of the gastric cardia frequently arises from a short segment of Barrett's epithelium. Given the similar epidemiologic and clinical associations of these two tumors, adenocarcinoma of the esophagus and gastric cardia probably involves the same disease process. Barrett's esophagus represents metaplastic transformation of the normal squamous mucosa to gastric-type glandular mucosa. The mechanisms by which gastroesophageal reflux of acid induces this metaplastic response are unknown, but medical or surgical treatment of gastroesophageal reflux usually does not lead to regression of Barrett's metaplasia. There are three histologic variants of Barrett's metaplasia: cardia-type, fundic-type, and intestinal-type. Only the intestinal-type metaplasia, also termed *specialized columnar epithelium*, is associated with an increased risk of adenocarcinoma.

Intestinal metaplasia follows a sequence of increasing dysplasia in the progression to malignancy. Genomic instability is common in dysplastic Barrett's mucosa. Aneuploid cell populations and deletions or alterations of tumor suppressor genes, particularly *p53*, are often observed in the mucosa of patients who eventually develop carcinoma. Further descriptions of the clinical associations of these genetic abnormalities may clarify the role of genetic analysis in identifying patients at extreme risk for adenocarcinoma.

Clinical Features

The clinical manifestations of esophageal adenocarcinoma are similar to those of squamous cell carcinoma, although chronic pyrosis, regurgitation, and chest pain caused by long-standing gastroesophageal reflux may be more common. Barrett's metaplasia does not produce symptoms, and the presence of Barrett's mucosa correlates poorly with the severity of reflux symptoms, suggesting that these patients may have an increased threshold for acid-induced symptoms. As with squamous cell tumors, symptoms attributable to adenocarcinoma occur in advanced stages when the tumor is large enough to interfere with swallowing.

Findings on Diagnostic Testing

Endoscopic Studies

Upper GI endoscopy with biopsy is the procedure of choice for diagnosing Barrett's metaplasia and early adenocarcinoma. Endoscopic examination of Barrett's metaplasia reveals circumferential, isolated islands (or tongues) of salmon-colored mucosa proximal to the normal site of the squamocolumnar junction at the lower esophageal sphincter. Because early adenocarcinoma may occur in regions of gastric metaplasia without any visible mucosal defects at endoscopic examination, biopsy specimens should be obtained of normal Barrett's tissue as well as of erosions, nodules, and strictures. The concurrent performance of brush cytologic examination may increase the yield of random biopsies in detecting malignant and premalignant tissue associated with Barrett's metaplasia. Symptomatic adenocarcinoma usually is characterized by an exophytic or ulcerated mass; however, benign peptic strictures often occur in patients with Barrett's mucosa. Distinguishing between benign and malignant strictures can require extensive mucosal sampling with biopsies and brush cytology specimens.

Histologic Evaluation

The interpretation of biopsy samples from patients with Barrett's metaplasia requires the expertise of an experienced GI pathologist. There is a high degree of interobserver variation in distinguishing low-grade dysplasia from no dysplasia. Similarly, identification of high-grade dysplasia is also subject to some interobserver variation. It may be difficult or impossible to distinguish high-grade dysplasia from invasive carcinoma if biopsy samples fail to include the lamina propria. Therefore, large or jumbo forceps should be used when sampling areas of Barrett's metaplasia. Flow cytometry has been used to identify aneuploid cell populations as well as other proliferative indices. However, the role of these variables in clinical practice is not clear.

Radiographic Studies

Advanced tumors often are obvious on barium swallow radiographic studies, appearing as apple core strictures or ulcerated mass lesions. Because Barrett's metaplasia tends to concentrate in the distal esophagus, adenocarcinomas are more likely to occur in the distal esophagus than are squamous cell tumors. Despite being useful for establishing the extent of advanced cancers, barium swallow radiography is clearly inferior to upper GI endoscopy for detecting uncomplicated Barrett's metaplasia and early adenocarcinoma.

Management and Course

The high incidence of progression to adenocarcinoma in patients with specialized columnar metaplasia has led to the implementation of endoscopic surveillance programs. Because medical and surgical antireflux therapy does not lead to regression of Barrett's metaplasia, surveillance programs usually are lifelong. Surveillance is indicated only for patients who are well enough and willing to undergo surgical resection once adenocarcinoma is detected. A reasonable strategy involves upper GI endoscopy every 1 to 2 years, with systematic, four-quadrant biopsy specimens obtained every 2 cm along the length of Barrett's metaplasia. In addition, any endoscopic abnormalities such as erosions or nodules should be biopsied. Patients with no dysplasia and no endoscopic abnormalities are reexamined in 2 years, whereas patients with endoscopic abnormalities or low-grade dysplasia should have a repeat examination in 6 to 12 months depending on the level of clinical concern. When high-grade dysplasia is documented and confirmed on review by an experienced pathologist, surgical resection should be considered. Several series have revealed a 40% to 50% incidence of invasive adenocarcinoma when endoscopic biopsy specimens document high-grade dysplasia. The decision to proceed with surgical resection should consider the high risk of coexisting malignancy against the operative risks and the desires of the patient. If patient preferences or comorbid conditions preclude surgical intervention in the absence of documented invasive cancer, endoscopic surveillance should continue every 3 months. If two consecutive sessions fail to demonstrate cancer, the interval can be increased to 6 months.

The staging and therapy of adenocarcinoma are essentially the same as the principles outlined for squamous cell carcinoma. Many trials evaluating the efficacy of surgery, chemotherapy, radiation therapy, and endoscopic therapy for esophageal cancer include both tumor types. Any curative resection should include the entire Barrett's segment given the 13% to 37% risk of multicentric tumors. The prognosis of adenocarcinoma of the esophagus is similar to squamous cell cancer with an overall 5-year survival of 7%. Aggressive endoscopic surveillance of Barrett's metaplasia may improve this outcome, but the efficacy and cost effectiveness of surveillance remain to be established.

OTHER MALIGNANT NEOPLASMS

Epithelial Tumors

Other histologic variants of esophageal cancer have been described. Some squamous cell carcinomas have a prominent spindle cell component. This lesion is termed *pseudosarcoma*. Another variant of squamous cell carcinoma is termed *verrucous carcinoma* because of the invasive nature of the primary lesion with only rare metastases. Adenoid cystic carcinoma appears to be derived from submucosal glands, whereas adenosquamous carcinomas combine features of the two common forms of esophageal cancer. Small cell carcinoma of the esophagus may be a primary esophageal tumor or it may represent a metastatic lesion from the lung. As with small cell tumors of the lung, esophageal lesions may be accompanied by paraneoplastic phenomena, including inappropriate antidiuretic hormone secretion and hypercalcemia. All of these histologic subtypes are rare, occur in the elderly, and have a poor prognosis, with the exception of verrucous lesions, which can often be cured because of the low incidence of distant disease.

Metastatic Carcinoma

Metastatic carcinomas constitute <1% of all malignant esophageal tumors. Malignant melanoma and breast cancer are the most common sources. Mediastinal adenopathy from a diverse group of tumors may mimic esophageal cancer on radiographic and clinical examination because of the extrinsic compression of the esophagus.

BENIGN ESOPHAGEAL TUMORS

Squamous Cell Papillomas

Squamous cell papillomas are small, sessile, polypoid lesions discovered incidentally during endoscopic examination for unrelated symptoms. Papillomas usually are solitary, and complete removal often is achieved with forceps biopsy, obviating the need for follow-up examination. The rare syndrome of esophageal papillomatosis has been associated with an increased risk of esophageal carcinoma; therefore, endoscopic surveillance in these patients may facilitate early detection of malignancy.

Submucosal Masses

Leiomyomas are the most common benign tumor of the esophagus. The majority are asymptomatic, but large tumors may cause dysphagia, chest pain, and hemorrhage. They most commonly occur in the distal esophagus. Barium swallow radiography and upper GI endoscopy readily detect symptomatic lesions. Large benign leiomyomas may be difficult to distinguish from rare malignant leiomyosarcomas. Other submucosal lesions of the esophagus are rare and include lipomas, fibromas, fibrovascular polyps, granular cell tumors, hemangiomas, and lymphangiomas. As with leiomyomas, the majority of these lesions are found incidentally and are not considered to be morbid.

CHAPTER 29

Structural Disorders and Miscellaneous Disorders of the Stomach

GASTRIC EMBRYOLOGY AND ANATOMY

The stomach first appears as a fusiform dilation of the primitive foregut. Over several weeks, it rotates 90 degrees clockwise around its longitudinal axis to project its left side anteriorly and its right side posteriorly. After rotation, the new left portion of the stomach elongates more rapidly than the right to form the greater and lesser curvatures, respectively. The cephalic aspect moves downward, and the caudal aspect moves upward and to the right, moving the stomach into its final position. The dorsal gastric mesentery forms the omental bursa, and the ventral mesentery attaches the stomach to the liver. The embryonic endoderm becomes the gastric epithelium and glands, whereas the mesoderm forms the connective tissue, muscle, and serosa of the stomach.

The size, shape, and position of the stomach vary greatly because of its distensibility; after a large meal, it may descend into the lower abdomen or pelvis. The stomach is separated into the cardia (the 1- to 2-cm segment distal to the esophagogastric junction), the fundus (the superior portion of the stomach above a horizontal plane that passes through the esophagogastric junction), the body (the large portion between the fundus and the antrum), the antrum (the distal one-fourth to one-third of the stomach), and the pylorus (the 1- to 2-cm channel that connects the stomach to the duodenum). Along the lesser curvature at the junction of the body and antrum is a bend that is accentuated during peristalsis (i.e., the angularis).

The celiac axis arises from the aorta and branches into the splenic artery (which branches to form the short gastric and left gastroepiploic arteries), left gastric artery, and hepatic artery (which branches to form the right gastric, gastroduodenal, and right gastroepiploic arteries) to form a dense anastomotic network that encircles the stomach. The inferior pancreaticoduodenal branch of the superior mesenteric artery serves the distal stomach as well. The venous drainage of the stomach generally accompanies the arterial supply and leads to the splenic, superior mesenteric, or portal veins.

The gastric enteric nervous system receives extrinsic sympathetic and parasympathetic input. Spinal sympathetic nerves pass through the thoracic sympathetic chain to form the splanchnic nerves that terminate in the celiac ganglia. Postganglionic fibers from the celiac ganglia terminate in the stomach wall. Afferent fibers from the stomach reach cell bodies in the dorsal root ganglia of the spinal cord. The vagus nerves provide parasympathetic innervation to the stomach, projecting from the dorsal motor nucleus of the vagus. Posterior and anterior gastric vagal trunks carry information from both vagi because the fibers interconnect at the level of the esophagus. After it enters the abdomen, the anterior vagus branches into the hepatic and anterior gastric branches; the posterior vagus divides into the celiac and posterior gastric branches. Vagal fibers from the gastric branches synapse within the myenteric and submucosal plexuses.

Lymphatics in the submucosa, muscularis, and serosa anastomose and drain to four main regions from the stomach: (1) The superior gastric lymph nodes receive lymph from the upper stomach; (2) the pancreaticolienal and splenic nodes receive lymph from the fundus and proximal body; (3) the inferior gastric and subpyloric nodes receive drainage from the distal greater curvature; and (4) the superior gastric, hepatic, and subpyloric nodes obtain lymph from the pylorus. Extensive communications exist between these four sites.

The layers of the stomach are the mucosa, the submucosa, the muscularis propria, and the serosa. The mucosa is further divided into the epithelium, lamina propria, and muscularis mucosae. The mucosal architecture consists of foveolae, or pits, that empty the gastric glands. An epithelium that is a single cell thick contains surface mucous cells and specialized cells depending on the gastric region. In the fundus, the pits are shallow. Beneath them are long, convoluted glands that are lined by parietal cells, which secrete hydrochloric acid and intrinsic factor, and by chief cells, which secrete pepsinogens. The proton pump, or H^+,K^+-adenosine triphosphatase, is located on the microvillous membranes of the parietal cells and mediates acid secretion. The antral glands contain G cells, which secrete gastrin intralumenally and into the bloodstream. Other endocrine cells are present that contain serotonin and somatostatin. The proliferative zone in gastric mucosa is located in the base of the pits and in the upper portion of the glands. Cells migrate from this zone to renew the surface epithelium in 2 to 6 days. Renewal of glandular epithelium from the same zone is slower, taking weeks to months. The lamina propria is less well developed than in the intestine and contains connective tissue, smooth muscle, lymphatics, blood vessels, nerves, lymphocytes, plasma cells, mast cells, fibroblasts, macrophages, and eosinophils. The submucosa is a layer of connective tissues that provides a loose framework for arterial, venous, and nerve passage. The muscularis propria consists of a uniform circular layer of smooth muscle surrounded by a variable longitudinal layer and bounded internally by a layer of oblique fibers most prominent in the upper stomach. Areolar tissue and a single layer of squamous mesothelial cells constitute the serosa.

DEVELOPMENTAL ABNORMALITIES OF THE STOMACH

Gastric Atresia

Etiology and Pathogenesis

With gastric atresia, the stomach may end blindly in an atretic segment, which may be absent altogether or may be occluded only with mucosal and submucosal tissue. Atresia may result from failed recanalization of the gut lumen during embryogenesis. The condition may be familial.

Clinical Features, Diagnosis, and Management

The presenting features include a large volume of amniotic fluid and nonbilious vomiting at birth. Abdominal radiography shows an air-distended stomach with no intestinal gas. Treatment is surgical excision of the atretic segment with pyloroplasty (for a short segment) or gastroenterostomy (for extensive disease).

Gastric Mucosal Membranes

Etiology and Pathogenesis

Nonocclusive mucosal membranes in the antrum or pylorus may contain squamous or columnar epithelium and probably result from the same factors that cause gastric atresia.

Clinical Features, Diagnosis, and Management

Nausea and vomiting may not develop until late childhood or adulthood. Abdominal radiographs are usually negative, and the diagnosis is usually made from upper gastrointestinal (GI) barium radiographic studies, which show a bandlike defect that may simulate a second pylorus. Treatment involves excision of the membrane with or without pyloroplasty.

Gastric Duplication

Etiology and Pathogenesis

Gastric duplications contain mucosa, submucosa, and muscularis and are separate from the stomach. Usually they are found as an extragastric mass, but they occasionally communicate with the stomach or pancreas.

Clinical Features, Diagnosis, and Management

Most patients present in infancy with an abdominal mass, pain, or obstruction. Occult or gross bleeding may result if communication is present. Rare perforations may produce peritonitis. Gastric duplications are usually found on upper GI barium radiographs and are amenable to surgical excision.

Microgastria

Etiology and Pathogenesis

Microgastria results from the failure of the stomach to develop from the foregut and is usually associated with fatal cardiac abnormalities.

Clinical Features, Diagnosis, and Management

Patients with microgastria present with vomiting, malnutrition, and anemia and usually die within weeks to months. If the patient survives, surgical construction of a jejunal pouch can be performed.

Gastric Teratoma

Etiology and Pathogenesis

Gastric teratomas are rare tumors composed of all three primary embryonic germ layers. They are found almost exclusively in males. Other associated congenital abnormalities are rare.

Clinical Features, Diagnosis, and Management

Patients present in childhood or adulthood with a mass, bleeding, or symptoms of obstruction. Abdominal radiography shows a calcific mass (resulting from the presence of teeth and bone), and upper GI barium radiography shows a gastric mass. Surgical resection is the preferred treatment; however, total gastrectomy with construction of a jejunal pouch may be needed for large tumors.

HYPERTROPHIC PYLORIC STENOSIS

Etiology and Pathogenesis

Neonatal hypertrophic pyloric stenosis, resulting from pyloric muscular edema and hypertrophy, causes gastric obstruction in 1 of 150 males and 1 of 750 females after birth. It has been suggested that a lack of nitric oxide synthase may produce pylorospasm. In contrast, most adult cases of hypertrophic pyloric stenosis result from peptic ulcer disease, gastritis, or malignancy.

Clinical Features, Diagnosis, and Management

Infants develop regurgitation, then projectile, nonbilious vomiting in the third or fourth week of life, which may continue and lead to malnutrition and weakness. Constipation, oliguria, and weight loss are complications of neonatal pyloric stenosis. On physical examination, the stomach is dilated, and gastric peristalsis may be visible. The hypertrophic pylorus usually is palpated as an olive-sized mass in the upper abdomen. Abdominal radiography shows a large gastric bubble with little intestinal gas; upper GI barium radiography may show a long, narrow pyloric canal. Ultrasound demonstration of the hypertrophied pylorus may obviate the need for contrast radiography. After correction of fluid and electrolyte deficiencies, surgical division of the pyloric muscle from the serosa to the submucosa is indicated and carries excellent long-term results.

Adults with acquired pyloric stenosis present with nausea, vomiting, early satiety, and pain. The diagnosis is made by upper GI barium radiography or upper endoscopy. Surgical resection is usually required, although endoscopic dilation is possible if a pneumatic dilator catheter can be passed to span the pylorus.

GASTRIC DIVERTICULA

Etiology and Pathogenesis

More than 75% of gastric diverticula occur on the proximal posterior wall and are thought to be congenital. More distal diverticula usually result from the scarring or dilation that accompanies peptic disease or malignancy.

Clinical Features, Diagnosis, and Management

Congenital diverticula usually are asymptomatic and are found incidentally on upper GI barium radiography. Rarely, bleeding or perforation may occur, requiring specific endoscopic or surgical therapy. In asymptomatic cases, no treatment is needed.

GASTRIC BEZOARS

Etiology and Pathogenesis

Bezoars are persistent concretions of gastric foreign matter and are composed of plant fibers (phytobezoars), hair (trichobezoars), medications (pharmacobezoars), and persimmons (disopyrobezoars). Most patients with phytobezoars have undergone prior gastric surgery, including vagotomy and pyloroplasty, antrectomy, and partial gastrectomy. Causes of postsurgical bezoar formation include impaired gastric motility, decreased secretion, increased mucus production from gastritis, and anastomotic stenosis. Gastroparesis from any cause can predispose to bezoar formation. Foods implicated in phytobezoars include grapes, oranges, raisins, figs, cherries, coconuts, peaches, apples, bran, oats, celery, pumpkins, sauerkraut, peanuts, cabbage, and potato peels. Phytobezoar development is enhanced by inadequate chewing, poor dentition, loose dentures, and rapid swallowing.

Trichobezoars are green-brown to black, mucus-covered masses of hair that occur most commonly in women who swallow their hair. Men with beards also may be at risk. Drug intoxication may result from medication trapped within the mass of hair. Pharmacobezoars may be composed of aluminum-containing antacids, enteric-coated aspirin, calcium preparations, magnesium carbonate, sucralfate, nifedipine, sodium polystyrene sulfonate (Kayexalate), and lecithin. Unripe persimmons contain a soluble tannin, shibuol, which forms a coagulum when mixed with gastric acid. Yeast bezoars may complicate gastric surgery, but they are often asymptomatic. Other nonfood substances that produce bezoars include furniture polish, cement, fruit pits, plastic, paper, string, cotton, Styrofoam, and toilet paper.

Clinical Features, Diagnosis, and Management

The signs and symptoms of bezoars depend on their size and the degree of disruption of gastric physiologic processes. Although many are asymptomatic,

TABLE 29-1
Therapy for Gastric Bezoars

TREATMENT TYPES	MECHANISM	SPECIFIC THERAPY
Enzymatic	Proteolysis	Papain, pancrelipase, pancreatin, Adolph's meat tenderizer
	Cellulolytic	Cellulase
	Mucolytic	Acetylcysteine
Medication	Prokinetic	Metoclopramide, cisapride
Mechanical	Removal	Endoscopic snare, basket, forceps
	Fragmentation	High-pressure water pulses, Nd:YAG laser
Surgical	Removal	

bezoars can produce nausea, vomiting, anorexia, bloating, halitosis, early satiety, dyspepsia, weight loss, and feelings of epigastric fullness or pain. Gastric obstruction, anemia, hemorrhage, ulceration, and perforation are complications of long-standing gastric bezoars. Abdominal radiography may show an ill-defined mass within the gastric air bubble. Upper GI endoscopy is the most sensitive test for diagnosis of a bezoar and can characterize its constituents. In contrast, upper GI barium radiography demonstrates the presence of gastric bezoars with a sensitivity as low as 24%.

The medical therapy for gastric bezoars includes enzymatic digestion, mechanical disruption, and other modalities (Table 29-1). Phytobezoars may respond to enzymatic agents, including papain (protease), Adolph's meat tenderizer, pancrelipase, pancreatin, cellulase, and acetylcysteine (mucolytic) as well as dilute hydrochloric acid. Gastric ulceration is felt to be a contraindication for enzyme therapy by some but not all clinicians. Insoluble bezoars must be removed mechanically with endoscopic baskets, forceps, and snares. An overtube can be used to reduce the potential for pulmonary aspiration. Alternatively, endoscopically directed water pulses may fragment some bezoars (usually phytobezoars) so that they may be lavaged from the stomach or pass spontaneously into the intestine. Nd:YAG lasers have also been used to fragment enzyme-resistant bezoars. Prokinetic medications (e.g., metoclopramide) may accelerate gastric emptying and help fragment loosely adherent bezoars. However, these agents are more likely to be useful as prophylactic agents after the bezoar has been fragmented, dissolved, or removed. Endoscopic dilation may be required for anastomotic or pyloric strictures, which predispose to bezoar formation. Certain bezoars, such as trichobezoars, are not amenable to medical management and require surgical excision. Surgery also is necessary for complications such as perforation.

GASTRIC FOREIGN BODIES

Etiology and Pathogenesis

Foreign bodies may be swallowed accidentally or intentionally. Small household items and toys are accidentally swallowed by children while playing. Gastric foreign bodies in adults include dental prostheses and toothbrushes, which are swallowed as a result of carelessness, rapid eating, poor eyesight, or ethanol intoxication. Intentional ingestion usually occurs in psychotic, demented, or incarcerated individuals. Illicit drugs may be concealed within the body by swallowing plastic or rubber bags that contain the drugs.

Clinical Features, Diagnosis, and Management

Although 80% to 93% of ingested foreign bodies pass spontaneously, symptoms may be caused by gastric penetration or perforation (leading to localized or generalized peritonitis), gastritis, mucosal tears or ulcers, abscess, hemorrhage, and fistulae. The clinician should consider removal of objects >2 cm in diameter or >5 cm in length (as they are unlikely to pass spontaneously), sharp objects with an increased risk of perforation, or potentially toxic objects. Button batteries that pass into the stomach do not require removal unless the patient has evidence of GI injury (hematochezia or abdominal pain). Most objects can be removed endoscopically with a snare or forceps and an overtube to prevent aspiration and additional injury. Surgery rather than endoscopy is indicated for large, jagged objects and packets of illicit drugs. Fluoroscopic removal of metallic foreign bodies using a magnet-tipped catheter is possible.

GASTRIC RUPTURE

Etiology and Pathogenesis

The stomach is relatively resistant to rupture because it is distensible and able to decompress through the pylorus and gastroesophageal junction. Gastric rupture may occur with emesis, blunt abdominal trauma, or in conditions of gastric overdistention. Disturbance of the normal pressure-release mechanisms (obstructing tumors of the esophagus, pancreas, pylorus, or duodenum, Nissen fundoplication, peptic ulcer disease, or congenital duodenal obstruction) can increase the likelihood of gastric rupture. Vomiting-induced gastric rupture usually develops along the greater curvature in the fundus as a consequence of gastric herniation into the chest and may occur during labor or the postpartum period, with pyloric stenosis, and after ipecac administration. Traumatic causes of gastric rupture include coughing, seizures, lifting of heavy objects, upper GI endoscopy, and the Heimlich maneuver. The site of rupture with overdistention is the lesser curvature near the cardia or fundus in 60% of cases. Nasal oxygen, mouth-to-mouth resuscitation, aerophagia, inadvertent gastric inflation during anesthesia, gas-producing food fermentation, gastric lavage, malfunctioning gastric tamponade balloons, sodium bicarbonate ingestion, and scuba diving have all been reported to cause gastric rupture through overdistention.

Clinical Features, Diagnosis, and Management

Symptoms appear abruptly after rupture (e.g., severe pain, abdominal distention, dyspnea, shock, and subcutaneous emphysema), and signs of peritonitis develop rapidly. Chest and abdominal radiographs show pneumoperitoneum. Additional diagnostic evaluation usually is limited by the life-threatening nature of the condition. Without surgery, mortality is 100% because of massive peritoneal soiling from the rupture, which usually is >5 cm. Even with surgery, mortality rates exceed 60% owing to peritonitis, air embolism, respiratory failure, mediastinitis, bleeding, and sepsis.

GASTRIC VOLVULUS

Etiology and Pathogenesis

Gastric volvulus is defined as an abnormal rotation of one part of the stomach around another and may be organoaxial (rotation around a line joining the pylorus and esophagogastric junction) or, less commonly, mesenteroaxial (rotation around a line from the center of the greater curvature to the porta hepatis). The distinction is unimportant because it has no prognostic importance, and mixed forms often exist. Complete volvulus may impair the gastric blood supply, leading to infarction. The condition is found in both sexes and patients of all ages. Predisposing factors are found in 50% of cases, including eventration of the diaphragm, hiatal hernia, phrenic nerve crush, prior trauma, adhesions, gastrostomies, Nissen fundoplications, and congenital abnormalities of mesenteric fixation.

Clinical Features, Diagnosis, and Management

Gastric volvulus manifests as an acute emergency or as a chronic recurrent gastric obstruction. Acute volvulus is characterized by the sudden onset of left upper quadrant pain and upper abdominal distention, with retching but an inability to vomit. A nasogastric tube cannot be passed because of the obstruction. The mortality of acute volvulus is 30% to 50%, owing to vascular occlusion infarction, perforation, and shock. In contrast, chronic gastric volvulus presents with mild, continuous or intermittent upper abdominal discomfort, postprandial bloating, dysphagia, and fullness. If a large amount of air or fluid is swallowed, thereby distending and tightening the twisted stomach, belching may be difficult. Self-induced vomiting or changes in position may temporarily relieve the symptoms of chronic gastric volvulus.

Abdominal or chest radiography may show a spherical stomach bubble with two air-fluid levels (fundus and antrum) in mesenteroaxial volvulus and a horizontal stomach with a single air-fluid level in organoaxial volvulus. Diaphragmatic eventration or a hiatal hernia may be noted on radiography or computed tomography. Upper GI barium radiography may reveal gastric dilation, the site of twist, and poor passage of the contrast agent distal to the obstruction.

In acute volvulus, immediate surgery is essential to reduce the volvulus. Anterior gastropexy should be performed if possible. Anatomic defects, such as hiatal hernias, should be corrected. If gastric necrosis has developed, local excision or gastrectomy may be needed. Endoscopic placement of dual percutaneous gastrostomies in the antrum and body has been reported. The role of surgery in chronic volvulus is less well defined. Some patients with minimal symptoms may do well without surgical intervention.

CHAPTER 30

Disorders of Gastric Emptying

DISORDERS WITH DELAYED GASTRIC EMPTYING

Incidence and Epidemiology

Many clinical conditions produce secondary delays in gastric emptying, or gastroparesis, by disrupting the normal neural or muscular function of the stomach. These include diseases that are localized to the stomach, disorders that involve the gastrointestinal tract diffusely, and nongastrointestinal diseases. The epidemiology of these conditions parallels that of the underlying disease. Patients may present with delayed gastric emptying that occurred either spontaneously or after a viral prodrome. Such idiopathic or viral cases of gastroparesis are most common in young women. Many cases of nonulcer dyspepsia (NUD) have associated abnormalities in gastric emptying and exhibit overlap with idiopathic gastroparesis.

Etiology and Pathogenesis

Disorders Involving the Stomach

Diabetic Gastroparesis. Patients with long-standing diabetes may experience periods of nausea, vomiting, early satiety, and fullness. In many of these patients, solid-phase gastric emptying is delayed significantly; however, symptoms do not always correlate with gastric motor abnormalities. In general, abnormal gastric emptying complicates diabetes (usually type I) of >10 years' duration and is associated with peripheral and autonomic neuropathy. In patients with recent-onset diabetes, gastric emptying may be accelerated. Motor abnormalities that contribute to delays in gastric emptying include loss of antral contractions, increased pyloric activity (pylorospasm), increased fundus compliance, and increased intestinal motor activity, which acts as a gastric brake. Most investigators believe that diabetic gastroparesis results from impaired intrinsic and extrinsic neural function of the stomach; however, impaired contractility at the smooth muscle level has been demonstrated in animal models.

Postoperative Gastroparesis. A small number of patients (<5%) who have undergone vagotomy and drainage for peptic ulcer disease or for malignancy experience nausea, vomiting, and early satiety secondary to postoperative stasis primarily of solid foods. Abnormalities in antral peristalsis and fundus tone have been demonstrated in this condition. Gastric stasis may also complicate gastroplasty or gastric bypass operations for morbid obesity, producing early satiety, anorexia, and weight reduction. A subset of patients undergoing fundoplication for gastroesophageal reflux develop gastroparesis by unknown mechanisms.

Idiopathic and Viral Gastroparesis. A number of patients (>25%) with gastroparesis have no predisposing factor for their disease. In many instances, fever, myalgias, nausea, and diarrhea precede the onset of gastroparesis, which suggests an underlying viral cause. The virus responsible in most cases is not identified; however, certain parvovirus-like agents (e.g., Norwalk agent) produce an acute gastroparesis pattern.

Nonulcer Dyspepsia. NUD is the most prevalent of the functional upper gastrointestinal tract syndromes. Delayed gastric emptying is reported in 30% to 82% of patients with NUD. Many patients with NUD also exhibit reduced antral contractions and increased sensitivity to mechanical distention of the stomach. Motor dysfunction in NUD is probably pathogenic for symptoms in some patients because prokinetic agents are effective therapy for many.

Gastric Slow Wave Dysrhythmias. A pacemaker area in the proximal gastric body generates rhythmic depolarizations at 3 cycles per minute (cpm). These are the gastric slow waves, which regulate contractile activity in the stomach. Disruptions in the slow wave rhythm that are too rapid (tachygastria) or too slow (bradygastria) as well as decreases in the electrical responses to meal ingestion are observed in many patients with nausea and vomiting, including those with idiopathic symptoms and those with symptoms secondary to systemic conditions (e.g., diabetes, pregnancy, motion sickness, and other causes of gastroparesis). Abnormal slow wave rhythm or amplitude responses are detected in approximately 70% of patients with delayed gastric emptying. However, up to one-third of nauseated patients with normal gastric emptying have abnormal gastric slow wave activity, which suggests that myoelectric disturbances are associated with symptom development independent of any motor disruption.

Medication-Induced Delays in Gastric Emptying. Many prescription and over-the-counter medications delay gastric emptying, including anticholinergics, β-adrenergic agonists, calcium channel antagonists, anti-parkinsonian agents, lithium, serotonin 5-HT$_3$ antagonists, opiates, progesterone, and tricyclic antidepressants (Table 30-1). Nonmedicinal compounds, including ethanol, tobacco, and marijuana, also inhibit gastric motor function. Total parenteral nutrition has been associated with delayed gastric emptying, which may relate in part to the induction of hyperglycemia.

Miscellaneous Gastric Disorders. Idiopathic cyclic nausea and vomiting syndrome is a disorder of unknown etiology. It is characterized by intermittent symptomatic periods that last for days followed by prolonged asymptomatic intervals that last for weeks to months. Many of these patients have delayed gastric emptying suggestive of underlying gastric motor dysfunction. Nausea, vomiting, and intolerance to solid and liquid meals are common after abdominal irradiation. Patients with upper abdominal malignancy (usually pancreatic) develop

TABLE 30-1
Effects of Medications on Gastric Emptying

Delay gastric emptying
    Ethanol (high concentration)
    Aluminum hydroxide antacids
    Atropine
    β-Adrenergic receptor agonists
    Calcitonin
    Calcium channel antagonists
    Dexfenfluramine
    Diphenhydramine
    Glucagon
    Interleukin-1
    L-Dopa
    Lithium
    Omeprazole
    Ondansetron
    Opiates
    Phenothiazines
    Progesterone
    Propantheline bromide
    Sucralfate
    Tetrahydrocannabinol
    Tobacco
    Tricyclic antidepressants
Accelerate gastric emptying
    β-Adrenergic receptor antagonists
    Cisapride
    Diazepam
    Domperidone
    Histamine H_2-receptor antagonists
    Metoclopramide
    Naloxone
    Prostaglandin E_2

symptomatic gastroparesis by unknown mechanisms, which can exacerbate nutritional deficits. Delayed emptying of solids is found with atrophic gastritis, which may relate to the decrease in gastric secretions that are necessary to process ingested food.

Disorders With Diffuse Gastrointestinal Involvement

Rheumatologic Disorders. Scleroderma produces dysphagia, heartburn, nausea, vomiting, bloating, abdominal pain, and bowel disturbances as a result of diffuse dysmotility involving the esophagus, stomach, small intestine, and colon. In most patients, gastroduodenal manometry demonstrates diffuse low-amplitude contractions that are consistent with myopathic involvement. However, a subset of patients with early disease exhibits high-amplitude, uncoordinated contractile activity, which is indicative of neuropathic disease. Rarely, polymyositis-dermatomyositis and systemic lupus erythematosus produce gastroparesis.

Chronic Intestinal Pseudo-obstruction.   Patients with this disorder may have associated gastric dysmotility with prominent nausea, vomiting, bloating, and early satiety. The presence of bladder dysfunction or orthostatic hypotension suggests diffuse neuromuscular disease. Pseudo-obstruction may be familial, it may occur after a viral prodrome, or it may be a paraneoplastic phenomenon with certain malignancies (usually small cell lung carcinoma).

Miscellaneous Diffuse Disorders.   Delayed gastric emptying may occur in diffuse muscle disorders (e.g., myotonic dystrophy and progressive muscular dystrophy) or with amyloidosis. Chagas' disease, resulting from an infection with *Trypanosoma cruzi*, can cause gastroparesis as part of a diffuse process involving smooth muscle tissues. Other infections that diffusely affect gut motor activity include varicella-zoster virus, Epstein-Barr virus, and *Clostridium botulinum*.

Nongastrointestinal Disorders

Eating Disorders.   Delayed gastric emptying with reduced antral contractility is a common manifestation of anorexia nervosa, a disorder that has associated symptoms of bloating, nausea, early satiety, heartburn, and epigastric pain. Causes of gastroparesis with anorexia nervosa include central nervous system inhibition and malnutrition, but no specific gastric pathology has been demonstrated. Some patients with bulimia nervosa exhibit delayed solid emptying. Rumination syndrome usually does not present with delayed emptying, although small reductions in postprandial antral motor activity have been documented.

Neurologic Disorders.   Nausea and vomiting are commonly reported by patients with neurologic disorders (e.g., cerebrovascular accidents, tumors, migraine headaches, seizures, Ménière's disease, and labyrinthitis). Altered gastric motility or emptying has been demonstrated after cerebrovascular accidents, with migraines, and after high cervical spinal injury. Gastric stasis may occur with disorders of autonomic function (e.g., Shy-Drager syndrome, Parkinson's disease, Guillain-Barré syndrome, and multiple sclerosis).

Endocrine and Metabolic Disorders.   Nausea, vomiting, and anorexia are frequently reported by patients with end-stage renal disease, even after adequate dialysis, but only a minority of these patients exhibit abnormal gastric emptying. Gastroparesis or intestinal pseudo-obstruction may develop in hypothyroidism, hyperparathyroidism, and hypoparathyroidism.

Biliary Tract Disease.   Some patients with gallbladder disease and those who have undergone a cholecystectomy have dyspepsia and delayed gastric emptying; however, the causal relationship between the biliary process and the gastric dysmotility is unproved.

Clinical Features

Patients with gastroparesis present with chronic or intermittent nausea, vomiting, bloating, early satiety, and postprandial abdominal pain. In mild cases, symptoms may be absent when the stomach is empty. As the disease progresses, bloating and nausea may increase slowly over several days because of incomplete gastric evacuation of multiple ingested meals, only to be relieved by voluminous vomiting of foul-smelling food ingested hours to days before. In severe gastroparesis, intractable retching may develop, even if no meal has been ingested in several hours. Other symptomatic manifestations of gastroparesis include heartburn resulting from delayed gastric acid clearance, hemorrhage secondary to Mallory-Weiss tears or stasis-induced mucosal irritation, and weight loss. Bezoar development may supervene and exacerbate symptoms of fullness and early satiety. Symptoms and signs of systemic diseases associated with gastroparesis or diffuse gastrointestinal dysmotility may be present—for example, neuropathic findings with diabetes and skin changes with scleroderma. Patients with diabetic gastroparesis may also report alterations in insulin requirements because of unpredictable intestinal nutrient delivery.

Findings on Diagnostic Testing

Laboratory Studies

Laboratory studies may assist in determining the severity and chronicity of the patient's disorder. Hypokalemia and contraction alkalosis result from severe vomiting, whereas anemia and hypoproteinemia are consistent with long-standing malnutrition. Specific serologic findings may suggest rheumatologic diseases such as systemic lupus erythematosus or scleroderma. Blood tests also can detect diabetes, uremia, or thyroid and parathyroid disease.

Radiographic and Endoscopic Studies

Most nauseated patients with presumed gastroparesis should undergo structural evaluation to exclude mechanical obstruction as a cause of symptoms. Abdominal radiography can be used to screen for obstruction of the small intestine, which can be followed by barium radiography, if clinically indicated. Upper gastrointestinal endoscopy is appropriate if gastric outlet obstruction secondary to peptic ulcer disease or malignancy is suspected.

Scintigraphic Studies

Gastric scintigraphic quantitation of gastric emptying has become the gold standard for diagnosis of gastroparesis. Liquid-phase gastric emptying scans involve ingestion of an aqueous-phase isotope such as ^{111}In-DTPA. These scans show first-order kinetics with a half-time of emptying of 8 to 28 minutes. Solid-phase gastric-emptying scintigraphic images using ^{99m}Tc-sulfur colloid mixed with a solid food such as scrambled eggs exhibit a biphasic emptying profile: an initial lag phase followed by a linear emptying phase, which persists until all digestible residue has been expelled by the stomach. In general, 40% to 80% of a solid meal is emptied within 2 hours of its ingestion. Gastroparesis is diagnosed when the times for emptying exceed the mean normal value by two standard deviations. Solid-phase scintigraphy is more sensitive for detection of gastroparesis than liquid-phase scans. The interpretation of a gastric-emptying scan as normal or abnormal should be made in conjunction with the clinical presentation, as many severely symptomatic patients will have apparently normal emptying, whereas completely asymptomatic individuals may have profound gastric retention.

Other methods of assessing gastric emptying, such as ultrasound, magnetic resonance imaging, gastric impedance, and applied potential tomography, do not appear to have significant advantages over gastric scintigraphy.

Gastroduodenal Manometry

Gastroduodenal manometry involves the peroral or transnasal placement of a catheter that monitors pressure changes over a 6- to 8-hour period. During the initial 4 to 5 hours, fasting motility is recorded, during which time one or more cycles of the migrating motor complex should be seen. Motor activity is then measured for 1 to 2 hours after a meal to detect the development of the characteristic fed motor pattern. Manometry affords the option of testing the acute motor effects of prokinetic drugs. Advances in the technique have provided the capability to record 24 hours of gastroduodenal motility in ambulatory patients. Manometry should be considered for patients with unexplained nausea and for patients who have not responded to prokinetic therapy. It should be used to exclude intestinal pseudo-obstruction in patients who are being considered for jejunostomy placement. Loss of fasting and fed control motor activities on manometry would indicate a diagnosis of gastroparesis. Manometry may also detect unsuspected intestinal pseudo-obstruction or findings suggestive of mechanical obstruction (e.g., minute rhythm).

Electrogastrography

Electrogastrography (EGG) measures gastric slow wave activity acquired from cutaneous electrodes placed over the stomach before and after a standard test meal. The signal is carefully filtered to exclude cardiac (60 cpm), respiratory (10 to 25 cpm), and intestinal (10 to 12 cpm) electrical activity. Tachygastria is the diagnosis if a significant fraction of the recording has a dominant frequency of >4 cpm, whereas the diagnosis is bradygastria if the signal is <2 cpm. After meal ingestion, the EGG signal increases in amplitude. In patients with gastroparesis, however, there is no change or there is a decrease in EGG amplitude after eating, which correlates with delays in gastric emptying. Indications for EGG are unexplained nausea and symptoms refractory to medical treatment. EGG is useful as a preoperative predictor of postoperative bloating after fundoplication in children. Currently, the performance of gastroduodenal manometry and EGG is limited to referral centers.

Management and Course

Dietary and Nonmedicinal Therapies

A patient with gastroparesis often benefits from nonmedicinal measures designed to compensate for the motor defect in the stomach. Medications that inhibit gastrointestinal motility should be discontinued if possible. The diet can be modified to reduce prolonged gastric distention. The patient with gastroparesis should be encouraged to eat several small meals per day rather than two to three large meals. Because liquids empty more rapidly than solids, the avoidance of solid foods with large amounts of indigestible residue is desirable. Because lipids are the most potent nutrient inhibitors of gastric emptying, a low-fat diet will benefit a patient with sluggish gastric emptying. However, it has been suggested that the reduction of indigestible dietary fiber is more useful in symptom control than the reduction of dietary fat.

TABLE 30-2
Drugs with Prokinetic Effects on the Stomach

MEDICATION	MECHANISMS OF ACTION	DOSAGE
Metoclopramide	Dopamine receptor antagonism 5-HT_4 facilitation of acetylcholine release from enteric nerves 5-HT_3 receptor antagonism	5–20 mg qid
Cisapride	5-HT_4 facilitation of acetylcholine release from enteric nerves Direct stimulant of smooth muscle contraction 5-HT_3 receptor antagonism	5–20 mg tid or qid
Erythromycin	Motilin receptor agonism	50–200 mg qid
Domperidone	Peripheral dopamine receptor antagonism (does not cross blood-brain barrier)	10–30 mg qid
Bethanechol	Muscarinic receptor agonism	25 mg qid

5-HT = serotonin.

Metabolic control is probably important in gastroparesis secondary to diabetes. Hyperglycemia delays solid gastric emptying and disrupts gastric myoelectrical activity in type I diabetes. Although no long-term studies have examined the effect of tight glycemic control on gastric function, the Diabetes Control and Complications Trial showed improvement in several neural functions with intensive insulin therapy. Therefore, it is recommended that diabetic patients should strive for near euglycemic levels.

Prokinetic Medication Therapy

Medical therapy of gastroparesis has focused on agents that promote gastric emptying (Table 30-2). Metoclopramide is a substitute benzamide that acts by serotonin (5-HT_4) receptor facilitation of cholinergic transmission in the gastric myenteric plexus as well as by dopamine and serotonin (5-HT_3) receptor antagonism. Metoclopramide acutely enhances gastric emptying, but a sustained prokinetic effect is not always attained. Despite this, patients report prolonged symptom improvement, indicating that the antiemetic effects of metoclopramide may be as important as its prokinetic action. Drowsiness, dystonias, galactorrhea, and nervous agitation caused by the central nervous system antidopaminergic actions limit the use of metoclopramide. Cisapride is a newer prokinetic agent without antidopaminergic effects that acts by 5-HT_4 facilitation of myenteric acetylcholine release as well as by 5-HT_3 antagonism and direct smooth muscle effects. In placebo-controlled trials, cisapride accelerates liquid and solid emptying and reduces symptoms for a year or more, although one study reported no improvement in symptoms or gastric emptying. Side effects from cisapride include headaches, cramping, and diarrhea. Erythromycin evokes striking changes in motility because it acts on receptors for motilin, a hormone that initiates migrating motor complex activity. At low doses, erythromycin is an effective prokinetic agent, but at high doses it causes vomiting and pain as a result of intense motor spasms. In a double-blind study of 10 diabetic patients with gastroparesis, intravenous erythromycin accelerated both liquid and solid gastric emptying. Little is known about the long-term efficacy of erythromycin; however, its prokinetic effects appear to exhibit desensitization similar to metoclopramide. A current area of pharmaceutical research focuses on the development of new prokinetic drugs. Domperidone is a peripheral dopamine-receptor antagonist with beneficial effects similar to metoclopramide, but because domperidone does not cross the blood-brain barrier, dystonias and agitation are rare. Potent derivatives of erythromycin without antimicrobial properties are being tested for prokinetic and symptomatic efficacy in treating gastroparesis.

The efficacy of prokinetic agents depends on their delivery into the bloodstream. Some clinicians have proposed giving drugs such as metoclopramide in liquid form to promote its delivery into the intestine. Metoclopramide given subcutaneously has been shown to improve symptoms and gastric emptying in patients with gastroparesis. It has also been documented to reduce chemotherapy-induced nausea when administered as a nasal spray. Cisapride in rectal suppositories also has potent prokinetic effects.

Therapy for Gastroparesis Refractory to Treatment with Prokinetic Agents

For patients resistant to diet and drug therapy, few treatment options exist. One study found endoscopic abnormalities, including *Candida* esophagitis and peptic disease, in 10 of 20 patients with exacerbations of diabetic gastroparesis. Symptoms decreased when these endoscopically defined problems were treated, which justifies endoscopy to evaluate unexplained clinical deterioration. Intermittent jejunostomy tube feedings reduce nausea and vomiting, decrease hospitalizations, and improve nutrition and overall health in diabetic patients. Surgical resections usually are of limited benefit, although total gastrectomy has resulted in symptom improvement in most patients with severe gastroparesis caused by prior vagotomy and gastric drainage.

DISORDERS WITH RAPID GASTRIC EMPTYING

Incidence and Epidemiology

Abnormally rapid gastric emptying is clearly clinically important in only one subset of patients, those who have undergone vagotomy and gastric drainage for ulcer disease or malignancy. The clinical manifestation of this complication, which occurs in 8% to 15% of surgeries, is the dumping syndrome. Other conditions are associated with accelerated emptying, but their clinical relevance is uncertain.

Etiology and Pathogenesis

Postvagotomy Dumping Syndrome

Any surgical procedure involving vagotomy may produce the dumping syndrome, which may be further exacerbated by gastric drainage procedures (e.g., pyloroplasty, antrectomy). Characteristically, these operations produce accelerated emptying of liquids with variable effects on solid-phase gastric emptying. This accelerated liquid emptying overwhelms the postprandial absorptive capabilities of the proximal intestine, leading to fluid shifts and massive release of vasoactive peptide hormones, including vasoactive intestinal polypeptide, serotonin, bradykinin, substance P, enteroglucagon, gastric inhibitory peptide, and neurotensin, which are responsible for the gastrointestinal and vasomotor symptoms of dumping syndrome. There may also be an excessive release of insulin that persists into the late postprandial period, producing hypoglycemia 1 to 4 hours after eating. Certain procedures (e.g., truncal vagotomy with antrectomy or pyloroplasty, and subtotal gastrectomy) accelerate the initial emptying of solids and impair gastric sieving. As a result, large quantities of larger-than-normal food particles are delivered to the intestine, where they are inefficiently digested and absorbed.

Other Causes of Rapid Gastric Emptying

Gastric emptying of fatty liquid meals is accelerated in patients with marked steatorrhea from pancreatic insufficiency. Some investigators have reported accelerations in liquid emptying in subsets of patients with duodenal ulcer disease. Patients with Zollinger-Ellison syndrome exhibit rapid liquid and solid emptying, which is probably not caused by gastric hypersecretion. Many newly diagnosed diabetics have accelerated rather than delayed gastric emptying. These findings probably are not clinically important in most patients.

Clinical Features

The early dumping syndrome, occurring 30 to 60 minutes after meal ingestion, is characterized by alimentary symptoms (abdominal pain, diarrhea, gas, bloating, borborygmi, and nausea) and vasomotor symptoms (flushing, palpitations, diaphoresis, lightheadedness, tachycardia, and even syncope). Physical examination of these patients may reveal orthostatic or even supine effects on pulse and blood pressure. When severe, dumping syndrome can be debilitating, producing a 30% weight loss. The late dumping syndrome occurs 1 to 4 hours after eating. Symptoms include diaphoresis, palpitations, tremulousness, hunger, weakness, confusion, and syncope and are believed to result from reactive hypoglycemia.

Findings on Diagnostic Testing

The diagnosis of dumping syndrome is based on a characteristic constellation of symptoms in a patient who has undergone gastric surgery. Diagnostic testing usually is not necessary. A hematocrit or plasma osmolarity determination in the early postprandial period after a glucose challenge may show hemoconcentration. Measures of packed cell volume and gastric scintigraphy are occasionally obtained, but they rarely provide critical information.

Management and Course

Dietary Management

Dietary recommendations for patients with dumping syndrome include ingestion of food high in proteins and fats and low in carbohydrates with minimal fluid intake during the meal. Non-nutritive fluids should be taken before or after ingestion of solids. In postvagotomy patients, liquid emptying is more rapid while sitting; therefore, some patients may benefit by assuming a supine position immediately after eating. Viscous guar and pectin have been recommended to thicken ingested liquids, but the efficacy of this practice is unproved.

Medication Therapy

The somatostatin analog octreotide reduces symptoms of early and late dumping syndrome. The effects of octreotide on gastric emptying are controversial, whereas the agent impressively blunts exaggerated postprandial hormone release. Despite the acute effects of octreotide on dumping syndrome, there is much less information on its long-term use. One study showed significant patient dropout because of the diarrheal side effects of the medication.

Surgical Therapy

Proposed surgical therapies for dumping syndrome include pyloric reconstruction, placement of a Roux-en-Y gastrojejunostomy, reversal of a gastrojejunostomy, construction of an antiperistaltic loop between the stomach and intestine, and retrograde electrical pacing of the small intestine. Each treatment has its enthusiasts; however, treatment fails in many patients, and postoperative gastroparesis develops in many more. Thus, it is difficult to recommend surgical therapy for the majority of patients with dumping syndrome.

CHAPTER 31

Acid-Peptic Disorders and Zollinger-Ellison Syndrome

ACID-PEPTIC DISEASE

Incidence and Epidemiology

Peptic ulcer disease (PUD), including duodenal and gastric ulcers, is a significant medical problem in the United States. There are 500,000 new cases per year and 4 million annual recurrences. The 1-year point prevalence of active PUD is 1.8%, and the lifetime prevalence is 11% to 14% for men and 8% to 11% for women. The incidence of duodenal ulcer peaked from 1950 to 1970, declined from 1970 to 1980, and has since stabilized, probably because of changes in the prevalence of *Helicobacter pylori*. Conversely, there has been a significant increase in hospitalizations of elderly patients with ulcer hemorrhage and perforation, which has been attributed to the increased used of NSAIDs. Genetic factors play a role in ulcer pathogenesis, as there is a threefold increase in lifetime prevalence among first-degree relatives and a 50% concordance among identical twins. Persons whose blood group is O and those who are nonsecretors of blood group antigens are at increased risk of PUD. Other causes of PUD include gastrinoms and systemic mastocytosis, and diseases that occur in both sporatic form and, less commonly, as genetically linked syndromes (multiple endocrine neoplasia type 1 and familial mastocytosis).

Etiology and Pathogenesis

Helicobacter pylori

H pylori infection causes most cases of histologic gastritis and PUD and may predispose to development of gastric carcinoma. *H pylori* is a curved, gram-negative rod that produces a characteristic highly active urease. *H pylori* culture requires a supplemented medium (chocolate agar) and grows within 3 to 5 days at 37°C. Evidence suggests that *H pylori* is transmitted by fecal-oral routes, based on increases in prevalence among family members, in chronic care facilities, and among endoscopy personnel and the demonstration of positive stool cultures for *H pylori* in affected individuals. Contaminated water may also be a source in some populations. The prevalence of *H pylori* gastritis increases from 10% at age 20 years to 50% at age 60 years. The annual infection rate is approximately 1%. These rates are higher among Latin Americans and blacks.

H pylori organisms reside in the gastric mucus layer adjacent to the epithelial cell surface; they occasionally penetrate into or between the epithelial cells. *H pylori* may also colonize ectopic gastric mucosa in the duodenum, esophagus (i.e., Barrett's metaplasia), Meckel's diverticula, and rectum. It has been postulated that gastric metaplasia in the duodenum secondary to acid production is necessary for development of duodenal ulcer disease. In the stomach, *H pylori* colonizes the fundus, body, and antrum and is found in 70% to 95% of patients with active chronic gastritis (i.e., increases in mucosal neutrophils and round cells). Histologic gastritis may be present only in the distal stomach, and with *H pylori* eradication, the lesion resolves. Patients who contract *H pylori* may progress from active superficial chronic gastritis to atrophic gastritis, which may then be associated with *H pylori* clearance. The prevalence of *H pylori* in pernicious anemia is only 3% to 21%. Patients undergoing surgery for PUD have a high prevalence of *H pylori* infection, which may decrease to 22% to 50% postoperatively, possibly secondary to duodenogastric bile reflux. Twenty-two percent to 63% of persons taking NSAIDs have *H pylori* infection; histologic gastritis in these patients is secondary to *H pylori*, with only 5% to 8% of *H pylori*–negative NSAID users exhibiting active chronic inflammation. It does not appear that *H pylori* predisposes to or worsens NSAID-induced injury.

Ninety percent to 100% of patients with duodenal ulcers and 70% to 90% of those with gastric ulcers have *H pylori* infection. The etiologic role of this organism is supported by numerous studies showing that *H pylori* eradication prevents ulcer recurrences. *H pylori* treatment also may produce more rapid ulcer healing and higher rates of ulcer healing. However, only 15% of *H pylori*–infected persons develop PUD, suggesting that specific factors are required for ulceration to occur. *H pylori* produces ammonia, which injures the gastric mucosal barrier; a protease, which degrades mucus glycoproteins, lipase, and phospholipase; and a cytotoxin. *H pylori*–positive patients have higher basal and meal-stimulated gastrin release, which has been postulated to be secondary to reduced antral somatostatin production. Gastrin levels decrease after *H pylori* eradication. Acid secretion is higher in *H pylori*–positive duodenal ulcer patients, and it does not decrease after *H pylori* eradication. Acid secretion is normal in *H pylori*–positive patients without PUD. *H pylori* releases a chemotactic factor for neutrophils and monocytes and elaborates cytokines and reactive oxygen metabolites, which may contribute to mucosal damage.

H pylori may be a predisposing factor for the development of gastric adenocarcinoma as well as for some gastric lymphomas. Chronic gastritis and *H pylori* infection are commonly associated with the development of adenocarcinoma, often in patients who acquired *H pylori* early in life. Cancers of the gastric cardia are not associated with *H pylori*. *H pylori* may be a risk factor for gastric lymphoma of mucosa-associated lymphoid tissue; regression of this low-grade lymphoma may occur after *H pylori* eradication.

Nonsteroidal Anti-Inflammatory Drugs

Two percent to 4% of persons taking NSAIDs develop serious complications, and 30% of ulcer deaths are attributable to the effects of NSAIDs. Acute and chronic NSAID ingestion causes subepithelial hemorrhages and erosions, but gastric adaptation lessens the prominence of these lesions over several days. Despite adaptation, gastric erosions are found at endoscopy in 30% to 50% of patients on chronic NSAID therapy. These superficial lesions bear little relation to subsequent ulcer development or to symptomatic dyspepsia. In case-controlled studies that have evaluated the risk of NSAID-induced ulceration relative to a matched control population, the relative risk of development of gastric ulcer is 4.0 and of duodenal ulcer is 1.7 to 3.2. About 25% of patients receiving chronic NSAID therapy develop gastric or duodenal ulcers at some point. Dyspepsia in patients taking NSAIDs is more common in the first few weeks of therapy and declines with time. The positive predictive value of dyspepsia for the presence of an ulcer is only 26%. Conversely, up to 40% of patients with NSAID-induced ulcers are asymptomatic; among patients who develop hemorrhage, 60% have no prior symptoms.

NSAID ingestion is associated with an increased risk of complications. It is estimated that 30% of cases of gastrointestinal bleeding and 29% of ulcer deaths are directly attributable to the effects of NSAIDs. For chronic NSAID therapy, the complication rate ranges from 1% to 4% per year. The incidence of NSAID-induced ulcer complications is increased up to 14-fold by a previous history of gastrointestinal bleeding or PUD. The relative risk of NSAID-related complications is greater than five in patients older than 60 years but is less than two in younger patients. NSAID complications also are dependent on the medication doses: There is a 1.7-fold higher rate of bleeding for patients taking 325 mg aspirin daily versus a 14-fold higher rate for patients taking 1200 mg per day. Concurrent use of corticosteroids and NSAIDs increases the risk of complications compared with using NSAIDs alone. Certain NSAIDs are associated with increased risks of complications compared with other agents. Nonacetylated salicylates (e.g., salsalate) minimally inhibit cyclo-oxygenase and produce fewer adverse side effects. Nabumetone and etodolac inhibit systemic prostaglandin production but spare gastroduodenal prostaglandin synthesis, leading to lower rates of ulceration and fewer gastrointestinal side effects. Other gastrointestinal NSAID side effects include ulceration and weblike strictures of the small intestine, acute colitis, exacerbations of inflammatory bowel disease, and ulcers, strictures, and perforation of the colon.

NSAIDs induce mucosal injury by direct damage and systemic effects. Many NSAIDs are weak acids that directly damage epithelial cells if absorbed. Other toxic local mechanisms include inhibition of mucosal prostaglandin secretion, reduced mucus secretion, and interference with cell turnover. The presence of ulcerations with chronic use of enteric-coated aspirin or the prodrug sulindac (which is not locally active) indicates the importance of systemic causes of NSAID-induced injury. Inhibition of cyclo-oxygenase with reduced prostaglandin production leads to reduced mucus and bicarbonate secretion, decreased mucosal blood flow, persistence of gastric acid secretion, and enhanced neutrophil adherence to vascular endothelial linings. Platelet cyclo-oxygenase inhibition also increases the risk of hemorrhage from mucosal lesions.

Miscellaneous Factors Associated with Ulcer Disease

After adjusting for other factors, current tobacco smokers are twice as likely to develop ulcers; the increased risk is directly related to the pack-years of smoking. Cigarette smoking has been postulated to increase susceptibility to *H pylori* infection by diminishing mucosal defensive factors and by providing a more favorable milieu for colonization. Cigarette smokers have higher pepsinogen I

TABLE 31-1
Diseases Associated with Duodenal Ulcers

Evidence strongly supports an association
    Zollinger-Ellison syndrome
    Systemic mastocytosis
    Multiple endocrine neoplasia type I
    Chronic pulmonary disease
    Chronic renal failure
    Cirrhosis
    Kidney stones
    α_1-Antitrypsin deficiency
Evidence only suggests an association
    Crohn's disease
    Hyperparathyroidism without multiple endocrine neoplasia type I
    Coronary artery disease
    Polycythemia vera
    Chronic pancreatitis

---

levels (because of *H pylori* infection), delayed solid and liquid emptying, reduced gastroduodenal prostaglandin production, decreased bicarbonate secretion, decreased mucosal blood flow, increased duodenogastric reflux, and increased free radical production.

The role of psychological factors in the pathogenesis of PUD is uncertain. Acute injury or disease may produce acute gastric erosions and ulcers independent of *H pylori* infection or NSAID use, but the importance of stress in this response is unknown. In a study of 4500 patients, emotional stress was associated with rises in PUD incidence, and with progressive degrees of stress the increases in the relative risk were 1.4 to 2.9.

Certain diseases are associated with increases in PUD (Table 31-1). The prevalence of PUD is increased threefold with chronic pulmonary disease, although the role of tobacco smoking in this association is uncertain. Patients with cystic fibrosis have an increased risk for PUD because of reduced bicarbonate secretion. α_1-Antitrypsin deficiency may lead to PUD because a lack of protease inhibitors. Cirrhosis and renal failure predispose to development of PUD by unknown mechanisms.

Seasonal variations have been reported for PUD development. The role of corticosteroid use in the absence of NSAID use is controversial. One review concluded that 1 month of steroid use resulting in an accumulative dose of >1 g prednisone (or its equivalent) increases the risk of PUD. There is no proven ulcerogenic effect of ethanol on the gastroduodenal mucosa in concentrations routinely ingested. There are no obvious dietary components that increase the risk of PUD, although foods that induce dyspepsia should be avoided.

Associated Factors in Pathogenesis

Mucosal Defenses.   Defensive elements that prevent gastroduodenal mucosal damage are divided into pre-epithelial, epithelial, and subepithelial factors. The pre-epithelial factors include the mucus-bicarbonate barrier, which serves as a modest barrier to H^+ and pepsin; the mucoid cap, which is a mucus and fibrin structure that forms in response to injury; and surface-active phospholipids, which enhance cell membrane hydrophobicity and increase mucus viscosity. Epithelial factors include restitution, which involves repair of epithelium by movement of existing cells over the damaged area; cellular resistance, which maintains an electrical gradient to prevent cellular acidification; acid-base transporters, which transport bicarbonate into the mucus and subepithelial tissues and extrude acid; growth factors; prostaglandins; and nitric oxide. Subepithelial factors include mucosal blood flow, which delivers nutrients and bicarbonate to the epithelium, and leukocyte adhesion and extravasation, which induce tissue injury and are suppressed by endogenous prostaglandins. Impairment of one or more of these defense mechanisms by *H pylori*, NSAIDs, or ischemia leads to mucosal injury and ulceration.

Duodenal Ulcer Pathophysiology.   Several abnormalities in gastroduodenal secretion, gastrin release, and gastric emptying have been observed in patients with duodenal ulcers. These patients secrete greater amounts of acid and pepsin at rest and after stimulation, which is associated with an increase in parietal cell mass, although, for both, there is significant overlap with normal persons. About one-third of patients with duodenal ulcers have abnormal responses to pentagastrin or histamine, whereas 60% have increased and abnormally prolonged acid responses to meal ingestion. When basal acid output (BAO) is expressed as a fraction of maximal acid output (MAO) stimulated by pentagastrin, only 10% to 20% of patients with duodenal ulcers are abnormal. An increase in nocturnal acid secretion is more important than BAO with duodenal ulcer, producing increases in the cumulative 24-hour acid secretion in this patient population. Despite these findings, it has been difficult to demonstrate reduced duodenal pH with duodenal ulcer disease. *H pylori* infection increases basal and meal-stimulated gastrin concentrations, but it remains uncertain whether patients with duodenal ulcers exhibit normal or increased sensitivity to circulating gastrin. Subpopulations of these patients may exhibit accelerated gastric emptying of liquids, which would increase the duodenal bulb acid exposure. The mucus gel covering the duodenum is weaker in patients with duodenal ulcers than in healthy individuals, and bicarbonate production in the duodenal bulb is reduced.

Gastric Ulcer Pathophysiology.   Most gastric ulcers are associated with *H pylori* infection or NSAID use, although 10% of patients have idiopathic ulcers. Type I ulcers occur in the gastric body, but are not associated with other gastroduodenal disease. Type II ulcers also occur in the body but are associated with duodenal scarring or ulcers, whereas type III ulcers occur in the prepyloric area. The pathophysiology of type II and type III ulcers is similar to that of duodenal ulcers, whereas type I ulcers are associated with reduced or normal acid secretion. Antral gastritis (usually caused by *H pylori*, but also by bile reflux) is prominent early in the course of gastric ulcer disease. It occasionally proceeds to gastric atrophy. Many proximal ulcers develop in areas of antral gland metaplasia. Resting and acid- and fat-stimulated pyloric contractions are reduced in gastric ulcer disease. This raises the possibility that sphincter dysfunction increases duodenogastric reflux, a phenomenon observed in some patients with gastric ulcers. Delayed gastric emptying, particularly of solids, is also seen. Although gastric acid secretion is not increased in most patients with gastric ulcers, some acid secretion is generally required for ulcerogenesis. Gastric ulcers tend to occur near the angularis, a region where the mucosa is supplied arterially, rather than by a rich submucosal plexus, which suggests an ischemic factor.

Clinical Features

Abdominal pain occurs in 94% of patients with PUD, but its sensitivity and specificity as markers for mucosal ulceration are low. The pain is usually epigastric in location, does not radiate, occurs 2 to 3 hours postprandially, and is relieved by food or antacids. The most discriminating symptom is pain that awakens the patient between midnight and 3 AM. This symptom affects two-thirds of patients with duodenal ulcers and one-third of those with gastric ulcers but is also reported in one-third of patients with nonulcer dyspepsia. Approximately 10% of patients with PUD, especially with NSAID-related disease, present with complications without a previous history of ulcer pain. It is probable that gastroduodenitis produces the same pain as PUD. One study showed that 90% of patients with classic ulcer symptoms had either an ulcer or endoscopic or histologic gastroduodenitis, although the percentage is much lower in patients with atypical pain.

Complications of PUD include hemorrhage, perforation, penetration, and obstruction. Hemorrhage occurs in 15% of patients with PUD and is most common after age 60 years, probably because of NSAID use in this age group. About one-third of patients treated with H_2-receptor antagonists have recurrent hemorrhage; however, eradication of *H pylori* may prevent these recurrences in *H pylori*–positive patients. Perforation occurs in 7% of patients and is increasing in incidence secondary to increased NSAID use. Duodenal ulcers perforate anteriorly, and gastric ulcers perforate along the anterior wall of the lesser curvature. Penetration differs from perforation in that the ulcer crater bores into an adjacent organ instead of leaking digestive contents into the peritoneal cavity. Gastric ulcers penetrate into the left lobe of the liver or the colon, causing a gastrocolic fistula, but duodenal ulcers penetrate into the pancreas, producing pancreatitis. Acute inflammation, edema, and scarring near the gastroduodenal junction can cause outlet obstruction in 2% of patients, producing heartburn, early satiety, weight loss, abdominal pain, and vomiting.

Findings on Diagnostic Testing

A number of disorders can produce dyspepsia, which mimics the clinical presentation of PUD, including nonulcer dyspepsia, upper gastrointestinal neoplasia, pancreaticobiliary diseases, mesenteric ischemia, and Crohn's disease.

Radiographic and Endoscopic Studies

Studies using air-contrast upper gastrointestinal barium radiography and upper gastrointestinal endoscopy show nearly equivalent sensitivity and specificity for the diagnosis of PUD, although single-contrast barium studies have high false-negative diagnostic rates. Upper gastrointestinal endoscopy has the advantage in that biopsy specimens can be obtained to document the presence of histologic gastritis or *H pylori* infection and to exclude malignancy in gastric ulcers. Radiographic demonstration of gastric ulcer healing is not a reliable indicator of benign histologic features; therefore, endoscopic biopsy is required for gastric ulcers found on barium radiography. In patients with gastric ulcers not secondary to the use of NSAIDs, four to eight biopsy specimens will yield a correct diagnosis in >95% of gastric malignancies. All suggestive ulcers should be examined at repeat upper gastrointestinal endoscopy 8 weeks after initiation of appropriate therapy. Although gastric ulcers that clearly develop in association with NSAID use do not always need biopsy, they should be observed until healed.

Helicobacter pylori Testing

A number of tests are available for documentation of *H pylori* infection. Histologic examination of endoscopic biopsy specimens with Giemsa, Warthin-Starry silver, or hematoxylin-eosin staining is the standard for diagnosis. To speed the diagnosis of *H pylori* infection, urease tests were developed in which biopsy specimens are placed in gels containing phenol red and urea (e.g., CLO-test). A change to red is indicative of *H pylori*–associated urease activity. Urease tests have 90% sensitivity and excellent specificity within 3 to 24 hours of biopsy. ^{13}C- and ^{14}C-urea breath tests, in which exhaled isotopic carbon dioxide concentrations after ingestion of ^{13}C- or ^{14}C-urea correlate with intragastric *H pylori* urease activity, offer 90% to 100% sensitivities and specificities for active *H pylori* infection without the need for endoscopic biopsy. Biopsy and breath test methods may give false-negative results in patients who have been given short courses of antibiotics. Enzyme-linked immunosorbent assays are available for detection of serum antibodies to *H pylori*, with sensitivities of 80% to 95% and specificities of 75% to 95%. Titers may decrease over 6 to 12 months but frequently remain abnormal; therefore, serologic testing is a poor means of assessing *H pylori* eradication.

The clinical indications for structural evaluation and *H pylori* testing of a patient with dyspepsia are a source of considerable debate. In patients younger than 40 years with mild or intermittent symptoms, empiric treatment with acid-suppressive drugs for 4 weeks is reasonable. If symptoms resolve and do not recur, no further evaluation is needed. Some clinicians advocate *H pylori* serologic testing in this population, and, if the test results are positive, treatment with antibiotics. However, this practice is not universally accepted for several reasons: Many patients with nonulcer dyspepsia are *H pylori*–positive but unresponsive to antibiotics; antibiotic therapy has definable adverse effects; and there is a concern about the development of antibiotic-resistant *H pylori* strains. Initial upper gastrointestinal endoscopy is recommended for patients older than 50 years, for those with long-standing or recurrent symptoms, for those with systemic symptoms (e.g., weight loss, anorexia, back pain), for those with hemorrhage, and for those with possible malignancy or other systemic disease. For endoscopically documented PUD, a biopsy specimen is obtained endoscopically for urease testing and histologic study. Urea breath testing is reserved for demonstration of *H pylori* eradication. Decision analyses have been conducted to determine the most cost-effective approach to patients with dyspepsia, but to date the results are highly dependent on the variable costs of diagnostic testing and do not consistently favor one diagnostic approach.

Serum Gastrin and Gastric Acid Secretion Testing

Serum gastrin measurements are indicated in patients with PUD and endocrine neoplasia (especially hyperparathyroidism), in patients with ulcers distal to the duodenal bulb, and in those with ulcers refractory to standard therapy, including *H pylori* eradication (Table 31-2). The indications for gastric acid secretion testing are to evaluate patients with hypergastrinemia in whom a gastrinoma is suspected, to document adequate acid suppression in patients with known gastrinoma, and, rarely, to evaluate refractory ulcer disease.

TABLE 31-2
Clinical Indications for Serum Gastrin Measurement

Multiple ulcers
Ulcers in unusual locations
Ulcers associated with severe esophagitis
Refractory ulcers that recur frequently
Patients with peptic ulcer disease awaiting surgery
Extensive family history of ulcer disease
Postoperative ulcer recurrence
Basal hyperchlorhydria
Unexplained diarrhea or steatorrhea
Hypercalcemia
Family history of pancreatic islet, pituitary, or parathyroid tumor
Prominent gastric or duodenal folds

Management and Course

Most ulcers are managed with medications—that is, drugs that suppress acid secretion, neutralize gastric acid, have cytoprotective effects, and eradicate *H pylori*. Endoscopy is indicated for control of hemorrhage and can be useful in some cases of gastric outlet obstruction. Surgery is required for other complications such as perforation and obstruction. Surgical management of PUD is discussed in Chapter 32.

Pharmacology of Antiulcer Medications

H$_2$-Receptor Antagonists.   Four H$_2$-receptor antagonists are approved for clinical use: cimetidine, ranitidine, famotidine, and nizatidine. These agents inhibit basal, histamine-stimulated, pentagastrin-stimulated, and meal-stimulated acid secretion in a linear, dose-dependent manner with a maximal 90% inhibition of vagal- and gastrin-stimulated acid production and near-total inhibition of nocturnal and basal secretion. Equipotent oral doses are 40 mg famotidine, 300 mg ranitidine, 300 mg nizatidine, and 1200 to 1600 mg cimetidine. Once daily bedtime dosing of H$_2$-receptor antagonists provides adequate control of acid secretion for treatment of PUD. Plasma concentrations of H$_2$-receptor antagonists are affected by renal insufficiency; doses should be halved when creatinine clearance is less than 15 to 30 ml per minute (cimetidine, famotidine) or <50 ml per minute (nizatidine, ranitidine). Side effects from these agents are rare but include cardiac rhythm disturbances with intravenous therapy, antiandrogenic effects resulting in gynecomastia and impotence (caused by cimetidine), hyperprolactinemia with galactorrhea, central neural effects (e.g., headache, lethargy, depression, memory loss), and hematologic effects (e.g., leukopenia, anemia, thrombocytopenia, and elevations in hepatic aminotransferases). Cimetidine (and less commonly ranitidine) bind to hepatic cytochrome P-450 enzymes, most seriously inhibiting metabolism of theophylline, phenytoin, lidocaine, quinidine, and warfarin.

Proton Pump Inhibitors.   The proton pump inhibitors, omeprazole and lansoprazole, inhibit H$^+$,K$^+$-adenosine triphosphatase activity in the gastric parietal cell canalicular membrane, leading to nearly complete inhibition of basal and stimulated acid secretion. Proton pump inhibitors have far greater effects on daytime (meal-stimulated) acid secretion than do H_2-receptor antagonists. Omeprazole is administered as enteric-coated granules because it degrades rapidly at acid pH. Its acid inhibition endures >24 hours because it permanently inactivates the proton pump. The optimal time for drug intake is before meals because proton pumps are maximally stimulated by food. By corollary, omeprazole is much less effective in fasting patients because most proton pumps are inactive. Proton pump inhibitor dosing is not modified by renal or hepatic disease. The frequency of adverse effects with the proton pump inhibitors is similar to that with H_2-receptor antagonists. Omeprazole inhibits certain cytochrome P-450 activities, altering the metabolism of diazepam, phenytoin, and warfarin; the metabolism of theophylline, lidocaine, and quinidine is unaffected. A 1-month course of omeprazole significantly increases gastrin concentrations, greater than is observed with H_2-receptor antagonists, with 12% of values exceeding the upper limits of normal. Three percent to 6% of patients on chronic omeprazole develop profound hypergastrinemia (>400 pg per ml). The consequences of this elevation are uncertain at this time. However, long-term omeprazole therapy (i.e., up to 7 years) is not associated with gastric dysplasia, carcinoid tumors, or carcinoma, although enterochromaffin-like cell hyperplasia has been noted. There is no agreement about the need to monitor serum gastrin levels with proton pump therapy, but some clinicians have advocated dose reduction or alternate therapies if serum gastrin levels are greater than 250 to 500 pg per ml.

Cytoprotective Agents.   Sucralfate, a complex salt of sucrose in which the eight hydroxyl groups of sucrose are replaced by sulfate and aluminum hydroxide, binds to tissue proteins, forming a protective barrier that absorbs bile salts and pepsin. Sucralfate may also stabilize gastric mucus and have trophic effects on the mucosa. Adverse effects of sucralfate include constipation and, in renal failure, the possibility of aluminum toxicity. The drug also binds several drugs, limiting their absorption.

Misoprostol is a prostaglandin E_1 analog that inhibits gastric acid secretion, stimulates bicarbonate and mucus secretion, enhances mucosal blood flow, and inhibits cell turnover. Dose-related diarrhea occurs in 10% to 30% of patients and may be associated with crampy discomfort. Women of child-bearing potential should be advised of the risk of fetal loss. Uterine bleeding can occur in women of any age.

Bismuth subsalicylate coats ulcer craters, possibly forming a protective layer against the effects of acid and pepsin. Bismuth compounds also stimulate mucosal prostaglandin E_2 production, increase bicarbonate secretion, and have anti–H $pylori$ activity. Toxicity of bismuth subsalicylate is extremely rare, although significant blood salicylate levels may occur. A new drug combination containing ranitidine and a bismuth compound has been released for treatment of H $pylori$ infection.

Antacids.   Antacids are used liberally by patients for symptomatic control of dyspepsia, although their role in primary management of PUD is limited. Antacids are effective because of their acid-neutralizing effects as well as their cytoprotective effects (e.g., increased prostaglandin release, mucus production, bicarbonate release) and their ability to bind bile salts and inhibit pepsin activity. Antacids containing sodium can cause significant sodium overload. Calcium carbonate may cause hypercalcemia, metabolic alkalosis, and renal insufficiency. Antacids that contain magnesium can cause diarrhea, whereas

TABLE 31-3
Eradication Rates of *Helicobacter pylori* with Various Regimens

REGIMEN	ERADICATION RATE (%)
Bismuth	
Bismuth subsalicylate	5–10
Colloidal bismuth subcitrate	10–35
Single antibiotics	
Amoxicillin	15–25
Clarithromycin	50
Other antibiotics	0–5
Proton pump inhibitors (omeprazole, lansoprazole)	0–15
Dual therapy	
Bismuth/amoxicillin	30–60
Bismuth/metronidazole	30–75
Amoxicillin/metronidazole	55–95
Omeprazole/amoxicillin or clarithromycin	55–85
Triple therapy	
Bismuth/metronidazole/tetracycline or amoxicillin	80–95

aluminum compounds may induce constipation and neurotoxicity in patients with renal failure.

Treatment of *H pylori*–Induced Peptic Ulcer Disease

Most peptic ulcers are caused by *H pylori* infection, and the presence of an *H pylori*–related duodenal or gastric ulcer is an indication for specific therapy to eradicate the organism (Table 31-3). Currently, eradication of *H pylori* to treat nonulcer dyspepsia or to prevent future development of gastric carcinoma is not recommended. A number of antibiotics are effective against *H pylori,* including ampicillin, amoxicillin, metronidazole, tetracyclines, quinolones, erythromycin, and clarithromycin. Bismuth compounds are also effective. Also, when antibiotics are given with acid-suppressing proton pump inhibitors (and to a lesser extent, H_2-receptor antagonists), eradication of the organism is enhanced. Because of therapeutic ineffectiveness and the development of drug resistance, single-agent regimens are rarely effective in *H pylori* eradication. The regimen of omeprazole (40 mg per day) and amoxicillin (2 g per day) was shown to eliminate *H pylori* in >80% of cases; however, many clinicians have not experienced this level of success. To increase the likelihood of *H pylori* eradication, most investigators recommend triple therapy with two antibiotics and either bismuth subsalicylate or a proton pump inhibitor. Numerous regimens have documented efficacy, but an inexpensive and effective program that has eradication rates of 80% to 95% and is considered the standard for treatment is a 2-week course of bismuth subsalicylate (2 tablets, four times daily), metronidazole (250 mg, four times daily), and tetracycline (500 mg, four times daily). Some clinicians advocate the addition of an antisecretory drug (e.g., an H_2-receptor antagonist or proton pump inhibitor) to accelerate ulcer healing, especially in patients with bleeding or penetration. For patients who fail this triple regimen, initiation of a metronidazole-free program of a high-dose proton pump inhibitor with clarithromycin and a second antibiotic for 2 weeks is indicated. Shorter courses have been proposed to enhance compliance, but the eradication rates decrease significantly if treatment is <10 days. The management of *H pylori* that is refractory to two courses of triple therapy is controversial; some clinicians recommend therapy with four to five drugs given in very high doses. However, these aggressive programs may produce adverse effects (e.g., antibiotic-associated colitis in up to 25% of cases), raising questions about their risk-benefit profiles. An alternative for these patients is maintenance acid-suppression therapy with H_2-receptor antagonists.

After treatment is concluded, no follow-up is needed in most cases unless the patient remains symptomatic. Urea breath testing 1 month after completion of therapy should be considered to document *H pylori* eradication in patients with complicated disease, who have severe underlying medical illness, or who have recurrent symptoms. After successful eradication, the rate of *H pylori* reinfection is approximately 1% per year. This explains the low (<10%) recurrence rate of gastric and duodenal ulcers in the first year. In contrast, PUD recurs 50% to 100% of the time within the first 2 years if no *H pylori*–directed therapy or chronic acid suppression is provided. Furthermore, chronic PUD carries a 2% to 3% per year risk of complications, with a lifetime risk of 20%. Risk factors predictive of duodenal ulcer recurrence include cigarette smoking, ethanol intake, early disease onset (<40 years of age), repeated duodenal ulcers, or endoscopic documentation of duodenal scarring or erosions.

Treatment and Prevention of NSAID-Related Peptic Ulcer Disease

Whenever possible, the inciting drug should be discontinued in a patient with an NSAID-induced ulcer. In these cases, antisecretory therapy with H_2-receptor antagonists, proton pump inhibitors, or cytoprotective agents should lead to ulcer healing in most cases within 8 weeks. If NSAIDs must be continued for their analgesic or anti-inflammatory effects, a number of regimens have demonstrated efficacy. Nonacetylated salicylates (e.g., salsalate) or newer NSAIDs (e.g., nabumetone, etodolac) may produce less gastrointestinal injury than other agents. H_2-receptor antagonists in conventional doses can heal small (<5 mm) gastric and duodenal ulcers within 8 weeks, but the healing of larger ulcers (especially gastric) is retarded (up to 47% failure rate). Omeprazole (40 mg per day) is more effective with continued NSAID use (95% rate of healing within 8 weeks). Misoprostol has limited efficacy in treating active ulcers in the presence of continued NSAID use; sucralfate has no role. The role of primary triple therapy for concurrent *H pylori* infection is undefined, but this regimen should be initiated for patients with recurrent ulcers who have discontinued NSAID use.

Because of the hazards of chronic NSAID use, medications to prevent ulcer development are given to some patients. Misoprostol is the only agent approved by the FDA for this purpose. At doses of 200 µg four times daily, misoprostol can reduce the 3-month incidence of gastric ulcers (>5 mm) from 8% to 12% down to 2%, and the incidence of duodenal ulcers from 5% to 1%. H_2-receptor antagonists prevent NSAID-induced duodenal ulcers but do not prevent gastric ulcers. It is not reasonable or cost effective to treat all NSAID users prophylactically; therefore, misoprostol prophylaxis should be reserved for patients with prior NSAID-induced disease or for elderly patients taking corticosteroids or anticoagulants or who have concurrent serious disease. The efficacy of proton pump inhibitors in preventing NSAID ulcers is undefined, but because they are so effective in treating acute NSAID ulcers, they may also be excellent prophylactic agents. Sucralfate has no prophylactic efficacy in this setting.

Management of Refractory Ulcers

Five percent to 10% of ulcers fail to heal after appropriate therapy and are considered refractory. Duodenal ulcers are considered refractory if 8 weeks of therapy is ineffective, whereas refractory gastric ulcers are defined by a lack of response to 12 weeks of treatment. Causes of refractory ulcers include patient noncompliance, surreptitious NSAID use, tobacco use, untreated *H pylori* infection, gastric acid hypersecretion (gastrinoma), and malignancy. Rare causes of chronic ulceration are Crohn's disease, amyloidosis, sarcoidosis, eosinophilic gastroenteritis, and infections (e.g., tuberculosis, syphilis, cytomegalovirus). For these cases, close endoscopic follow-up is indicated with performance of multiple biopsies to exclude malignancy or nonpeptic causes. High-dose proton pump inhibitors, omeprazole (40 mg per day) and lansoprazole (60 mg per day), can heal 90% of refractory ulcers after 8 weeks, reducing the need for surgical intervention. However, surgery should be considered for diagnosis and treatment of patients who do not respond to this aggressive regimen.

ZOLLINGER-ELLISON SYNDROME

Incidence and Epidemiology

Zollinger-Ellison syndrome (ZES) is a disorder of acid hypersecretion secondary to a gastrin-secreting tumor or gastrinoma. Estimates of the incidence of ZES range from 0.1% to 1% of patients with PUD. The age range of affected individuals is from 7 to 90 years, with the majority of patients being diagnosed between ages 30 and 50 years. The male-to-female ratio ranges from 2:1 to 3:2. Gastrinomas may be sporadic or they may be genetically transmitted and associated with multiple endocrine neoplasia type I (MEN I). Sporadic gastrinomas often are malignant, whereas MEN I–associated gastrinomas follow a more benign course.

Etiology and Pathogenesis

Gastrin is produced by non–beta-cell endocrine tissue in ZES, which is thought to arise from pancreatic ductular epithelium rather than from pancreatic islet cells. In ZES, unregulated hypergastrinemia leads to overstimulation of acid production by parietal cells and an increase in the mass of parietal cells susceptible to overstimulation. In addition to high circulating concentrations of gastrin, there is evidence that post-translational processing of gastrin is altered in patients with ZES, which may correlate with the level of dedifferentiation of the gastrinoma tumor tissue. More than 80% of gastrinomas are localized to the gastrinoma triangle, which is bounded by the confluence of the cystic duct and common bile duct superiorly, the junction of the second and third duodenal portions inferiorly, and the junction of the pancreatic neck and body medially. Although classically considered a pancreatic tumor, up to 40% of gastrinomas arise within the duodenal wall, whereas primary tumors occasionally originate in the stomach, bones, ovaries, liver, and lymph nodes. One-half of gastrinomas are malignant, and 30% to 55% of patients present with multiple tumors or metastatic disease.

Gastrinoma cells are heterogeneous; generally well differentiated; and contain chromogranin, neuron-specific enolase, and tyrosine hydroxylase. Various secretory granules are observed that do not appear to correlate with malignant potential. Other peptides produced by gastrinomas include somatostatin, pancreatic polypeptide, adrenocorticotropic hormone, and vasoactive intestinal polypeptide (VIP). Cushing's syndrome may occur in association with ZES.

Clinical Features

More than 90% of ZES patients develop ulcers at some point, most commonly in the duodenal bulb (75%). These ulcers usually are <1 cm in diameter, but they may be giant lesions. Other sites include the distal duodenum (14%) and the jejunum (11%). PUD refractory to medications; recurrent ulcers after surgery; PUD with diarrhea; or PUD with obstruction, perforation, or hemorrhage should raise suspicion of ZES. Two-thirds of patients with ZES experience gastroesophageal reflux symptoms, which may be severe. Diarrhea is present in >50% of cases and can occur in the absence of ulcer symptoms. Diarrhea is ameliorated by nasogastric suction or potent acid suppression, providing evidence for the causative role of acid hypersecretion. Features of diarrhea in ZES include high-output secretion (often several liters per day resulting from the acid itself and resulting from the effects of other peptides, such as VIP), maldigestion with steatorrhea secondary to acid inactivation of pancreatic enzymes, a sprue-like state caused by acid-induced villous damage, and reduced micelle formation caused by insoluble bile salts.

One-fourth of ZES patients have MEN I syndrome involving the parathyroid (85%), pancreas (81%), pituitary (65%), and, less commonly, the adrenal cortex and thyroid in autosomal dominant fashion. Patients with ZES as part of MEN I present at a younger age than those with sporadic ZES; some clinical manifestation (usually hyperparathyroidism) appears by age 40 years. Hypercalcemia with hyperparathyroidism may exacerbate the hypergastrinemia and acid hypersecretion of ZES and may have additional manifestations that provide clues to the diagnosis, including a history of nephrolithiasis. Other findings include visual field defects resulting from pituitary tumor development and hyperprolactinemia. Thirteen percent of patients with ZES and MEN I develop gastric carcinoid tumors.

Findings on Diagnostic Testing

Serum Gastrin Determination

Fasting gastrin levels in normal individuals and PUD patients are usually <150 pg per ml. A serum gastrin level of >1000 pg per ml in a person who secretes gastric acid is virtually diagnostic of ZES. Pernicious anemia also rarely produces gastrin levels of >1000 pg per ml, but these persons are achlorhydric. Many patients with ZES have gastrin levels between 150 pg per ml and 1000 pg per ml. These levels may also occur with retained gastric antrum after gastrojejunostomy, G-cell hyperplasia, renal insufficiency, resection of the small intestine, gastric outlet obstruction, rheumatoid arthritis, vitiligo, diabetes, and pheochromocytoma (Table 31-4).

TABLE 31-4
Differential Diagnosis of Hypergastrinemia

Hypochlorhydria, and achlorhydria with or without pernicious anemia
Retained gastric antrum
G-cell hyperplasia
Renal insufficiency
Massive resection of the small intestine
Gastric outlet obstruction
Rheumatoid arthritis
Vitiligo
Diabetes mellitus
Pheochromocytoma

Provocative Testing

The secretin stimulation test is the easiest and most reliable provocative test to distinguish between the possible causes of hypergastrinemia. After secretin injection (2 mg per kg intravenously), serum gastrin levels increase by 200 pg per ml within 15 minutes in >90% of ZES patients, with few false-positive results (occasionally with achlorhydria). In contrast, PUD and G-cell hyperplasia produce decreases, no change, or only small increases in serum gastrin levels. The calcium infusion test (5 mg per kg per hour intravenously) produces a >400 pg per ml increase in the serum gastrin level within 3 hours in >80% of ZES patients. Many false-positive results occur, however, and adverse effects secondary to systemic hypercalcemia may also occur. Calcium testing is reserved for patients with negative findings on secretin stimulation tests who are strongly suspected of having ZES. Most patients with ZES have >50% increases in gastrin levels after meal ingestion, compared with >200% increases in patients with G-cell hyperplasia, but the sensitivity and specificity of the standard meal test is low.

Gastric Acid Secretion Testing

A BAO of >15 mEq per hour is found in >90% of ZES patients, and a BAO of >5 mEq per hour is found in 55% of patients with ZES after surgery. However, 12% of patients with duodenal ulcers also exhibit a BAO of >15 mEq per hour. A BAO-to-MAO ratio of >0.6 is highly specific for ZES, but many patients with ZES have lower ratios. Because secretin stimulation testing is not 100% specific, some clinicians advocate performing gastric acid secretion testing before secretin stimulation testing to confirm acid hypersecretion. If the specialized equipment for acid analysis is not available, a gastric pH of >3 essentially rules out ZES.

Tumor Localization

Gastrinomas may be difficult to localize, with no tumor found in 30% to 50% of patients with ZES. Computed tomographic (CT) scanning appears to be the most effective initial diagnostic study in patients with confirmed ZES, with a sensitivity of 59% for extrahepatic gastrinoma and 72% for liver metastases and specificities of 95% to 98%. If metastatic disease is found, no further evaluation is needed. Abdominal ultrasound has a much lower sensitivity and is less useful.

Endoscopic ultrasound appears to provide a more sensitive means of detecting primary gastrinomas in the pancreas, but this diagnostic modality is not widely available. Selective angiography is useful in detecting an additional 16% of primary tumors and 24% of hepatic metastases with high specificity (84% to 100%) if the CT scan is interpreted as negative. Selective portal venous sampling can detect step-ups in gastrin levels at the site of a primary or metastatic gastrinoma with high sensitivity (70% to 90%), but numerous false-positive studies raise questions about the technique's usefulness. Selective arterial secretin injection into the celiac, splenic, gastroduodenal, hepatic, and superior mesenteric arteries with measurement of hepatic venous gastrin concentrations may replace portal venous sampling. Other localization techniques include magnetic resonance imaging, octreotide scanning, and intra-arterial methylene blue injection. Intraoperative techniques such as ultrasound, endoscopic illumination, and palpation may be useful in selected cases.

Management and Course

A primary gastrinoma in the absence of metastatic disease should be surgically resected. This may be possible in up to 30% of cases. Because of the trophic effects of the elevated gastrin levels, mild acid hypersecretion may persist for several years postoperatively. Gastrinomas in MEN I are often multicentric; surgical resection is usually not possible unless a clear single tumor is identified. When curative surgical resection cannot be performed, a number of medical, surgical, and chemotherapeutic options exist. The 5-year survival is >90% for patients who have undergone curative resection or who have had negative findings on diagnostic laparotomy but is <20% in patients with hepatic metastases. Primary duodenal or lymph node tumors have a favorable prognosis.

Medical Treatment

The primary aim of medical therapy in ZES is control of acid hypersecretion. The most potent agents in ZES are the proton pump inhibitors omeprazole and lansoprazole, which inhibit acid secretion, reduce dyspepsia, and promote ulcer healing. The median dose of omeprazole required for control of acid hypersecretion is 60 mg per day; little tachyphylaxis or toxicity has been observed with long-term proton pump inhibitor therapy. H_2-receptor antagonists may also be used; however, high doses are required, tachyphylaxis often develops, and side effects are common.

Surgical Treatment

In rare instances, total gastrectomy is indicated for patients with unresectable gastrinoma who have failed or cannot tolerate aggressive medical therapy. Before the introduction of proton pump inhibitors, proximal gastric vagotomy was occasionally performed as an adjunct to H_2-receptor antagonist therapy. Parathyroidectomy may reduce hypercalcemia in patients with MEN I, affording easier medication control of acid hypersecretion.

Chemotherapy

Chemotherapy for metastatic gastrinoma is of limited use, with modest initial response rates of <40% to combination regimens (e.g., streptozocin, 5-fluorouracil, and doxorubicin [Adriamycin]) but no change in survival. The decision to begin chemotherapy is based on the growth rates of the metastases and symptomatic response to medical treatment. Other approaches that have been evaluated include interferon therapy, hepatic artery embolization, hepatic arterial chemotherapy infusion, and octreotide injections.

CHAPTER 32

Surgery for Peptic Ulcer Disease and Postgastrectomy Syndromes

SURGERY FOR DUODENAL ULCER DISEASE

Effective antisecretory medications have made surgery for duodenal ulcer disease a rare event, although certain disease complications require emergency or elective surgical intervention. Several surgical techniques have been developed to acutely manage these complications and prevent their recurrence.

Surgical Techniques

Subtotal Gastrectomy

Resection of 60% to 65% of the stomach, including the antrum and a portion of the parietal cell mass, cures peptic ulcer disease in most patients. The gastric remnant may be joined to the intestine in a Billroth I anastomosis, in which the duodenum is sewn directly to the stomach, or a Billroth II anastomosis, in which a blind duodenal afferent limb is constructed and gastric drainage is through a gastrojejunostomy. The choice between these anastomoses depends on the condition of the duodenum and the amount of stomach resected.

Truncal Vagotomy and Drainage

Truncal vagotomy reduces basal acid secretion by 85%, stimulated acid output by 50%, and pepsin secretion by 80%. After vagotomy, the sensitivity of parietal cells to gastrin is also reduced. Vagal sectioning removes the tonic inhibitory effect of the vagus on pyloric motor activity; therefore, a drainage procedure must be performed with truncal vagotomy procedures to prevent gastric retention. The commonly performed Heineke-Mikulicz pyloroplasty is a longitudinal incision of the pyloroduodenum, which is then closed transversely. Alternatively, a gastrojejunostomy is performed if severe duodenal disease or an inflammatory mass is present. Rarely, Jaboulay gastroduodenostomy and Finney pyloroplasty procedures are performed to promote more rapid gastric emptying.

Selective and Highly Selective Gastric Vagotomy

With selective vagotomy, the stomach is denervated but the extragastric vagal branches are preserved; thus, a drainage procedure is required. The highly selective or proximal gastric vagotomy severs only the vagal branches that supply the proximal stomach, leaving antropyloric innervation intact; thus, gastric drainage is not necessary. The reduction in acid and pepsin secretion after highly selective vagotomy is similar to that after truncal vagotomy.

Laparoscopic Ulcer Surgery

Perforated duodenal ulcers can be closed and patched with omentum using laparoscopic techniques. Laparoscopy or thoracoscopy may be used to perform truncal vagotomy with endoscopic pneumatic pyloric dilation in patients who have had prior incomplete vagotomy and pyloroplasty. However, these techniques have not been adequately evaluated for primary therapy. Highly selective vagotomy may be accomplished during laparoscopy, but the procedure is time consuming. The Taylor II procedure involves laparoscopic anterior seromyotomy with section of the anterior proximal vagal branches, which produces a significant reduction in acid secretion.

Indications for Surgery

Intractable Duodenal Ulcer Disease

Intractable duodenal ulcer disease has become rare since the introduction of potent antisecretory agents, particularly the proton pump inhibitors. It is defined by the persistence of severely symptomatic (e.g., pain, blood loss) and endoscopically proven persistent ulceration. The operations that appear to be most useful in this setting are highly selective gastric vagotomy and truncal vagotomy with antrectomy (with resection of 30% to 40% of the stomach). Highly selective vagotomy has a very low incidence of postoperative dumping syndrome, diarrhea, maldigestion, anemia, and weight loss, but it has a higher ulcer recurrence rate. Truncal vagotomy and antrectomy has a 10% to 20% incidence of dumping syndrome as well as increased reports of diarrhea, anemia, and weight loss, but ulcer recurrence is <1%. If possible, a Billroth I anastomosis is chosen, although a Billroth II procedure is indicated for severe scarring of the duodenal bulb. Vagotomy and pyloroplasty should be reserved for ill, elderly patients for whom an expedient operation is indicated.

Ulcer Perforation

Emergency surgery is indicated for duodenal ulcer perforation. It has two goals: to close the perforation and to perform definitive surgery to prevent ulcer recurrence. If the ulcer edges are friable, a tongue of vascularized omentum may be sewn over the perforation. If the edges are nonedematous and nonfriable, the ulcer margins may be approximated before omental patching. Addition of highly selective vagotomy significantly reduces postoperative ulcer recurrence without increasing the mortality and morbidity of the surgery. Such definitive ulcer surgery should be performed if the perforation has existed for >24 hours, if the abdomen is not contaminated, and if the patient is otherwise in good health. If bleeding occurs in association with perforation, suture ligature of the ulcer bed may be needed in addition to closure of the perforation and definitive ulcer surgery.

Hemorrhage

The indications for emergency surgery to control duodenal ulcer hemorrhage are massive exsanguination when maintenance of vital signs is impossible; the necessity of transfusing 6 to 8 units of blood to maintain blood pressure in the first 24 hours; slow, continued bleeding for 48 hours; recurrent bleeding while on medications; and a visible vessel that cannot be managed endoscopically. The first step during surgery is to open the duodenum and suture the bleeding vessels in the ulcer bed. Occasionally, ligation of the gastroduodenal artery may be required to treat persistent oozing. The second step is the performance of definitive ulcer surgery. Vagotomy with pyloroplasty is indicated for a patient with massive hemorrhage in which a shorter operative time is desired. Highly selective vagotomy or vagotomy and antrectomy may be performed in healthier, more stable patients in whom a more prolonged operation does not increase mortality or morbidity.

Obstruction

Chronic duodenal and pyloric channel ulcers cause 80% of cases of gastric outlet obstruction. Preoperative hydration, electrolyte supplementation, and intravenous hyperalimentation may be needed for the fluid and nutritional deficits resulting from gastric obstruction. Nasogastric suction for several days can restore gastric tone, and gastric instillation of nonabsorbable antibiotics can minimize bacterial colonization of the stomach. If possible, truncal vagotomy with drainage or antrectomy should be performed. If the pylorus is severely inflamed or scarred, the safest procedure is a truncal vagotomy with gastrojejunostomy. Construction of a feeding jejunostomy and a draining gastrostomy at the time of surgery is often performed to afford enteral feeding and gastric decompression should a protracted course of delayed gastric emptying follow the operation.

Penetration

Duodenal ulcer penetration is a common cause of intractable ulcer symptoms. It is usually treated with vagotomy and antrectomy rather than highly selective vagotomy because of the postulated increased virulence of the ulcer disease.

Fistulae

Rarely, fistulae develop between the duodenum and common bile duct or gallbladder. Vagotomy and antrectomy with Billroth II anastomosis treats the ulcer and excludes the fistula. However, if the duodenal stump cannot be closed, nonresectional therapy with vagotomy should be considered, leaving the fistula intact.

SURGERY FOR BENIGN GASTRIC ULCERS

In many cases of benign gastric ulcer disease, a procedure that reduces gastric acid secretion is less likely to be successful than surgery that resects the target tissue because acid hypersecretion usually is not present. Surgical intervention also must take into account the rare presentation of a gastric malignancy as an apparently benign ulceration.

Operative Techniques

Type I ulcers occur in the gastric body, usually along the lesser curvature of the stomach, and are not associated with acid hypersecretion. The operation of choice for these patients is antrectomy (removal of 40% to 50% of the stomach), including excision of the ulcer with Billroth I anastomosis, but no vagotomy. This procedure has a low ulcer recurrence rate (<2%) and preserves normal gastroduodenal continuity. Type II ulcers are gastric ulcers that occur in association with duodenal ulcers and are associated with acid hypersecretion. Vagotomy with antrectomy is the preferred operation, although vagotomy and drainage or highly selective vagotomy are used in rare cases. Type III ulcers are prepyloric in location. They occur in the setting of acid hypersecretion and are best managed by vagotomy and antrectomy. Highly selective vagotomy is associated with frequent ulcer recurrence in type III ulcers (35% to 40%). Type IV ulcers appear at or near the gastroesophageal junction. Ulcers >2 cm distal to the junction may be removed with antral resection extending up the lesser curvature. With more proximal ulcers, antrectomy may be performed, leaving the ulcer behind. In this instance, surgical biopsy specimens are obtained to exclude malignancy. Alternatively, the resection line may include the ulcer and distal esophagus with construction of a Roux-en-Y esophagogastrojejunostomy (i.e., Csendes' procedure).

Indications for Surgery

Hemorrhage from gastric ulcers is often more serious than from duodenal ulcers. The treatment of choice is distal gastric resection to include the ulcer with gastroduodenal anastomosis, although ulcer excision with either vagotomy and drainage or highly selective vagotomy may be performed in high-risk

TABLE 32-1
Causes of Postoperative Recurrent Ulcer

Inadequate operation
    Incomplete vagotomy
    Inadequate drainage
    Inadequate resection
        Insufficient gastric resection
        Retained gastric antrum
    Long afferent limb in Billroth II resection
Poor selection of primary operation
    Gastroenterostomy alone
    Vagotomy for gastric ulcer
Hypersecretory states
    Zollinger-Ellison syndrome
    Multiple endocrine neoplasia type I
    G-cell hyperplasia
    Retained gastric antrum
    Hypercalcemia
    Other endocrinopathies (e.g., Cushing's syndrome, adrenal cortical tumor)
Ulcerogenic medications
    Salicylates
    NSAIDs
    Corticosteroids
    Reserpine

patients. Perforated gastric ulcers are also treated with antrectomy that includes the ulcer, but local excision or omental patching may be performed in unstable patients. Obstruction caused by a prepyloric ulcer is a rare complication that is managed by antrectomy with Billroth I anastomosis.

POSTGASTRECTOMY COMPLICATIONS

Recurrent Ulcer After Surgery

The causes of recurrence include an inadequate operation, a poor selection of operative technique, a hypersecretory state, and use of ulcerogenic drugs such as NSAIDs (Table 32-1). The most common cause of disease recurrence is incomplete vagotomy, usually of the posterior trunk. With highly selective vagotomy, inadequate clearance of vagal fibers over the distal 6 to 8 cm of esophagus, failure to resect the criminal nerve of Grassi, or failure to divide the vagal distribution at the greater gastric curvature may be the cause. Poor antral drainage may also promote ulcer recurrence because gastric retention can stimulate acid production. The retained gastric antrum syndrome may develop with anatomic isolation of gastrin-producing tissue in the afferent limb of a Billroth II anastomosis, a region that is not subject to acid-regulated feedback inhibition. The recurrence rate for a gastric ulcer after any type of vagotomy is high if the vagotomy is not accompanied by resection. Particularly high recurrence rates are reported after highly selective vagotomy for pyloric and prepyloric ulcers.

The incidence of Zollinger-Ellison syndrome (ZES) is 2% in patients with postoperative recurrent ulcer. Therefore, fasting serum gastrin levels are obtained in all patients undergoing surgery for a duodenal ulcer. A second rare cause of hypergastrinemia is G-cell hyperplasia, an autosomal dominant condition that is effectively treated by antrectomy. Ulcers recur in this condition if the initial operation is a vagotomy only, without resection. Hypercalcemia and Cushing's syndrome are rare causes of acid hypersecretion.

The diagnosis of recurrent ulcers is best made with upper gastrointestinal endoscopy. Fasting gastrin levels should be obtained and, if elevated, a secretin stimulation test should be performed to screen for ZES. Gastric acid secretion testing can be used to assess completeness of vagotomy, which is suggested by a basal acid output of >5 mEq per hour or by a significant increase in acid output after modified sham feeding (in which the patient chews meat and spits it out without swallowing). Retained gastric antrum syndrome is diagnosed by hypergastrinemia, negative findings on secretin stimulation testing, a dilated duodenal stump on upper gastrointestinal barium radiography, and positive findings on a technetium pertechnetate scan.

The therapy for a recurrent ulcer is dependent on its cause; surgery is recommended for retained gastric antrum or resectable gastrinomas. If medications (e.g., proton pump inhibitors) do not relieve recurrent ulcers that are secondary to other causes, surgical revision may be necessary. If recurrence follows highly selective vagotomy, antrectomy is the procedure of choice, whereas antrectomy with repeat vagotomy is performed after initial vagotomy and drainage.

Postgastrectomy Syndromes

Dumping Syndrome

Surgery that impairs distal vagal function and includes drainage or resection may allow rapid passage of hyperosmolar gastric contents into the intestine, producing fluid shifts and release of vasoactive hormones (Table 32-2). The early dumping syndrome exhibits abdominal symptoms (pain, borborygmi, and diarrhea) and vasomotor symptoms (flushing, weakness, palpitations, diaphoresis, lightheadedness, and syncope). These symptoms occur in the first 30 to 60 minutes after a meal. The late dumping syndrome, which is postulated to result from excessive postprandial insulin release, produces reactive hypoglycemia 1 to 4 hours after meal ingestion. Dumping syndrome can be prevented by preserving pyloric innervation and smooth muscle function, as in highly selective vagotomy. Treatment of dumping syndrome relies on low-carbohydrate diets, with separation of solids and liquids. Assuming a supine position after eating may delay gastric emptying of nutrients. Increasing nutrient viscosity with pectin or other compounds may have efficacy in rare cases. The somatostatin analog octreotide alleviates symptoms by inhibiting the release of vasoactive peptides and insulin and by slowing intestinal transit. Surgical procedures may be attempted, but they are often unsuccessful.

Diarrhea

Postvagotomy diarrhea occurring 1 to 3 hours postprandially may result from a combination of factors: rapid gastric emptying and intestinal transit, increased ileal fluid and bile salt delivery to the colon, and intestinal bacterial overgrowth.

TABLE 32-2
Chronic Sequelae of Surgery for Peptic Ulcer Disease

	RATE AFTER VARIOUS OPERATIONS (%)			
COMPLICATION	PGV	TV+D	V+A	SG
Dumping syndrome	5	10–15	10–20	10–20
Diarrhea	2–5	15–30	5–40	2–18
Anemia	0.5	3–15	7	10–40
Bone disease			20	30
Weight loss	2–10	5–20	10–30	20–40

PGV = proximal gastric vagotomy; TV+D = truncal vagotomy plus drainage; V+A = vagotomy plus antrectomy; SG = subtotal gastrectomy.

Treatment includes antidumping dietary measures as well as bile acid–binding agents (e.g., cholestyramine) or oral antibiotics, both of which are frequently unsuccessful. Similarly, surgical intervention for postvagotomy diarrhea often does not produce improvement in symptoms.

Gastroparesis

Severe gastric retention, usually of solid foods, is a rare complication of gastric surgery. Affected patients should avoid poorly digestible foods. The condition is treated with prokinetic agents, although refractory cases may require total gastrectomy to achieve improvement in symptoms.

Alkaline Reflux Gastritis

Excessive duodenogastric reflux of bile, pancreatic enzymes, and intestinal secretions is thought to produce a characteristic syndrome of burning epigastric pain unresponsive to antacids and aggravated by eating and recumbency. The diagnosis is one of exclusion of recurrent ulcer and is often uncertain. Surgical construction of a Roux-en-Y gastrojejunostomy to direct intestinal fluid distally produces symptom relief in only 30% to 60% of cases.

Maldigestion

Maldigestion may result from rapid gastric emptying and intestinal transit, inadequate food particle dispersion owing to reduced trituration, impaired pancreatic and gallbladder responses to food, intestinal bacterial overgrowth, and dyscoordination of intestinal nutrient and pancreaticobiliary delivery. Maldigestion is rarely a significant problem alone, but it may aggravate other postgastrectomy complications.

Anemia

Chronic anemia frequently occurs secondary to iron, folate, or vitamin B_{12} deficiency. Iron deficiency results from impairment of the dissociation of ferric iron from food; thus, ferrous iron supplements should be given. In rare instances of vitamin B_{12} deficiency (usually after subtotal or total gastrectomy), monthly vitamin B_{12} injections are given.

Bone Disease

Bone disease is more common after gastrectomy than after vagotomy, and it takes years to develop. Osteomalacia is caused by calcium and vitamin D malabsorption and is manifested by loss of bone radiodensity, reduced serum calcium levels, retention of infused calcium, and elevated parathyroid hormone levels.

Weight Loss

Severe weight loss is usually seen only after removal of large portions of the stomach and results from reduced intake, malabsorption, and maldigestion. Other diagnoses, such as celiac sprue or infections (e.g., tuberculosis) may be unmasked by the gastric procedure.

Gastric Cancer

There is an increased incidence of gastric adenocarcinoma that manifests 15 to 20 years after surgery; the incidence is greater after gastrectomy than after vagotomy.

CHAPTER 33

Nonulcer Dyspepsia

INCIDENCE AND EPIDEMIOLOGY

Dyspepsia refers to persistent or recurrent upper abdominal pain or discomfort characterized by postprandial fullness, early satiety, nausea, and bloating. Patients with dyspepsia and no definable structural or biochemical abnormality are classified as having functional, or nonulcer, dyspepsia (NUD). Approximately 25% of the United States population reports recurrent symptoms each year, but only 10% to 20% of this subset seeks medical attention because of symptom severity, fear of malignancy, and underlying anxiety or other psychosocial factors. NUD is at least twofold to threefold more common than peptic ulcer disease. Approximately 30% of persons with dyspepsia experience spontaneous symptom resolution with time.

ETIOLOGY AND PATHOGENESIS

Gastric Acid and Helicobacter pylori Infection

Acid secretion is normal in most patients with NUD. Moreover, most do not exhibit hypersensitivity to acid perfusion of the stomach, suggesting that acid-related dysfunction plays a role only in a minority of cases. Similarly, there is no clear association of *Helicobacter pylori* infection with symptoms of NUD. Furthermore, *H pylori* eradication clearly alleviates symptoms only in a small subset of patients with NUD.

Gastric Motor Activity

Twenty-five percent to 50% of patients with NUD exhibit postprandial antral hypomotility or delayed gastric emptying, which does not correlate with any specific symptom complexes and has an unclear etiology. Additional rhythm disturbances of the gastric slow wave have been reported with NUD. Acute stress can produce motor abnormalities similar to those found in NUD, but it is not established that symptoms of NUD are explained by such effects.

Gastric Afferent Sensitivity

Although gastric compliance is normal in most patients with NUD, at least 50% experience discomfort with gastric distention, suggesting that an afferent neural defect produces visceral hyperalgesia. The lack of altered peripheral pain thresholds in these patients indicates that the defect is specific to the gut and is not generalized.

Psychological Factors

Patients with NUD are more psychologically distressed than healthy controls. One study reported that affected patients had a higher frequency of lifetime psychiatric diagnoses. Dyspeptic patients have been reported to perceive negative life events more strongly than controls.

Diet and Environmental Factors

When carefully evaluated, dyspeptic symptoms cannot be attributed to specific foods. Coffee may aggravate symptoms, but it is unknown if this is secondary to gastric irritation or to induction of gastroesophageal reflux. There is no evidence that smoking tobacco or ingesting ethanol cause NUD. Although NSAIDs can produce dyspeptic symptoms, there is no clear association between NUD and NSAID use.

CLINICAL FEATURES

NUD has been classified into subcategories based on the dominant symptoms. Ulcerlike NUD is characterized by episodes of epigastric pain that is relieved by antacids or food, whereas refluxlike NUD manifests with heartburn and regurgitation. Dysmotility-like NUD is characterized by discomfort that is aggravated by food or associated with early satiety, fullness, nausea, retching, vomiting, or bloating. There is a fourth, nonspecific NUD subtype with symptoms that does not fit the other categories. There is extensive overlap between the subgroups, and studies of motor and sensory function have shown no distinctive physiologic differences between them. Neither is there a clear difference in responses to drug therapy between the distinct subcategories of NUD. The clinician should consider patient use of medications that may produce dyspepsia, including iron, potassium, digoxin, theophylline, erythromycin, and ampicillin. Other conditions that can mimic dyspepsia include chronic pancreatitis, intestinal angina, malignancies, Ménétrier's disease, infiltrative diseases (e.g., Crohn's disease, sarcoidosis, eosinophilic gastroenteritis, tuberculosis, and syphilis), and abdominal wall pain from muscle strain, nerve entrapment, or myositis. Therefore, specific findings of these diagnoses should be assessed by a careful history and physical examination.

FINDINGS ON DIAGNOSTIC TESTING

Peptic ulcer is one of the most common diagnoses to exclude in patients who present with dyspepsia. Unfortunately, the sensitivity and specificity of the history and physical examination in distinguishing NUD from peptic ulcer disease are low. Upper gastrointestinal endoscopy should be performed in patients older than 50 years or in those with alarm symptoms (e.g., weight loss, hemorrhage, dysphagia, vomiting, and NSAID use). Ideally, it is performed when the patient is symptomatic and not taking acid-suppressing medications to enhance detection of ulcer disease. Although double-contrast upper gastrointestinal barium radiography has a high sensitivity for detection of ulcer disease, it does not afford the capability of biopsy for detection of *H pylori* or exclusion of malignancy in suggestive lesions. For younger patients with no alarming symptoms, empiric therapy may be offered instead, reserving endoscopy for those who remain symptomatic. Serology tests for *H pylori* may be useful as part of the initial evaluation because a negative result makes a diagnosis of peptic ulcer disease less likely in the absence of NSAID use. Gastric scintigraphy may demonstrate gastroparesis in subsets of patients with NUD; however, symptoms and responses to therapy with prokinetic agents often correlate poorly with gastric scintigraphic test results. If systemic disease is the suspected cause of gastroparesis, blood testing can detect diabetes, thyroid disease, and rheumatologic conditions. Twenty-four-hour esophageal pH monitoring may produce positive results in many patients with refluxlike NUD and in up to one-third of patients with NUD of other subtypes in whom gastroesophageal reflux is not suspected. Ultrasound, computed tomography, and gastric acid secretion tests have extremely low yields in dyspeptic patients and should not be performed unless indicated by specific findings on examination or laboratory studies.

MANAGEMENT AND COURSE

A positive clinical diagnosis and confident reassurance by the clinician are key steps in the management of patients with NUD and may obviate the need for medication therapy in many patients. A firm diagnosis of NUD after appropriate investigation is usually safe, and progression to severe structural disease is rare. Patients should avoid aggravating medications (e.g., NSAIDs) if possible. Postprandial symptoms may be reduced by avoiding irritating foods or by eating low-fat meals or more frequent but smaller meals throughout the day.

Medication Therapy

No medications have been approved by the U.S. Food and Drug Administration for treating NUD. Furthermore, placebo response rates in NUD range from 30% to 70%, making the interpretation of any therapeutic response difficult. A meta-analysis of H_2-receptor antagonists showed a response rate that was 20% greater than placebo, but these trials may have included many patients with predominant gastroesophageal reflux. Three trials with metoclopramide showed efficacy superior to placebo, although side effects were common. Cisapride produces global symptom improvement in 60% to 90% of patients with dysmotility-like NUD, although many of these patients also had features of gastroesophageal reflux. Sucralfate and anticholinergic agents have not convincingly shown efficacy in NUD. Similarly, eradication of *H pylori* does not provide significant symptom improvement over placebo in most NUD trials. Agents that reduce visceral hyperalgesia in NUD are being tested. The kappa opioid agonist fedotozine has shown efficacy in placebo-controlled trials of patients with NUD. However, this drug remains investigational.

Therapeutic Approach

Drug therapy should be tailored to treat the dominant symptoms. Patients with ulcerlike NUD should be given a 4-week trial of an H_2-receptor antagonist. Dysmotility-like NUD should initially be managed with a prokinetic agent (e.g., cisapride) for 4 weeks. If these trials are ineffective, switching to the prokinetic agent in ulcerlike NUD and the acid-suppressing agent in dysmotility-like NUD may be attempted. Long-term medication use should be avoided. Patients who do not respond to this approach may be given antispasmodic agents, especially if there is a suggestion of symptom overlap with irritable bowel syndrome (IBS). Alternatively, a trial of antidepressant medications may be given, even in the absence of depression, because they have been shown to have efficacy in some IBS subtypes, although no controlled studies have been performed in NUD. If anxiety is present, specific behavioral therapy (e.g., relaxation training) may reduce symptoms and encourage health-promoting behavior. Repeated diagnostic testing should be avoided. The physician should set realistic expectations for the affected patient and make the patient aware that complete symptom control may not be possible.

CHAPTER 34

Gastritis, Duodenitis, and Associated Ulcerative Lesions

ACUTE GASTRITIS

Etiology and Pathogenesis

Acute hemorrhagic and erosive gastritis begins as damage to the epithelium caused by mucosal hypoxia or by the direct action of NSAIDs or other injurious agents or conditions (e.g., bile acids; central nervous system disease [Cushing's ulcer]; reduced blood flow caused by stress, trauma, burns, or sepsis). When mucosal defenses are breached, acid, proteases, and bile acids penetrate into the lamina propria, where they cause vascular injury, stimulate nerves, and activate the release of histamine and other mediators. *Helicobacter pylori* is a small, curved, gram-negative rod that is associated with duodenal and gastric ulcers. Acute *H pylori* gastritis is defined as primary infection in association with severe acute inflammation, abrupt symptom onset, and hypochlorhydria.

Clinical Features and Diagnosis

Acute hemorrhagic and erosive gastritis comes to clinical attention in the evaluation of patients with acute upper gastrointestinal bleeding. It appears on endoscopic examination as petechiae and as small red or black erosions. Stress-induced lesions begin in the fundus and body of the stomach, whereas NSAID-evoked hemorrhagic gastritis involves all portions of the stomach, including the antrum. Histologic findings correlate poorly with endoscopically defined abnormalities and may show regenerating epithelium and sparse inflammation. Acute ulcers may occur in association with gastritis, especially with stress, and are usually multiple, large (0.5 to 2.0 cm in diameter), and located in the fundus and body.

Patients with acute *H pylori* gastritis present with acute epigastric pain, nausea, and vomiting. Endoscopic evaluation shows striking antral abnormalities that mimic the appearance of lymphoma or carcinoma. Histologically, there is intense neutrophilic infiltration, edema, and hyperemia; these features clear with appropriate antibiotic therapy.

CHRONIC GASTRITIS

Helicobacter pylori *Gastritis*

Etiology and Pathogenesis

Although *H pylori* is present in many patients with nonulcer dyspepsia, it is doubtful that it has a major role in the generation of symptoms in most of these patients. However, the majority of patients with chronic *H pylori* infection have neither symptoms nor endoscopic findings, although chronic gastritis may be found on gastric mucosal biopsy specimens. There is a close correlation between chronic inflammation and the immune response to *H pylori*. Serum IgG anti-*H pylori* titers correlate with the intensity of inflammation and the number of lymphoid follicles. Lymphoid follicles that accompany *H pylori* gastritis may play a role in mucosa-associated lymphoid tissue lymphomas, which are low-grade B-cell tumors that infiltrate glandular epithelium.

Clinical Features and Diagnosis

Symptoms attributable to *H pylori* infection are reliably present only with peptic ulcer disease. Endoscopic findings in *H pylori* gastritis are variable and typically involve the entire stomach, although biopsies directed at the antrum alone may miss the diagnosis in up to 10% of cases. Techniques to detect *H pylori* organisms include Giemsa and silver stains and the less reliable hematoxylin and eosin preparation. *H pylori* organisms occur in the mucus overlying the mucosa and adjacent to epithelial cells at the mucosal surface and in the pits. Gastric glands are rarely involved. *H pylori* gastritis is characterized by chronic superficial inflammation with lymphocytes, plasma cells, macrophages, and eosinophils, usually accompanied by acute inflammation consisting of neutrophilic infiltration of the surface and foveolar epithelium and lamina propria. Lymphoid follicles, which are aggregates of lymphocytes with a central germinal center of pale mononuclear cells, are often seen and are virtually pathognomonic of *H pylori* gastritis. Acute inflammation is more common in antral than in proximal tissues. Other means of detecting *H pylori* infection with serologic tests or functional tests of urease activity are discussed in Chapter 31.

Chronic Chemical Gastritis

Etiology and Pathogenesis

NSAIDs and bile are the principal causes of chronic chemical gastritis, although iron and potassium supplements may also be injurious. Persons exposed to NSAIDs for several weeks exhibit an adaptive phenomenon that protects mucosal integrity, but in many patients this adaptation is often short-lived. Bile gastritis is a chronic condition in which bile-containing intestinal contents reflux into the

TABLE 34-1
Comparison of Autoimmune and Environmental Metaplastic Atrophic Gastritis

FINDINGS	AUTOIMMUNE	ENVIRONMENTAL
Gross distribution	Gastric body only; diffuse	Antrum more than body; multifocal
Cause	Genetic; autoimmunity	Dietary and external agents, possible *Helicobacter pylori*
Affected populations	Mainly Northern Europeans	Worldwide, all races; regional high incidences
Gastric acid secretion	Absent to low	Low to normal
Serum antibodies		
Parietal (oxyntic) cell	Yes	No
Intrinsic factor	Yes	No
Pernicious anemia	Yes (late)	No
Associated conditions		
Gastric ulcer	Rare	Yes
Gastric cancer	Probable	Definite
Hyperplastic polyps	Yes	Yes
Endocrine hyperplasia	G cell in antrum, ECL cell in body	No
Carcinoid tumors	Yes	Yes

ECL = enterochromaffin-like.

stomach. It is most commonly diagnosed in patients who have undergone pyloroplasty or partial gastric resection. Bile acids and lysolecithin are known to induce acute gastric mucosal injury, which is enhanced by pancreatic enzymes.

Clinical Features and Diagnosis

Dyspeptic symptoms prompt an evaluation of a patient with presumed chronic chemical gastritis. The gastric mucosa in chemical gastritis exhibits minimal inflammation, but foveolar hyperplasia, edema, increased lamina propria smooth muscle fibers, and vascular dilation and congestion may be present. Foveolae may have a tortuous corkscrew appearance, especially if biopsy specimens are taken near a gastroenterostomy. Foveolar hyperplasia secondary to bile reflux may regress if bile is diverted from a gastroenterostomy by means of a Roux-en-Y gastrojejunostomy. Although eosinophils may be prominent, only 30% of NSAID users exhibit neutrophils.

Atrophic Gastritis

Etiology and Pathogenesis

The principal types of metaplastic atrophic gastritis are autoimmune and environmental (Table 34-1). Autoimmune metaplastic atrophic gastritis (AMAG) is an autosomal dominant disorder in which an immune response is directed against parietal cells and intrinsic factor in the proximal gastric mucosa, producing vitamin B_{12} deficiency and pernicious anemia. The mucosal changes of AMAG closely parallel elevations in serum antibodies to parietal cells (possibly against H^+,K^+-adenosine triphosphatase) and intrinsic factor. Loss of parietal cell mass produces profound hypochlorhydria. Affected patients may also exhibit other autoimmune diseases, including Hashimoto's thyroiditis, endocrine abnormalities, and vitiligo. In AMAG, antral G cells release large amounts of gastrin, which causes an increase in the number of endocrine cells and may produce hyperplastic endocrine cell nodules in and around the gastric glands. This hyperplasia centers on the enterochromaffin-like (ECL) cell, which is the endocrine cell responsible for histamine secretion. In some patients, ECL hyperplasia progresses to carcinoid tumor. The malignant potential of these tumors is low, and only 9% metastasize. The risk of carcinoma in pernicious anemia, which usually is associated with AMAG, is 3- to 18-fold higher than in the general population, whereas the risk for AMAG alone is probably somewhat less. AMAG generally has a negative association with *H pylori*.

Environmental metaplastic atrophic gastritis (EMAG) is most prevalent in Japan, South America, and China and is believed to result from *H pylori* infection, gastric bacterial overgrowth, coal dust exposure, tobacco smoking, or dietary salt, nitrate, or nitrite consumption. Nitroso compounds generated by the gastric bacterial metabolism of nitrates may be important in EMAG, in the formation of intestinal metaplasia, and in the subsequent development of gastric carcinoma. Similarly, chronic *H pylori* infection is correlated with intestinal metaplasia and may be a risk factor for development of gastric carcinoma, although it is likely that other cofactors are also required to induce mutagenesis and carcinogenesis.

Nonmetaplastic atrophic gastritis can result from antral resection, in which the loss of oxyntic cells in the proximal gastric remnant is prominent and may be so severe that vitamin B_{12} deficiency results from insufficient intrinsic factor secretion. These patients have reduced circulating gastrin levels, which in turn fail to maintain the trophic effect on the oxyntic glands.

Clinical Features and Diagnosis

In general, atrophic gastritis is asymptomatic unless one of its sequelae (e.g., vitamin B_{12} deficiency or gastric malignancy) supervenes. Gastric biopsy specimens from patients with atrophic gastritis show a variety of patterns. Two types of metaplasia are seen with AMAG and EMAG. Pseudopyloric metaplasia represents replacement of parietal and chief cells with mucus-secreting and endocrine (gastrin) cells that are similar to those found in prepyloric antral mucosa. Intestinal metaplasia is characterized by the replacement of the surface, foveolar, and glandular epithelium in the oxyntic or antral mucosa by intestinal epithelium, which is recognizable because of the presence of goblet cells. Type I intestinal metaplasia involves complete replacement of gastric mucosa by intestinal epithelium, whereas in type II and III metaplasia, the replacement is incomplete, with persistent gastric-type mucin cells. Goblet cells in type II metaplasia show acidic sialomucins, whereas in type III metaplasia, goblet cells show acidic sulfomucin. Incomplete intestinal metaplasia (especially type III) is associated with the greatest risk of gastric adenocarcinoma.

In AMAG, the metaplasia, glandular atrophy, and inflammation (e.g., lymphocytic destruction of oxyntic glands) are limited to the gastric body and fundus. On upper gastrointestinal endoscopic examination, the rugae are inconspicuous and the submucosal vessels are clearly visible under the thinned mucosa. The early stage of AMAG, termed *active autoimmune gastritis*, is characterized by patchy involvement; there are multiple retained islands of normal mucosa that resemble pseudopolyps. Pseudohypertrophy of parietal cells may be present and findings of chemical gastritis may be seen on antral biopsy specimens. In end-stage AMAG, metaplastic replacement is complete, and in extreme degrees of intestinal metaplasia, the mucosa may exhibit villi and appear identical to tissue from the small intestine. Serum tests, which are useful to confirm AMAG, include elevations in the levels of antibodies to parietal cells and to intrinsic factor and a reduction in the ratio of pepsinogen I to pepsinogen II.

EMAG is characterized by multiple localized areas of atrophy, metaplasia, and inflammation, which are most prominent in the antrum and present, but to a lesser degree, in the gastric body. For a definitive diagnosis of EMAG, at least 20% of the available antral mucosa must be replaced by metaplasia or atrophy. There often is a proximal migration of the transitional zone from normal mucosa to metaplastic tissue. Thinning of body and fundus mucosa may occur secondary to reduced gastrin levels. Pepsinogen ratios are abnormal in some but not all cases of EMAG, and some patients will exhibit evidence of *H pylori* infection. In addition, gastric ulcers that are not related to the use of NSAIDs may be present in the areas of intestinal metaplasia, regions of atrophy in the antrum, and the transitional zone between oxyntic and antral mucosa.

In postantrectomy mucosal atrophy, there is overall mucosal thinning associated with shortening of oxyntic glands. Intestinal metaplasia may be prominent around the anastomosis, but it is not excessive in the more proximal gastric remnant.

Miscellaneous Forms of Chronic Gastritis

Eosinophilic Gastritis

Eosinophilic gastritis is characterized by eosinophilic infiltration into any or all layers of the stomach, often in association with peripheral eosinophilia and allergic conditions. Eosinophilic infiltration of the mucosa is most common and the only form that can be diagnosed from findings of endoscopic biopsy. Gastric mucosal involvement is most prevalent in the antrum (up to 100%), especially in children. Other biopsy findings include epithelial necrosis and regeneration.

Infectious Gastritis

Except for infections with *H pylori*, healthy individuals rarely develop chronic infectious gastritis. Some dyspeptic patients are infected with a urease-positive, spirochete-like organism, *Gastrospirillum hominis*, which is similar to organisms found in the stomachs of cats, dogs, monkeys, and other animals. However, alterations of gastric mucosal defenses as occurs in atrophic gastritis or in acquired immunodeficiency syndrome (AIDS) may predispose to bacterial, viral, parasitic, or fungal gastric infection.

Phlegmonous gastritis is an overwhelming bacterial gastritis that produces acute epigastric pain, fever, and peritonitis in alcoholics, the elderly, and AIDS patients. The gastric wall and mucosa are grossly thickened as a result of intense diffuse and suppurative inflammation. Causative organisms include streptococci, *Escherichia coli*, staphylococci, *Haemophilus* species, and gas-forming bacteria that may produce emphysematous gastritis. Risk factors include gastric polypectomy and India-ink injection. The diagnosis is usually made at laparotomy, and treatment involves gastric resection and antibiotics. Gastric tuberculosis typically manifests with symptoms related to gastric obstruction and ulceration because of antropyloric involvement, although it may involve atypical sites in patients with

AIDS. Cultures of endoscopic biopsy specimens are required because acid-fast bacilli are rarely seen. The stomach may also be involved in infection with *Mycobacterium avium* complex in patients with AIDS. Syphilitic gastritis in secondary syphilis is characterized by erosive antral gastritis, ulcers, or thickened rugae, which produce symptoms of anorexia, epigastric pain, and vomiting. Biopsy specimens show prominent spirochetes, acute and chronic inflammation with mucosal destruction, and mononuclear vasculitis in the submucosa and muscularis. The diagnosis is made in the appropriate clinical setting of positive findings on syphilis serologic tests. Rarely, gummata and fibrosis in tertiary syphilis may produce obstruction and the appearance of an infiltrating mass.

Cytomegalovirus (CMV) is the most common viral cause of infectious gastritis and is especially common in patients with AIDS who present with acute pain, nausea, vomiting, ulceroerosive disease that mimics neoplasia, and nonulcerative nodules of the body and fundus of the stomach. Atypical lymphocytosis may be present; biopsy specimens show enlarged nuclei with intranuclear inclusions in glandular cells, macrophages, and endothelial cells. In children, CMV infection produces gastric fold enlargement with protein-losing enteropathy (i.e., childhood Ménétrier's disease) and is characterized by intense eosinophilic infiltration of the lamina propria. Rarely, herpes simplex virus causes gastric mucosal erosions.

Parasitic infections that cause gastritis include cryptosporidiosis, anisakiasis, ascariasis, strongyloidiasis, and hookworm. Gastric cryptosporidiosis produces antral narrowing, erythema, edema, and inflammation. It is a common infection in AIDS patients. Anisakiasis is the most common helminthiasis affecting the stomach. It occurs after ingestion of raw fish and is reported most frequently in Japan and the Netherlands. The *Anisakis* worm burrows into the mucosa, producing severe pain, nausea, and vomiting. The histologic findings include eosinophilic infiltration, necrosis, and multinucleated giant cells.

The stomach can be affected with disseminated histoplasmosis, exhibiting ulceration and rugal-thickening, organism-laden macrophages. *Cryptococcus* species may infect the stomach in AIDS. *Candida* organisms commonly colonize gastric ulcers, but invasive gastric candidiasis is rare in immunocompromised patients.

Crohn's Disease

One percent to 5% of patients with Crohn's disease have severe upper gastrointestinal involvement with erythema, edema, nodularity, cobblestoning, erosions, ulcers, strictures, and obstruction. The antrum is most frequently involved, exhibiting linear ulcerations and aphthous erosions. Biopsy specimens show focal, nonspecific, neutrophilic and mononuclear infiltration; therefore, the diagnosis often is dependent on other clinical manifestations of Crohn's disease. Histologic proof of Crohn's gastritis is provided only by the demonstration of granulomas, which are found in only 7% to 34% of patients.

Granulomatous Gastritis

Symptomatic gastric disease with gross alterations (e.g., nodularity, ulcers, thickened rugae, and obstruction) is extremely rare with sarcoidosis, although noncaseating granulomas are not uncommonly found in asymptomatic individuals. Isolated granulomatous gastritis may affect the distal stomach, producing obstruction as a result of wall thickening, lumenal narrowing, and the presence of transmural noncaseating granulomas. The cause of the disease is unknown. It may respond to treatment with corticosteroids, or surgery may be required.

TABLE 34-2
Classification of Conditions with Large Gastric Folds

Hypertrophic gastropathies
    Ménétrier's disease
    Zollinger-Ellison syndrome
Other conditions associated with large gastric folds
    Infections
        Helicobacter pylori
        Cytomegalovirus
        Syphilis
        Histoplasmosis
    Neoplasia
        Carcinoma
        Lymphoma
        Carcinoid
    Miscellaneous
        Lymphocytic gastritis
        Sarcoidosis
        Eosinophilic gastroenteritis
        Cronkhite-Canada syndrome

Lymphocytic Gastritis

Lymphocytic gastritis, characterized by T-lymphocyte infiltration of the surface and foveolar epithelium, may be isolated, or it may occur in association with celiac sprue, lymphocytic and collagenous colitis, or *H pylori* gastritis, or after use of the antithrombotic agent ticlopidine. Hypertrophic lymphocytic gastritis produces large rugal folds, but it is distinct from Ménétrier's disease. Varioliform gastritis manifests an endoscopic finding in the gastric body that consists of erosions overlying elevated lesions that resemble octopus suckers.

Hypertrophic Gastropathies

Hypertrophic gastropathies include those conditions with enlarged rugae of the gastric body and fundus that exhibit increased numbers of mucosal epithelial cells, including Ménétrier's disease (i.e., epithelial hyperplasia of the surface and foveolar mucous cells with atrophic or normal oxyntic glands); Zollinger-Ellison syndrome (i.e., increased parietal cells with normal numbers of mucous cells); and mixed hyperplastic gastropathy (i.e., increased numbers of mucous and oxyntic glandular cells) (Table 34-2). Patients with Ménétrier's disease present with epigastric pain, weight loss (up to 25 kg), nausea, vomiting, gastrointestinal hemorrhage, and diarrhea, and are diagnosed by biopsy findings of extreme foveolar hyperplasia. Hypoalbuminemia is found in 20% to 100% of patients with Ménétrier's disease. Basal and stimulated acid secretion is low or normal, and gastrin levels may be slightly elevated. The risk of progression to gastric carcinoma is controversial; sepsis and vascular and thromboembolic complications are probably a greater threat to affected patients. No medications consistently improve Ménétrier's disease, although anticholinergics have been reported to increase albumin levels. Subtotal or total gastric resection may relieve pain and correct hypoalbuminemia. Transforming growth factor alpha is markedly increased in gastric mucous cells in Ménétrier's disease and may play a pathogenic role. Acute and chronic *H pylori* gastritis may cause rugal thickening so striking as to suggest Ménétrier's disease and may produce glandular hyperplasia, gastric hypersecretion with or without hypoalbuminemia, and edema. Enlarged gastric folds may be caused by malignant neoplasms (e.g., lymphoma, adenocarcinoma), carcinoid tumors, or Cronkhite-Canada syndrome.

CHRONIC DUODENITIS

Peptic Duodenitis

Etiology and Pathogenesis

Peptic duodenitis refers to duodenal mucosal changes resulting from chronic exposure to gastric acid. Acute or chronic inflammation may be present, especially with *H pylori* infection. Gastric mucous cell metaplasia (GMCM) is characterized by the replacement of duodenal mucosa with gastric-type mucus-secreting cells. It is an adaptive response to acid exposure and is most common in patients with duodenal ulcer, in men, and in tobacco smokers. With Zollinger-Ellison syndrome, GMCM may extend into the distal duodenum and jejunum. The association of *H pylori* organisms with GMCM is very strong in active duodenitis and may represent a precursor to duodenal ulcer development. Brunner's gland hyperplasia also occurs in the duodenal bulb in response to acid exposure and is an adaptive response that leads to increased bicarbonate secretion.

Clinical Features and Diagnosis

Patients with peptic duodenitis may be asymptomatic, or they may present with dyspeptic symptoms identical to those of peptic ulcer disease. Endoscopic evaluation may reveal erythema, edema, and erosions. Brunner's gland hyperplasia gives a nodular appearance to the mucosa of the duodenal bulb. Although rarely obtained, duodenal biopsy specimens may show neutrophilic and mononuclear infiltration. GMCM is characterized by the presence of gastric mucous cells as well as by metaplastic chief cells and parietal cells, which have acid secretory capability, as demonstrated by the Congo red staining technique. *H pylori* colonization of metaplastic but not normal duodenal mucosa may be observed. Brunner's gland acini are visible with hyperplasia but are rarely seen in normal histologic resection specimens.

Miscellaneous Forms of Chronic Duodenitis

Crohn's Disease

Duodenal Crohn's disease may produce erosions, aphthous ulcers, linear ulcers, cobblestoning, nodules, fold thickening, and stenosis. Histologic findings may be indistinguishable from those of peptic ulcer disease.

Celiac Sprue

Blunting of the villi and chronic inflammation occur with peptic duodenitis as well as with celiac sprue; therefore, if sprue is a diagnostic consideration, biopsy specimens should be obtained from the distal duodenum or jejunum.

Infectious Duodenitis

Infectious duodenitis caused by *M avium* complex or *Enterocytozoon bieneusi* may be seen in AIDS and in other forms of immunodeficiency.

CHAPTER 35

Tumors of the Stomach

ADENOCARCINOMA

Incidence and Epidemiology

Adenocarcinoma of the stomach occurs more commonly in men than in women, usually during the sixth and seventh decades. China, Japan, Chile, the former Soviet Union, and Eastern European countries have very high incidences of gastric adenocarcinoma, whereas India and Africa have exceptionally low rates of gastric carcinoma. In the United States, the annual incidence is 10 cases per 100,000 population, which is one-tenth of the incidence in Japan and one-fifth of the incidence in the former Soviet Union. There has been a dramatic, unexplained decline in the rate of this disease during the past 30 years in both high- and low-incidence countries.

Etiology and Pathogenesis

Risk Factors

Gastric adenocarcinoma has been linked to diets that are high in carbohydrates and salt-preserved foods but deficient in fresh fruits and vegetables. A high dietary intake of nitrates, which are used to preserve vegetables and meats, has also been associated with gastric adenocarcinoma. Dietary nitrates serve as a source of *N*-nitrosamines, which are carcinogenic. Differences in nitrate intake between countries correlate with mortality from gastric adenocarcinoma, suggesting a possible explanation for the geographic variation in disease rates.

An epidemiologic association of *Helicobacter pylori* with the development of gastric adenocarcinoma has been reported. Patients infected with *H pylori* are three to six times more likely to develop gastric adenocarcinoma than uninfected persons. This risk is higher in women and black Americans. In contrast, *H pylori* is not linked to proximal or gastroesophageal junction adenocarcinoma, indicating that other pathogenic mechanisms lead to the development of these tumors. A carcinogenic effect of *H pylori* infection remains unproved. One possible mechanism involves a progression from chronic gastritis to the premalignant condition of atrophic gastritis with intestinal metaplasia and eventually to cancer. The validity of this hypothesis has not been established. Studies are under way to determine if *H pylori* eradication reduces the risk of gastric adenocarcinoma.

Gastric cancer is strongly associated with chronic atrophic gastritis and co-existent intestinal metaplasia. In regions at highest risk of gastric adenocarcinoma, atrophic gastritis is nearly universal, and intestinal metaplasia is found in one-third of the population. Intestinal metaplasia is present in the stomach of 70% of gastric adenocarcinoma patients. Conversely, only 10% of patients with intestinal metaplasia and atrophic gastritis may eventually develop gastric cancer, even when followed for 20 years. Chronic atrophic gastritis may result from type B antral gastritis associated with *H pylori* or type A fundic gastritis associated with autoimmune disease. Patients with pernicious anemia and type A atrophic gastritis have an increased risk of gastric adenocarcinoma, but the magnitude and timing associated with this increased risk are poorly defined.

Patients with a prior gastrectomy, especially a Billroth II gastrojejunostomy, have a two-fold increased risk of gastric adenocarcinoma, which manifests >20 years after the gastrectomy. The anastomotic stoma is the primary site of gastric tumors. Intestinal metaplasia with dysplasia may precede tumor development. The mechanism of carcinogenesis in postgastrectomy patients remains unclear, but increased concentrations of *N*-nitroso compounds and bile acids in the stomach have been implicated.

Tumors of the proximal stomach, particularly the gastroesophageal junction, have distinct risk factors. Gastroesophageal junction adenocarcinomas constitute 25% of gastric cancers and, unlike distal stomach tumors, have been increasing in incidence in recent decades. Many proximal tumors occur in the setting of Barrett's metaplasia of the esophagus and represent a variant of esophageal adenocarcinoma. Proximal stomach tumors are more likely to be associated with tobacco use; they are not associated with *H pylori* infection. Based on these differences, adenocarcinoma of the gastroesophageal junction is often considered separately from tumors of the fundus, body, and antrum.

Histopathology

Gastric adenocarcinoma has the morphologic appearance of an ulcerated mass in 40% to 50%, a polypoid mass in 40% to 50%, a diffusely infiltrating mass, termed *linitis plastica*, in 7%, and a superficial spreading mass in 2%. *Early gastric cancer* is a term that applies to tumors limited to the mucosa and submucosa. In some cases, there may be associated lymph node involvement. Early gastric cancer has a favorable prognosis and is most commonly diagnosed during screening of asymptomatic high-risk populations. Several clinical and pathologic features of gastric cancer cor-

TABLE 35-1
TNM Staging of Gastric Carcinoma

STAGE	T STAGE	N STAGE	M STAGE	5-YEAR SURVIVAL (%)
IA	T1	N0	M0	91
IB	T1	N1	M0	82
	T2	N0	M0	
II	T1	N2	M0	65
	T2	N1	M0	
	T3	N0	M0	
IIIA	T2	N2	M0	49
	T3	N1	M0	
	T4	N0	M0	
IIIB	T3	N2	M0	28
	T4	N1	M0	
IV	T4	N2	M0	5
	Any T	Any N	M1	

relate with survival. Younger patients, patients with linitis plastica, or patients with proximal tumors have a poor prognosis. The two best predictors of survival are depth of invasion (T stage) and metastases to lymph nodes (N stage) or distant sites (M stage). The T staging is defined as follows: Tumors limited to the mucosa or submucosa are T1; invasion of the muscularis propria is T2; extension beyond the serosa is T3; and invasion of adjacent structures defines T4. Perigastric lymph nodes <3 cm from the primary tumors are classified as N1, whereas all lymph nodes associated with major blood vessels or distant nodes are classified as N2. Based on these pathologic features, gastric tumors are categorized by a TNM staging system into four stages that correlate with long-term survival (Table 35-1).

Histologically, gastric cancer is divided into an intestinal type, which is characterized by epithelial cells that form glandular structures, and a diffuse type, which is characterized by sheets of undifferentiated cells. The intestinal type is more common in countries where gastric cancer is endemic, whereas the diffuse type is more common in low-risk populations, such as in the United States. The intestinal type is more likely to be associated with intestinal metaplasia and atrophic gastritis and has a more favorable prognosis than the diffuse type. Rarely, gastric malignancies exhibit adenomatous and squamous features. This adenosquamous variant has a poor prognosis.

Clinical Features

Patients with gastric adenocarcinoma are often asymptomatic until the tumor reaches an advanced stage. Symptoms usually are nonspecific and include epigastric pain, early satiety, bloating, nausea, vomiting, and weight loss. Rarely, gastrointestinal hemorrhage or gastric outlet obstruction are the initial manifestation of a gastric tumor. The physical examination findings may be normal, show occult or gross gastrointestinal blood loss, or exhibit lymphadenopathy or hepatomegaly with disease dissemination.

Findings on Diagnostic Testing

Laboratory Studies

Laboratory evaluation of a patient with gastric adenocarcinoma may reveal nonspecific abnormalities. Anemia may be present secondary to chronic blood loss, chronic disease, or vitamin B_{12} deficiency with pernicious anemia. Hypoalbuminemia reflects poor nutrition, and abnormal liver chemistry values suggest hepatic involvement.

Upper Gastrointestinal Endoscopy

Patients with suggestive symptoms or physical examination findings should be evaluated with upper gastrointestinal endoscopy or double-contrast upper gastrointestinal barium radiography. Upper gastrointestinal endoscopy may provide evidence that strongly suggests a neoplasm, but endoscopic biopsy is necessary to confirm the diagnosis. The overall sensitivity and specificity of upper gastrointestinal endoscopy with biopsy are 95% and 99%, respectively. Obtaining brushings of endoscopic abnormalities before forceps biopsy may improve the sensitivity. The highest yield is achieved by obtaining brush cytologic specimens and a total of seven biopsy specimens from the lesion; ulcers are sampled at the base and the four quadrants of the edge. Because the sensitivity of biopsy is not 100%, all suggestive gastric ulcers should be re-evaluated with upper gastrointestinal endoscopy performed after therapy to confirm healing, and a biopsy of any persistent mucosal defects should be performed. Some tumors appear as thickened gastric folds with normal overlying mucosa, which are caused by infiltration of the tumor into the submucosa. These cancers can be diagnosed with cautious use of a snare to obtain a biopsy specimen that samples the submucosa.

Radiographic Studies

When performed by an experienced radiologist, upper gastrointestinal radiography detects >90% of gastric adenocarcinomas. Characteristic radiographic findings include an asymmetric ulcer crater, distorted or nodular folds radiating from an ulcer, a lack of distensibility, and a polypoid mass. However, radiography does not have the capability to obtain histologic samples.

Staging Evaluation

The most accurate means of determining T and N stages of gastric cancer is endoscopic ultrasound (EUS), although the ability of EUS to differentiate inflammatory from malignant adenopathy is limited. EUS is unable to detect the majority of distant metastases; computed tomographic (CT) scanning provides the best means of determining M stage. Occasionally, the M stage is overstaged on CT scans; therefore, all suspected metastases should be confirmed with operative or CT-guided biopsy.

Management and Course

Surgical Therapy

Complete surgical resection is the only therapeutic option that offers a potential cure of gastric adenocarcinoma. Detection at an early stage is critical. The importance of surgical resection is reflected in the 5-year survival rate of 40% to 60% in patients with resectable tumors, compared with the 5-year survival rate of <5% in patients who undergo palliative resection. In Japan, mass screening programs for the detection of early gastric cancer have resulted in a resectability rate of nearly 90% and an overall 5-year survival rate of 37%. In low-incidence regions such as the United States, where no screening programs exist, the resectability rate is only 40% and the overall 5-year survival rate is 10% to 15%. Operative mortality rates are also lower in Japan because of the increased surgical experience and improved diagnosis of patients with early stage disease.

There is no consensus on the optimal curative surgical procedure for gastric adenocarcinoma. The superiority of total gastrectomy over stage-dependent subtotal gastrectomy remains to be established. If the latter procedure is performed, disease-free surgical margins of at least 5 cm beyond the tumor are recommended; total gastrectomy is often required to achieve this goal if the tumors are advanced or infiltrating. Splenectomy usually is performed if tumors are located along the greater curvature. Adenocarcinomas of the proximal fundus are treated by proximal gastric resection. Tumors of the gastroesophageal junction require en bloc resection of the distal esophagus and proximal stomach, often by a combined thoracic and abdominal approach. In any surgical resection of a gastric adenocarcinoma, extensive nodal dissection may improve survival and assist in planning postoperative adjuvant therapy. The role of resection of isolated hepatic metastases at the time of gastrectomy has not been determined in controlled clinical trials.

Patients with tumors that are not amenable to complete resection may require surgical resection or bypass to palliate obstructive symptoms. Although there are no controlled trials, palliative resection is generally preferred to bypass because of lower operative morbidity and mortality. The operative mortality for palliative resection is as low as 8% in specialized centers, and the 2-year survival rate is 25%. Stent placement or Nd:YAG laser tumor ablation may be performed endoscopically in patients who are poor surgical candidates. Nd:YAG laser coagulation necrosis can successfully treat acute or chronic transfusion-requiring gastrointestinal hemorrhage associated with gastric adenocarcinoma.

Nonsurgical Therapy

The role of chemotherapy and radiation therapy in the treatment of gastric adenocarcinoma is evolving. Combination therapy with 5-fluorouracil, doxorubicin, and cisplatin is superior to single-agent therapy; however, response rates are only 30% to 50%, and there is no evidence of improved survival. Combined radiation therapy and chemotherapy may improve survival of patients undergoing a potentially curative resection. Further clinical trials of preoperative neoadjuvant therapy and the introduction of new therapeutic agents may further define the role of cytoreductive therapy in gastric cancer.

Screening in High-Risk Populations

In Japan, the incidence of gastric adenocarcinoma exceeds all other tumors. Screening asymptomatic adults every 1 to 2 years with upper gastrointestinal barium radiography or upper gastrointestinal endoscopy has resulted in earlier detection and decreased mortality. The low incidence of gastric adenocarcinoma and the high cost of mass screening prohibit adopting this strategy in low-risk populations, although certain high-risk groups may benefit from surveillance. Patients with pernicious anemia, those who had gastric surgery >20 years previously, or persons with gastric adenomatous polyps represent high-risk populations. Currently, however, there is no evidence that surveillance improves survival in these patients.

GASTRIC LYMPHOMA

Incidence and Epidemiology

Non-Hodgkin's lymphoma is the second most common malignancy of the stomach, constituting 5% of malignant gastric tumors. Forty percent of gastrointestinal lymphomas occur in the stomach, and one-third have no associated lymph node involvement.

Etiology and Pathogenesis

Similar to adenocarcinoma of the stomach, gastric lymphomas often occur in the setting of chronic atrophic gastritis and intestinal metaplasia. The tumors most commonly infiltrate the submucosal layers, producing thickened rugal folds or submucosal masses with overlying ulceration. There is evidence that >90% of low-grade gastric B-cell tumors, termed *mucosal-associated lymphoid tissue (MALT) lymphomas*, are caused by *H pylori* infection. The critical role of *H pylori* in the genesis of these tumors is supported by reports of complete regression of early stage tumors with antibiotic therapy.

Clinical Features

Gastric lymphoma can mimic adenocarcinoma of the stomach clinically. Patients present with nonspecific symptoms of early satiety, epigastric pain, anorexia, and vomiting. Gastrointestinal hemorrhage and perforation resulting from extensive ulceration are less common manifestations. Physical examination may reveal an abdominal mass or peripheral adenopathy.

Findings on Diagnostic Testing

Upper gastrointestinal endoscopy and double-contrast upper gastrointestinal barium radiography are the primary means of detecting gastric lymphoma, but the ability to obtain biopsy specimens makes upper gastrointestinal endoscopy the procedure of choice. CT scans demonstrate evidence of associated adenopathy in two-thirds of patients. Occasionally, lymphoma appears as a thickened fold, which on endoscopic biopsy may reveal a submucosal mass with normal overlying mucosa. In this setting, EUS may define the wall layers involved and may direct snare resection to confirm the diagnosis. Laparotomy may be necessary to define the extent of disease.

Management and Course

Gastric lymphoma has a favorable prognosis compared with gastric adenocarcinoma. The 5-year survival rate is 50%. The Ann Arbor staging system for gastric

TABLE 35-2
Ann Arbor Staging System for Gastric Lymphoma

STAGE	EXTENT OF DISEASE	RELATIVE INCIDENCE (%)
I	Limited to stomach	26–38
II	Involvement of abdominal lymph nodes	43–49
III	Involvement of lymph nodes above the diaphragm	13–31
IV	Disseminated disease	

non-Hodgkin's lymphoma is based on the extent of disease, which, once established, helps in planning the appropriate therapy (Table 35-2). Patients with stage I tumors limited to the stomach have cure rates of >80% and should undergo total gastrectomy or limited gastrectomy with adequate margins. Postoperative chemotherapy and radiation therapy may improve survival in patients with this early stage disease. Patients with stage II to stage IV disease are best treated with combination chemotherapy, but if bulky transmural stomach tumors are present, prophylactic gastrectomy is often performed to prevent treatment-related perforation. Patients with disseminated non-Hodgkin's lymphoma rarely survive 2 years. The majority of MALT lymphomas are stage I, and early mucosal tumors may respond to antibiotic therapy directed at *H pylori* eradication. More advanced MALT lymphomas require systemic chemotherapy. MALT lymphomas, in particular, have a relatively favorable outcome.

METASTATIC TUMORS

Malignant neoplasms from distant sites may metastasize to the stomach. Common sources include melanoma, ovarian, colon, lung, and breast cancer. Tumors may be mucosal or submucosal with associated ulceration. Patients may experience epigastric pain, vomiting, and gastrointestinal hemorrhage.

MISCELLANEOUS BENIGN AND MALIGNANT GASTRIC TUMORS

Gastric Polyps

Gastric polyps are rare, and the vast majority are hyperplastic with no malignant potential. They usually are <1 cm and rarely produce symptoms. Adenomatous polyps account for 10% to 20% of gastric polyps and are premalignant lesions. Adenomas should be resected, and a program of endoscopic surveillance should be instituted to detect recurrence. Large numbers of fundic hyperplastic polyps may be observed in some patients with Ménétrier's disease (i.e., hypertrophic gastropathy). Similarly, patients with familial adenomatous polyposis (FAP) or Gardner's syndrome may have fundic gland polyposis. These polyps usually are hamartomas, although some are adenomatous. Gastric adenomas in patients with FAP have the potential for malignant degeneration, necessitating endoscopic surveillance and excision.

Gastric Carcinoid

Carcinoid tumors of the stomach represent 0.3% of all gastric tumors. Gastric carcinoids are endocrine tumors that produce multiple bioactive substances, including serotonin, histamines, somatostatin, and kinins, but they rarely produce the flushing, diarrhea, and cardiopulmonary symptoms characteristic of the carcinoid syndrome. Carcinoids usually are submucosal lesions, although they can cause ulceration of the overlying mucosa. They are often multicentric in conditions associated with hypergastrinemia, such as atrophic gastritis and Zollinger-Ellison syndrome. In this setting, carcinoids are rarely malignant. Sporadic carcinoids behave more aggressively, and complete excision is recommended. Metastatic tumors may require systemic chemotherapy to control tumor bulk. The somatostatin analog octreotide can improve symptoms in many patients with the carcinoid syndrome.

Leiomyoma and Leiomyosarcoma

Leiomyomas are the most common gastric submucosal masses. They usually cause no symptoms and are often detected incidentally during upper gastrointestinal endoscopy. Rarely, a leiomyoma undergoes a malignant transformation to a leiomyosarcoma, which accounts for <1% of gastric malignancies. A leiomyosarcoma is a highly vascular tumor that may produce massive gastrointestinal hemorrhage. The differentiation of a leiomyoma from a leiomyosarcoma is often problematic and is based on the number of mitotic figures and invasiveness seen on histologic examination. The 5-year survival rate of patients after resection of a leiomyosarcoma is approximately 50%.

CHAPTER 36

Structural Anomalies and Miscellaneous Diseases of the Small Intestine

EMBRYOLOGY AND ANATOMY

The foregut is the progenitor of the proximal duodenum up to the ampulla of Vater. The midgut gives rise to the distal duodenum, jejunum, and ileum. The midgut initially communicates freely with the yolk sac and then narrows to be connected by the omphalomesenteric or vitelline duct. The primitive gut forms a U-shaped loop that herniates into the umbilical cord in the sixth week of gestation. The proximal limb of the loop then rotates around the superior mesenteric artery axis and at 10 weeks returns to the abdominal cavity, with an additional counterclockwise rotation. The small intestine is attached to the posterior abdominal wall by a broad-based mesentery from the duodenojejunal junction to the ileocecal region.

The adult small intestine is approximately 600 cm long, including the duodenum (the terminus of which is demarcated by the ligament of Treitz), and the jejunum and ileum (40% and 60% of the length after the ligament of Treitz, respectively). The jejunal loops settle into the left upper quadrant; the distal ileum settles into the right lower quadrant. The duodenal bulb is invested with intra-abdominal mesentery, whereas much of the rest of the length is retroperitoneal, re-entering the peritoneal cavity at the ligament of Treitz. The jejunum is thicker than the ileum and has more prominent plicae circulares, which are mucosal and submucosal invaginations.

The arteries, veins, and lymphatics of the small intestine travel through the mesentery. The hepatic artery gives rise to the gastroduodenal artery, which branches into the anterior and posterior superior gastroduodenal arteries. These arteries communicate with the inferior pancreaticoduodenal artery, which arises from the superior mesenteric artery to supply the duodenum. The jejunum and ileum receive their supply from branches of the superior mesenteric artery. The veins draining the small intestine usually follow the arterial supply. Small lymph channels (i.e., lacteals) drain into mesenteric lymph nodes, which subsequently drain into the cisterna chyli and thoracic duct.

The small intestine has a rich intrinsic innervation supplied by the myenteric plexus, which lies between the longitudinal and circular muscle layers and the submucosal plexus. The extrinsic neural supply arises from the superior mesenteric ganglion (sympathetic) and the vagus nerve (parasympathetic). A rich sensory innervation consists of different nerves from the dorsal root ganglia and nodose ganglia.

The small intestine is composed of four concentric layers: the mucosa, the submucosa, the muscularis propria, and the serosa. The mucosa consists of an epithelial layer overlying the lamina propria and muscularis mucosae. The epithelium is a continuous sheet of columnar cells overlying the villi and forming the crypts. These epithelial cells transport the products of digestion into the capillaries and lymphatics, through which they are distributed to other areas of the body. Tight junctions between adjacent epithelial cells restrict water and ion flow. In a process of cellular renewal lasting 3 to 5 days, undifferentiated stem cells in the crypts give rise to four differentiated cell types: enterocytes and mucus-secreting goblet cells, which migrate to the villus; Paneth's cells, which migrate to the crypt bases; and enteroendocrine cells, which are broadly distributed. Undifferentiated crypt cells also secrete the secretory component–IgA complex into the intestinal lumen. Villus enterocytes exhibit prominent microvilli and possess numerous enzymes for digestion (e.g., disaccharidases, peptidases); genes involved in lipid absorption (e.g., apolipoproteins, fatty acid–binding proteins); and many receptors, carriers, and transporters. Several cytoskeletal filaments contribute to the structural rigidity of the brush border in differentiated villus cells; some extend from the cell membrane to produce a surface coat, the glycocalyx. Goblet cells are present throughout the entire gastrointestinal tract, but they are most numerous in the ileum, producing the mucus that serves as a lubricant and a cytoprotective agent. Paneth's cells are believed to be involved in host defense because of abundant expression of lysozyme and defensins and the ability to degranulate in response to bacteria. Enteroendocrine cells produce hormones and include D cells (somatostatin); L cells (glucagon-like immunoreactivity); enterochromaffin cells (serotonin); and cholecystokinin-, substance P–, and motilin-secreting cells. Other cell types include the "tuft," or caveolated, cells, the M cells overlying Peyer's patches, and intraepithelial lymphocytes. M cells serve as antigen sampling cells and engulf macromolecules, viruses, and bacteria by endocytosis and deliver them to immune tissues.

The lamina propria contains immune cells (e.g., lymphocytes, macrophages, neutrophils, plasma cells, and mast cells). Plasma cells are responsible for IgA synthesis before complexing with secretory component from the enterocyte. Lymphoid follicles are collections of lymphocytes in the mucosa and submucosa. Peyer's patches are collections of follicles in the lamina propria and submucosa that drain into lymph vessels and then to mesenteric lymph nodes. Other components of the lamina propria include fibroblasts, smooth muscle cells, arterioles, venules, and a central lacteal for delivery of nutrients into the vascular system.

The submucosa contains connective tissue, blood vessels, the submucosal plexus, and, in the duodenum only, Brunner's glands, which secrete mucus and bicarbonate. The muscularis propria consists of an outer longitudinal layer and an inner circular muscle layer, which generate peristalsis. The serosa is composed of mesothelial cells overlying loose connective tissue. This outer layer is continuous with the mesentery.

DEVELOPMENTAL ABNORMALITIES

Atresia, Stenosis, and Membranes

Etiology and Pathogenesis

During embryologic development, the lumen of the small intestine is occluded by epithelium. Failure of recanalization and intrauterine ischemic events can result in stenosis, which may result from simple membranes to lesions as complex as atresias involving all layers. Stenosis and atresia can be associated with other congenital abnormalities (e.g., Down's syndrome, malrotation, anorectal malformations, and cardiac, pulmonary, renal, and pancreatic malformations). Type I atresia is characterized by a membranous septum of mucosa and submucosa with intact bowel wall and mesentery. Type II atresia exhibits two blind loops of small intestine connected by a fibrous cord. In type IIIa atresia, two blind loops are separated by a gap. In type IIIb atresia, the distal superior mesenteric artery is absent; the condition may be hereditary. Type IV denotes multiple atresias. Other factors in the development of atresia and stenosis include maternal ergotamine use, fetal methylene blue exposure, and neonatal immunodeficiency.

Clinical Features, Diagnosis, and Management

With intestinal stenosis and atresia, vomiting begins soon after birth and is devoid of bile if the obstruction is proximal to the ampulla of Vater. Polyhydramnios may be present before birth, and maternal ultrasound studies may detect proximal bowel dilation, fetal ascites, and extralumenal calcifications. Very rarely in adults, duodenal membranes produce symptoms of fullness, vomiting, and weight loss. Duodenal obstruction distal to the bulb gives a typical "double-bubble" sign on abdominal radiography. Upper gastrointestinal barium radiography can confirm the site of obstruction, but often it is not necessary. Barium enema radiography is recommended to exclude Hirschsprung's disease and malrotation with volvulus. Gastrojejunostomy is performed for proximal duodenal obstructions; duodenojejunostomy is used for distal duodenal blockage. Type IIIb and type IV atresias may require extensive resection. Endoscopic laser or cautery techniques may be performed in adults with duodenal membranes. All patients are given total parenteral nutrition postoperatively until normal intestinal function returns.

Duplications

Etiology and Pathogenesis

Duplications of the small intestine contain all layers of the wall. They may or may not communicate with the lumen. In some cases, they may be lined with heterotopic mucosa of gastric, pancreatic, esophageal, thyroid, or bronchial origin. Most duplications of the small intestine are found in the ileum.

Clinical Features, Diagnosis, and Management

Patients with duplications often present with symptoms of obstruction in infancy or childhood, and less commonly, with perforation into the head of the pancreas causing pancreatitis, hemorrhage, or malignancy (e.g., adenocarcinoma, carcinoid, squamous cell carcinoma). Obstructions result from a mass effect or from intussusception. The diagnosis is seldom made preoperatively, although barium radiography of the small intestine or enteroclysis may demonstrate the duplication if it communicates with the gut lumen. Computed tomographic (CT) or ultrasound studies may show a cystic mass, whereas radiolabeled technetium scans (i.e., a Meckel scan) may produce positive findings if gastric mucosa is present. Treatment is surgical: complete resection, if possible, or drainage into the adjacent intestinal lumen.

Malrotation

Etiology and Pathogenesis

Abnormal rotation of the small intestine is the most common cause of intestinal obstruction in childhood. Patients with nonrotation present with the entire small intestine in the right peritoneum and the colon in the left abdomen. There is a high risk of volvulus. Malrotation or incomplete rotation is characterized by subpyloric or subhepatic positioning of the cecum with attachment of the small intestine by a narrow vascular pedicle (instead of a broad mesentery), a situation favoring volvulus formation. Ladd's bands, which are peritoneal bands passing from the cecum across the duodenum to the right upper quadrant, may produce duodenal obstruction. Reversed rotation produces a condition in which the mesentery of the small intestine passes in front of the transverse colon, producing colonic obstruction. Failure of the cecum to descend into the right lower quadrant causes a mobile cecum, predisposing to volvulus. Half of the patients have other congenital anomalies, including duodenal atresia, annular pancreas, or Hirschsprung's disease.

Clinical Features, Diagnosis, and Management

Patients usually present within weeks of birth with bilious vomiting and distention with visible peristalsis. The course may be complicated by intestinal or cecal volvulus that leads to ischemia and perforation. Older children, adolescents, and adults may experience intermittent vomiting, failure to thrive, recurrent pain, or volvulus with acute abdominal pain, bloody stools, and distention. Abdominal radiography shows gastric and proximal intestinal dilation. Upper gastrointestinal barium radiography may demonstrate the site of obstruction and characterize the degree of malrotation. CT scans may show abnormal positioning of the superior mesenteric artery and vein. Treatment involves surgical division of the obstructing bands, resection of any infarcted segments, and fixation of the cecum to prevent volvulus. Most patients do well postoperatively, but a subset of children experience persistent nausea, vomiting, and pain because of dysmotility and damage to the small intestine from long-standing obstruction.

Meckel's Diverticulum

Library Resource Center
Renton Technical College
3000 N.E. 4th St.
Renton, WA 98056

Etiology and Pathogenesis

A Meckel's diverticulum, the most common gastrointestinal congenital anomaly, results if the vitelline duct fails to completely resorb. Usually, the duct remnant persists as a diverticular sac. A thick, fibrous band connected to the umbilicus occasionally persists, however, leading to volvulus or strangulation of bowel loops. Diverticula are often located within 100 cm of the ileocecal valve and are usually 1 to 10 cm in length. One-half contain heterotopic tissue: gastric, pancreatic, colonic, hepatobiliary, or Brunner's glands. *Helicobacter pylori* may colonize heterotopic gastric mucosa and produce inflammation.

Clinical Features, Diagnosis, and Management

Gastrointestinal bleeding may result from ileal ulceration secondary to acid production from heterotopic diverticular gastric mucosa. Other manifestations include obstruction of the small intestine, diverticulitis (from enterolith impaction), perforation, and malignancies (e.g., carcinoid, sarcoma, and adenocarcinoma). Obstruction is caused by intussusception, volvulus, entrapment in hernias, or inflammation and scarring. Children most commonly present with gastrointestinal bleeding, whereas obstruction is by far the most common complication in adults. In children, radiolabeled technetium scanning is highly sensitive and specific; in adults, the technique has high false-negative and false-positive rates (e.g., in Crohn's disease) even in bleeding patients. The sensitivity of the test may be enhanced by administration of cimetidine, which decreases secretion of the radiolabeled anion by ectopic gastric mucosa, and of pentagastrin, which enhances technetium uptake. Barium radiography of the small intestine may visualize the diverticulum, although rapid intestinal transit may cause false-negative results. Enteroclysis has an improved sensitivity for detection. Angiography may demonstrate active bleeding and document the persistent vitelline artery and its branches. Surgical resection is indicated for hemorrhage, obstruction, or perforation and may need to include adjacent small intestine if it is ulcerated, inflamed, or obstructed. Most asymptomatic Meckel's diverticula need no therapy. Resection of diverticula found incidentally during laparotomy has been advocated if the diverticula are large, if they have persistent fibrous bands, or if they have a palpable mass.

Superior Mesenteric Artery Syndrome

Etiology and Pathogenesis

In rare instances, the superior mesenteric artery compresses the third portion of the duodenum against fixed retroperitoneal structures, possibly because the artery is positioned at an acute angle to the aorta.

Clinical Features, Diagnosis, and Management

The typical clinical presentation is occasional epigastric distress with vomiting. The symptoms may be acute or chronic and may date back to childhood. Abdominal radiography may be normal or show a "double-bubble" sign. Upper gastrointestinal barium radiography reveals an abrupt cutoff of barium flow in the third duodenal portion. A narrowed angle of the superior mesenteric artery to the aorta may be seen on angiography. Initial therapy involves small liquid feedings; postprandially, the patient lies prone or on the left side. Duodenojejunostomy is reserved for refractory cases.

Preduodenal Portal Vein

Etiology and Pathogenesis

The embryonic preduodenal portal vein normally atrophies before birth, but rarely it persists. This anomaly may be associated with a preduodenal common bile duct, intestinal stenosis, annular pancreas, malrotation, and biliary tract abnormalities.

Clinical Features, Diagnosis, and Management

The patient typically presents with obstructive symptoms that require surgical attention.

STRUCTURAL ABNORMALITIES

Duodenal Diverticula

Etiology and Pathogenesis

Congenital duodenal diverticula predominately occur most often within 2 cm of the ampulla of Vater and may represent the site of ampullary drainage in some cases. Acquired duodenal diverticula usually develop in the duodenal bulb.

Clinical Features, Diagnosis, and Management

Most duodenal diverticula are found incidentally on upper gastrointestinal barium radiography or endoscopy (i.e., upper gastrointestinal endoscopy or endoscopic retrograde cholangiopancreatography). They are usually asymptomatic, although in rare cases they lead to common bile duct obstruction because of extrinsic compression or ampullary distortion. Cases of obstruction are managed by choledochoduodenostomy or Roux-en-Y choledochojejunostomy.

Volvulus

Etiology and Pathogenesis

Volvulus is an abnormal twisting of the intestine around its mesentery and may produce strangulation and gangrene. In the United States, most cases of volvulus of the small intestine are caused by a pre-existing defect such as an anomaly of rotation, postoperative adhesion, or congenital bands.

Clinical Features, Diagnosis, and Management

Most patients present with symptoms of acute obstruction and possibly an acute abdomen. Signs include a distended abdomen, guarding and rigidity, and occasionally a palpable mass. Abdominal radiography may show distention with air-fluid levels consistent with obstruction. Upper gastrointestinal barium radiography may define anomalies of rotation. Angiography may show twisting of the superior mesenteric artery, confirming the diagnosis. The treatment involves surgery; the ischemic or gangrenous bowel is resected, although occasionally derotation alone is sufficient.

Intussusception

Etiology and Pathogenesis

Intussusception occurs when a segment of bowel telescopes into adjacent distal bowel, causing obstruction and possibly ischemia. Intussusception in children usually is idiopathic, but a pathologic lead point caused by a mass (e.g., leiomyoma, lymphoma), a duplication, or an intramural hematoma, as with Henoch-Schönlein purpura, is present in 8% to 12% of cases. In contrast, a causative factor can be identified in 90% of adult patients in the form of an intestinal or extraintestinal mass (e.g., leiomyoma, neurofibroma, lipoma, lymphoma, polyp, metastatic tumor, Kaposi's sarcoma), Meckel's diverticulum, or intussusception after a Billroth II gastrojejunostomy.

Clinical Features, Diagnosis, and Management

Children present with acute abdominal pain, vomiting, hematochezia, a palpable mass, diarrhea, and somnolence. Adults may present with subtle intermittent or chronic abdominal pain, nausea and vomiting, weight loss, and an abdominal mass. Abdominal radiography may show a crescent of gas capping the intussusception, a gas-free area corresponding to the intussusception itself, or a target sign outlining the intussusception. Barium enema radiography is indicated for children because of the frequent localization in the ileocecal region, where the test may be diagnostic and reduce the intussusception as well. If the lesion fails to reduce or if perforation is present, surgery is required. Ultrasound may be of use in some children; CT scanning usually is not needed. Upper gastrointestinal barium radiography is not used in children if perforation is suspected. The diagnosis is more challenging in adult patients and may require a combination of abdominal radiography, upper gastrointestinal and barium enema radiography, ultrasound, and CT studies. Adults should undergo surgical resection, as most cases are associated with mass lesions. Manual reduction of adult intussusception is not recommended if a malignancy is present because this maneuver may facilitate tumor metastases.

Lymphangiectasia

Etiology and Pathogenesis

Intestinal lymphangiectasia is characterized by obstruction of lymph drainage that leads to malabsorption of chylomicrons and fat-soluble vitamins and to protein-losing enteropathy (PLE). Lymphenteric fistulae may develop, and proteins, chylomicrons, and lymphocytes may drain directly into the intestinal lumen. Lymphangiectasia may be a primary congenital disease (Milroy's disease) or secondary to retroperitoneal carcinoma or lymphoma, retroperitoneal fibrosis, chronic pancreatitis, mesenteric tuberculosis or sarcoidosis, Crohn's disease, Whipple's disease, scleroderma, celiac disease, or heart disease.

Clinical Features, Diagnosis, and Management

Patients present with malabsorption, steatorrhea, and lymphocytopenia with hypogammaglobulinemia. Edema and hypoproteinemia may be prominent. Milroy's disease presents at any age with asymmetric lymphedema of an extremity.

Rarely, opportunistic infections (e.g., atypical mycobacteria, warts, cellulitis), pain, distention, nausea, chylous ascites or pleural effusions, and gastrointestinal bleeding occur. Laboratory studies can show increased amounts of fecal fat, a prolonged prothrombin time, and reduced calcium or vitamin A levels. The diagnosis of lymphangiectasia rests on demonstration of dilated lymphatic lacteals, which may appear endoscopically as white opaque spots but are definitively shown on intestinal biopsy specimens. Biopsy specimens may also show villous atrophy and mild inflammation. Fecal levels of α_1-antitrypsin are usually elevated, which is indicative of PLE. Barium radiography of the small intestine may show only nonspecific fold thickening as a result of hypoalbuminemia. A CT scan may be diagnostic in patients with lymphangiectasia secondary to malignancy. With secondary lymphangiectasia, therapy should be directed at the underlying cause. Otherwise, medium-chain triglycerides may be given to supplement low dietary fat intake to reduce steatorrhea. Peripheral edema is reduced by postural drainage and elastic stockings.

ULCERS OF THE SMALL INTESTINE

Primary Ulcers

Etiology and Pathogenesis

The diagnosis of a primary ulcer of the small intestine is made after secondary causes are excluded (Table 36-1). Therefore, the etiology and pathogenesis of primary ulcers are unknown. Most primary ulcers are located in the ileum, although perforated ulcers usually occur in the jejunum. They are solitary in 70% of cases, varying in diameter from 0.3 to 5.0 cm. Eosinophilic infiltration and granulation tissue with fibrosis and stenosis may be present.

Clinical Features, Diagnosis, and Management

Primary ulcers of the small intestine can bleed, obstruct, or perforate. Histories may include symptoms of partial small intestine ulceration over a 3-day to 20-year period. One-half of the patients exhibit iron deficiency anemia. Primary ulcers are detected by contrast radiography, upper gastrointestinal endoscopy or small intestine enteroscopy, or laparotomy, which is necessary for diagnosis in a large percentage of cases. Enteroclysis has a higher sensitivity for detection of primary ulcers than upper gastrointestinal barium radiography and is the procedure of choice. Abdominal radiography without contrast detects ulcers only in cases of obstruction or perforation. Red cell scintigraphy and angiography are useful if significant hemorrhage is present. In addition to its diagnostic utility, surgical intervention is indicated for treatment of complications (e.g., perforations, significant hemorrhage, and obstruction).

Medication-Induced Ulcers

Etiology and Pathogenesis

The most prevalent causes of medication-induced ulcers of the small intestine are NSAIDs and potassium supplements. Multiple small bowel ulcers (in 8.4% of patients), mucosal diaphragms, strictures, and perforations are associated with

---

TABLE 36-1
Causes of Ulceration of the Small Intestine

Infection
    Tuberculosis
    Typhoid
    Cytomegalovirus
    Syphilis
    Parasitic diseases
    Strongyloidiasis
    Campylobacteriosis
    Yersiniosis
Inflammatory causes
    Crohn's disease
    Systemic lupus erythematosus
    Diverticulitis
Mucosal lesions
    Ulcerative jejunoileitis
Tumors
    Malignant histiocytosis
    Lymphoma
    Adenocarcinoma
    Melanoma
    Kaposi's sarcoma
Vascular causes
    Mesenteric insufficiency
    Giant cell arteritis
    Vasculitis
    Vascular abnormality
    Amyloidosis
Hyperacidity
    Zollinger-Ellison syndrome
    Meckel's diverticulum
    Stomal ulceration
Metabolic causes
    Uremia
Medications
    Potassium chloride
    NSAIDs
    Antimetabolites
Radiation therapy
Idiopathic ulcers
    Primary ulcer
    Behçet's syndrome

NSAID use. NSAID-induced ulcers of the small intestine typically involve the distal intestine. Mucosal diaphragms can narrow the intestinal lumen to 1 mm, and they can be multiple. Submucosal fibrosis replacing or merging with the muscularis mucosae is characteristic. Independent risk factors for NSAID-induced gastrointestinal complications include age exceeding 60 years, previous NSAID complications, and concomitant corticosteroid use. However, because small bowel effects have not been examined independently, it is unknown if these risk factors apply to small bowel enteropathy alone. Small intestine ulceration also can result from use of enteric-coated potassium drugs. The risk is increased by several factors: delayed intestinal transit, advanced age, and concurrent systemic illness. Other drugs that cause small bowel ulcers or perforation include corticosteroids, cytarabine, digoxin, and ferrous sulfate preparations.

Clinical Features, Diagnosis, and Management

Patients with medication-induced ulcers of the small intestine present with acute or chronic blood loss, obstruction, perforation, weight loss, hypoalbuminemia, and vague abdominal pain. Barium radiography (small intestine barium radiography or enteroclysis) and endoscopy (including enteroscopy) are commonly used for diagnosis, although detection of subtle mucosal diaphragms may require surgical enterotomy. If possible, the offending medication should be discontinued. Alternatively, use of a prodrug (e.g., nabumetone or sulindac) or a less potent cyclo-oxygenase inhibitor may decrease local injury. Surgical intervention is necessary to treat complications such as hemorrhage, stricture, or perforation. The therapeutic role of prostaglandin analogs (e.g., misoprostol) is unproved.

Ulcers Associated with Systemic Disease

Etiology and Pathogenesis

Behçet's syndrome affects the skin, joints, vascular system, central nervous system, and intestinal tract. Intestinal ulceration affects <1% of patients. Deep ulcers surrounded by a minimally inflamed mucosa are characteristic and found most often in the ileocecal region. Patients with systemic lupus erythematosus may present with ulcers of the small intestine as a result of microthrombosis and vasculitis.

Clinical Features, Diagnosis, and Management

The optimal treatment of Behçet's syndrome is not established, although intestinal resection may be necessary. No medical treatment consistently alters its course, and postoperative ulcer recurrence is common.

Diffuse Ulcers and Concurrent Malabsorption

Etiology and Pathogenesis

Chronic ulcerative jejunoileitis may complicate long-standing celiac sprue in patients older than 60 years of age. It is characterized by multiple superficial or deep ulcers in the small intestine (gastric and colonic ulcers occur rarely) in the setting of villous atrophy, mucosal inflammation, and crypt hyperplasia. Rarely, chronic ulcerative jejunoileitis occurs in patients who have no history of celiac sprue. Splenic atrophy is found with both celiac sprue and chronic ulcerative jejunoileitis. The condition is often difficult to distinguish from T-cell lymphoma of the small intestine, which complicates both celiac sprue and chronic ulcerative jejunoileitis. Non–T-cell lymphomas (e.g., immunoproliferative small intestinal disease, Mediterranean [B-cell] lymphoma) may resemble chronic ulcerative jejunoileitis. Therefore, determination of lymphocyte cell surface markers is essential for proper diagnosis and management. Lymphomatous infiltration of lymph nodes, liver, spleen, and bone marrow is common with concurrent lymphoma.

Clinical Features, Diagnosis, and Management

Patients present with chronic symptoms of malabsorption including abdominal pain, fever, weight loss, diarrhea, and steatorrhea. Twenty percent to 30% have complications (e.g., obstruction, melena, and perforation). The diagnosis is considered in patients with celiac sprue who have worsening malabsorption despite adherence to a gluten-free diet. Barium radiography of the small intestine may show strictures and intestinal fold thickening. CT scans may show mesenteric lymphadenopathy or splenic atrophy, but these findings are nonspecific. Upper gastrointestinal endoscopy with biopsy is essential in a patient suspected of having chronic ulcerative jejunoileitis. Adequate tissue must be obtained to exclude the diagnosis of lymphoma. Therapeutic options are limited, and most patients survive <2 years. Prednisone should be considered for patients without lymphoma. Surgical resection may be necessary to treat complications or lymphomatous involvement. Disseminated T-cell lymphoma is treated with aggressive chemotherapy.

DRUG-INDUCED DISEASE OF THE SMALL INTESTINE

Drugs Causing Ischemia

Etiology and Pathogenesis

Drug-induced intestinal ischemia can result from arterial vasoconstriction, systemic or splanchnic hypotension, or mesenteric thrombosis. Antihypertensives (including diuretics) promote hypotension and hypovolemia, whereas catecholamines (e.g., dopamine, vasopressin, norepinephrine) produce vasoconstriction. Digoxin reduces splanchnic blood flow. Cocaine-evoked peripheral vasoconstriction causes ischemia, which may be exacerbated by rebound vasodilation. Ergot alkaloids for treatment of migraines rarely cause splanchnic vasospasm with bowel infarction. Oral contraceptive use predisposes to mesenteric arterial or venous thrombosis, which is fatal in 50% of severe cases. The risk of thromboembolism decreases to normal within 1 month of discontinuation of oral contraceptives.

Clinical Features, Diagnosis, and Management

Drug-induced ischemia carries a 70% to 90% mortality because of delays in presentation and coexistent health problems. Patients present with poorly localized pain, fever, hematochezia, distention, and ileus. Abdominal radiography may show perforation, obstruction, or ileus. CT studies may assist in the diagnosis of mesenteric infarction. Angiographic studies may appear normal with nonocclusive ischemia, but may also show thrombosis or spasm secondary to digoxin or ergot alkaloids. Supportive measures, including fluids, electrolytes, and correction of acid-base disturbances, should be provided. Nitroprusside may be useful for vasoconstriction secondary to digoxin or ergot alkaloids. Surgical resection of infarcted segments is often required.

Anticoagulants

Etiology and Pathogenesis

Gastrointestinal hemorrhage may result from the use of anticoagulants. The incidence of this complication is dependent on intensity of therapy, adequacy of dosage monitoring, route of administration, concurrent drug therapy, and the age and underlying clinical condition of the patient. Most episodes of gastrointestinal bleeding in patients taking anticoagulants are attributable to pre-existing intestinal lesions.

Clinical Features, Diagnosis, and Management

The most prominent symptom is hemorrhage, which manifests as hematemesis, melena, or hematochezia. If possible, anticoagulants should be discontinued, or reduced. Endoscopic evaluation may locate and treat the bleeding site. Clinical findings of intramural hematoma formation include symptoms of obstruction and biliary symptoms or pancreatitis as a result of the obstruction at the ampulla of Vater by a hematoma. Intramural hematomas are detected on barium radiography or ultrasound examinations. Conservative medical management usually is sufficient, although surgery may be needed to treat persistent obstruction or perforation.

Drugs Causing Intestinal Dysmotility

Etiology and Pathogenesis

Drug-induced intestinal pseudo-obstruction results from anticholinergic drugs, phenothiazines, tricyclic antidepressants, opioids, calcium channel antagonists, clonidine, and cyclosporin. The chemotherapeutic agent vincristine may have neurotoxic effects on intestinal motor function.

Clinical Features, Diagnosis, and Management

In most instances, intestinal function returns soon after discontinuation of the offending drug. The narcotic bowel syndrome results from chronic opiate use and is characterized by pain, intermittent vomiting, or weight loss. These symptoms are initially relieved by narcotic use. Abdominal radiography shows a pattern consistent with ileus. On narcotic withdrawal, patients may experience vomiting, diarrhea, and cramping, which may be reduced by clonidine, 0.1 mg two to four times daily.

Drugs Causing Malabsorption

Etiology and Pathogenesis

Nutrient assimilation may be impeded by tetracycline (chelates calcium), cholestyramine (binds iron and vitamin B_{12}), mineral oil (reduces solubilization of carotene and fat-soluble vitamins in bile salt mixed micelles), thiazide diuretics (impair ileal sodium transport), and aluminum and magnesium hydroxide (precipitate calcium and phosphate ions). Prokinetics and cathartics can accelerate intestinal transit. Colchicine, neomycin, methotrexate, methyldopa, and allopurinol can cause mucosal injury.

Clinical Features, Diagnosis, and Management

Clinicians must be aware of the malabsorptive capabilities of certain medications that may exacerbate the poor nutritional status of a patient. For some drugs, prophylactic supplementation may be reasonable—for example, folate administration to patients taking sulfasalazine and folate and vitamin D supplements for patients taking phenytoin or colestipol.

Chemotherapeutic Agents

Etiology and Pathogenesis

Many chemotherapeutic agents produce cytotoxic effects on the mucosal cells in the small intestine because these cells have a high turnover rate.

Clinical Features, Diagnosis, and Management

Nausea and vomiting are common side effects of chemotherapeutic drugs and patients often exhibit these symptoms early in the course of therapy. Erosive enteritis manifests as pain, bleeding, vomiting, ileus, and diarrhea. This syndrome is seen in patients who are being treated with methotrexate, 5-fluorouracil, actinomycin D, doxorubicin, cytosine arabinoside, bleomycin, or vincristine. Preconditioning for bone marrow transplantation with cyclophosphamide and total body irradiation produces diffuse intestinal injury. Pain, diarrhea, and anorexia are common symptoms. Neutropenic enterocolitis or typhlitis can result from chemotherapy for leukemia or lymphoma. The clinical manifestations include fever, vomiting, right lower quadrant pain, and hematochezia.

NECROTIZING ENTEROCOLITIS

Acute Jejunitis

Etiology and Pathogenesis

Acute jejunitis is a problem of nonindustrialized nations. The disease results from infection with *Clostridium perfringens* type C. This organism, which is present in tissues, stool, and food of affected persons, produces a characteristic beta-toxin.

Clinical Features, Diagnosis, and Management

Acute jejunitis occurs sporadically and in epidemics. The patient's presenting symptoms are bloody diarrhea, fever, and abdominal pain caused by full-thickness intestinal necrosis. Mortality rates may approach 60%. Immunization against the beta-toxin reduces hospital admissions by >80%.

Neonatal Necrotizing Enterocolitis

Neonatal necrotizing enterocolitis (NEC) is a disease of unknown etiology that manifests as focal or diffuse intestinal ulceration and necrosis in premature or

TABLE 36-2
Classification of Protein-Losing Enteropathy

Increased interstitial pressure
   Congenital intestinal lymphangiectasia
   Mesenteric lymphatic obstruction
      Tuberculosis
      Sarcoidosis
      Lymphoma
      Retroperitoneal fibrosis
   Increased right heart pressure
      Constrictive pericarditis
      Congestive heart failure
   Whipple's disease
   Crohn's disease
Breakdown of the enterocyte barrier
   Ulcerative diseases
      Erosive gastroenteritis
      Neoplasia
      Crohn's disease
      Pseudomembranous enterocolitis
      Acute graft-versus-host disease
   Nonulcerative diseases
      Ménétrier's disease
      Viral gastroenteritides
      Bacterial overgrowth
      Parasitic diseases (malaria, giardiasis, schistosomiasis)
      Whipple's disease
      Eosinophilic gastroenteritis
      Celiac sprue
      Tropical sprue
      Systemic lupus erythematosus

low-birth-weight infants. There is a high prevalence of NEC in children whose mothers used cocaine during pregnancy, which is supportive of ischemia as a pathogenic factor. Bacterial colonization is a requirement for the development of NEC in experimental models; the occurrence of NEC epidemics in neonatal units is consistent with an infectious cause. In 95% of cases, enteral feedings were initiated before the onset of NEC, suggesting a possible source of infection.

PROTEIN-LOSING ENTEROPATHY

Etiology and Pathogenesis

PLE is the gastrointestinal loss of plasma protein in abnormal amounts. Under normal conditions, intestinal loss of serum proteins accounts for <10% of daily protein catabolism. This may increase fivefold in patients with PLE, leading to hypoproteinemia. Enteropathies resulting in PLE include ulcerating malignancies, ulcerative colitis, Crohn's disease, and diseases that disrupt lymphatic drainage (Table 36-2). Nonulcerating diseases associated with PLE include

Ménétrier's disease, atrophic gastritis, tropical sprue, celiac sprue, eosinophilic gastroenteritis, collagenous colitis, and colonic polyposis syndromes. Acute and chronic intestinal infections and bacterial overgrowth may produce PLE. Rheumatologic disorders such as systemic lupus erythematosus and mixed connective tissue disease can be complicated by PLE.

Clinical Features, Diagnosis, and Management

PLE causes severe dependent edema, although steatorrhea and lymphopenia may be present. The diagnosis is made by observing elevations in quantitative fecal α_1-antitrypsin concentrations or clearance. Radiolabeled albumin scintigraphy occasionally localizes the source. The α_1-antitrypsin clearance is calculated by dividing the product of daily stool volume and stool α_1-antitrypsin concentrations by the serum α_1-antitrypsin concentration. Gastric sources cannot be detected with α_1-antitrypsin testing because the protein is degraded at a pH of <3; false-positive results may occur if hematochezia or meconium is present or if laxatives have been ingested. The therapy for PLE is the same as that described for lymphangiectasia. Dependent edema is controlled mechanically, and dietary fat is replaced with medium-chain triglycerides. Rarely, surgical lymphovenous anastomosis is helpful.

CHAPTER 37

Dysmotility and Bacterial Overgrowth of the Small Intestine

DYSMOTILITY OF THE SMALL INTESTINE

Incidence and Epidemiology

The incidence of dysmotility of the small intestine varies according to the underlying disease, but overall it is less common than motor disturbances of the esophagus, stomach, and colon. As manometric and electromyographic techniques are more widely used, increased numbers of small intestine motor disturbances will be identified.

Etiology and Pathogenesis

Small intestine dysmotility can result from primary diseases of smooth muscle and enteric nerve tissue. The cause may be secondary to diseases involving smooth muscle, neurologic diseases, endocrine disorders, or other diseases, or it may be secondary to medications (Table 37-1).

Primary Causes

Familial Visceral Myopathies. Familial visceral myopathies (FVMs) are genetic diseases that produce degeneration and fibrosis of smooth muscle cells. The disease can involve the entire muscularis propria, but it may be confined to the longitudinal layer. Type I FVM is an autosomal dominant disorder characterized by esophageal dilation, megaduodenum, redundant colon, and megacystis. Megaduodenum manifests in adolescence; >75% of patients are girls who become symptomatic after menarche. Ten percent develop symptomatic intestinal pseudo-obstruction. Gastroparesis is rare. Of symptomatic cases, 75% have abnormal findings on esophageal manometry, and only

---

TABLE 37-1
Causes of Dysmotility in the Small Intestine

Primary causes
  Familial types
    Familial visceral myopathies (types I, II, III)
    Familial visceral neuropathies (types I, II)
    Childhood visceral myopathies (types I, II)
  Nonfamilial or sporadic types
    Visceral myopathies
    Visceral neuropathies
    Irritable bowel syndrome (?)
Secondary causes
  Smooth muscle diseases
    Rheumatologic disease (e.g., scleroderma, polymyositis and dermatomyositis, systemic lupus erythematosus, mixed connective tissue disease)
    Muscular dystrophies (e.g., myotonic dystrophy, Duchenne's muscular dystrophy)
    Amyloidosis
  Neurologic diseases
    Chagas' disease
    Intestinal ganglioneuromatosis
    Paraneoplastic pseudo-obstruction
    Parkinson's disease
    Spinal cord injury
  Endocrine disorders
    Diabetes mellitus
    Thyroid disease
    Hypoparathyroidism
  Medications
    Phenothiazines
    Tricyclic antidepressants
    Antiparkinsonian drugs
    Ganglionic blockers
    Clonidine
    Opiates
  Miscellaneous
    Celiac sprue
    Small intestine diverticulosis
    Radiation enteritis
    Jejunoileal bypass
    Diffuse lymphoid infiltration of the small intestine
    Postgastrointestinal viral infection
    Anorexia nervosa and bulimia nervosa

20% report dysphagia. Constipation occurs in one-half of cases and volvulus has been reported. Megacystis rarely leads to urinary infection. Type II FVM is an autosomal recessive disorder. Patients present in adolescence to middle age with gastroparesis, small intestine dilation and diverticula, striated muscle degeneration, peripheral neuropathy, deafness, ptosis, and ophthalmoplegia. Symptomatic intestinal pseudo-obstruction often necessitates long-term parenteral nutrition. Type III FVM probably is an autosomal recessive condition characterized by diffuse intestinal dilation from the esophagus to the rectum. All patients have chronic intestinal pseudo-obstruction and require parenteral nutrition.

Familial Visceral Neuropathies.   Familial visceral neuropathies (FVNs) are genetic diseases of myenteric plexus degeneration. Type I FVN is an autosomal dominant disease characterized by dilation of the distal small intestine and colon. Patients present with postprandial abdominal pain, distention, and diarrhea or constipation. One-fourth of patients have gastroparesis. Histologic study reveals marked reductions in argyrophilic myenteric neurons and nerve fibers. Most patients have mild malnutrition but require parenteral nutrition. Type II FVN is an autosomal recessive disease with hypertrophic pyloric stenosis, dilation, malrotation of the small intestine, associated central nervous system malformations, and patent ductus arteriosus. All patients present in infancy with fatal intestinal pseudo-obstruction. Other FVNs have been reported that exhibit associated neurologic symptoms, ptosis, ophthalmoplegia, mental retardation, and intestinal diverticula.

Childhood Visceral Myopathies.   Childhood visceral myopathies (CVMs) are diseases distinct from FVMs. Patients with type I CVM present before 5 years of age with symptomatic dilation from the stomach to the rectum. Volvulus of the colon or occasionally the stomach or small intestine occurs in some cases. The disease usually is fatal but long-term parenteral nutrition may prolong life. Type II CVM is a more common autosomal recessive condition with intestinal pseudo-obstruction, microcolon with malrotation and malfixation in the left abdomen, intestinal and colonic shortening, and megacystis with recurrent urinary infection. The disease occurs predominantly in female infants. Most patients die in infancy, although parenteral nutrition may prolong life. The prune-belly syndrome may be the male counterpart.

Nonfamilial Visceral Myopathies and Neuropathies.   Rare cases of primary visceral myopathy appear to have no genetic predisposition. Histologically, there are no differences between the familial and nonfamilial types. Non-FVNs are more common than non-FVMs. They are caused by chemical, medication, or viral damage to the myenteric plexus. Patients with nonfamilial neuropathies exhibit active but nonperistaltic intestinal motor activity. Clinical manifestations are consistent with intestinal pseudo-obstruction. Histologic studies show reduced numbers of myenteric neurons, and those that remain are abnormal. Hypertrophy of the muscularis propria may also be observed.

Secondary Causes

Scleroderma.   The small intestine is the second most frequently involved gastrointestinal organ in scleroderma, after the esophagus. Forty percent of patients exhibit gastric or intestinal stasis. Wide-mouth diverticula may be present, as may pneumatosis cystoides intestinalis, a finding that signifies a poor prognosis. Smooth muscle degeneration and collagen replacement, most prominently of the circular muscle layer, characterizes the disorder. Manometric evaluation reveals a hypomotility pattern. Conventional stains do not detect myenteric plexus damage, but some patients exhibit a manometric pattern of uncoordinated intense contractions of the small intestine, suggesting neuropathy in the early stages of disease.

Other Rheumatologic Disorders.   Dermatomyositis and polymyositis involve the gastrointestinal tract in 50% of cases. The common presentation is dysphagia. Megaduodenum and delayed intestinal transit may be prominent; intestinal pseudo-obstruction is rare. Smooth muscle dysfunction in systemic lupus erythematosus results in dilation of the small intestine and ileus, which is postulated to be secondary to vasculitis-related ischemia. Gastrointestinal involvement in mixed connective tissue disease, which is detected by high titers of antinuclear antibody against ribonucleoprotein, resembles that of scleroderma.

Myotonic Dystrophy.   Myotonic dystrophy is characterized by difficulty in muscle relaxation, a nasal voice, cataracts, and cardiac conduction defects. Dysphagia is the most common gastrointestinal motor symptom, although diarrhea, constipation, and intestinal pseudo-obstruction may occur. Radiographic findings include dilation of the small intestine, hypomotility, and delayed transit, whereas manometry shows low-amplitude contractions, retrograde fasting motility, and increased tonic contractions. Histologic evaluation shows swollen degenerated smooth muscle cells with fatty replacement as well as rare degenerative changes in the colonic myenteric plexus.

Duchenne's Muscular Dystrophy.   Duchenne's muscular dystrophy is an X-linked recessive disorder that causes gastrointestinal smooth muscle degeneration and atrophy and separation of smooth muscle fibers with connective tissue. Symptoms are usually related to esophageal or gastric dysmotility rather than intestinal motor disruption, although intestinal pseudo-obstruction can occur.

Amyloidosis.   Amyloid protein is deposited in the small intestine in primary, secondary, myeloma-associated, or hereditary (familial Mediterranean fever) amyloidosis. In primary and myeloma-associated amyloidosis, muscle involvement predominates, resulting in dysmotility, whereas mucosal deposition in secondary and hereditary amyloidosis produces malabsorption. Amyloid is rarely deposited in the myenteric plexus, but when it is, a visceral neuropathic pattern is produced.

Other Neuromuscular Diseases.   Chagas' disease is characterized by myenteric plexus destruction secondary to infection with *Trypanosoma cruzi*. Common manifestations are megaesophagus and megacolon, although megaduodenum and megajejunum may occur. Symptoms include constipation, diarrhea, and intestinal pseudo-obstruction. Chronic intestinal pseudo-obstruction may be a paraneoplastic consequence of small cell lung carcinoma, epidermoid lip carcinoma, or other malignancies. It is characterized by widespread myenteric and submucosal neuronal and axonal degeneration with mononuclear infiltration. Pheochromocytoma may produce intestinal pseudo-obstruction as a consequence of excess catecholamine production. Small bowel dysmotility with dilation and hypomotility occur with Parkinson's disease. Medications used to treat the disease may exacerbate these symptoms. Histologic studies show cytoplasmic hyaline inclusions (e.g., Lewy bodies) in the myenteric neurons of the esophagus and colon. Gastrointestinal neurofibromas occur in 10% of patients with neurofibromatosis and have very rarely been associated with intestinal pseudo-obstruction. Spinal cord injury produces minimal chronic effects on small intestine motor activity, although constipation and postprandial distention are prevalent and pseudo-obstruction has been reported. However, immediately after spinal damage, ileus and distention are common.

Endocrine Disorders.   The small intestine is not as severely involved in diabetes mellitus as the stomach and colon. There are no morphologic abnormalities of the myenteric or submucosal plexuses. Some patients experience symptomatic intestinal dysmotility with and without concurrent bacterial overgrowth. Although smooth muscle thickening with eosinophilic hyaline body deposition has been observed, myopathy does not occur in most diabetics. Hyperthyroidism enhances intestinal transit, causing diarrhea and malabsorption, whereas hypothyroidism retards transit, producing constipation, ileus, and pseudo-obstruction. Hypoparathyroidism may lead to intestinal pseudo-obstruction because hypocalcemia can impair contractile activity.

Medication-Induced Dysmotility of the Small Intestine.   Although medications most often affect the motor activity of the colon, motility of the small intestine can be inhibited by phenothiazines, antiparkinsonian agents, tricyclic antidepressants, anticholinergics, opiates (including loperamide), and calcium channel antagonists. Conversely, cisapride, erythromycin, cholinergic agonists, and octreotide can stimulate small bowel contractile activity.

Miscellaneous Causes of Dysmotility of the Small Intestine.   Intestinal pseudo-obstruction has been reported in patients with celiac sprue. Jejunal diverticulosis results from altered small bowel motility. It complicates scleroderma, celiac sprue, Fabry's disease, type II FVM, and Cronkhite-Canada syndrome. Abdominal irradiation can produce acute dysmotility of the small intestine and chronic motor disruption, with development of bacterial overgrowth, diarrhea, malabsorption, and intestinal pseudo-obstruction. Diffuse lymphoid infiltration of the lamina propria, muscularis propria, and myenteric plexus of the small intestine resulting in intestinal pseudo-obstruction has been reported. Recurrent episodes of pseudo-obstruction occur after jejunoileal bypass for morbid obesity; bacterial overgrowth in the bypassed segment is believed to be the cause. Intermittent antibiotic courses may benefit patients with chronic symptoms. The eating disorders anorexia nervosa and bulimia nervosa exhibit delayed intestinal transit, although the clinical significance of this finding is uncertain.

Clinical Features

Most patients with dysmotility of the small intestine have similar clinical manifestations, regardless of the underlying disease. At one end of the spectrum patients are asymptomatic; at the other end they suffer from chronic intestinal pseudo-obstruction, which is defined as the presence of symptoms and signs of obstruction without mechanical blockage. Most patients, however, have an intermediate pattern of postprandial, crampy abdominal pain, bloating, nausea, and vomiting. Diarrhea and malabsorption can result from bacterial overgrowth. The abdomen may be silent with smooth muscle dysfunction or it may exhibit hyperactive, high-pitched bowel sounds characteristic of neuropathic disease. Extraintestinal manifestations involving the urinary tract and peripheral or central nervous structures may be evident with primary intestinal dysmotility; specific organ systems may be involved in secondary disease (e.g., sclerodactyly with scleroderma).

Findings on Diagnostic Testing

Laboratory Studies

Numerous blood tests provide evidence of malnutrition or malabsorption, including anemia (iron, folate, or vitamin B_{12} deficiency), low cholesterol, hypocalcemia, and hypoalbuminemia. Blood tests can also detect secondary causes of intestinal dysmotility: hyperglycemia with diabetes, abnormal thyroid chemistry values with hyperthyroidism or hypothyroidism, hypocalcemia with hypoparathyroidism, positive serologic findings with rheumatologic disease, elevated creatine phosphokinase levels with muscular dystrophy, the presence of antimyenteric neuronal antibodies with paraneoplastic intestinal dysmotility, and positive findings on hemagglutination and complement fixation studies in Chagas' disease.

Radiographic Studies

Abdominal radiographs may show diffuse or localized intestinal dilation with or without air-fluid levels. Barium radiography of the small intestine may confirm dilation with delayed transit and altered motor patterns on fluoroscopy. Enteroclysis may be necessary to confidently exclude mechanical obstruction in some cases. Barium enema radiography and intravenous pyelography may detect colonic or urinary motor dysfunction. Chest radiography and chest and abdominal computed tomographic (CT) scans may confirm a diagnosis of paraneoplastic intestinal dysmotility.

Small Intestine Manometry

Small intestine manometry characterizes abnormal motor patterns during fasting and after a meal. The migrating motor complex is a stereotypical pattern consisting of three phases that recur every 90 to 120 minutes during fasting. The fed motor pattern is characterized by irregular phasic contractions in the small intestine that begin soon after meal ingestion and persist for >2 hours until the digested nutrients pass the intestine. Myopathic disease produces diffuse reductions in contractile amplitude, but the migrating motor complex and fed patterns usually are preserved. Visceral neuropathies produce abnormal or absent migrating motor complex activity, abnormal migration of contractions, or loss of the normal fed pattern. The amplitude and frequency of contractions may be increased with neuropathic disease. A manometric pattern of clustered contractions separated by periods of motor quiescence lasting >1 minute has been described in association with mechanical obstruction. Some clinicians use manometry along with negative findings on radiographic testing to diagnose intestinal obstruction.

The Role of Surgery in Diagnosis

The gold standard for diagnosis of visceral myopathy and neuropathy is surgical full-thickness intestinal biopsy with trichrome staining of the specimen, which detects smooth muscle fibrosis, and silver staining, which assesses the myenteric plexus. Surgery is also necessary in rare cases in which small intestinal obstruction is still a consideration after negative findings on barium radiography of the small intestine. Biopsy specimens of striated muscle may diagnose muscular dystrophy.

Management and Course

Dietary Therapy

Postprandial symptoms may respond to dietary supplements that provide 1500 to 1800 kcal per day in three to four feedings of equal size. Liquid supplements (e.g., Ensure, Isocal, Vivonex) are emptied faster from the stomach and progress through the small intestine more easily than solid food. Vivonex is low in fat content, elemental in nature (i.e., it does not require digestion), lactose free, and well absorbed. Carbonated beverages produce gaseous distention and should be avoided. For severe pseudo-obstruction, feedings should be withheld, and intravenous hydration and nasogastric suction should be instituted. If symptoms are prolonged, total parenteral nutrition may be necessary, often on a permanent basis.

Medication Therapy

Prokinetic medications are often prescribed for intestinal dysmotility, but they often are less effective in treating dysmotility than gastroparesis. Cisapride can accelerate small intestinal transit, but its effectiveness in treating intestinal pseudo-obstruction is unproved. Octreotide may reduce nausea, vomiting, bloating, and pain over the short term in patients with bacterial overgrowth secondary to intestinal pseudo-obstruction with scleroderma. Erythromycin has propulsive effects in the small intestine and has shown efficacy in treating some patients with intestinal dysmotility. Pain control with narcotics is discouraged because they inhibit gut motor activity and have a potential for drug dependence. Constipation may respond to osmotic laxatives (e.g., milk of magnesia) or tap water enemas. Bulk laxatives may exacerbate symptoms and are not recommended.

Surgical Therapy

In patients with dysmotility limited to short intestinal segments (e.g., megaduodenum), the duodenum may be drained with side-to-side duodenojejunostomy, or it may be partially resected. Surgery should be avoided if the dysfunctional segments are longer because adhesions may develop that could exacerbate obstructive symptoms.

SMALL INTESTINE BACTERIAL OVERGROWTH

Incidence and Epidemiology

Bacterial overgrowth in the small intestine is a syndrome characterized by nutrient malabsorption associated with excessive numbers of bacteria in the small bowel lumen. Various structural and functional disorders of the gastrointestinal tract predispose to the development of bacterial overgrowth.

Etiology and Pathogenesis

Causes of Bacterial Overgrowth

Conditions favoring bacterial overgrowth include intestinal stasis, abnormal proximal connections to the colon, reduced acid secretion, immunodeficiency, or advanced age (Table 37-2). Chronic strictures from Crohn's disease, lymphoma, and radiation injury cause stasis, as do intestinal diverticula and blind loops resulting from Billroth II anastomoses, Roux-en-Y gastrojejunostomy, jejunoileal bypass for morbid obesity, and Kock continent ileostomy. Primary and secondary causes of intestinal hypomotility as described earlier in this chap-

---

TABLE 37-2
Conditions Favoring Development of Bacterial Overgrowth

Intestinal stasis
    Anatomic
        Strictures
        Diverticulosis of the small intestine
        Surgery (e.g., enteroenteric anastomosis, Billroth II gastrojejunostomy, jejunoileal
            bypass, Kock continent ileostomy)
    Dysmotility of the small intestine
        Scleroderma
        Idiopathic intestinal pseudo-obstruction
        Diabetic autonomic neuropathy
Abnormal connection between proximal and distal intestine
    Fistulae
        Gastrocolic
        Gastrojejunocolic
    Resection of the ileocecal junction
Hypochlorhydria
    Atrophic gastritis
    Hypochlorhydric medications
    Surgery for peptic ulcer disease
Immunodeficiency
    Primary immunodeficiency
    Acquired immunodeficiency syndrome
    Malnutrition
Age

---

ter predispose to bacterial overgrowth. Abnormal connections that cause bacterial overgrowth include gastrocolic and gastrojejunocolic fistulae and resected ileocecal junctions. Gastric acid is responsible for decreasing the bacterial inoculum reaching the proximal small intestine. Therefore, hypochlorhydria resulting from atrophic gastritis, ulcer surgery, and possibly acid-suppressive medication therapy may predispose to bacterial overgrowth, especially if conditions promoting stasis are also present. Bacterial colonization of the small intestine may occur with common variable immunodeficiency and acquired immunodeficiency syndrome; however, its clinical significance in these conditions is uncertain. The incidence of bacterial overgrowth increases in elderly patients. It probably is secondary to a combination of several conditions, including hypochlorhydria, stasis, and malnutrition, which itself can cause bacterial colonization.

Consequences of Bacterial Overgrowth

Bacterial overgrowth results in malabsorption of fats, carbohydrates, and protein in the absence of intestinal invasion. Bacterial deconjugation of bile acids, particularly by anaerobic organisms, is the primary mechanism for malabsorption of fats and fat-soluble vitamins (vitamins A, D, and E). The synthesis of vitamin K by lumenal bacteria accounts for the absence of coagulopathy. Bacterial metabolites (e.g., hydroxylated fatty acids, unconjugated bile acids) may have a toxic effect on the intestinal mucosa. Reduction of brush border disaccharidases by bacterial proteases (especially anaerobic) and decreased monosaccharide uptake may produce carbohydrate malabsorption. Diarrhea results from the generation of osmotically active carbohydrate fragments. Bacterial formation of hydrogen and carbon dioxide can produce abdominal gas and pain. Hypoproteinemia is seen with bacterial overgrowth and is a consequence of bacterial competition for ingested proteins, decreased amino acid and peptide uptake, decreased levels of pancreatic enterokinase, and protein-losing enteropathy. Anaerobic bacteria compete with the host for vitamin B_{12}, which leads to macrocytic anemia in some patients. In contrast, lumenal bacteria synthesize folate, leading to normal or increased serum folate levels. Bacterial overgrowth can also produce thiamine and nicotinamide deficiency.

Bacteria-Induced Intestinal Mucosal Injury

Histologic evidence of mucosal damage has been observed in some cases of bacterial overgrowth, with subtotal villous atrophy and increased numbers of inflammatory cells within the lamina propria. Focal ulcerations and erosions have been seen, especially in cases of pouchitis secondary to ileal pouch–anal canal anastomosis or Kock continent ileostomy.

Clinical Features

Diarrhea and weight loss are prominent symptoms of bacterial overgrowth as a result of malabsorption, maldigestion, and reduced oral intake. Vitamin B_{12} deficiency may produce macrocytic anemia or neurologic changes. Other manifestations of vitamin deficiencies include night blindness, osteomalacia, tetany, peripheral neuropathy, and edema. Extraintestinal consequences of bacterial overgrowth include dermatitis, hepatic injury, nephrotoxicity, and arthritis.

Findings on Diagnostic Testing

Microbiological Studies

Microbiological cultures of small intestine aspirates are the gold standard for diagnosis of bacterial overgrowth. Fluid samples are obtained using fluoroscopically placed catheters or capsules or using endoscopic suction. The aspirates are transferred immediately to an anaerobic transport vial and plated for aerobic and anaerobic organisms. Symptomatic bacterial overgrowth is usually associated with detection of anaerobes. The presence of $>10^5$ colony-forming units per milliliter in the duodenum is diagnostic of bacterial overgrowth.

Breath Tests

Breath tests measure excretion of hydrogen or carbon dioxide produced by intralumenal bacterial metabolism of an administered substrate. These tests were devised as a less invasive alternative to intubation of the small intestine. The hydrogen breath test is advantageous because no radiolabeled compounds are ingested. However, 15% to 20% of normal subjects harbor flora that do not produce hydrogen; therefore, false-negative results are significant. Carbohydrate substrates, including lactulose and glucose, have been used for hydrogen breath tests. They provide 62% to 68% sensitivity and 44% to 83% specificity for diagnosis compared with intestinal fluid culture. Elevated levels of fasting breath hydrogen have been observed in a minority of patients with bacterial overgrowth. The radiolabeled pentose ^{14}C-D-xylose is a good substrate for breath testing because of its minimal metabolism by the host. It exhibits a 30% to 100% sensitivity and 89% to 100% specificity for diagnosis of bacterial overgrowth. Radiolabeled bile acid breath tests are no longer used because of poor sensitivity and specificity.

Other Tests

Other diagnostic tests that suggest bacterial overgrowth include blood levels of certain vitamins (e.g., vitamin B_{12}) and the Schilling's test. If not already known, the underlying cause of bacterial overgrowth may be diagnosed with specific endoscopic, radiographic, and manometric techniques.

Management and Course

Initial management of bacterial overgrowth consists of fluid and nutritional support, including vitamin replacement. Numerous antibiotics have efficacy in treating bacterial overgrowth, including tetracycline, chloramphenicol, ampicillin, erythromycin, clindamycin, metronidazole, oral aminoglycosides, and quinolones. Most patients respond to a single 7- to 10-day course, but some require intermittent antibiotic therapy or a continuous course of alternating antibiotics to minimize the development of resistant organisms. Prokinetic agents have limited efficacy in intestinal dysmotility as described earlier in this chapter. Surgical correction of anatomic causes of intestinal stasis can be considered.

CHAPTER 38

Infections of the Small Intestine with Bacterial and Viral Pathogens

ILLNESS FROM BACTERIAL TOXINS

Bacterial pathogens frequently elaborate toxins that cause gastrointestinal symptoms, including diarrhea and vomiting. Most of these organisms are acquired through contaminated food or water supplies (Table 38-1).

Staphylococcus aureus

Etiology and Pathogenesis

Staphylococcus aureus is a gram-positive coccus that is carried by 30% to 50% of healthy individuals. The organism produces at least seven enterotoxins and a delta-toxin that cause fluid secretion in the intestine. *S aureus* is the second most common cause of bacterial food poisoning, which occurs in epidemics during warm weather, probably because of its association with large gatherings (e.g., picnics). The high sugar or salt content of certain foods (e.g., salads, pastries, meats) allows selective growth of the organism.

Clinical Features, Diagnosis, and Management

The clinical features of food poisoning with *S aureus* include nausea, vomiting, and abdominal cramps. These symptoms occur with an attack rate of 80% to 100% within 8 hours after ingestion of preformed enterotoxin. Diarrhea often follows. Full recovery usually occurs within 48 hours. The diagnosis is clinical and sometimes confirmed by culturing the organism from the food or food handler.

TABLE 38-1
Features of Agent-Specific Food-Borne Disease

ORGANISM/AGENT	INCUBATION (HOURS)	DIARRHEA	FEVER	VOMITING	ENTEROTOXIN	IMPLICATED FOODS
Staphylococcus aureus	1–8	+	–	+++	++	Salad, pastry, meat
Bacillus cereus						
Emetic disease	1–6	+	–	+++	++	Fried rice
Diarrheal illness	6–14	+++	–	+	+	Meat, vanilla sauce, creamed foods, salad, chicken soup
Clostridium botulinum	12–36	±	–	±	++	Raw honey (infants), improperly canned foods
Clostridium perfringens	8–24	+++	–	±	++	Meat, pasta salad, dairy products, Mexican food
Vibrio cholerae	12–72	+++	–	+	+++	Seafood, contaminated water
Enterotoxigenic *Escherichia coli*	24–72	+++	+	–	+	Salad, fruit, meat, pastry
Puffer fish	<2	+	–	+	+	Puffer fish, South American frogs, blue-ringed octopus
Paralytic shellfish	1–3	–	–	+	+	Bivalved mollusks
Ciguatera	1–6	+	–	+	+	Barracuda, grouper, snappers, jacks, reef sharks
Scombroid	<2	±	–	+	–	Tuna, albacore, mackerel, skip jacks
Salmonella species	8–48	+++	++	+	+	Eggs, poultry, beef, dairy products
Yersinia species	24–72	+++	++	±	+	Milk, tofu
Vibrio parahaemolyticus	4–96	++	±	±	+	Oysters, crabs, shellfish
Non-O:1 *Vibrio cholerae*	6–72	++	±	±	–	Seafood, eggs, potatoes
Rotavirus	48–72	+++	+	++	–	Fresh water, seafood
Norwalk virus	24–48	++	+	++	–	Shellfish, drinking water

+ to +++ = severity of symptom (or production of enterotoxin), usually present; – = usually absent; ± = minimal severity/variable presence.

Bacillus cereus

Etiology and Pathogenesis

Bacillus cereus is an aerobic, motile, spore-forming gram-positive rod. It is the fifth most common bacterial pathogen responsible for food poisoning. *B cereus* causes vomiting if it is consumed in fried rice, and diarrhea if it is ingested in meats, vanilla sauce, cream-filled baked goods, salads, and chicken soup. These two symptoms appear to be caused by different toxins.

Clinical Features, Diagnosis, and Management

Two forms of illness have been characterized. Patients with the emetic illness present with vomiting and cramping. Diarrhea occurs in one-third of the cases, and fever is rare. Symptoms appear 1 to 6 hours after ingestion and persist for 2 to 10 hours. The diarrheal illness is characterized by profuse watery diarrhea, cramping, and, rarely, vomiting. The illness has an incubation period of 6 to 14 hours and a duration of 16 to 48 hours. The diagnosis is based primarily on clinical information. Both syndromes are self-limited. Prevention of *B cereus* infection involves proper food handling and storage.

Clostridium botulinum

Etiology and Pathogenesis

Clostridium botulinum is a ubiquitous, anaerobic, spore-forming gram-positive bacterium that produces a neurotoxin capable of blocking acetylcholine at the neuromuscular junction. Ingestion of improperly canned food can cause disease. Infection from raw honey has been reported in infants younger than 6 months.

Clinical Features, Diagnosis, and Management

Patients present with mild nausea, vomiting, diarrhea, and abdominal pain 12 hours to 8 days after ingestion. Neurologic symptoms include diplopia, ophthalmoplegia, dysarthria, dysphagia, dysphonia, descending weakness, paralysis, postural hypotension, and respiratory muscle paralysis that can be fatal if mechanical ventilation is not provided. Full recovery may take months. The diagnosis is confirmed by detection of botulinum toxin in the stool and vomitus of infected patients or in the contaminated food. Electromyography is sometimes helpful in distinguishing this illness from Guillain-Barré syndrome. Patients should receive antitoxin early in the course of disease. However, allergic reactions may occur in up to 10% of cases.

Clostridium perfringens

Etiology and Pathogenesis

Clostridium perfringens is a nonmotile, obligate anaerobe that is one of the four most common causes of bacterial food poisoning worldwide. The organism produces a heat-labile enterotoxin that binds to mucosal cell surfaces, causing structural damage and leading to loss of electrolytes, fluids, and proteins. Most outbreaks occur in the autumn and winter after ingestion of improperly stored beef, fish, poultry, pasta salads, dairy products, and Mexican foods.

Clinical Features, Diagnosis, and Management

C perfringens causes watery diarrhea, cramping, and pain 8 to 24 hours after ingestion of contaminated food. The disease is self-limited, and recovery is expected within 24 hours. The organism may cause diarrhea in the elderly and in patients in chronic care facilities. It has also been implicated as a cause of antibiotic-associated diarrhea. A rare colitis-like illness with hemorrhage has been reported. Other toxins (e.g., alpha- and beta-toxin) can produce necrotizing enterocolitis, ileus, and pneumatosis intestinalis. Definitive diagnosis is made by demonstration of $>10^5$ organisms per gram in contaminated food or $>10^6$ spores per gram in stools of affected individuals, or by detection of *C perfringens* enterotoxin in assays. In general, *C perfringens* diarrhea is treated supportively, although oral metronidazole may be given to patients with prolonged *C perfringens* antibiotic-associated diarrhea.

Vibrio cholerae

Etiology and Pathogenesis

Cholera, which is caused by *Vibrio cholerae*, is endemic in southern Asia, Africa, and Latin America. *V cholerae* is a motile, monoflagellated, gram-negative, curved rod that classically produces voluminous watery diarrhea through elaboration of an enterotoxin. Other toxins (e.g., zonula occludens toxin, accessory cholera toxin), enzymes (e.g., mucinase), and extracellular proteins (e.g., hemagglutinin, neuraminidase) may also have roles in disease pathogenesis. Cholera, acquired from seafood or fecally contaminated water, primarily affects children (2 to 9 years of age) and women of childbearing age who live in crowded conditions with poor water and waste sanitation. Other persons at increased risk of infection include those with hypochlorhydria and those with impaired immune function. Person-to-person transmission is not thought to be important. Cholera toxin consists of an "A" subunit, which is internalized and irreversibly activates mucosal adenylate cyclase, thus producing massive electrolyte and fluid secretion, and a "B" subunit, which binds to specific surface receptors and enables the A subunit to obtain entry into the cell. The inoculum size required to produce illness is $>10^6$ organisms.

Clinical Features, Diagnosis, and Management

Although mild to moderate illness from cholera may occur, severe complicated cholera is characterized by staggering fluid loss in the feces (up to 10% to 15% of body weight in several hours), vomiting, metabolic acidosis, hyponatremia, hypokalemia, hypoglycemia, lethargy, altered sensorium, and seizures. Paralytic ileus, muscle cramps, weakness, and cardiac arrhythmias may herald death. Diarrhea, which is described as having the consistency of rice water, begins abruptly after an incubation period of a few hours to 7 days and peaks within 24 hours. The diagnosis is presumed from the characteristic clinical presentation, but direct stool examination or careful stool culturing using thiosulfate-citrate-bile salt agar can definitively identify the organism. Therapy involves prompt initiation of oral rehydration with glucose and electrolyte solutions endorsed by the World Health Organization. Intravenous lactated Ringer's solution may be required to treat severe dehydration or concomitant vomiting. Antibiotics shorten the period of excretion of *V cholerae* and reduce diarrhea volume and duration. Tetracycline (250 to 500 mg four times daily for 3 days) is commonly used, but streptomycin, chloramphenicol, trimethoprim-sulfamethoxazole, nalidixic acid, ampicillin, and furazolidone are also effective. Primary infection with *V cholerae* confers immunity to subsequent infection for at least 3 years. Parenteral and oral vaccines are being evaluated.

Enterotoxigenic Escherichia coli

Etiology and Pathogenesis

Enterotoxigenic *Escherichia coli* (ETEC) produces disease by adherence to the gut mucosa and elaboration of a heat-labile toxin and two heat-stable toxins. The heat-labile toxin is similar to cholera toxin and activates intestinal adenylate cyclase, producing secretory diarrhea. One of the heat-stable toxins activates guanylate cyclase. Mucosal adherence is dependent on the attachment of fimbriae. ETEC is a major cause of diarrhea in children in developing countries and accounts for most cases of traveler's diarrhea after ingestion of contaminated salads, peeled fruits, meats, and pastries.

Clinical Features, Diagnosis, and Management

Patients with ETEC present with watery diarrhea, cramping, pain, headache, arthralgias, myalgias, vomiting, and low-grade fever. If untreated, the symptoms persist for 3 to 5 days. Dehydration is severe only in the very young or very old. Fluid and electrolyte replacement is emphasized. Vaccine trials have met with variable success.

Toxins Associated with Seafood Consumption

Etiology and Pathogenesis

Three toxins associated with fish produce neurologic abnormalities. These are tetrodotoxin (puffer fish), saxitoxin (shellfish), and ciguatoxin (ciguatera, including barracuda, grouper, snappers, jacks, and reef sharks). Saxitoxin and ciguatoxin are produced by unicellular organisms called dinoflagellates. Scombroid fish poisoning results from the ingestion of *Proteus* species– or *Klebsiella* species–generated saurine present in spoiled tuna, albacore, mackerel, and skip jacks.

Clinical Features, Diagnosis, and Management

Tetrodotoxin, saxitoxin, and ciguatoxin produce paresthesias, ataxia, hypotension, seizures, cardiac arrhythmias, and respiratory and skeletal muscle paralysis. These symptoms may be fatal in 5% to 18% of saxitoxin ingestions and 30% to 60% of tetrodotoxin ingestions. An enzyme-linked immunosorbent assay is available for the detection of ciguatoxin. Therapy for these syndromes is generally supportive; IV mannitol has been suggested to counter the effects of ciguatoxin, a sodium channel agonist. Patients with scombroid fish poisoning exhibit flushing, erythema, vertigo, and a generalized burning sensation caused by histamine-like properties of saurine. Elevated histamine levels may be detected in contaminated fish. Antihistamines effectively treat persons with scombroid poisoning.

ILLNESS FROM INVASIVE BACTERIAL PATHOGENS

Enteropathogenic Escherichia coli

Etiology and Pathogenesis

Enteropathogenic *E coli* (EPEC) produces illness in part because of its enteroadherent properties. It affects primarily children younger than 2 years of age who are hospitalized. Older children and adults may serve as reservoirs for this illness. Enteroinvasive and enterohemorrhagic *E coli* infections primarily affect the colon and are discussed in Chapter 46.

Clinical Features, Diagnosis, and Management

EPEC produces watery diarrhea, which may be associated with vomiting, fever, failure to thrive, metabolic acidosis, and life-threatening dehydration. Bloody stools rarely occur. The diagnosis is made by stool culture with serotyping, documentation of tissue culture adherence, or detection of the adherence factor by DNA probe techniques. Therapy relies on fluid and electrolyte replacement, as the illness is usually self-limited.

Nontyphoidal Salmonella species

Etiology and Pathogenesis

The genus *Salmonella* is divided into three species: *S typhi*, *S choleraesuis*, and *S enteritidis*. Outbreaks of infection tend to be during the summer and autumn. Nontyphoidal *Salmonella* species account for 25% to 40% of food-borne enteric illness in the United States. These organisms may have a propensity to infect infants younger than 1 year. Other persons at risk include adolescents and elderly individuals (older than 70 years); patients with malignancy, immunosuppression, alcoholism, hypochlorhydria, sickle cell anemia, cardiovascular disease, hemolytic anemia, or schistosomiasis; and those who have recently undergone surgery. *Salmonella* organisms are acquired from infected eggs, poultry, beef, dairy products, pet turtles, carmine red dye, aerosols, fomites, marijuana, thermometers, endoscopes, and platelet transfusions. Person-to-person transfer is important only in institutional settings where fecal contamination is prevalent. The production of diarrhea depends on invasion of the mucosa of the small intestine. Toxigenic and inflammatory mechanisms are involved. Occasionally, intense colitis with ulceration, hemorrhage, and microabscesses may occur. Nontyphoidal *Salmonella* species rarely invade beyond the mesenteric lymph nodes, and blood cultures that are positive occur in <10% of cases. The risk of *Salmonella* bacteremia increases in men older than 50 years of age and in patients with sickle cell anemia, aortic aneurysms, neoplasms, hemolysis, acquired immunodeficiency syndrome, and valvular heart disease.

Clinical Features, Diagnosis, and Management

Nontyphoidal *Salmonella* species produce diarrhea ranging from infrequent loose stools to a cholera-like illness. Dysentery is rare. Fever, abdominal pain, malaise, headache, nausea, and vomiting are present in up to 50% of cases. Symptoms begin within 8 to 48 hours of exposure and persist for 2 to 3 days. Complications include osteomyelitis, bacteremia, focal abscesses, infected aneurysms, and sepsis. Diagnosis is made by stool culture and treatment is supportive for mild to moderate disease. Antimicrobials are not used for such disease because they may prolong intestinal and biliary tract carriage of the organism and do not shorten the duration of symptoms. Indications for antibiotics include extremes of age, immunodeficiency, sepsis, abscess, osteomyelitis, and chronic typhoid carrier states. Antibiotics with efficacy include ampicillin, amoxicillin, chloramphenicol, quinolones, and trimethoprim-sulfamethoxazole for 10 to 14 days orally or parenterally. For typhoid carriers, norfloxacin or ciprofloxacin is given orally for 3 weeks.

Salmonella typhi

Etiology and Pathogenesis

The pathogenesis of *S typhi* resides with the Vi antigen, which appears to prevent antibody binding and subsequent phagocytosis by the host. The organism is transmitted by human feces or by contact with asymptomatic carriers. Initially, transient bacteremia results from organism release from dying macrophages in the Peyer's patch. Persistence of *S typhi* in the circulating macrophages leads to seeding of distant sites and a second phase of bacteremia that coincides with enteric fever.

Clinical Features, Diagnosis, and Management

The clinical presentation of typhoid fever is an acute febrile illness lasting 3 to 5 weeks associated with headache, malaise, mental confusion, anorexia, abdominal discomfort, bloating, constipation (early), diarrhea (late), and upper respiratory symptoms. After an incubation period of 3 to 60 days, fever (temperature of 39°C to 40°C) develops and persists for 2 to 3 weeks. The liver and spleen may be enlarged, abdominal tenderness may mimic appendicitis, and clusters of rose spots appear on the skin of the anterior trunk. Blood cultures are positive in >90% of patients. Three percent to 13% of patients experience a symptomatic relapse. Complications include intestinal perforation (which can be fatal) and hemorrhage, jaundice, acute cholecystitis, and hepatic necrosis. Oral and parenteral vaccines are effective in prevention of illness (see Chapter 23).

Yersinia *Organisms*

Etiology and Pathogenesis

Yersinia species are gram-negative, non–lactose-fermenting coccobacilli that cause gastrointestinal illness primarily in children. In the United States, *Y enterocolitica* has become more common since 1980, whereas *Y pseudotuberculosis* is reported in Europe. *Y enterocolitica* is transmitted by the fecal-oral route; by animals (e.g., dogs); and by contaminated milk (raw or chocolate), ice cream, tofu, and water.

Clinical Features, Diagnosis, and Management

Y enterocolitica produces diarrhea, which may be blood streaked. Abdominal pain often occurs in the right lower quadrant in persons older than 5 years and may mimic appendicitis. Other symptoms include fever, vomiting, dysentery, arthritis, and pharyngitis. Most cases resolve over 2 to 3 days, although diarrhea can persist for months in children. Rarely, a fulminant course develops with ulcerative enterocolitis, mesenteric adenitis, peritonitis, small bowel gangrene, and hemorrhage. Sepsis may occur in patients with iron overload states (e.g., hemochromatosis, cirrhosis, and hemolysis). Focal *Yersinia* infections may involve the meninges, joints, bone, sinuses, and pleural spaces. Patients who are HLA-B27–positive may develop postinfectious thyroiditis, glomerulopathy, Reiter's syndrome, carditis, arthritis, rashes, erythema nodosum, ankylosing spondylitis, and inflammatory bowel disease. Stool examination shows leukocytes and erythrocytes, and stool cultures will be positive if special techniques specific for *Yersinia* species are used. Antibiotics (e.g., aminoglycosides, tetracycline, chloramphenicol, trimethoprim-sulfamethoxazole) are given only for septicemic illness; they have no effect on disease course in other patients and do not prevent postinfectious complications.

Listeria monocytogenes

Etiology and Pathogenesis

L monocytogenes causes gastrointestinal illness after ingestion of unpasteurized milk products. Populations at risk include pregnant women, infants, immunosuppressed individuals, the elderly, veterinarians, and laboratory workers.

Clinical Features, Diagnosis, and Management

Listeria may cause an illness ranging from mild fever to sepsis, with diarrhea, meningoencephalitis, perinatal listeric septicemia (granulomas and abscesses in multiple organs), cervical adenitis, endocarditis, arthritis, osteomyelitis, brain abscess, peritonitis, and cholecystitis. Early treatment with ampicillin (or trimethoprim-sulfamethoxazole) is indicated because of the seriousness of the illness.

Aeromonas *Species and* Plesiomonas shigelloides

Etiology and Pathogenesis

Aeromonas species and *Plesiomonas shigelloides* are important pathogens responsible for gastroenteritis (including traveler's diarrhea), wound infection, and meningitis. *Aeromonas* species are acquired from contaminated water. They produce illness through elaboration of an enterotoxin and cytotoxic activity. *P shigelloides* is present in contaminated oysters and seafood. Disease is caused by the organism's invasion of the small intestine and by production of heat-labile and heat-stable enterotoxins.

Clinical Features, Diagnosis, and Management

A hydrophila produces diarrhea (watery with blood and mucus), fever, and vomiting in the warmer months. Symptoms usually last <1 week, but rare cases may persist for >1 year. The role of antibiotics for treating infections from *Aeromonas* species is undefined, but the organisms are sensitive to quinolones, aminoglycosides, trimethoprim-sulfamethoxazole, tetracycline, third-generation cephalosporins, and chloramphenicol. Infections with *P shigelloides* most commonly produce vomiting, dehydration, fever, and bloody diarrhea for 1 to 14 days. Extraintestinal manifestations include sepsis, meningitis, endophthalmitis, arthritis, cellulitis, and cholecystitis. *P shigelloides* is susceptible to chloramphenicol, aminoglycosides, trimethoprim-sulfamethoxazole, tetracycline, imipenem, third-generation cephalosporins, and quinolones.

Other Vibrio Species

Etiology and Pathogenesis

Noncholera vibrios are acquired from contaminated water or seafood. *Vibrio parahaemolyticus* is a halophilic vibrio found in salt water or its inhabitants. It elaborates an enterotoxin and produces inflammation in the small intestine. Non-O:1 cholera vibrios cause gastroenteritis (including traveler's diarrhea), wound and ear infections, pneumonia, biliary tract disease, and bacteremia after ingestion of oysters, grated eggs, and potatoes, or after exposure to dogs. Other vibrios (e.g., *V fluvialis, V furnissii, V hollisae, V mimicus*) may also cause diarrheal illness.

Clinical Features, Diagnosis, and Management

V parahaemolyticus produces a range of illness from mild diarrhea to dysentery after an incubation of >24 hours, with associated nausea, vomiting, headache, and fever. Because most cases are self-limited, antibiotics are generally not needed; they do not shorten the course of illness. Non-O:1 cholera vibrios produce diarrhea, which lasts 1 to 6 days and may be severe (>20 stools per day) or bloody, as well as cramping, fever, nausea, and vomiting after a 12-hour incubation. Most cases are self-limited, but severe diarrhea due to non-O:1 vibrio may be treated with tetracycline. The diagnosis is confirmed with selective culture techniques for non-O:1 cholera vibrios (e.g., thiosulfate-citrate-bile salts agar).

VIRAL GASTROENTERITIS

Five classes of viruses produce human illness (rotavirus, Norwalk virus, adenovirus, calicivirus, and Norwalk-like [other small round viruses]), whereas others are suspected pathogens (astrovirus, breda-like virus, corona-like virus).

Rotavirus

Etiology and Pathogenesis

Rotavirus is a nonenveloped, spherical, 70-nm RNA virus that is the single most important cause of infant death in non–cholera-endemic areas. Rotavirus affects children from 6 to 24 months, usually during the winter in temperate climates and year-round in the tropics. Rarely, the agent affects adults. Transmission is by fecal-oral transfer, most likely person to person, with children and asymptomatic adults serving as the major reservoirs. Eighty percent to 100% of children have antibodies to rotavirus by age 2 years. Antibodies are present in breast milk, providing a possible explanation for the lower incidence of infection in breast-fed children. Recurrent infections with differing serotypes are not uncommon. Infection with rotavirus produces shortened villi, hypertrophied crypts, mitochondrial swelling, microvillous abnormalities, and mononuclear infiltration of the lamina propria. Disaccharidase activity is reduced, leading to osmotic diarrhea, and gastric emptying may be delayed.

Clinical Features, Diagnosis, and Management

Children may present after a 48- to 72-hour incubation with profound dehydration, metabolic acidosis, and electrolyte disturbances as a result of severe diarrhea and associated vomiting. Other symptoms including low-grade fever, pharyngitis, and otitis media may be reported. The disease persists for 4 to 5 days, and recovery is complete within 14 days. Stools are devoid of red or white blood cells. Antibody-dependent assays can detect viral particles shed into the stool, although some rare subgroups are not diagnosed with these techniques. The therapy for rotaviral diarrhea involves prevention of exposure and rehydration and replacement of electrolytes through oral or intravenous fluid supplements. Milk intake should be temporarily reduced or eliminated because of viral-induced lactase deficiency. A live, quadrivalent rhesus rotavirus vaccine is currently being tested and appears partially effective.

Norwalk Virus

Etiology and Pathogenesis

Norwalk virus is a 27-nm, nonenveloped, round viral particle that causes epidemic diarrhea in both developed and underdeveloped countries. Norwalk-induced diarrhea exhibits high attack rates, a high propensity for secondary transmission (usually person-to-person by fecal-oral or airborne routes), a lack of seasonal variability in attack rates, and water as a frequent common source. Norwalk virus may be acquired from swimming pools, lakes, and municipal water supplies, as well as from shellfish, schools, nursing homes, cruise ships, travelers, and family members. Biopsy specimens of the small intestine reveal decreased height of intestinal epithelial cells, increased epithelial vacuolization, and increased lamina propria and villous leukocyte infiltration. Brush border enzymes are reduced and gastric emptying may be delayed.

Clinical Features, Diagnosis, and Management

After a 24- to 48-hour incubation, Norwalk virus produces an illness in older children and adults lasting 2 hours to several days and characterized by diarrhea with associated nausea, vomiting, cramping, low-grade fever, myalgias, anorexia, and headache. There are no commercially available diagnostic tests for Norwalk virus infection. Confirmation of the diagnosis can be made by detection of viral particles in the stool or vomitus or by demonstrating a fourfold increase in antibody titers; these tests usually require research laboratories. Therapy centers on fluid and electrolyte replacement and symptomatic treatment of diarrhea.

DIARRHEA OF UNCERTAIN ETIOLOGY

The etiology of most nonepidemic diarrheal illness remains undefined despite careful fecal analysis. Bacterial enteropathogens such as cytotoxigenic *Bacteroides fragilis*, *Klebsiella pneumoniae*, and miscellaneous gram-negative bacilli may be identified by research laboratories in many of these cases. Small, round viruses resembling Norwalk or astroviruses may also be found. Parasites such as *Cyclospora* species or *Cryptosporidia* organisms may cause diarrheal illness after ingestion of contaminated fruit or water supplies.

CHAPTER 39

Chronic Infections of the Small Intestine

TROPICAL SPRUE

Incidence and Epidemiology

Tropical sprue is a disease of the entire small intestine that causes malabsorption in persons who visit or reside in certain tropical areas (e.g., Africa, the Middle East, Central America, Puerto Rico, Cuba, Haiti, and the Dominican Republic). It occurs predominantly in adults, sporadically, and as a sequel to large outbreaks of acute undifferentiated diarrhea. Poor sanitation has been associated with tropical sprue. Visitors may be afflicted within weeks of arrival to an endemic area, but the disease usually occurs in those who have lived there >1 year. In rare instances, tropical sprue does not become clinically apparent for months or years after the patient's return to a temperate climate.

Etiology and Pathogenesis

Most studies suggest that tropical sprue results from persistent contamination of the small intestine by toxigenic strains of coliform bacilli. Most affected patients have bacterial overgrowth with *Klebsiella pneumoniae*, *Enterobacter cloacae*, or *Escherichia coli*. These organisms produce toxins that increase net water secretion, reduce solute absorption, and cause structural abnormalities. In contrast to the syndrome of bacterial overgrowth in the small intestine, the bacterial population in tropical sprue consists of only one or two species. Most non-native residents develop tropical sprue after an attack of acute watery diarrhea. Acute infectious diarrhea is often associated with transient jejunal colonization with coliform bacilli; the basic defect in tropical sprue may be a permanent colonization with these bacteria that would otherwise be cleared. In some regions (e.g., South India, South Africa), tropical sprue is not associated with bacterial colonization of the small intestine, indicating the involvement of other etiologic agents, possibly viral. Although some patients with tropical sprue respond therapeutically to folate supplements, the role of folate deficiency in the pathogenesis of tropical sprue is undefined.

Clinical Features

The onset of tropical sprue is marked by an episode of acute watery diarrhea with associated cramping and gas. After a week, these symptoms become milder and chronic. Patients develop intolerance as a result of the loss of brush border lactase activity; some also develop ethanol intolerance. Within 2 to 4 months, jejunal folate malabsorption leads to anorexia, reduced oral intake, and weight loss. After 6 months, folate and vitamin B_{12} deficiency lead to megaloblastic anemia, which is characterized by weakness and glossitis. Other findings of advanced disease include pallor, edema, stomatitis, hyperpigmentation, and neurologic disorders.

Findings on Diagnostic Testing

Laboratory Studies

Tropical sprue may result in megaloblastic anemia, which is caused by reduced serum levels of folate and vitamin B_{12}. Levels of carotene, vitamin A, vitamin D, albumin, cholesterol, and calcium are also reduced. A marked prolongation of prothrombin time is unusual.

Studies of Intestinal Function

D-Xylose absorption is uniformly reduced. Steatorrhea is present in 50% to 90% of cases. Glucose tolerance test results are abnormal in 50%, whereas tests of protein loss such as fecal α_1-antitrypsin levels may show elevated values. Antibiotic therapy can improve vitamin B_{12} absorption, whereas the addition of intrinsic factor has no effect.

Radiographic Studies

Thickening and coarsening of mucosal folds may be evident on barium radiography of the small intestine, but this finding is not diagnostic. Contrast radiography can be used to exclude other causes of diarrhea in a patient with presumed tropical sprue.

Small Intestine Histology

Histologic changes in tropical sprue include lengthening of the crypt area, broadening and shortening of the villi, and infiltration of the lamina propria by chronic inflammatory cells. A completely flat mucosa is present in 10% of cases.

Management and Course

Spontaneous remissions of tropical sprue rarely occur. Therefore, treatment should be initiated in patients who exhibit the appropriate symptoms, laboratory findings, and small intestine biopsy results. Pharmacologic doses of folate may produce remission of megaloblastic anemia, return of appetite, weight gain, and resolution of intestinal histologic abnormalities. This therapy alone may be curative in early disease, although treatment for 2 years may be required for normalization of intestinal structure and function. Folate therapy usually is insufficient for chronic disease. These patients require antibiotics (e.g., tetracycline or nonabsorbable sulfonamides) to eradicate the intestinal coliform bacilli. Combination therapy with folate, 5 mg per day; vitamin B_{12} injections, 1000 µg per week; and tetracycline, 250 mg four times daily, usually results in complete healing, although 6 months of therapy may be needed. Recurrence is common among native residents but is unlikely for visitors who return to a temperate climate.

WHIPPLE'S DISEASE

Incidence and Epidemiology

Whipple's disease results from infection with the Whipple bacillus *Tropheryma whipellii*, which is observed free and within macrophages in the intestinal mucosa, liver, mesenteric and peripheral lymph nodes, heart, central nervous system, eye, kidney, synovium, and lung. Most cases have been reported in the United States and Europe, and affected patients are more commonly male and white. The mean age at diagnosis is 50 years.

Etiology and Pathogenesis

Whipple's bacillus has not been cultured, nor does it cause a disease in animal models. However, the bacilli are clearly detected using special staining techniques (e.g., periodic acid–Schiff [PAS], Gram's, and Giemsa). A polymerase chain reaction technique identifies the characteristic ribosomal sequence of Whipple's bacillus. Electron microscopy demonstrates that the bacillus core is enclosed within a plasma membrane, which is surrounded by a cell wall consisting of three layers. The inner layer contains polysaccharides that stain positively with PAS. The outer layer resembles a plasma membrane and may be of host origin, which possibly accounts for the failure of the host to mount a humoral antibody response to the infection. The inflammatory response to the organism is muted and consists primarily of macrophages. Whipple's bacillus shares antigenic similarity with streptococcal groups B and G and with *Shigella flexneri*. There is clear evidence that a clinically well patient has impaired cellular immunity, including lymphocytopenia and diminished responses to nonspecific mitogens and antigens, suggesting a role for immune factors in disease pathogenesis. Approximately one-fourth of patients with Whipple's disease are HLA-B27 positive, which is indicative of a genetic predisposition.

Clinical Features

Whipple's disease is characterized by myriad findings referable to infectious involvement of several organ systems. The prominent symptoms are weight loss (usually 20 to 30 pounds, but possibly >100 pounds), diarrhea, arthralgias, fever, and abdominal pain. Diarrhea has the usual features of steatorrhea but may be watery. Occult gastrointestinal bleeding is common, and gross bleeding is occasionally seen. Arthralgias are migratory and nondestructive, involving the large joints. They often precede the intestinal manifestations. The articular attacks usually are acute in onset and last for hours to days. Sacroiliitis is common (20% to 30%), but ankylosing spondylitis is rare. Weight loss, diarrhea, and fever precede the diagnosis by 1 to 4 years, whereas arthralgias typically develop 9 years before the diagnosis. Pericarditis and endocarditis are common (50% to 75%) but rarely produce significant symptoms. Apical systolic murmurs are detected in 25% of patients. Friction rubs and congestive heart failure develop in 10% of patients or fewer. Central nervous system manifestations include dementia, personality change, hemiparesis, seizures, insomnia, hypersomnia, hyperphagia, polydipsia, ataxia, ophthalmoplegia, nystagmus, myoclonus, and Wernicke's encephalopathy. Rhythmic convergence of the eyes associated with synchronous contractions of the masticatory muscles—oculomasticatory myorhythmia—is unique to Whipple's disease. Eye findings include uveitis, vitreitis, retinitis, retrobulbar neuritis, and papilledema. Chronic nonproductive cough and pleuritic chest pain are common.

Physical examination usually reveals significant weight loss and hypotension. Low-grade fever is present in 40% to 50% of patients. Hyperpigmentation, hyperkeratosis, and purpura are cutaneous manifestations. Joint examination rarely shows swelling, effusions, or warmth. Peripheral lymphadenopathy is present in 50%, and 25% have mesenteric adenopathy, which may exhibit a palpable abdominal mass. Abdominal tenderness and distention are common. Hepatosplenomegaly is rare. Neurologic features can be prominent and in some cases strongly suggest the diagnosis (e.g., oculomasticatory myorhythmia).

Findings on Diagnostic Testing

Laboratory Studies

Anemia is present in 90% of patients and results from chronic disease, iron deficiency, and folate or vitamin B_{12} deficiency. Neutrophilia is present in one-third of patients. Mild lymphocytopenia is common. Eosinophilia and thrombocytosis rarely occur. Hypoalbuminemia (mean of 2.7 g per dl) is prevalent, whereas serum globulin levels are usually normal. The prothrombin time is often prolonged. Steatorrhea occurs in 93% of cases. D-Xylose test results are abnormal in 78% of patients. Malabsorption of vitamin B_{12} occurs in 13%. Analysis of the cerebrospinal fluid is rarely useful, but occasionally it detects PAS-positive macrophages. Polymerase chain reaction testing for the Whipple's bacillus ribosomal sequence may become a specific diagnostic test for the disease in the future.

Radiographic Studies

Upper gastrointestinal barium radiographic studies may appear normal, or they may demonstrate coarsening of duodenal and jejunal folds. Enlarged retroperitoneal lymph nodes may widen the duodenal loop or displace the stomach. Abdominal or retroperitoneal lymphadenopathy may also be visualized with

TABLE 39-1
Differential Diagnosis of Periodic Acid–Schiff (PAS)-Positive Macrophages

DISORDER	LIGHT MICROSCOPY	ELECTRON MICROSCOPY
Normal small intestine	Occasional, nonsickled PAS-positive inclusions	No organisms
Whipple's disease	Frequent, round, and sickle-shaped PAS-positive inclusions	Bacilli 0.25 × 1–2 μm
Mycobacterium avium complex	Frequent, round PAS-positive inclusions with acid-fast bacilli	Mycobacteria
Histoplasmosis	Frequent, large, round PAS-positive inclusions with encapsulated organisms	Encapsulated fungi
Macroglobulinemia	Faint, homogeneously stained PAS-positive macrophages	No organisms

ultrasound, computed tomographic (CT), or magnetic resonance imaging (MRI) studies. Chest radiographs occasionally will show fibrosis, focal infiltrates, or pleural effusions. Joint radiographs usually appear normal, but bone erosions and narrowing of joint spaces may be seen. Similarly, sacroiliitis may be seen on bone radiographs, but ankylosing spondylitis is unusual. CT and MRI scans are essential for detection of central nervous system lesions.

Small Intestine Histology

The diagnostic procedure of choice for Whipple's disease is biopsy of the small intestine, including samples taken for electron microscopy; four to six biopsy specimens should be obtained because of the patchy nature of the disorder. On upper gastrointestinal endoscopy, the duodenal folds appear thickened and are coated with yellow-white granular material. The lamina propria is packed with macrophages containing PAS-positive, round or sickle-shaped inclusions that represent bacilli in varying stages of digestion. Free extracellular bacilli may also be observed below the epithelial basal lamina. Other causes of numerous PAS-positive macrophages in the lamina propria are easily distinguished from Whipple's disease; these include *Mycobacterium avium* complex in acquired immunodeficiency syndrome (AIDS), macroglobulinemia, and systemic mastocytosis (Table 39-1). In rare instances, the results of the examination of biopsy specimens of the small intestine are normal. In such cases, the diagnosis may be established by electron microscopic detection of bacilli in cerebrospinal fluid or by biopsy of brain tissue or lymph node.

Management and Course

Whipple's disease is treated with trimethoprim-sulfamethoxazole twice daily for 1 year. This regimen should eradicate central nervous system disease. Parenteral penicillin is used for patients who are too ill to tolerate oral medications. Oral penicillin for 1 year is used for patients who are allergic to sulfonamides. Supplemental folate, vitamin B_{12}, fat-soluble vitamins, and iron may be necessary for severely malnourished patients.

After treatment, patients should have periodic clinical and laboratory evaluation because relapse, especially in the central nervous system, is not uncommon and can lead to irreversible dementia and death. Follow-up biopsy of the intestine is of little use because PAS-positive macrophages may persist for years after successful treatment. However, in suspected relapse, detection of free bacilli in the biopsy specimen is definitive. The spinal fluid should be examined for PAS-positive macrophages if central nervous system relapse is suspected. A repeat 1-year course of trimethoprim-sulfamethoxazole is recommended for treatment of central nervous system relapse. Chloramphenicol is used if trimethoprim-sulfamethoxazole fails. For non-central nervous system relapses, a second course of trimethoprim-sulfamethoxazole is given, and penicillin is administered if there is no response.

TUBERCULOSIS

Etiology and Pathogenesis

Enteric tuberculosis may be the primary infection, or it may be secondary to pulmonary tuberculosis (in 10% of cases). The populations at risk are alcoholics, Asians, and patients with AIDS. Swallowing infected sputum, miliary spread, and direct infection from adjacent organs can lead to intestinal involvement. Gastrointestinal tuberculosis primarily affects the ileocecal area and colon, and, rarely, the duodenum, stomach, and esophagus. It may mimic Crohn's disease or colonic carcinoma. Intestinal atypical mycobacteriosis must also be considered in the differential diagnosis because it exhibits similar symptoms in immunocompromised patients (e.g., AIDS).

Clinical Features, Diagnosis, and Management

Symptoms of tuberculous enteritis include fever, night sweats, weight loss, anorexia, nausea, abdominal pain, and diarrhea. A right lower quadrant abdominal mass is palpable in one-half of the patients. Complications include obstruction, hemorrhage, and malabsorption (because of bacterial overgrowth). A positive intradermal test and active pulmonary disease on chest radiographs suggest the diagnosis. Barium radiography of the small intestine may show an ulcerated nodular ileocecal area with multiple short strictures resembling Crohn's disease, lymphoma, or ameboma. Circumferential ulcerations characterize tuberculosis, whereas longitudinal ulcerations occur in Crohn's disease. Colonoscopy, CT scans, and laparoscopy with peritoneal biopsy are useful in some cases. Laparotomy reveals a thickened bowel wall and a serosa studded with tubercles. Regional lymph nodes may show caseating necrosis. Treatment involves a multidrug regimen—for example, isoniazid (300 mg per day), ethambutol (15 mg per kg per day), and rifampicin (600 mg per day).

HISTOPLASMOSIS

Etiology and Pathogenesis

Histoplasmosis can cause an ulcerative enteritis, most commonly in the terminal ileum or colon. It can occur in normal hosts and in patients with AIDS. In most cases, various regions of the gastrointestinal tract are involved.

Clinical Features, Diagnosis, and Management

Intestinal histoplasmosis presents with fever, chills, malaise, anorexia, and weight loss and may be complicated by hemorrhage, obstruction, perforation, or malabsorption. Rarely, the disease presents as protein-losing enteropathy. The diagnosis is confirmed by demonstration of *Histoplasma capsulatum* in biopsy specimens from the rectum or involved gastrointestinal segments. Increases in complement fixation titers may be useful in some cases. Therapy with amphotericin B (2 g over 10 weeks) or ketoconazole (200 to 400 mg daily for 6 months) has been proposed.

CHAPTER 40

Celiac Sprue

INCIDENCE AND EPIDEMIOLOGY

Celiac sprue, also known as celiac disease and gluten-sensitive enteropathy, is characterized by intestinal mucosa damage and malabsorption secondary to dietary intake of wheat, rye, barley, or oats. Symptoms may appear with the introduction of cereal into the diet in the first 3 years of life. A second peak in incidence occurs in adults during their third or fourth decade, although disease onset as late as the eighth decade has been reported. The true incidence of celiac sprue is uncertain because many cases are asymptomatic. Clinically evident disease affects 1 in 3000 to 1 in 10,000 adults in the United States. In western Ireland, the incidence approaches 1 in 300. The disease is rare in Japan, Southeast Asia, and Africa.

ETIOLOGY AND PATHOGENESIS

Environmental Factors

Celiac sprue results from an interplay of environmental factors, genetic predisposition, and immunologic interactions. The alcohol-soluble gliadin fraction of wheat gluten and similar alcohol-soluble proteins (*prolamins*) in rye, barley, and oats contain the disease-promoting moieties in these grains. A single variety of wheat may contain 40 or more different, closely related gliadins. A-gliadin, the major α-gliadin that activates celiac sprue, has amino acid sequence similarity to the E1b protein of human adenovirus serotype 12, suggesting that molecular mimicry is involved in the immunopathogenesis of the disease.

Genetic Factors

Symptomatic or asymptomatic celiac disease can occur in 5% to 15% of first-degree relatives of patients with defined celiac sprue. Three-fourths of identical twins are concordant for the disorder. Celiac sprue is strongly associated with HLA class II D region genes, which may be important determinants of disease susceptibility. Among siblings who share one or two HLA haplotypes, 28% to 40% develop celiac disease. The difference between this incidence and the 75% concordance noted in identical twins indicates the presence of genetic factors outside the HLA locus. Genes that code for immunoglobulin heavy-chain allotype markers on human IgG heavy chain, for T-cell receptors, and for the host immune response may be markers for other regions associated with disease susceptibility.

Immune Factors

Humoral and cellular immune factors influence the manifestations of celiac sprue. Significant elevations in IgA antigliadin antibodies are more common in untreated than treated patients with celiac disease, and they are unusual in healthy individuals. Because antigliadin antibodies are found in the serum and intestinal secretions of patients with other intestinal diseases, however, they are not specific for celiac disease. Patients with celiac sprue have increased numbers of IgM-, IgG-, and IgA-producing cells in the lamina propria of the small intestine, which may release immunoglobulin on gliadin challenge. Antigliadin antibodies may induce disease by activating the complement cascade and cell-mediated cytotoxicity. Patients with celiac disease may also have additional antibodies to milk, egg, and soy proteins. Proinflammatory cytokines secreted by T cells and mononuclear cells may contribute to tissue injury. Numbers of intraepithelial lymphocytes are increased in active celiac sprue and remain increased during remission. CD4 T cells in the lamina propria are thought to contribute to epithelial cell damage and alterations in crypt cell growth through the release of cytokines; CD8 T cells may have impaired suppressor function.

CLINICAL FEATURES

The clinical presentation of celiac sprue can vary markedly, especially in adults. Progressive weight loss, diarrhea, flatulence, and distention are classic gastrointestinal symptoms. Malaise and weakness may be the only manifestations of mild disease. Patients with minimal disease may have no gastrointestinal symptoms and present simply with anemia or osteopenic bone disease. In some cases, symptoms develop only after an infectious disease, metabolic stress, or gastric surgery. Stools can be bulky and foul-smelling, watery, soft, or nearly normal. Diarrhea results from malabsorption of carbohydrates, proteins, and fats; stimulation of colonic secretion by hydroxy-fatty acids and bile acids. Alterations in motility can be caused by the loss of small intestinal hormone-producing cells in the small intestine, small numbers of patients may even be constipated. Some patients report anorexia, whereas others experience voracious appetites. The magnitude of weight loss depends on the extent (lesions begin proximally in the duodenum), the severity of the intestinal lesion and the degree to which the patient increases dietary intake. Children with celiac sprue typically present in the first to third years of life. Symptoms often disappear during adolescence but may recur during early adulthood.

Patients with celiac sprue may present with extraintestinal manifestations. Anemia may be secondary to iron or folate malabsorption or, in the case of severe ileal disease, vitamin B_{12} deficiency. Osteopenic bone disease results from calcium and vitamin D malabsorption. Hypocalcemia (and hypomagnesemia) may be associated with tetany and may lead to secondary hyperparathyroidism. Cutaneous bleeding, epistaxis, hematuria, and gastrointestinal hemorrhage may result from vitamin K malabsorption. Neurologic manifestations include peripheral sensory neuropathy, patchy demyelination of the spinal cord, and cerebellar atrophy with ataxia. Psychiatric findings include mood changes, irritability, and depression. The cause of the neurologic and psychiatric manifestations is unknown; furthermore, these symptoms may not resolve with the exclusion of gluten from the diet. Muscle weakness may result from a proximal myopathy. Vitamin A deficiency may lead to night blindness. Women may experience amenorrhea, delayed menarche, and disturbed fertility. Men may report impotence and infertility.

Physical findings depend on disease severity. Patients with mild disease exhibit no abnormal physical symptoms. In more severe disease, emaciation, clubbed nails, dependent edema, ascites, ecchymoses, pallor, cheilosis, glossitis, decreased peripheral sensation, and a positive Chvostek or Trousseau sign may be detected. Hyperkeratosis follicularis may result from vitamin A deficiency. The abdomen may be distended and tympanitic and have a doughy consistency.

FINDINGS ON DIAGNOSTIC TESTING

Laboratory Studies

Screening tests for celiac sprue are the same as those used to assess other malabsorptive conditions. Nonspecific findings include anemia (microcytic resulting from iron deficiency or macrocytic resulting from folate or vitamin B_{12} deficiency), hypocalcemia, hypophosphatemia, hypomagnesemia, metabolic acidosis, hypoalbuminemia, hypoglobulinemia, low serum vitamin A levels, a prolonged prothrombin time, and an elevated serum alkaline phosphatase level. Fecal fat levels may be increased on qualitative (i.e., Sudan stain) or quantitative assessment. D-Xylose absorption usually is abnormal. Other tests of absorption or intestinal permeability (e.g., uptake of chromium ethylenediaminetetraacetic acid, urinary sugar excretion ratios) are used only as research tools. HLA typing is used in some centers for patients in whom biopsy of the small intestine, antibody testing, and absorption testing are nondiagnostic. HLA typing is also useful for identifying family members at risk of developing celiac disease.

Antibody Testing

Several antibody tests are useful adjuncts in the diagnosis of celiac sprue. They also are used to screen family members of affected patients. Serum antigliadin antibodies are detected in 90% of symptomatic patients and in many asymptomatic patients, but they may also be found in patients with other diseases of the small intestine (e.g., Crohn's disease). Direct assay of antigliadin antibodies in the intestinal fluid does not add to the utility of antibody testing. The IgA antibody is more specific than the IgG antigliadin antibody. Reduction in IgA antigliadin titers may be observed with dietary gluten restriction. IgA antiendomysial antibodies are elevated in 95% of patients with active celiac disease, and they are somewhat more specific than antigliadin antibodies. Antireticulin antibodies have low sensitivity in detecting celiac sprue (40% to 50%) but are more specific than antigliadin antibodies. Combinations of these antibody tests provide a higher degree of sensitivity and specificity for the detection of celiac disease than any single test.

Small Intestine Histology

Biopsy of the small intestine mucosa is the gold standard for the diagnosis of celiac sprue. In patients with active disease, endoscopic inspection may reveal a loss of duodenal folds with scalloping that is suggestive of villous atrophy. Celiac sprue specifically involves the mucosa, sparing the submucosa, muscularis propria, and serosa, with more severe involvement of the proximal intestine (duodenum, proximal jejunum) and less intense ileal involvement. In active disease, there may be complete loss of villi, resulting in a flat absorptive surface of the mucosa and crypt elongation. Columnar epithelial cells that line the surface of the mucosa are replaced by cuboidal or squamoid cells, which have basophilic cytoplasms. The surface epithelium is heavily infiltrated with intraepithelial lymphocytes. Increased numbers of plasma cells, lymphocytes, eosinophils, and mast cells infiltrate the lamina propria. Subtotal villous atrophy may be observed in milder disease or in disease that has been treated with a gluten-restricted diet. It should be recognized that other infectious or inflammatory diseases produce similar histologic findings; therefore, the diagnosis of celiac sprue is contingent on the appropriate clinical scenario and response to a gluten-free diet. In some patients, colonic or gastric biopsy specimens may reveal lymphocytic infiltration, which is consistent with the diagnoses of lymphocytic colitis and gastritis, respectively.

MANAGEMENT AND COURSE

Therapy

The mainstay of treatment of celiac sprue is a gluten-free diet. Commitment to this diet is lifelong, requiring the complete elimination of wheat (including triticale, spelt, and semolina), rye, barley, and oat products from the diet. Corn, rice, sorghum, buckwheat, and millet do not activate the disease. Gluten is not present in distilled liquor; therefore, whisky and other spirits are well tolerated. However, barley-containing beer and ale should be avoided. Because of the loss of brush border lactase activity, dairy products should initially be avoided, but these substances can be reintroduced after symptom improvement is achieved on a gluten-restricted diet. Symptomatic improvement with these dietary recommendations may be reported as soon as 48 hours after their initiation. Recovery of normal intestinal histologic features often takes much longer (i.e., months), and in 50% of patients abnormalities persist despite strict adherence to the diet.

The distal intestinal mucosa heals more rapidly than the proximal mucosa. Supplemental iron or folate (and rarely vitamin B_{12}) may be needed to treat anemia early in the course of therapy. Vitamin K may be required to treat a coagulation deficit. Osteopenic bone disease is treated with vitamin D replacement. Corticosteroid therapy should be reserved for patients unresponsive to dietary gluten restriction or for patients with complications. The role of cyclosporine in rare cases of atypical sprue is uncertain. If dietary measures are instituted early, the prognosis of celiac sprue is good. Untreated disease can lead to malnutrition, debilitation, and complications.

Complications

Intestinal and extraintestinal complications may occur in celiac sprue. Ten percent to 15% of patients with celiac sprue develop malignancy, usually after 20 to 40 years of disease. Lymphoma of the small intestine is often multifocal and diffuse, constituting 50% of the neoplasms that complicate celiac disease. It is usually of T-cell origin. The diagnosis of lymphoma may be difficult because of the insidious onset of symptoms in many patients. Carcinoma of the small intestine as well as of the mouth, pharynx, and esophagus are more common in patients with celiac sprue than in the normal population. Evidence strongly suggests that adherence to a gluten-free diet reduces the subsequent incidence of malignancy. Chronic ulcerative jejunoileitis is characterized by multiple ulcers and strictures of the small intestine. Patients with celiac disease who have this complication often are refractory to gluten restriction and further predisposed to development of lymphoma. Other causes of refractoriness to dietary therapy include refractory sprue and collagenous sprue in which a thick band of collagen-like material is deposited under the intestinal epithelial cells. Collagenous colitis has also been associated with celiac sprue. Some refractory patients respond to corticosteroids or other immunosuppressive drugs (e.g., azathioprine, cyclophosphamide, cyclosporine); however, some require permanent parenteral hyperalimentation to maintain adequate nutrition and hydration.

The main extraintestinal complication of celiac sprue is dermatitis herpetiformis, a skin disease with intensely pruritic papulovesicular lesions on the elbows, knees, buttocks, sacrum, face, scalp, neck, and trunk. Approximately 5% of patients with celiac disease report symptomatic dermatitis herpetiformis. Most patients who present initially with dermatitis herpetiformis exhibit celiac sprue-like findings on intestinal biopsy specimens and may respond slowly to a gluten-free diet, although this is not universal. A granular or speckled pattern of IgA deposits is noted at the epidermal-dermal junction of uninvolved skin in most patients; a linear pattern is less common. Complement components (C3, C5) may also be found in association with the IgA deposits. Dapsone therapy can result in rapid improvement of skin lesions but has no effect on intestinal mucosal lesions. Celiac sprue exhibits clinical associations with other immune-mediated diseases such as insulin-dependent diabetes mellitus, thyroid disease, IgA deficiency, Sjögren's syndrome, systemic lupus erythematosus, mixed cryoglobulinemia, vasculitis, pulmonary disease, pericarditis, mesenteric lymph node cavitation, inflammatory bowel disease, neurologic disorders, ocular abnormalities, IgA mesangial nephropathy, primary sclerosing cholangitis, and primary biliary cirrhosis. Some patients exhibit hyposplenism, which may increase the risk of bacterial infection. These persons should be given prophylactic antibiotics before invasive procedures or dental work.

CHAPTER 41

Disorders of Epithelial Transport in the Small Intestine

DISORDERS OF CARBOHYDRATE ABSORPTION

Starch, sucrose, and lactose are the major dietary carbohydrates. Their assimilation requires hydrolysis to and subsequent small intestine mucosal uptake of monosaccharide components. In conditions of malabsorption, intralumenal carbohydrate draws fluid into the small intestine by an osmotic process. On delivery to the colon, the sugars become substrates for bacterial fermentation and are converted from oligosaccharides or disaccharides to monosaccharides, further increasing the osmotic load. Bacterial conversion of carbohydrates to short-chain fatty acids that are absorbed across the colon wall partially compensates for this increased load.

Lactase Deficiency

Etiology and Pathogenesis

Adult lactase deficiency is the most prevalent genetic deficiency syndrome worldwide, affecting >50% of the population. It is viewed as an autosomal recessive trait. The condition, which results in decreases in lactase levels during childhood and adolescence to 5% to 10% of those at birth, primarily affects black American, Asian, Mediterranean, Native American, and Mexican American populations and spares all but 5% to 15% of people of Northern European descent (Table 41-1). A second disorder, congenital lactase deficiency, is a rare autosomal recessive condition that is characterized by watery diarrhea in infancy. Lactose intolerance also may develop after insults to the intestine, such as infections or inflammatory disease (e.g., celiac sprue) that result in reduced absorptive surface area, insufficient contact time, and reduced mucosal enzyme levels. In many of these conditions, recovery of nor-

TABLE 41-1
Ethnic Distribution of Lactase Deficiency

POPULATION	PREVALENCE OF LACTASE DEFICIENCY (%)
Northern European	5–15
Mediterranean	60–85
African black	85–100
American black	45–80
American white	10–25
Native American	50–95
Mexican American	40–75
Asian	90–100

Source: Data from FJ Simoons. The geographical hypothesis and lactose malabsorption: a weighing of the evidence. Am J Dig Dis 1978;23:963.

mal lactase activity is prolonged after adequate treatment of the primary disorder. Milk intolerance also can result from sensitization to a protein component of cow's milk rather than reduced lactase levels. This sensitivity can follow an infection (e.g., with rotavirus in infants).

Clinical Features, Diagnosis, and Management

Lactase-deficient adults report distention, bloating, abdominal pain, flatulence, and diarrhea after ingestion of more than 12 to 18 g of lactose (i.e., 1 to 1½ glasses of milk). Historically, the lactose tolerance test has been relied on for diagnosis, which in normal individuals is characterized by an increase in the blood glucose level of >20 mg per dl after ingestion of 50 g of lactose in water. False-positive results may be observed with diabetes, and gastroparesis may cause false-negative results. Breath hydrogen testing is an alternative noninvasive method involving gas chromatographic analysis of expired breath to detect hydrogen after the ingestion of lactose. Lactase deficiency is diagnosed if the rise in breath hydrogen is >20 ppm. The magnitude of the rise correlates semiquantitatively with the degree of malabsorption. False-positive tests may occur in patients with bacterial overgrowth, whereas persons who have colonic bacteria that do not produce hydrogen gas may have false-negative test results. In infants, the finding of an acidic pH and the presence of reducing substances on stool analysis suggest the diagnosis. Response to a low lactose diet is very supportive of a diagnosis suggested by the history. The gold standard for diagnosis of lactase deficiency in any person is an assay of disaccharidase activity on intestinal biopsy specimens, but this test is rarely necessary.

The management of lactase deficiency involves dietary reduction of lactose supplemented with exogenous lactase. Many individuals need only to reduce their intake of dairy products. In such cases, strict dietary exclusion is not recommended because milk represents a valuable source of calcium. Milk products are available in which the lactose is prehydrolyzed by supplemental lactase. Substitute milk products in which other carbohydrates are substituted for lactose are widely sold. Lactase supplements in the form of tablets may be consumed with each lactose-containing meal (two to four tablets). Although yogurt contains lactose, it is well tolerated because the bacteria in the active culture possess intrinsic lactase activity.

Sucrase-Isomaltase Deficiency

Etiology and Pathogenesis

Sucrase-isomaltase deficiency is an autosomal recessive disorder characterized by undetectable intestinal sucrase activity and reduced isomaltase activity. The diagnosis is made in patients ranging in age from infants to young adults. The disorder may result from impaired processing of the enzyme or inappropriate transport to sites other than the brush border, probably because of distinct mutations in the sucrase-isomaltase gene.

Clinical Features, Diagnosis, and Management

In infants, symptoms develop with introduction of sucrose-containing formulas. The diagnosis is made by oral sucrose tolerance testing, breath hydrogen testing after sucrose challenge, or by assay of intestinal mucosal enzyme levels. Institution of a sucrose-free diet is associated with cessation of diarrhea and weight gain. Dietary starch is usually well tolerated. Oral sucrase supplements are being tested.

Trehalose Deficiency

Etiology and Pathogenesis

Trehalose intolerance is a rare condition of carbohydrate malabsorption in the United States, probably because young mushrooms are the only significant dietary source of this sugar. Relative trehalose deficiencies are common in Greenland.

Clinical Features, Diagnosis, and Management

Affected individuals develop abdominal pain, bloating, and diarrhea after ingestion of the mushrooms. Mucosal biopsy specimens show an absence of trehalose activity. Treatment is avoidance of young mushrooms.

Glucose-Galactose Malabsorption

Etiology and Pathogenesis

Congenital glucose-galactose malabsorption is an autosomal recessive condition characterized by impaired sodium-coupled glucose-galactose transport caused by a mutation in the transporter protein. Transient glucose malabsorption may develop in infants after gastrointestinal surgery or gastroenteritis (caused by rotavirus). It usually resolves rapidly.

Clinical Features, Diagnosis, and Management

Affected infants present with watery diarrhea and dehydration in the first week of life. Fecal analysis reveals a low pH and the presence of reducing substances. Replacement of dietary glucose and galactose with fructose produces immediate symptomatic improvement.

Intolerance to Other Carbohydrates

Etiology and Pathogenesis

Fructose and sorbitol are poorly absorbed carbohydrates. Malabsorption of these two sugars may produce symptoms in the absence of any hereditary enzyme deficiency. Fructose is prevalent in fruits, sucrose, and soft drinks, and sorbitol is contained in fruits, dietetic candies, and chewing gum. Malabsorption of starch from wheat, corn, oat, potato, and bean sources has been reported in susceptible populations. Rice generally does not provoke symptoms. Starch from refined or gluten-free flour is better absorbed, suggesting that fiber or protein components rather than the starch itself may be responsible for the symptoms.

Clinical Features, Diagnosis, and Management

Susceptible patients may present with bloating, flatulence, pain, or diarrhea after ingestion of relatively small amounts of these carbohydrates (e.g., two cans of soda or four sticks of gum). Hydrogen breath testing after ingestion of fructose, sorbitol, or starch has been used in research settings to document malabsorption. This test is rarely used in clinical settings. When suspected or documented, reduction of dietary consumption of the offending carbohydrate is recommended. Simethicone is often given, but its efficacy is limited. The effectiveness of charcoal compounds is controversial. Similarly, the administration of supplemental α-galactosidase (Beano) to hydrolyze dietary oligosaccharides has met with limited success in alleviating symptoms.

DISORDERS OF PROTEIN AND AMINO ACID ABSORPTION: ENTEROKINASE DEFICIENCY

Etiology and Pathogenesis

Congenital enterokinase deficiency produces low proteolytic activity in the duodenal juice despite normal levels of amylase and lipase. The addition of exogenous enterokinase converts trypsinogen to trypsin, resulting in activation of other proteolytic enzymes.

Clinical Features, Diagnosis, and Management

Infants with enterokinase deficiency present with diarrhea, growth retardation, and hypoproteinemia with edema. Steatorrhea may result from secondary mucosal changes and pancreatic insufficiency. The diagnosis is confirmed by enzyme assay of a mucosal biopsy specimen or by activation of proteolytic activity in the duodenal fluid by adding enterokinase. Patients are treated with pancreatic enzyme supplements.

DISORDERS OF AMINO ACID TRANSPORT

Etiology and Pathogenesis

The capacity of the intestine to absorb dipeptides and tripeptides provides insurance against the development of nutritional insufficiency even though intestinal transport of amino acids may be impaired. Hartnup disease is an autosomal recessive condition characterized by a defect in the transport of neutral amino acids. Cystinuria is an autosomal recessive defect of cystine and dibasic amino acid transport. Other disorders of amino acid transport include lysinuric protein intolerance (dibasic amino acids), blue diaper syndrome (tryptophan), oasthouse urine disease (methionine), Lowe's syndrome (lysine, arginine), and Joseph's syndrome (glycine, proline, hydroxyproline).

Clinical Features

Disorders of intestinal amino acid transport generally present with extraintestinal manifestations: pellagra-like rash and neuropsychiatric symptoms in Hartnup disease; renal calculi and chronic pancreatitis in cystinuria; growth retardation and hepatosplenomegaly in lysinuric protein intolerance; hypercalcemia and nephrocalcinosis in blue diaper syndrome; mental retardation and seizures in oasthouse urine disease; aminoaciduria in Joseph's syndrome; and mental retardation, cataracts, and renal failure in Lowe's syndrome.

DISORDERS OF FAT ABSORPTION: ABETALIPOPROTEINEMIA

Etiology and Pathogenesis

Abetalipoproteinemia is an autosomal recessive disorder in which plasma apolipoprotein B–containing lipoproteins (B100 and B48) are absent, producing very low plasma cholesterol and triglyceride levels. The disorder results from a defect in the intestinal microsomal transfer protein responsible for triglyceride, cholesteryl ester, and phosphatidylcholine transfer. Variants of abetalipoproteinemia include chylomicron retention disease (or Anderson's disease, B48 is absent), normotriglyceridemic abetalipoproteinemia (B100 is absent), and the autosomal codominant disorder, familial hypobetalipoproteinemia.

Clinical Features, Diagnosis, and Management

The initial clinical manifestations of abetalipoproteinemia are fat malabsorption and erythrocyte acanthosis at birth. Long-term sequelae include fat-soluble vitamin deficiency and development of retinopathy and spinocerebellar degeneration. A biopsy specimen from the intestine of a fasted patient shows the mucosa to be engorged with fat droplets, reflecting the inability to synthesize and secrete chylomicrons. Anderson's disease and normotriglyceridemic abetalipoproteinemia are not associated with acanthosis or low triglyceride levels. The clinical manifestations of familial hypobetalipoproteinemia are milder and may occur at a later age. Management of these conditions includes dietary fat restriction and vitamin A, E, and K supplementation.

MISCELLANEOUS DEFECTS

Disorders of Electrolyte and Mineral Transport

Etiology and Pathogenesis

Congenital chloridorrhea is an autosomal recessive defect of Cl^-/HCO_3^- exchange in the small intestine and colon that results in the loss of chloride absorption, intestinal acidification, and secondary impairment of sodium absorption. Isolated cases of congenital defects in intestinal sodium absorption have been reported. Familial hypomagnesemia is characterized by impaired intestinal magnesium absorption in the intestine. Acrodermatitis enteropathica is an autosomal recessive disorder of altered zinc uptake. Menkes' (steely hair) syndrome is a generalized X-linked recessive disorder of cellular copper transport.

Clinical Features, Diagnosis, and Management

Patients with congenital chloridorrhea present at birth with watery diarrhea, hyponatremia, hypochloremia, dehydration, metabolic alkalosis, and hypokalemia. The diagnosis is confirmed by documenting elevated levels of fecal chloride (>100 mEq per liter). Patients are treated with oral sodium chloride and potassium chloride solutions. Patients with congenital sodium absorptive defects present with metabolic acidosis and watery diarrhea characterized by fecal sodium losses exceeding those of chloride and by increased fecal bicarbonate. Therapy consists of fluid and sodium citrate supplements. Patients with familial hypomagnesemia present with tetany and seizures in infancy and are treated with oral magnesium therapy. Acrodermatitis enteropathica is an illness associated with diarrhea, alopecia, failure to thrive, and a rash of the perioral and perianal regions and extremities; it is treated with oral zinc. Menkes' syndrome is characterized by growth retardation, abnormal hair, hypopigmentation, bone changes, and cerebral degeneration, and usually is fatal by the age of 3 years.

Microvillous Inclusion Disease

Etiology and Pathogenesis

Microvillous inclusion disease results from defective brush border assembly and differentiation caused by abnormal cytoskeletal elements that produce villous atrophy. The enterocytes lack microvilli, or they have disordered microvilli as well as vesicular bodies and intracytoplasmic vacuoles.

Clinical Features, Diagnosis, and Management

Infants present after birth with severe diarrhea. The diagnosis is made by jejunal biopsy or by electron microscopic demonstration of microvillous inclusions in biopsy specimens from the rectal mucosa. Lifelong total parenteral nutrition is required in most cases, although the somatostatin analog octreotide and a subtotal colectomy may reduce stool volume and electrolyte loss in some cases. Intestinal transplantation has had some success and may become standard therapy for this disease.

Disorders of Vitamin B$_{12}$ Absorption

Etiology and Pathogenesis

Congenital vitamin B$_{12}$ malabsorption is an autosomal recessive disorder with an unknown pathogenesis. Investigators have postulated defects in the ileal intrinsic factor-vitamin B$_{12}$ receptor or in postreceptor pathways. Transcobalamin II deficiency is characterized by absence of the vitamin B$_{12}$ transport protein. Congenital intrinsic factor deficiency may be secondary to no intrinsic factor synthesis, to altered intrinsic factor that binds less efficiently to ileal receptors, or to synthesis of intrinsic factor that is abnormally sensitive to acid or proteolytic degradation.

Clinical Features, Diagnosis, and Management

Congenital vitamin B$_{12}$ malabsorption is characterized by megaloblastic anemia and neurologic disease with low serum vitamin B$_{12}$ levels in childhood. Schilling's test shows impaired absorption of vitamin B$_{12}$ despite administration of intrinsic factor, pancreatic enzymes, and antibiotics. Therapy involves monthly injections of vitamin B$_{12}$. Patients with transcobalamin II deficiency develop megaloblastic anemia in infancy and have normal levels of vitamin B$_{12}$. This disorder is treated with massive doses of vitamin B$_{12}$ to ensure that the vitamin will enter tissues by passive diffusion. The laboratory findings of congenital intrinsic factor deficiency are similar to those of pernicious anemia but without achlorhydria, atrophic gastritis, or parietal cell antibodies.

Primary Bile Salt Malabsorption

Etiology and Pathogenesis

Primary bile salt malabsorption in children is characterized by the in vitro finding of impaired taurocholic acid uptake in ileal biopsy specimens. In adults, primary bile salt malabsorption is associated with subtotal villous atrophy of the ileal mucosa and mononuclear infiltration of the lamina propria. There are also findings suggestive of immunologic mediation.

Clinical Features, Diagnosis, and Management

Patients present with chronic diarrhea with exaggerated fecal losses of bile salts. Diagnostic tests include measurements of radioactivity in the breath and stool after ingestion of ^{14}C-cholylglycine, quantitation of fecal radioactivity after administration of radiolabeled taurocholate, and measurement of total excretion and aqueous concentrations of fecal bile acids. Alternatively, a total body count after ingestion of the taurine conjugate of a synthetic bile acid containing an isotope of selenium (the SeHCAT test) may be diagnostically useful. Regardless, confirmation of the diagnosis relies on a therapeutic response to oral cholestyramine.

CHAPTER 42

Short Bowel Syndrome

INCIDENCE AND EPIDEMIOLOGY

An increasing number of patients undergo resection of an extensive amount of the small intestine and survive because of improvements in perioperative and postoperative techniques. The consequences of small bowel resection are variable, but in general the presence of short bowel syndrome depends on the length and intestinal region removed.

ETIOLOGY AND PATHOGENESIS

Causes of Short Bowel Syndrome

The most common disorders in adults that lead to massive resection of the small intestine are a vascular insult and Crohn's disease (Table 42-1). Risk factors for vascular disease include advanced age, congestive heart failure, atherosclerotic and valvular heart disease, chronic diuretic use, hypercoagulable states, and oral contraceptive use. Less common adult causes include jejunoileal bypass, abdominal trauma, neoplasm, and radiation enteropathy. Pediatric causes of short bowel syndrome are intestinal atresia, midgut or segmental volvulus, abdominal wall defects, necrotizing enterocolitis, Hirschsprung's disease, hypercoagulable states, cardiac valvular vegetations, Crohn's disease, and abdominal trauma.

TABLE 42-1
Causes of Short Bowel Syndrome

Adult causes
    Intestinal vascular insults
        Superior mesenteric artery embolus or thrombosis
        Superior mesenteric vein thrombosis
        Volvulus of the small intestine
        Strangulated hernia
    Postsurgical causes
        Jejunoileal bypass
        Abdominal trauma with resultant resection
        Inadvertent gastroileal anastomosis for peptic ulcer disease
    Miscellaneous
        Crohn's disease
        Radiation enteritis
        Neoplasms
Pediatric causes
    Prenatal causes
        Vascular accidents
        Intestinal atresia
        Midgut or segmental volvulus
        Abdominal wall defect
    Postnatal causes
        Necrotizing enterocolitis
        Trauma
        Inflammatory bowel disease
        Midgut segmental volvulus
        Hirschsprung's disease
        Radiation enteritis
        Venous thrombosis
        Arterial embolus or thrombosis

Factors That Influence Absorption
After Intestinal Resection

Factors that influence nutrient absorption after small bowel resection include the extent and site of resection, the presence of the ileocecal junction, the condition of the remaining bowel and of other organs, and the degree of adaptation in the residual intestine. The amount of small intestine remaining after resection determines the absorptive surface area and the transit time. Approximately one-half of the small intestine may be resected without significant nutritional sequelae, but resections of 75% or more almost invariably produce severe malabsorption. Long-term survival has been reported with only 15 to 48 cm of residual jejunum in addition to the duodenum. Although the ileum can assume absorption of the nutrients, vitamins, and minerals normally absorbed in the duodenum and jejunum, the loss of enteroendocrine cells from the proximal intestine may result in decreased pancreaticobiliary secretion, thereby exacerbating malabsorption. Ileal resection can lead to bile salt diarrhea and vitamin B_{12} deficiency (after resections of <100 cm) and significant steatorrhea (after resections of >100 cm). As ileal nutrients regulate gastric emptying and small bowel transit, ileal resection may shorten intestinal transit times, magnifying the absorptive defect. A combined resection of the small intestine and colon usually increases dehydration and sodium and potassium depletion compared with a resection of the small intestine alone.

Surgical removal of the ileocecal junction accelerates transit time in the small intestine and increases bacterial colonization of the residual intestine, producing bile salt deconjugation, fat and fat-soluble vitamin malabsorption, vitamin B_{12} malabsorption, and bile salt diarrhea.

Conditions that impair the function of the residual intestine, such as Crohn's disease, lymphoma, and radiation enteritis, also increase the severity of absorptive defects. Pancreatic enzyme activity may be reduced if patients are severely malnourished. Gastric hypersecretion may result from a massive resection.

Animal models suggest that intestinal villi become taller and thicker after small bowel resection, whereas in human biopsy specimens, mucosal hyperplasia has been demonstrated. Increased ileal absorption of glucose, maltose, sucrose, bile acids, vitamin B_{12}, and calcium after proximal resection has been documented in animals, as has increased activity of the enzymes involved in DNA and pyrimidine synthesis. In humans, there is a gradual improvement in absorption of fat, nitrogen, and carbohydrate after extensive resection of the small intestine. In contrast, functional adaptation of the colon after intestinal resection is poorly documented. Adaptation of the small intestine depends on the presence of intralumenal nutrients; intestinal hypoplasia may result from complete reliance on parenteral nutrition. Lumenal nutrients also evoke pancreaticobiliary secretions, which produce mucosal hyperplasia directly. Increased levels of hormones stimulated by intralumenal nutrients may play a role in these mucosal responses. The role of polyamines (e.g., putrescine, spermidine, and spermine) in adaptive mucosal growth is undefined.

CLINICAL FEATURES

The clinical presentation of short bowel syndrome is divided into three phases: early, intermediate, and late. In the immediate postoperative period after 75% or more of the small bowel has been resected, diarrhea, dehydration, and electrolyte deficiencies (hyponatremia, hypokalemia, hypocalcemia, and hypomagnesemia) supervene. An intermediate phase follows, with malabsorption, weight loss, and malnutrition. During the late phase, weight often stabilizes despite ongoing diarrhea and steatorrhea. However, some patients who have had extensive resection require supplemental therapy to prevent life-threatening nutritional sequelae.

Diarrhea results from decreased transit time, increased osmolarity of the lumenal contents (as a result of carbohydrate malabsorption), bacterial overgrowth, gastric hypersecretion, and increased water and electrolyte secretion. In the early postoperative phase, fluid losses may exceed 5 liters per day, especially with concomitant colectomy. Nutritional deficiencies produce weight loss, lassitude, weakness, fatigue, and growth retardation (in children). Fatty acid malabsorption also may lead to hypocalcemia and hypomagnesemia, which subsequently produce tetany, osteomalacia, and osteoporosis. Fat-soluble vitamin deficiency is common, as is vitamin B_{12} deficiency, but other water-soluble vitamins and trace metals are generally well absorbed even if the resection is extensive. Folate deficiency and zinc deficiency rarely occur.

Gastric hypersecretion may occur after massive resection of the small intestine, leading to peptic ulcer disease and anastomotic breakdown. Increased diarrhea occurs secondary to intestinal mucosal damage, impaired micelle formation, and inhibition of pancreatic enzyme function. Gastric hypersecretion is maximal the first day after small bowel resection and usually lessens with time. The mechanisms of gastric hypersecretion development are unclear, but gastrin-dependent and gastrin-independent pathways may be involved.

Calcium oxalate renal calculi may develop in patients with short bowel syndrome because of increased absorption of dietary oxalate in the colon, decreased urinary concentrations of calcium-binding anions (e.g., phosphate and citrate), and reduced urinary volume. The incidence of gallstones is increased twofold to threefold by ileal resection. This rise classically has been believed to be the result of bile salt malabsorption, which results in cholesterol supersaturation of gallbladder bile. However, calcium-containing cholesterol stones and pigment stones are also prevalent after small bowel resection, indicating that other mechanisms may be involved as well.

Complications specific to jejunoileal bypass for morbid obesity include bypass enteritis, L-lactic acidosis, and encephalopathy secondary to bacterial D-lactate production; immune-mediated skin disease; arthritis; myalgias; focal interstitial nephritis; renal tubular acidosis; and hemolytic anemia. Cirrhosis is a late complication and is believed to result from bacterial overgrowth in the blind loop.

FINDINGS ON DIAGNOSTIC TESTING

Laboratory Testing

Laboratory studies may exhibit abnormalities that are dependent on the severity of nutrient, vitamin, and mineral deficiencies. Electrolyte determinations may reveal hyponatremia, hypokalemia, hypocalcemia, and hypomagnesemia, whereas a complete blood count may show anemia caused by vitamin B_{12} deficiency and, less commonly, folate and iron deficiencies. Fat-soluble vitamin deficiencies (i.e., A, D, E, and rarely K) may be evident. Urine oxalate levels may be elevated in patients predisposed to oxalate calculi. Fecal analysis would reveal elevated fat levels. The gold standard for detection of bacterial overgrowth is quantitative culture of intestinal fluid obtained endoscopically or from a fluoroscopically placed aspiration catheter.

Radiographic Studies

In most cases, radiographic evaluation of a patient with short bowel syndrome is unnecessary. However, barium radiography of the small intestine may be performed if the length of residual bowel is uncertain. Bone radiography and bone densitometry can be used to assess for osteomalacia and osteoporosis in a patient with calcium and vitamin D malabsorption. Ultrasound may be of value in detecting gallstones, and intravenous pyelography or renal ultrasound may detect renal calculi.

MANAGEMENT AND COURSE

Medical Therapy

The primary goal of medical therapy for short bowel syndrome is to control diarrhea. Opiate agents are the most effective antidiarrheal agents for this condition and act by delaying transit in the small intestine and increasing intestinal capacity. Loperamide may be effective in some cases, but many patients require more potent agents such as codeine or tincture of opium to control symptoms. Kaolinpectin and fiber preparations are useful for patients with mild diarrhea. In patients with limited ileal resection, cholestyramine may be effective for treatment of bile salt diarrhea. Subcutaneous octreotide has been demonstrated to reduce fluid and electrolyte losses in patients with short bowel syndrome as a result of antimotility effects, decreased digestive juice secretion, and influences on mucosal fluid and electrolyte transport. Potential risks of octreotide therapy include development of gallstones, impaired release of gut hormones necessary for intestinal mucosal adaptation, and tachyphylaxis. H_2-receptor antagonists and proton pump inhibitors may reduce gastric hypersecretion, thereby minimizing peptic ulcer complications and inhibiting the gastric secretory component of the patient's diarrhea. Oral broad-spectrum antibiotics are warranted if intestinal bacterial overgrowth is suspected. Pancreatic enzyme supplements are given to patients with proximal intestinal resections because of the loss of cholecystokinin and secretin release and to those with severe protein-calorie malnutrition.

Nutritional Therapy

During the initial postoperative phase of short bowel syndrome, total parenteral nutrition is required to prevent diarrhea, dehydration, and fluid and electrolyte losses. The length of time a patient requires parenteral nutrition varies. It has been reported that patients with 30 to 50 cm of healthy small intestine and most of the colon remaining can often be weaned from parenteral nutrition within 1 year, whereas patients with concomitant colectomy generally need at least 60 cm of small bowel to avoid permanent intravenous feeding. Patients receiving long-term parenteral nutrition at home require a permanent intravenous catheter that must be placed surgically. Abnormalities of hepatic function are described in patients on permanent intravenous hyperalimentation, including gallbladder sludge, gallstones, steatonecrosis, and cirrhosis. Metabolic bone disease may also complicate prolonged parenteral nutrition because of aluminum contamination of protein hydrolysates or toxic effects of parenteral vitamin D.

Limited oral intake should be resumed when stool output is <2 liters per day to stimulate intestinal adaptation. Elemental or semielemental formulas are recommended initially. These formulas contain sucrose or glucose polymers, easily digested proteins, or free amino acids or short peptides, vitamins and minerals, and minimal amounts of fat. They also contain glutamine, which is a purported stimulant of intestinal adaptation. Elemental diets are well absorbed in the proximal jejunum. Because of their poor taste, these formulas are often administered in slow infusions through nasogastric or nasoenteric tubes.

After stabilization of nutritional and fluid status is achieved, the patient with short bowel syndrome may resume food intake. It is common practice to use a low-fat, high-carbohydrate diet because of the adverse effects of steatorrhea (e.g., colonic secretion, binding of divalent cations to fatty acids, hyperoxaluria and renal calculus formation). Most clinicians recommend restricting fat to the extent necessary to avoid mineral and fat-soluble vitamin deficiency. Patients with preservation of the colon often require more significant fat restriction (<60 g per day) to control diarrhea and reduce oxalate absorption. Medium-chain triglycerides, which are efficiently hydrolyzed and absorbed in the proximal intestine, may be given as caloric supplements; however, they have an unpleasant taste, produce diarrhea if given in doses of >35 g per day, and do not contain essential fatty acids. Restriction of dietary lactose or supplementation with lactase is necessary in many patients to avoid worsening of diarrhea, cramping, and bloating. Patients with hyperoxaluria should avoid high oxalate foods (e.g., chocolate, cola, tea, carrots, celery, spinach, pepper, nuts, plums, figs, strawberries) in addition to restricting fat intake. Cholestyramine has been used to treat hyperoxaluria, but it may worsen fat and fat-soluble vitamin malabsorption. Rarely, lactic acidosis may produce metabolic encephalopathy; these patients are managed with dietary carbohydrate restriction and nonabsorbable antibiotics.

Clinical deficiency of water-soluble vitamins are rare in patients with short bowel syndrome (except for vitamin B_{12}), whereas fat-soluble vitamin deficiencies are common. Patients are advised to take multiple-vitamin preparations containing two to five times the recommended dietary allowances. Patients with ileal resections of >90 cm should receive intramuscular vitamin B_{12}, 100 µg per month. Serum retinol, calcium, 25-hydroxyvitamin D, and urinary calcium should be monitored to assess the adequacy of vitamin A and D supplementation. Calcium intake of 1000 to 1500 mg per day is encouraged. Postmenopausal women should be given supplemental estrogen to reduce bone demineralization. Symptomatic hypomagnesemia may mandate intravenous magnesium replacement, as oral magnesium supplements can worsen diarrhea. Iron and zinc deficiency occasionally develop, requiring specific supplementation. Deficiencies of other minerals usually are prevented by multiple-vitamin preparations.

Surgical Therapy

Surgical procedures have been devised to slow intestinal transit in patients with short bowel syndrome, including antiperistaltic intestinal segments, colonic interposition, construction of intestinal valves, creation of recirculating loops, and retrograde electrical pacing. However, these operations have not achieved significant success in clinical trials. Tapering enteroplasty may improve intestinal function in patients with short bowel syndrome who have had a dilated small intestine. Transplantation of the small intestine represents an important new treatment option. Some patients have been able to discontinue parenteral nutrition and maintain excellent nutrition after a successful transplant. Enteral feeding usually is possible within a few weeks of surgery. Complications of intestinal transplantation include acute rejection (e.g., cryptitis, villous blunting, vasculitis, mononuclear cell infiltration of the lamina propria, mucosal sloughing), chronic rejection (e.g., villous atrophy, subintimal vascular thickening, muscular fibrosis), graft-versus-host disease, and lymphomas.

CHAPTER 43

Tumors and Other Neoplastic Diseases of the Small Intestine

Neoplasms of the small intestine are rare, accounting for only 1% of all gastrointestinal malignancies (Table 43-1). Fifty percent to 80% are benign (most commonly adenomas, leiomyomas, and lipomas). Hamartomatous lesions also occur in the small intestine and frequently are seen in patients with Peutz-Jeghers and Cronkhite-Canada polyposis syndromes. Malignant tumors include adenocarcinomas, carcinoids, lymphomas, and leiomyosarcomas.

ADENOMA AND ADENOCARCINOMA

Incidence and Epidemiology

The incidence of adenomas of the small intestine is unknown because most patients are asymptomatic. The annual incidence of adenocarcinoma is 4 per 1 million. Adenocarcinoma of the small intestine is more common in developed countries; the regional variation in the incidence of this tumor parallels the incidence of colon cancer. Adenomas and adenocarcinomas occur more frequently in patients with familial adenomatous polyposis (FAP), and most develop in the duodenum and periampullary region. Other conditions associated with an increased frequency of adenocarcinoma include long-standing Crohn's disease, celiac sprue, and urologic ileal conduits.

Etiology and Pathogenesis

Although the molecular and genetic events leading to dysplasia and carcinoma of the small intestine remain unknown, the adenoma-to-carcinoma model characteristic of colorectal cancer appears to be operative in the pathogenesis of adenocarcinoma of the small intestine. The 50% to 90% incidence of duodenal adenomas and 5% incidence of duodenal carcinomas in patients with FAP suggest that the genetic and molecular mechanisms of carcinogenesis in the small

---

TABLE 43-1
Classification of Tumors of the Small Intestine

Benign epithelial tumors
  Adenoma
Malignant epithelial tumors
  Primary adenocarcinoma
  Metastatic carcinoma
  Carcinoid tumors
Lymphoproliferative disorders
  Lymphoid hyperplasia
  Immunoproliferative disease
  Malignant lymphoid tumors
    Lymphoma
    Plasma cell tumors
    Leukemias
    Primary macroglobulinemia
Benign and malignant mesenchymal tumors
  Myogenous
  Lipomatous
  Fibromatous
  Neurogenic
Hamartomas
  Peutz-Jeghers syndrome
  Brunner's gland
  Cronkhite-Canada syndrome
  Neurofibromatosis

---

intestine are similar to those of colorectal cancer. As with colorectal polyps, there is a spectrum of dysplasia, from the diminutive tubular adenoma to large villous polyps exhibiting high-grade dysplasia and invasive carcinoma. Up to 30% to 50% of small intestinal villous polyps contain foci of invasive adenocarcinoma, providing further evidence of the adenoma-to-carcinoma sequence.

Clinical Features

The majority of adenomas in the small intestine are asymptomatic, but polyps of >1 cm may cause intermittent abdominal pain or occult gastrointestinal hemorrhage. The duodenum is the most common site for both sporadic and FAP-associated adenomas. Large villous adenomas in the duodenum and peri-ampullary region may cause gastric outlet obstruction, obstructive jaundice, and pancreatitis.

Patients with adenocarcinoma are more likely to exhibit symptoms, including intermittent abdominal pain, weight loss, and occult or gross gastrointestinal bleeding. Patients with periampullary duodenal carcinomas may manifest jaundice. Patients with celiac sprue may present with new-onset weight loss and abdominal pain after years of quiescent disease. Similarly, patients with Crohn's disease exhibit symptoms of obstruction that may mistakenly be attributed to a flare of their underlying disease.

TABLE 43-2
Distribution of Malignant Tumors of the Small Intestine

TUMOR	DUODENUM (%)	JEJUNUM (%)	ILEUM (%)
Primary adenocarcinoma	40	38	22
Malignant carcinoid	18	4	78
Primary lymphoma	6	36	58
Leiomyosarcoma	3	53	44

The physical examination findings in patients with adenomas and adenocarcinomas of the small intestine are often normal. A minority of patients have specific findings such as an abdominal mass, but nonspecific findings, including fecal occult blood loss, are common. Patients with gastric outlet obstruction may exhibit abdominal distention or a succussion splash.

Findings on Diagnostic Testing

Routine upper gastrointestinal endoscopy identifies up to 50% of sporadic adenomas and adenocarcinomas in the small intestine. The vast majority of adenomas in patients with FAP occur in the proximal duodenum and periampullary region. Approximately 50% of sporadic adenomas and carcinomas occur in the jejunum and ileum, which may be accessible to enteroscopy (Table 43-2). Lesions in the proximal or middle jejunum can be visualized with push enteroscopy and a biopsy can be done. More distal lesions are not accessible with this technique. Sonde enteroscopy relies on peristalsis to propel the tip of the instrument into the distal intestine. Although a near complete examination of the small intestine is possible, sonde enteroscopy is limited by the inability to obtain a biopsy specimen and the lack of widespread availability. Most distal lesions can be identified with barium radiography of the small intestine. Enteroclysis, which is more sensitive for detecting diminutive mass lesions, may be used after normal barium radiography if there is a high clinical suspicion of a tumor in the small intestine. Angiography is used in patients with gastrointestinal hemorrhage, when no source can be identified on upper gastrointestinal endoscopy or colonoscopy. Adenocarcinomas appear as hypovascular masses with associated encasement of the surrounding vessels. Computed tomographic (CT) scans are helpful in staging tumors of the small intestine by identifying lymph node and hepatic metastases.

Management and Course

The majority of small tubular adenomas in the proximal duodenum can be removed endoscopically. Because villous adenomas have a 30% to 50% incidence of invasive carcinoma, surgical resection is usually indicated. If preoperative or intraoperative histologic examination suggests invasive adenocarcinoma within a villous adenoma, pancreaticoduodenectomy (i.e., the Whipple procedure) should be performed. Patients with high operative risks or discrete pedunculated polyps may be treated initially in specialized centers with endoscopic snare resection. However, pathologic evidence of invasive carcinoma or incomplete excision may alter the risk-benefit profile in favor of surgical therapy. Local excision involves a 30% risk of recurrence within 12 months. Therefore, all endoscopically excised polyps require repeat upper gastrointestinal endoscopic evaluation 3 to 6 months later.

The only option for long-term survival for patients with adenocarcinoma is complete surgical resection. Even with resection, the 5-year survival rate for this condition is 10% to 20%; most patients survive <6 months. Surgical therapy for tumors in the jejunum and proximal ileum involves segmental resection. A right hemicolectomy is required to treat adenocarcinoma of the distal ileum. When preoperative or intraoperative staging suggests the tumor is unresectable, palliative resection usually is performed, given the high rate of intestinal obstruction. Neither chemotherapy nor radiation therapy is effective for small bowel adenocarcinoma.

CARCINOIDS

Incidence and Epidemiology

The small intestine represents the second most common anatomic site for development of carcinoid tumors; nearly 80% of small bowel carcinoids occur in the ileum. Carcinoids account for 20% to 40% of all malignant small bowel tumors, with an annual incidence of 3 per 1 million. As with adenocarcinoma, the incidence increases with age. Carcinoids are more common in men and in black Americans.

Etiology and Pathogenesis

The molecular and genetic mechanisms responsible for carcinoid tumor formation are unknown. These neoplasms are members of the family of endocrine tumors termed *amine precursor uptake and decarboxylation tumors* (APUDomas). Histologically, carcinoids resemble other neuroendocrine tumors and are characterized by clumps of uniform cells with hyperchromatic nuclei. In general, carcinoids of the small intestine produce clinical signs and symptoms caused by the local effects of the tumor mass, but a small percentage of patients manifest a constellation of systemic symptoms, termed the *carcinoid syndrome*, attributable to overproduction of peptide hormones. Serotonin is responsible for the majority of symptoms in the carcinoid syndrome, but prostaglandins, gastrin, bradykinin, and other substances also produced by carcinoid tumors may affect the clinical presentation.

Seventy percent of carcinoids in the small intestine are detected incidentally at upper gastrointestinal endoscopy, surgery, or autopsy. Although the natural history of these asymptomatic lesions remains unclear, the 5% risk of metastatic disease among lesions <1 cm in diameter suggests that all small bowel carcinoids are potentially malignant. With symptomatic tumors, the incidence of distant disease is as high as 30%.

Clinical Features

The most common clinical presentation of a symptomatic carcinoid tumor of the small intestine is intermittent abdominal pain caused by intestinal obstruction.

Carcinoids also produce an intense desmoplastic response that contributes to the obstruction by causing the mesentery to retract and angulate. Rarely, patients with large carcinoids present with hemorrhage caused by overlying mucosal ulceration.

Ten percent of patients with symptomatic small bowel carcinoids develop the carcinoid syndrome. Although localized foregut carcinoids may produce the carcinoid syndrome, carcinoids of the small intestine cause this syndrome only after hepatic metastasis. The most common symptoms are flushing and diarrhea, which may be mild and intermittent. Flushing is precipitated by emotional stress, exertion, and meal or ethanol ingestion, or it occurs spontaneously. Less common features of the syndrome include bronchospasm and right-sided heart failure. Carcinoid heart disease usually occurs after several years of the disease and results from tricuspid regurgitation and pulmonic stenosis. Patients with carcinoid syndrome may experience a hypotensive crisis during the induction of general anesthesia.

Findings on Diagnostic Testing

Imaging Studies

Because most carcinoids occur in the ileum, upper gastrointestinal endoscopy and colonoscopy have limited roles in identifying these tumors. The majority of symptomatic lesions are demonstrated on barium radiographs of the small intestine. The desmoplastic distortion of the mesentery may be evident as kinking and tethering of the intestine. A CT scan is also helpful in demonstrating these mesenteric changes. It is the procedure of choice for documentation of hepatic metastases. As with other neuroendocrine tumors, scintigraphy with ^{123}I-labeled octreotide may identify primary and metastatic carcinoids not detected by conventional imaging techniques.

Laboratory Testing

Diagnosis of the carcinoid syndrome relies on detection of elevated urinary levels of 5-hydroxyindoleacetic acid (5-HIAA), the major metabolite of serotonin. Excretion of >10 mg of 5-HIAA in a 24-hour urine sample is consistent with excess circulating serotonin. False-positive tests may be caused by phenothiazines, malabsorption, and chronic intestinal obstruction. Plasma serotonin levels can be used for diagnosis and to monitor for tumor recurrence.

Management and Course

Surgical excision is the procedure of choice for all carcinoid tumors of the small intestine. Asymptomatic lesions <1 cm in diameter may be treated with local excision, but lesions of >1 cm require a wide surgical excision comparable with that for adenocarcinomas. Duodenal lesions require a Whipple procedure; distal ileal lesions require ileocecectomy; and lesions in the jejunum and proximal ileum require segmental resection with 10-cm margins. When localized disease is resected, the overall 5-year survival is 75%, compared with 20% for metastatic disease.

Patients with metastatic disease and the carcinoid syndrome may benefit from debulking surgery. The somatostatin analog octreotide is >90% effective in palliating symptoms of the carcinoid syndrome. Initial doses range from 50 to 250 µg subcutaneously two to three times daily, but as the disease progresses, larger doses may be necessary. Carcinoid tumors have a 40% response rate to combination chemotherapy with streptozocin and 5-fluorouracil, but this regimen does not improve survival.

LYMPHOMA

Incidence and Epidemiology

Primary lymphoma accounts for 10% to 20% of the malignancies of the small intestine, with an annual incidence of 2 per 1 million. The small intestine is second to the stomach as a site for development of primary gastrointestinal lymphoma. There are two major variants of lymphoma with distinct epidemiologic associations. In Western countries, lymphomas of the small intestine are discrete tumors of the non-Hodgkin's variety, occurring most commonly in patients older than 50 years, in association with celiac sprue, nodular lymphoid hyperplasia of the small intestine, and immunodeficiency syndromes including acquired immunodeficiency syndrome. The other variant is termed *immunoproliferative small intestine disease* (IPSID) and occurs almost exclusively in developing countries. Patients usually present in young adulthood with diffuse intestinal involvement.

Etiology and Pathogenesis

The etiology of the non-Hodgkin's variant of small bowel lymphoma is unknown. The majority are B-cell lymphomas, with histologic features similar to those of lymphomas in the salivary gland, lung, and thyroid. This has prompted the theory that these lymphomas arise from common mucosa-associated lymphoid tissue. In contrast to sporadic lymphomas in the small intestine, those associated with celiac sprue usually are of T-cell origin.

Evidence suggests that the IPSID variant of lymphoma of the small intestine is dependent on an infection with a micro-organism. The disease occurs almost exclusively in geographic regions where parasitic and other enteric infections are endemic. Tetracycline given early in the course of the disease can induce a complete remission. Although the putative infectious agent has not been identified, it clearly has a role in the early stages of disease. A lack of response to antibiotics in patients with later-stage disease, however, suggests that other factors are also involved.

Clinical Features

Non-Hodgkin's lymphoma of the small intestine produces a discrete mass lesion. The clinical presentation is similar to that of other tumors of the small intestine. Intermittent abdominal pain caused by obstruction is the most common complaint. Weight loss is often profound, and a small percentage of patients present with acute abdominal pain caused by perforation. Diarrhea, abdominal pain, and weight loss are symptoms of lymphoma in patients with celiac sprue after years or decades of quiescent disease. Misinterpreting these symptoms as a flare of celiac sprue may delay diagnosis.

TABLE 43-3
Staging of Primary Non-Hodgkin's Lymphoma of the Small Intestine

Stage IE	Intestinal involvement without nodal involvement
Stage IIE	Intestinal involvement with involvement of regional lymph nodes
Stage IIIE	Involvement of intestine and lymph nodes on both sides of the diaphragm, without or with splenic involvement (stage IIIES)
Stage IV	Diffuse involvement of >1 extralymphatic organ, with or without nodal involvement

Patients with IPSID present earlier than those with non-Hodgkin's lymphomas. Patients report profound diarrhea and weight loss in addition to obstructive symptoms. Many patients have associated clubbing of the digits. Unlike non-Hodgkin's lymphoma, a palpable abdominal mass is uncommon.

Findings on Diagnostic Testing

Barium radiography of the small intestine is the primary means of detecting small bowel lymphomas. The majority of non-Hodgkin's lesions occur in the ileum; therefore, endoscopy is of limited value. Lesions within the distal 5 to 10 cm of the terminal ileum are accessible to colonoscopic biopsy. A CT scan provides invaluable staging information including the detection of intra-abdominal and intrathoracic malignant lymph nodes. There are no specific laboratory features of non-Hodgkin's lymphoma, but serum protein electrophoresis demonstrates an α-heavy chain paraprotein in 20% to 70% of patients with IPSID.

Management and Course

The staging of lymphomas of the small intestine is similar to that of gastric lymphomas (Table 43-3). Patients with disease limited to the small intestine and intra-abdominal lymph nodes should undergo resection with curative intent. Even if curative resection is not possible, palliative resection is often used to prevent perforation resulting from chemotherapy-induced tumor necrosis. Combination chemotherapy is indicated for unresectable disease, but the role of adjuvant therapy after curative resection is undefined. The 5-year survival rate after curative resection is 35%, whereas the corresponding survival rate for unresectable disease is <25%. Patients who develop lymphoma as a complication of celiac sprue have a 5-year survival rate of 10%. This may in part be because of the inability to distinguish symptoms of lymphoma in the setting of underlying disease of the small intestine.

MYOGENIC TUMORS

Leiomyomas are benign neoplasms of intestinal smooth muscle. They usually remain asymptomatic and are discovered only incidentally. A small percentage of these submucosal tumors may grow to several centimeters in diameter, however, and obstruct the intestinal lumen or cause intussusception. In addition, ulceration of the overlying mucosa may result in gastrointestinal hemorrhage. Barium radiography of the small intestine may demonstrate a ball-shaped mass with normal overlying mucosa or an ulcerated mass. Symptomatic lesions require surgical resection because imaging procedures cannot distinguish benign leiomyomas from malignant leiomyosarcomas.

Leiomyosarcomas are extremely rare tumors of the small intestine, with an annual incidence of 1 per 1 million, usually occurring in individuals older than 50 years. The clinical presentation is identical to that of other tumors of the small intestine, with the exception that patients with leiomyosarcomas tend to present with gastrointestinal hemorrhage. Although submucosal in origin, leiomyosarcomas frequently become necrotic. Ulceration of the overlying mucosa predisposes these vascular tumors to significant bleeding. Angiography often reveals a vascular mass, and a CT scan may demonstrate invasion of adjacent structures or distant metastasis. In the absence of distant spread or local invasion, leiomyosarcomas may be difficult to differentiate from leiomyomas, but histologic examination reveals that leiomyosarcomas have more mitotic figures. Aggressive surgical therapy with resection of isolated liver or pulmonary metastases is the only option for long-term survival. Prognosis is directly related to tumor size and resectability. The 5-year survival rate is 20% to 50%.

CHAPTER 44

Structural Anomalies and Diverticular Disease of the Colon

COLONIC EMBRYOLOGY AND ANATOMY

The colon is composed of the embryonic midgut (appendix, cecum, ascending colon, and proximal transverse colon) and the hindgut (distal transverse colon, descending colon, sigmoid colon, and rectum), which develop during the fourth gestational week. The cloaca, located at the distal end of the hindgut, is separated into the ventral urogenital sinus and the dorsal rectum by the anorectal septum. The anal membrane ruptures in the eighth week, forming the anal canal. Development of the colonic epithelium is similar to that of the small intestine and occurs with the formation of a slitlike lumen at 8 to 9 weeks. Epithelial ridges form at 10 to 11 weeks, resulting in the formation of broad villi. Cystlike spaces develop at 12 to 15 weeks that divide these broad villi into secondary villi. Epithelial cells proliferate, leading to the formation of the colonic crypts. The colonic villi disappear between the twenty-ninth week and term, leaving only the colonic crypts. The fetal colonic epithelium contains many small intestinal cell types, including goblet cells, columnar epithelial cells with microvilli, and enteroendocrine cells, which appear to secrete trophic factors. Neural crest cells, precursors of enteric ganglia, migrate from the transverse colon to the anus from weeks 12 to 16, forming the enteric nervous system. Smooth muscle cells and muscular structures such as the taenia coli and haustra appear in the tenth week.

The adult colon is 3 to 5 feet in length, extending from the ileocecal junction to the proximal rectum. The lumenal diameter progressively decreases from the cecum (7.5 to 8.5 cm) to the sigmoid colon (2.5 cm). The ascending and descending colons, rectum, and posterior surfaces of the hepatic and splenic flexures are fixed retroperitoneal structures, whereas the cecum, transverse colon, and sigmoid colon are intraperitoneal. The circular muscle envelops the full circumference of the colon, while the outer longitudinal muscle layer is confined to three bands, the taenia coli, located 120 degrees apart around the circumference. The haustra are sacculations separated by the plicae semilunares. The rectum is a 12- to 15-cm-long structure extending from the sigmoid colon to the anus. It is composed of mucosal, submucosal, and circumferential inner circular and outer longitudinal layers. In contrast to the colon, the rectum has no serosal layer. The anal canal is a slitlike structure, 4 cm in length, which is lined by highly sensitive squamous epithelium lacking hair follicles, sebaceous glands, and sweat glands. The dentate line is a mucocutaneous junction located 1.0 to 1.5 cm above the anal verge. A 6- to 12-mm transitional zone from squamous to columnar epithelium exists above the dentate line. The columns of Morgagni are mucosal folds above the dentate line. The anorectal ring is the palpable upper border of the anal sphincter, 1.0 to 1.5 cm above the dentate line.

The cecum, ascending colon, and transverse colon receive arterial blood from the superior mesenteric artery, which branches into the ileocolic, right colic, and middle colic arteries. The inferior mesenteric artery supplies the descending colon, sigmoid colon, and upper rectum through its left colic, sigmoidal, and superior rectal branches. The marginal artery of Drummond runs along the mesenteric border of the colon, connecting these arterial branches. The arc of Riolan is a tortuous vessel that connects the middle colic to the left colic artery. The remainder of the rectum is supplied by the middle and inferior rectal arteries, which originate from the internal iliac and internal pudendal arteries, respectively. The venous drainage of the colon parallels the arterial supply except for the inferior mesenteric vein, which runs retroperitoneally before entering the splenic vein. Hemorrhoidal tissue receives blood from the rectal arteries. The internal hemorrhoids drain into the superior rectal vein, and the external hemorrhoids drain into the pudendal veins. Lymphatic capillaries encircle the colon in the submucosa and muscularis mucosae. Lymph nodes are located on the bowel wall (epicolic), along its inner margin (paracolic), around the mesenteric arteries (intermediate), and at the origin of the superior mesenteric artery and the inferior mesenteric artery (main). Lymph from the lower rectum and anal canal above the dentate line enters the inferior mesenteric nodes and iliac nodes and subsequently drains to the periaortic nodes. Below the dentate line, lymph drains to the inguinal nodes and to the rectal lymph nodes.

The sympathetic and parasympathetic nerves to the colon follow the course of the blood vessels. The sympathetic nerves project from the superior mesenteric plexus, which supplies the proximal colon, and the inferior mesenteric plexus, which supplies the left colon and rectum. The parasympathetic supply to the right colon comes from the vagus, and the pelvic nerve supplies the distal colon. Distal sympathetic and parasympathetic fibers also innervate the bladder, prostate, and sexual organs, all of which may be injured during dissection of the rectum. Afferent fibers from the pudendal nerve innervate the anal epithelium, contributing to the exquisite sensitivity of this structure.

The mucosa of the colon is similar histologically to that of the small intestine in that both are lined by simple columnar epithelium, but the colonic mucosa lacks villi. The lamina propria contains plasma cells, macrophages, lymphocytes, and abundant lymphoid nodules, which often extend into the submucosa. Subepithelial fibroblasts produce many of the components of the basal lamina. The epithelial cells undergo rapid renewal every 6 days and are replaced by descendants of stem cells from the lower third of the crypts. There are three main epithelial cell types: absorptive colonocytes, goblet cells, and enteroendocrine cells. Colonocytes are capable of absorbing sodium, chloride, and water but not glucose or amino acids. These cells have a limited ability to absorb fatty acids and package them into chylomicrons. Goblet cells secrete mucus that lubricates and protects the epithelium against adherence of pathogens. Enteroendocrine cells secrete enteroglucagon, peptide YY, serotonin, substance P, leu-enkephalin, pancreatic polypeptide, and somatostatin. These cells are more numerous in the rectum and appendix, which may explain the frequent occurrence of neuroendocrine tumors at these sites.

DEVELOPMENTAL ABNORMALITIES OF THE COLON

Hirschsprung's Disease

Etiology and Pathogenesis

Hirschsprung's disease results from the failure of the neural crest cells to complete their caudal migration to the anus during fetal development. The aganglionic segment does not relax, and the normal proximal bowel hypertrophies and dilates. The rectosigmoid is involved in 75% to 80%, whereas the entire colon and parts of the small intestine are involved in 5% to 10% of cases.

Clinical Features, Diagnosis, and Management

Delayed passage of meconium and distention are presenting symptoms in newborns, whereas older children may present with chronic constipation, distention, volvulus, and perforation. Adults with very short segment involvement may report a history of constipation dating back to childhood. Digital examination may show an empty rectal vault in Hirschsprung's disease compared with voluminous stool with idiopathic megacolon. Abdominal radiography may show colonic dilation and a paucity of gas. Barium enema radiography may show a short, narrow transition zone. Falsely negative barium enema exaiminations may occur in patients with total colonic aganglionosis, very short segment involvement, or neonatal Hirschsprung's disease. Anorectal manometry may demonstrate loss of the rectoanal inhibitory reflex (i.e., relaxation of the internal anal sphincter in response to rectal distention). Deep rectal biopsy specimens that include the mucosa and submucosa are necessary for diagnosis of Hirschsprung's disease, and in some patients full-thickness operative biopsy specimens may be needed. Biopsy specimens from affected persons exhibit hyperplastic or hypertrophic nerve fibers. Routine and acetylcholinesterase staining reveal an absence of ganglion cells and increased acetylcholinerase staining, respectively. A colostomy is frequently performed before definitive surgical repair to allow the bowel to stabilize and resume a normal caliber. Pull-through operations (Swenson, Duhamel, Soave) can anastomose normally innervated bowel to the anus with or without resection of affected bowel. Rectal myotomy may be curative in patients with short segment involvement.

Colonic Duplications

Etiology and Pathogenesis

The colon and rectum account for 5% to 10% of gastrointestinal duplications. They are thought to result from failure of the colon to recanalize in utero, caudal twinning, or incomplete separation of the notochord from the ectoderm. Duplications may communicate with the colonic lumen, or they may be closed cysts.

Clinical Features, Diagnosis, and Management

Duplications produce symptoms of obstruction, volvulus, and hemorrhage. They can be complicated by infection and malignant degeneration. Abdominal radiography, barium enema radiography, or computed tomographic (CT) scanning may reveal masses or show communication with the colon. Rectal duplications are resected when possible because of the risk of malignancy. Tubular duplications elsewhere can be treated by dividing the common wall.

Malrotation

Etiology and Pathogenesis

Malrotation occurs when the midgut fails to complete the 270-degree rotation before re-entering into the abdomen at 10 to 12 weeks of gestation. The cecum and right colon overlie the duodenum in the right upper quadrant and Ladd's bands form over the duodenum to peritonealize the cecum. Malrotation is associated with intestinal atresia, intussusception, Hirschsprung's disease, and abdominal wall defects.

Clinical Features, Diagnosis, and Management

Infants present with bilious vomiting, a flat abdomen, and bloody stools indicative of proximal intestinal obstruction, volvulus, or ischemia. Rarely, malrotation presents later in life. Abdominal radiography may show gastric or duodenal obstruction. Upper gastrointestinal barium radiography may reveal displacement of the ligament of Treitz on the right, whereas barium enema radiography may demonstrate the cecum in the right upper quadrant. Surgery for malrotation involves reducing any volvulus, severing the Ladd bands, removing the appendix, and fixing the duodenum in the right upper quadrant and the cecum in the left upper quadrant.

Imperforate Anus

Etiology and Pathogenesis

Imperforate anus is classified according to its anatomic level. The bowel with high lesions (more common in males) terminates above the levator ani muscles, the rectum in low lesions (more common in females) terminates below the levator ani and may be accompanied by fistulous connections to the perineum, vagina, or other organs. Imperforate anus is associated with congenital genitourinary, sacral, cardiac, or gastrointestinal anomalies in 50% of cases.

Clinical Features, Diagnosis, and Management

Infants present with failure to pass meconium unless a fistula is present. Characterization of the defect relies on air invertograms (to identify the location of the rectum), fistulograms, CT scans or magnetic resonance imaging studies, intravenous pyelography, and voiding cystourethrograms. Low lesions can be treated by dilation of fistulous tracts with or without anoplasty. High lesions are treated with an initial diverting colostomy followed by a pull-through operation—for example, the Pena and deVries procedure—which has a 70% to 80% success rate.

VOLVULUS

Etiology and Pathogenesis

A dilated, redundant colon is required for the development of volvulus, which causes <10% of colonic obstructions in the United States. Sigmoid volvulus (60% of cases) occurs in elderly and institutionalized persons and in patients with neuropsychiatric disease, chronic constipation, or colonic atony and after laxative abuse. Cecal volvulus (<20% of cases) occurs in younger patients and is thought to be caused by anomalous right colon fixation and a mobile cecum, prior adhesions, pregnancy, or left colon obstruction. Most patients with cecal volvulus have full axial twisting of the associated mesentery and blood vessels, but in some, the cecum is folded in an anterior cephalad direction (cecal bascule). The resulting tension on the colonic wall may produce gangrene. Failure of the mesentery to fuse normally or a narrowing of the mesenteric attachments may rarely lead to volvulus of the transverse colon.

Clinical Features, Diagnosis, and Management

Patients with sigmoid volvulus present with abdominal pain, distention, and obstipation. Gangrene is suggested by fever, signs of peritoneal irritation, or leukocytosis. Abdominal radiography demonstrates an inverted U-shaped loop with a dense line running to the point of torsion. In uncomplicated cases, radiography enhanced with meglumine (Gastrografin) or barium enema may define the site of volvulus and lead to therapeutic reduction of the twisted loop. These techniques are avoided in patients with possible peritonitis, however. In the absence of peritonitis, sigmoidoscopy with placement of a rectal tube may result in dramatic decompression. Elective resection of the involved colon should follow. Emergency surgery is indicated if there is evidence of ischemia, gangrene, or unsuccessful detorsion.

Cecal volvulus is characterized by pain, nausea, vomiting, and obstipation. In many patients, the symptoms are intermittent. Abdominal radiography may show a kidney-shaped, air-filled structure in the left upper quadrant and multiple air-fluid levels in the small intestine. Barium or Gastrografin enema radiography may show the site of torsion but is not indicated if plain radiography provides the diagnosis. Right hemicolectomy with primary anastomosis or cecopexy and cecostomy is recommended if gangrene is not present. Resection, ileostomy, and mucous fistula construction are indicated for cases complicated by gangrene.

Patients with volvulus of the transverse colon manifest symptoms of colonic obstruction. Barium enema radiography provides a diagnosis. Most patients require operative detorsion and resection of the involved colonic segment.

UNCOMPLICATED DIVERTICULOSIS

Etiology and Pathogenesis

Diverticulosis is defined as the presence of diverticula. In the colon, diverticula are of the false or pseudodiverticula type, consisting only of mucosa and serosa with no intervening muscularis. In industrialized nations, 33% to 50% of the population older than 50 years of age has colonic diverticula, which may relate to low levels of dietary fiber. Ninety-five percent of patients with diverticulosis have diverticula in the sigmoid colon. Involvement of the sigmoid and other colonic regions occurs in 24% and of the entire colon in 7%. Sigmoid diverticulosis is accompanied by thickening of the circular muscle, shortening of the taenia coli, and narrowing of the lumen. Diverticula tend to form at points of weakness in the colon wall, usually adjacent to the taenia coli. Most diverticula are 0.1 to 1.0 cm in diameter, whereas larger diverticula may be the consequence of prior diverticulitis. Rectal diverticula are rare because of the presence of the circumferential longitudinal muscle layer.

Development of diverticulosis depends on the strength of the colon wall and the pressure difference between the lumen of the colon and the peritoneal cavity. Muscle thickening in the sigmoid colon likely represents a prediverticular condition resulting from development of high intralumenal pressure in an area of small diameter, with no corresponding increase in wall strength. The elasticity and tensile strength of the colon decrease with age, an effect that is most marked in the sigmoid colon. Deterioration in colonic structural proteins in Ehlers-Danlos and Marfan syndromes may explain the premature development of diverticula in these conditions. The role of primary colonic motor disorders in the pathogenesis of diverticulosis is undefined, and the association of diverticulosis and irritable bowel syndrome is controversial.

Clinical Features, Diagnosis, and Management

Eighty percent to 85% of persons with diverticulosis never develop significant symptoms, although some have mild, intermittent abdominal pain, bloating, flatulence, and altered defecation. The coexistence of irritable bowel syndrome is possible in these patients. Three-fourths of the remaining patients develop diverticulitis and one-fourth report hemorrhage. On barium enema radiography, diverticula appear as contrast-filled colonic protrusions, which may persist after evacuation. The presence of diverticula may reduce the accuracy of barium enema radiography to 50% in the detection coexisting colonic neoplasia. Colonoscopy may reveal diverticular orifices, sigmoid tortuosity, and thickened folds consistent with prior diverticulitis. Therapy for symptomatic but uncomplicated diverticular disease relies on increased intake of dietary fiber or use of fiber supplements.

DIVERTICULITIS

Etiology and Pathogenesis

Diverticulitis or diverticular inflammation begins as peridiverticulitis caused by a microperforation of the colon. As for uncomplicated diverticulosis, the incidence of diverticulitis increases with age. Most cases of diverticulitis occur in sigmoid diverticula, but inflammation of diverticula at other sites, including the rectum and appendix, may occur.

Clinical Features, Diagnosis, and Management

Early manifestations of diverticulitis include pain and tenderness over the site of inflammation (usually in the lower abdomen or pelvis), nausea and vomiting, ileus, fever, a possible palpable mass, and tenderness or a mass effect on rectal examination. Complications of progressive inflammation include abscess, perfo-

TABLE 44-1
Stages of Diverticulitis

Pericolic abscess
Pelvic abscess
Generalized suppurative peritonitis
Fecal peritonitis

ration, fistulization, and obstruction (Table 44-1). CT scans may reveal thickening of the colon wall, pericolic inflammation, fistulae, sinuses, abscess cavities, and obstruction. A CT scan is indicated if the diagnosis is uncertain, abscess or fistula formation is suspected, medical therapy has not produced improvement, or the patient is immunocompromised. Ultrasound is occasionally useful for detection and directed drainage of pericolonic fluid collections. Barium enema radiography is not recommended during the acute attack, although water-soluble contrast enemas may be performed if the diagnosis is in doubt. Careful flexible sigmoidoscopy is used during an episode of suspected diverticulitis to differentiate a neoplasm from an inflammatory diverticular mass, but colonoscopy is contraindicated in cases of acute diverticulitis.

Management of diverticulitis includes fluid replacement, nasogastric suction for ileus or obstruction, and broad-spectrum antibiotics to treat infection with anaerobes, gram-negative bacilli, and gram-positive coliform organisms. Unstable patients should receive ampicillin, gentamicin, and metronidazole, whereas more stable patients with local peritoneal signs may be given ampicillin/sulbactam, imipenem/cilastatin, or ticarcillin/clavulanate for 7 to 10 days. When necessary, clindamycin may substitute for metronidazole, vancomycin for penicillin, and aztreonam for gentamicin. Oral quinolones, amoxicillin/clavulanate, or a cephalosporin may be given to patients who have no peritoneal signs. Indications for surgery are perforation, abscess, fistula, obstruction, recurrent diverticulitis, and inability to exclude carcinoma. In the case of urgent surgery, primary anastomosis is not attempted because anastomotic breakdown is possible. In these cases, elective closure of the colostomy is performed 3 months after recovery. However, a one-stage operation with anastomosis can be performed in the absence of advanced age, sepsis, hemodynamic instability, an unprepared colon, local contamination, friable tissues, malnutrition, steroid use, and poor blood supply. Percutaneous CT-guided abscess drainage may be beneficial preoperatively in patients who are stable and without signs of sepsis. Fistulae usually can be resected in a one-stage procedure, whereas obstruction usually mandates a two-stage operative approach. Surgical resection can reduce the likelihood of recurrent diverticulitis from 30% to between 5% and 10%. In most cases, distal sigmoid resection must be complete to minimize recurrent diverticular inflammation.

DIVERTICULAR HEMORRHAGE

Etiology and Pathogenesis

Massive bleeding from colonic diverticula occurs in 5% of patients; minor bleeding occurs in up to 47%. Hemorrhage from diverticular disease originates from an arterial source (vasa recta), usually within one diverticulum. Although most diverticula are sigmoid in location, half of diverticular hemorrhages emanate from right colonic sources. It has been suggested that traumatic factors induce intimal proliferation, scarring, and rupture of the vasa recta in the absence of inflammatory change.

Clinical Features, Diagnosis, and Management

Passage of large amounts of bright red blood from the rectum with hypotension, tachycardia, or syncope are the usual clinical manifestations of diverticular hemorrhage. A blood transfusion may be required. Spontaneous cessation of bleeding occurs in 80% of patients. Complications of diverticular hemorrhage are related to hypovolemia and involve the heart, brain, kidneys, and lungs. The means of localizing the site of colonic hemorrhage depend on the extent of bleeding. Slow, intermittent hemorrhage is best approached with colonoscopy, whereas torrential bleeding necessitates scintigraphic and angiographic evaluation. Methods to increase the accuracy of colonoscopy include high-flux irrigation and intraoperative colonoscopy with antegrade colonic lavage through a cecostomy. Successful localization of the bleeding site by these methods enables limited resection of the appropriate colonic segment. Scintigraphy with ^{99m}Tc sulfur colloid or ^{99m}Tc-tagged erythrocytes in conjunction with angiography confirms the presence of active bleeding and helps to localize the approximate site of hemorrhage. Selective mesenteric angiography may show extravasation of the contrast agent if the bleeding rate is >0.5 ml per minute. In such cases, the angiocatheter may also be used to deliver intra-arterial vasopressin or synthetic emboli to stop the bleeding in patients who are not surgical candidates.

Minor hemorrhage (<2 units transfused) with spontaneous cessation is managed conservatively. Persistent hemorrhage (2 to 4 units transfused) mandates use of scintigraphy and angiography to localize the site of bleeding and to reduce the rate of blood loss so that surgical resection of the involved segment may be done on a semielective basis. More urgent surgery is necessary for major hemorrhage (>4 units transfused) that does not stop. If the site of bleeding cannot be determined, total abdominal colectomy may be needed.

CHAPTER 45

Motility Disorders of the Colon and Irritable Bowel Syndrome

IDIOPATHIC CONSTIPATION

Etiology and Pathogenesis

Constipation may be reported when the patient experiences infrequent defecation, straining on defecation, hard stools, or a sensation of incomplete fecal evacuation. Difficult evacuation of stools of normal consistency more commonly results from pelvic floor or anal sphincter dysfunction, which is discussed in Chapter 13. Infrequent passage of hard stools is more consistent with colonic inertia or slow-transit constipation, in which motor activity is diffusely impaired throughout the colon. The pathogenesis of idiopathic colonic inertia is uncertain, but the condition has been associated with reduced numbers of high-amplitude peristaltic contractions in the colon. These contractions are believed to be the motor precursor to defecation. Other persons exhibit increased rather than decreased motility, but the contractions are stationary or retrograde, thereby retarding aboral propagation of fecal material. Histologic examination of resected colon specimens from patients with idiopathic constipation often reveals that neurons in the myenteric plexus are absent or abnormal, which suggests overlap with neuropathic intestinal pseudo-obstruction.

Clinical Features, Diagnosis, and Management

Idiopathic colonic inertia is characterized by infrequent defecation and stools that are desiccated and difficult to pass. Severe forms of slow-transit constipation may result in defecation frequencies of less than once per week.

In such patients, other causes of constipation should be excluded. Blood tests for levels of thyroid stimulating hormone and serum calcium are obtained to exclude hypothyroidism and hyperparathyroidism. Structural evaluation of the colon should be performed to exclude mechanical obstruction. Barium enema radiography can exclude blockage and may detect colonic dilation and loss of haustra. Prolonged barium retention suggests diffuse colonic hypomotility. If patients are older than 40 to 45 years of age, colonoscopy should be considered to exclude malignancy, especially with symptoms of recent onset. Demonstration of the rectoanal inhibitory reflex on anorectal manometry, which is the relaxation reflex of the internal anal sphincter with rectal distention, can be used to screen for Hirschsprung's disease in an adult with constipation since childhood. Defecography is a cineradiographic technique in which thick barium paste is placed in the rectum and the process of defecation is recorded. This technique can identify structural problems (e.g., rectoceles or rectal prolapse) or functional disorders (e.g., rectosphincteric dyssynergia) that may manifest as constipation. For patients with colonic inertia, demonstration of delayed colonic transit is mandatory if surgical therapy is considered. The standard assessment of colonic transit is with serial abdominal radiographs obtained after the patient ingests radiopaque markers. The radiopaque marker technique can also be used to estimate regional transit, which will determine if motor function is diffusely or locally impaired. Another technology available in referral centers is colonic transit scintigraphy, which can assess regional and total colonic transit of an orally ingested or intestinally perfused radioisotope. Many clinicians using these methods have observed that a sizable subset of patients reporting constipation have normal colonic transit. Many of these patients exhibit abnormal psychometric profiles and should not be considered for surgical management.

In mild cases of idiopathic constipation, laxative regimens with or without fiber supplements are successful (see Chapter 13). Patients with pelvic floor or anal sphincter dysfunction may respond to biofeedback techniques that retrain coordinated defecation. Structural abnormalities (e.g., rectoceles or rectal prolapse) may be treated surgically. These findings may be secondary to constipation rather than its cause, however; care must be taken in selecting patients for operative intervention. For patients with severe colonic inertia unresponsive to standard laxative therapy and who report worse symptoms after taking fiber supplements, other medical and surgical options exist. Oral isotonic colonic lavage solutions containing polyethylene glycol can be ingested on a daily basis to increase defecation frequency and improve stool consistency. To date, prokinetic agents (e.g., cisapride) have had limited use in treating severe colonic inertia, but this remains an area of active investigation. The prostaglandin E analog misoprostol produces diarrhea in healthy persons—a side effect that has been used to advantage in treating severe idiopathic constipation. Small studies suggest that this agent may increase defecation frequency in patients with constipation refractory to other agents. Subtotal colectomy with ileorectal anastomosis is occasionally necessary for carefully selected patients who have colonic inertia confirmed by colonic transit testing. The long-term results are generally good. In such cases (<10% of referrals to tertiary centers), defecation frequency increases, and stools become softer, although other symptoms (e.g., pain) improve with less reliability. Many centers advocate gastroduodenal manometry to exclude diffuse gastrointestinal dysmotility, which has been reported to decrease response rates to subtotal colectomy.

CHRONIC DIARRHEA

Etiology and Pathogenesis

It has been postulated that diarrhea in the absence of definable inflammatory or infectious disease may result from disordered colonic motor activity. Early descriptions of irritable bowel syndrome (IBS) defined subsets of patients with painless diarrhea, although, in fact, many of these patients may have had lactase deficiency or microscopic/collagenous colitis. In cases of idiopathic diarrhea, transit through the proximal colon may be accelerated, and fecal weights may increase with rapid emptying of the ascending and transverse colon. In carcinoid syndrome, transit through the small intestine, ascending colon, and transverse colon is markedly accelerated, which contributes to diarrhea. Postprandial colonic tone is increased, with carcinoid syndrome potentially reducing the capacity of the colon.

Clinical Features, Diagnosis, and Management

The approach to a patient with diarrhea is discussed in detail in Chapter 12, whereas the evaluation and management of diarrhea-predominant IBS are discussed here. Many of the therapies that reduce diarrhea act by inhibiting motor activity. This includes opiates, which retard transit in the colon and small intestine; anticholinergics and calcium channel antagonists, which blunt increases in postprandial colonic motility; and the somatostatin analog octreotide, which delays transit in the small intestine in addition to exerting antisecretory effects.

ACUTE MEGACOLON

Etiology and Pathogenesis

Acute megacolon occurs in patients with fulminant inflammatory bowel disease, severe infectious colitis, or conditions that produce colonic dilation without evidence of intrinsic colonic disease or obstruction (e.g., trauma, orthopedic surgery, obstetrical procedures, pelvic and abdominal surgery, metabolic imbalance, and neurologic disorders).

Clinical Features, Diagnosis, and Management

Most patients with noninflammatory acute megacolon are middle-aged or older, presenting with abdominal distention and reduced bowel sounds. Fever, peritoneal signs, and leukocytosis usually are absent. Abdominal radiography may show gaseous colonic distention, which is maximal in the cecum. With such a presentation, oral feedings should be stopped, intravenous fluids started, and a nasogastric tube inserted. When colonic obstruction is a consideration, a diatrizoate (Hypaque) enema can be diagnostic and can further stimulate colonic evacuation, thereby reducing distention. Colonic decompression can also be accomplished by passage of a rectal tube or by frequent tap water enemas. Underlying metabolic abnormalities should be corrected. The therapeutic value of medications such as guanethidine, neostigmine, cisapride, and erythromycin is undefined. When the cecal diameter is >11 cm, colonoscopic decompression is attempted to aspirate intralumenal gas. For patients who are refractory to medical and colonoscopic management and who exhibit persistent cecal dilation of >11 cm, tube cecostomy may be efficacious. Exploratory laparotomy is indicated for patients manifesting fever, leukocytosis, or peritoneal signs.

CHRONIC INTESTINAL PSEUDO-OBSTRUCTION

Etiology and Pathogenesis

Chronic intestinal pseudo-obstruction may result from various systemic and hereditary disorders, or it may be idiopathic (see Chapter 37). The pathophysiologic features of pseudo-obstruction may be myopathic, characterized by diffuse intestinal and colonic hypomotility, or neuropathic, characterized by uncoordinated, intense intestinal contractile bursts. Causes of colonic myopathy include familial visceral myopathies, scleroderma, amyloidosis, myotonic and muscular dystrophy, and nonfamilial visceral myopathy. Causes of colonic neuropathy include familial visceral neuropathies, early scleroderma or amyloidosis, diabetes, porphyria, brain stem tumor, multiple sclerosis, dysautonomias, paraneoplastic phenomena, Chagas' disease, and Hirschsprung's disease. The differential diagnosis of colonic pseudo-obstruction in children, other than Hirschsprung's disease, includes Kawasaki's disease, Duchenne's muscular dystrophy, and familial visceral myopathies and neuropathies.

Clinical Features, Diagnosis, and Management

Patients with colonic dysmotility secondary to generalized chronic intestinal pseudo-obstruction usually have symptoms referable to numerous organs. Esophageal involvement produces dysphagia, heartburn, and regurgitation; gastric and small bowel involvement produces nausea, vomiting, bloating, distention, constipation, and diarrhea if there is concurrent bacterial overgrowth in the small intestine. Colonic involvement characteristically produces distention and constipation. Specific causes of intestinal pseudo-obstruction may be associated with bladder dysfunction or autonomic or peripheral neuropathy.

The diagnosis of chronic intestinal pseudo-obstruction depends on recognition of the clinical syndrome and exclusion of mechanical obstruction and mucosal disease by barium enema radiography or colonoscopy. Myopathic disease may produce increased colonic caliber with loss of haustra and poor to nonexistent contractions. In contrast, fluoroscopic inspection during barium enema radiography may show disorganized contractility with neuropathic conditions. Radiography of the urinary tract may define extraintestinal manifestations in some disorders that produce intestinal pseudo-obstruction. Gastroduodenal manometry may demonstrate diffuse hypomotility with myopathic disease or disorganized, intense intestinal bursts with neuropathic disease. Delays in gastric emptying and intestinal and colonic transit are demonstrable using scintigraphic techniques, whereas radiopaque marker techniques are useful for detection of colonic inertia in association with intestinal pseudo-obstruction. In many patients, surgical full-thickness biopsy specimens of the small intestine are necessary to confirm a diagnosis of chronic intestinal pseudo-obstruction.

The goals of treatment of chronic intestinal pseudo-obstruction are to maintain adequate nutrition and restore intestinal propulsion. In mild to moderate disease, diet should be modified: smaller and more frequent meals, liquid or soft foods, and less indigestible fiber. Supplemental iron, folate, calcium, and vitamins (D, K, B_{12}) may be needed. Some patients may benefit from enteral feedings through a nasoenteric tube or jejunostomy. Severely affected patients may need prolonged total parenteral nutrition, which carries long-term risks of infection and liver disease. Oral antibiotics may produce immediate dramatic improvement in patients with bacterial overgrowth in the small intestine. Prokinetic drugs have generally produced disappointing results in treating chronic intestinal pseudo-obstruction. Cisapride has been demonstrated to accelerate intestinal transit in patients with pseudo-obstruction, but its clinical efficacy is unproved. The somatostatin analog octreotide can reduce symptoms and bacterial overgrowth in patients with pseudo-obstruction secondary to scleroderma. Reports from studies of small numbers of patients suggest that this agent may have long-term clinical benefit in patients with pseudo-obstruction secondary to various conditions. Other proposed therapeutic agents include erythromycin, the gonadotropin-releasing hormone analog leuprolide, naloxone, and metoclopramide. In patients with localized pseudo-obstruction, surgical bypass may produce symptomatic improvement (e.g., duodenojejunostomy for megaduodenum, colectomy for isolated colonic pseudo-obstruction). Venting enterostomies may provide relief of gaseous distention and bloating in selected patients who are dependent on total parenteral nutrition.

COLONIC DYSMOTILITY IN OTHER CONDITIONS

Various clinical conditions can have secondary effects on colonic motor activity, contributing to symptoms in affected patients. In malabsorptive conditions, fat delivery to the cecum and ascending colon can induce vigorous high-amplitude contractions and rapid aboral transit. Advanced ulcerative colitis can result in loss of fasting phasic contractions, as observed on manometry, and the loss of haustra, evident on radiography. Colonic transit in colitis is rapid, perhaps reflecting the lack of retarding pressure waves. In contrast, ulcerative proctitis is associated with high-amplitude rectal contractions, which may explain complaints of tenesmus by affected patients. Numerous medications accelerate (laxatives and prokinetics) or delay (opiate antidiarrheals) colonic transit.

IRRITABLE BOWEL SYNDROME

Incidence and Epidemiology

The IBS is a disorder characterized by altered bowel habits with or without abdominal pain in the absence of organic disease. The most widely accepted definition is provided by the Rome criteria: (1) the presence of at least 3 months of continuous or recurrent abdominal pain or discomfort relieved by defecation or associated with a change in the frequency or consistency of the stool; and (2) two of the following symptoms at least 25% of the time: altered stool frequency, altered stool form, altered stool passage, passage of mucus, and bloating or distention (Table 45-1). Using these criteria, 9% to 22% of the United States population reports symptoms that would be diagnostic for IBS. Only a small fraction of this number seek medical attention, however, suggesting that other factors determine the decision to obtain the advice of a physician. Patients with IBS

TABLE 45-1
Criteria for Diagnosing Irritable Bowel Syndrome

At least 3 mos of the following continuous symptoms:
Abdominal pain or discomfort that is relieved by defecation or associated with a
change in frequency or consistency of stool
Disturbed defecation involving two or more of the following characteristics at least
25% of the time:
Altered stool frequency
Altered stool form (e.g., lumpy, hard, loose, or watery)
Altered stool passage (e.g., straining, urgency, or feeling of incomplete evacuation)
Passage of mucus
Bloating or feeling of abdominal distention

---

usually present before 45 years of age. The disease is more common in women
and is now recognized as a significant problem in the elderly.

Etiology and Pathogenesis

The pathogenesis of IBS is poorly understood, but it probably involves altered
gastrointestinal motor and sensory function and psychological disturbances.

Gastrointestinal Motor Abnormalities

Studies have not convincingly demonstrated abnormalities of myoelectric and
motor activity in the colon under basal conditions; however, colonic motility
may be significantly disturbed with stimulation. The gastrocolonic response, the
increase in colon motor activity after meal ingestion, may be more intense and
prolonged in IBS. Similarly, exaggerated colonic motor responses may be
observed in patients with IBS after cholecystokinin injection, rectal balloon inflation, or colonic bile acid perfusion. Minor abnormalities in migrating motor
complex activity and postprandial motor activity in the small intestine are
demonstrable in IBS but likely have little pathogenic role, whereas increases in
clustered contractions and intense propagating contractions in the small intestine have been reported. As with the colon, the small intestine exhibits increased
contractile responses to cholecystokinin and neostigmine. Abnormalities in
esophageal motility, gastric motor and myoelectric activity, and gallbladder contractile function have been reported in subsets of patients with IBS.

Gastrointestinal Sensory Abnormalities

The most active area of investigation into the pathogenesis of IBS is in the field
of visceral hypersensitivity. Under basal conditions, patients with IBS often perceive physiologic motor activity in the small intestine that healthy controls do not
sense. A major complaint of patients with IBS is that of a sensation of increased
gas. After rigorous investigation, patients were found not to exhibit increased gastrointestinal gas, but rather sense lower volumes of gas infusion than asymptomatic persons. Studies of balloon inflation in the rectum, colon, and other regions

demonstrate abnormal perception of distention in 60% to 94% of patients (especially those with diarrhea), including increased discomfort and abnormal referral patterns in which inflation in one region is perceived to be at a distant anatomic site. Conversely, patients with IBS have normal sensitivity to noxious cutaneous stimulation, localizing the defect to the visceral nervous system.

Abnormal Psychological Factors

The central nervous system can have potent effects on gastrointestinal motor function. In healthy volunteers, painful somatic stimulation and induction of emotional stress can increase rectal contractions, alter physiologic motor patterns in the small intestine, and delay gastric emptying. It has been postulated that the presence of psychological disturbances is a major determinant of a patient's decision to seek medical care, whereas the majority of persons with IBS-like symptoms and normal psychosocial functioning recognize the functional nature of symptoms without reliance on the care of a physician. Abnormal psychiatric features, including major depression, somatization disorder, anxiety disorder, panic disorder, neuroticism, hostility, hypochondriasis, and phobias, are reported in up to 80% of patients with IBS. Psychiatric features predate or occur simultaneously with the onset of bowel symptoms, indicating that IBS is not the cause of psychological dysfunction. Studies have reported that women with IBS have a high prevalence (30% to 50%) of physical or sexual abuse in childhood, a rate three to eleven times that of the control population.

Other Proposed Pathogenic Factors

Other factors in the genesis of symptoms of IBS may be carbohydrate malabsorption, food intolerance, bile salt–induced colonic secretion and dysmotility, and altered gastrointestinal hormone release. None of these factors has been shown convincingly to relate to symptom development in more than a very small subset of patients with IBS, however.

Clinical Features

The intensity, location, and timing of abdominal pain in patients with IBS are highly variable. The pain may be so intense as to interfere with daily activities. Pain is most often described as crampy or achy, but sharp, dull, and gaslike pains are also reported. Abdominal pain in IBS may be exacerbated by meal ingestion or by stress and may be relieved by defecation or passage of flatus. Despite this, the pain rarely leads to significant weight loss or malnutrition, and it does not interrupt sleep.

By definition, patients with IBS present with alterations in bowel function, including constipation, diarrhea, or constipation alternating with diarrhea. With constipation-predominant IBS, patients report stools that are hard or pelletlike and difficult to pass, often resulting in a sensation of incomplete fecal evacuation. In patients who have diarrhea, stools are loose and frequent but of normal daily volume; movements often occur early in the morning, after a meal, and with stress. Passage of fecal mucus is reported by 50% of patients. The passage of blood, nocturnal diarrhea, malabsorption, or weight loss warrants an aggressive search for organic disease.

Patients with IBS frequently report symptoms referable to other organs. Up to 50% report heartburn, early satiety, nausea, and vomiting, whereas 87% experience dyspepsia. High incidences of dysfunction of the genitourinary organs (dysmenorrhea, dyspareunia, impotence, urinary frequency, incomplete urinary evacuation), fibromyalgia, low back pain, headaches, fatigue, insomnia, and impaired concentration have been reported with IBS.

Physical examination of patients with IBS is usually unimpressive. The patient may appear anxious and have cold, clammy hands. Abdominal palpation may reveal mild, diffuse tenderness or a tender bowel loop. The presence of organomegaly, adenopathy, or occult fecal blood is not consistent with a diagnosis of IBS.

Findings on Diagnostic Testing

The diagnosis of IBS involves the careful exclusion of organic disease and is tailored to the individual patient based on the presenting symptoms and age. Patients with constipation-predominant, diarrhea-predominant, or pain-predominant patterns are managed differently.

Laboratory Studies

Most patients should undergo a minimal laboratory evaluation to help exclude inflammatory or neoplastic disease. Anemia, leukocytosis, or leukopenia determined by a complete blood cell count suggest organic disease, as does an elevated sedimentation rate.

Structural Studies

Sigmoidoscopy should be performed in most patients with suspected IBS. In constipated patients, sigmoidoscopy helps to exclude obstructive lesions, and in patients with diarrhea-predominant IBS, it helps to assess for inflammatory bowel disease or other forms of colitis. In patients with diarrhea and a normal sigmoidoscopic appearance, random biopsies of the colon can exclude microscopic or collagenous colitis as diagnostic possibilities. In patients older than 40 to 45 years with new onset of symptoms, complete evaluation of the colon with barium enema radiography or colonoscopy should be performed to exclude malignancy.

Approach to Patients with Constipation-Predominant Irritable Bowel Syndrome

Selected patients should undergo blood tests to exclude hypothyroidism and hyperparathyroidism. If constipation is refractory to medical management, function tests of colonic motor activity with radiopaque marker techniques, anorectal manometry, and defecography can exclude colonic inertia, pelvic floor abnormalities, and anal sphincter dysfunction.

Approach to Patients with Diarrhea-Predominant Irritable Bowel Syndrome

For patients who have recently traveled, used antibiotics, or ingested well water, stool samples should be obtained for leukocyte count, examination for ova and parasites, and culture for *Clostridium difficile*. In some cases, duodenal aspiration to test for *Giardia* may be needed. Biopsy of the small intestine and upper gastrointestinal barium radiography are useful if inflammatory diseases (e.g., celiac sprue or Crohn's disease) are suspected. Hyperthyroidism should be considered in anxious patients with weight loss or palpitations. Lactase deficiency can be excluded with a hydrogen breath test or a trial on a lactose-free diet. Persistence of diarrhea during fasting warrants a search for secretory processes. Screening for laxative use should be considered, as laxative abuse is common in patients with unexplained diarrhea.

Approach to Patients with Pain-Predominant Irritable Bowel Syndrome

Most patients with pain-predominant IBS require only a screening workup, but a rare patient may need further evaluation. Upper gastrointestinal endoscopy is indicated for severe dyspepsia or heartburn. Liver chemistry studies and ultrasound are performed for suspected biliary tract disease. Computed tomographic scans are obtained if malignancy is a concern, whereas gastric scintigraphy or gastroduodenal manometry may be indicated in a patient with prominent nausea, vomiting, or early satiety. In very rare instances, screening for porphyria or heavy metal intoxication is performed.

Management and Course

Once the diagnosis of IBS is secured, the physician should offer reassurance and education to the patient, imparting an awareness that IBS is a functional disorder without long-term health risks. In 25% of cases, this approach is sufficient. Nonetheless, 75% of patients with IBS receive medications to reduce their symptoms, even though no medication has been shown convincingly to have positive therapeutic effects in the IBS population as a whole.

Medical Therapy

Medication regimens for patients with IBS should be customized to treat the predominant symptoms of each individual. The key to managing constipation-predominant IBS is to increase stool water and bulk, thereby reducing the effort needed for defecation. A high-fiber diet is prescribed, and often bulking agents (e.g., bran, psyllium, methylcellulose, or polycarbophil) are introduced gradually. Patients should be cautioned that fiber supplementation may take several weeks to produce a satisfactory result and that gas and distention may result if large doses are ingested rapidly. Those patients who respond inadequately are given osmotic laxatives such as milk of magnesia or a poorly absorbed sugar (e.g., lactulose, sorbitol). Prokinetic agents (e.g., cisapride) may be useful in some patients, but their action usually is weak.

The management of diarrhea-predominant IBS centers on reducing defecation frequency and urgency and improving stool consistency. Opiate agents (e.g., loperamide, diphenoxylate with atropine) are most effective. Fiber supplements are often given, but controlled trials demonstrate little benefit for patients prone to diarrhea. Antispasmodic drugs such as anticholinergics and calcium channel antagonists inhibit the gastrocolonic response and are useful in treating patients with postprandial diarrhea. Other efficacious medications for diarrhea-predominant IBS include tricyclic antidepressants, cholestyramine, serotonin

TABLE 45-2
Foods and Flatus Production

Normoflatulogenic foods
  Meat, poultry, and fish
  Vegetables (e.g., lettuce, cucumber, broccoli, pepper, avocado, cauliflower, tomato, asparagus, zucchini, okra, olives)
  Fruits (e.g., cantaloupe, grapes, berries)
  Carbohydrates (e.g., rice, corn chips, potato chips, popcorn, graham crackers)
  Nuts
  Miscellaneous (e.g., eggs, nonmilk chocolate, gelatin, fruit ice)
Moderately flatulogenic foods
  Pastries
  Potatoes
  Eggplant
  Citrus
  Apple bread
Extremely flatulogenic foods
  Milk and milk products
  Vegetables (e.g., onions, beans, celery, carrots, Brussels sprouts)
  Fruits (e.g., raisins, bananas, apricots, prune juice)
  Miscellaneous (e.g., pretzels, bagels, wheat germ)

antagonists (e.g., ondansetron), and disodium cromoglycate for rare cases of food hypersensitivity.

Severe abdominal pain represents the most difficult symptom to treat in patients with IBS. Addictive narcotics should not be administered. Fiber supplements are often given for this indication, although the data supporting the practice are unconvincing. Patients with excess gas may be offered dietary advice (Table 45-2). Antispasmodics are useful in some patients, especially those with postprandial pain. Tricyclic antidepressants (and possibly serotonin reuptake inhibitors) may benefit a sizable subset of patients with pain-predominant IBS. Dyspepsia may respond to prokinetic agents (e.g., cisapride) or acid-suppressive medications (e.g., H_2-receptor antagonists).

Other classes of medications have been advocated for treating IBS. Antigas products, such as simethicone, activated charcoal, and α-galactosidases (Beano), have been proposed for patients with significant distention, but controlled trials of these agents have not been performed. The gonadotropin-releasing hormone analog leuprolide has been recommended for patients with severe pain. However, this agent induces amenorrhea and osteoporosis and should be used with care. Tranquilizers, including benzodiazepines, have been prescribed for patients with IBS for decades, but their use is not recommended because of the potential for abuse, development of tolerance, and worsening of underlying depression. The area of most active pharmacologic research involves agents that reduce the visceral hypersensitivity present in most patients with IBS. To date, granisetron ($5-HT_3$ antagonist) and octreotide (somatostatin analog) have been shown to reduce perception of rectal distention, but their efficacy has not been shown convincingly in placebo-controlled trials. A peripheral opiate agonist, fedotozine, has shown efficacy in placebo-controlled trials in Europe, but it is not yet available in the United States. Alternative medical approaches to treatment of IBS, including oral lactobacillus, herbal treatments, and ayurvedic preparations have not proven effective.

Psychotherapy, Biofeedback, and Hypnosis

The involvement of psychiatrists and psychologists has been reserved for patients with IBS exhibiting clear psychosocial dysfunctional behavior; some clinicians advocate a broader role for such specialists. Some studies of psychotherapy report reductions in abdominal pain, diarrhea, and somatic symptoms as well as anxiety. Biofeedback and relaxation training may reduce symptoms. Hypnosis has been effective in selected patients with medically refractory symptoms. Consistent problems with most of these investigations include poor definitions of symptom response or lack of appropriate control populations.

Patient Outcome

IBS usually persists in a waxing and waning fashion for many years. Despite this, the quality of life for patients with IBS can be improved by appropriate physician involvement; patients can cope with their symptoms and experience an improved sense of well-being. Patients likely to report good outcomes include those who are male, have a brief history of symptoms, have an acute symptom onset, exhibit predominant constipation, and have a good initial response to therapy.

CHAPTER 46

Bacterial Infections of the Colon

INFECTION WITH *SHIGELLA* SPECIES

Incidence and Epidemiology

Approximately 15,000 cases of shigellosis are reported annually in the United States. Of these, 90% result from infection with *Shigella sonnei* or *Shigella flexneri*. Shigellosis is most common in children between the ages 6 months and 5 years. *S sonnei* usually is the cause, whereas *S flexneri* is the more common isolate in persons older than 15 years. The organism is transmitted by fecal-oral contact; via infected food or water; during travel; or in chronic care institutions, day care centers, or nursing homes. *S dysenteriae* has produced epidemic shigellosis.

Etiology and Pathogenesis

Shigella species are aerobic, nonmotile, glucose-fermenting, gram-negative rods that are highly contagious, causing diarrhea after ingestion of as few as 180 organisms. Host resistance factors include gastric acidity and normal colonic microflora. *Shigella* species cause damage by two mechanisms: invasion of colonic epithelium, which is dependent on a plasmid-mediated virulence factor, and production of enterotoxin, which is not essential for colitis but which enhances virulence. Acute shigellosis produces an intense neutrophilic and mononuclear cell lamina propria infiltrate, hemorrhage, ulcers, mucus depletion, and occasional crypt abscesses. The infection most severely affects the rectosigmoid, but pancolitis is observed in 15% of cases. *Shigella* toxin has an A-B subunit structure that binds to specific cell receptors. After binding, the toxin is internalized, where it inhibits cellular protein synthesis and elicits fluid secretion. Serum and secretory antibodies to *Shigella* organisms are produced after exposure to the organism. They appear to have some protective effect against subsequent clinical attacks.

Clinical Features

Patients with dysentery caused by *Shigella* species present with acute bloody diarrhea and tenesmus; passage of mucus and development of fever occur 1 to 3 days after exposure. The infection may exhibit a two-phase pattern: an initial small bowel phase of severe watery diarrhea followed by a colonic phase of passage of smaller volumes of blood-tinged mucus or a few small blood clots. Symptoms may be more severe in malnourished children or debilitated adults, whereas some healthy individuals may note only mild diarrhea. The clinical course usually is self-limited, with resolution of diarrhea within 1 week (2 to 3 days in children), but some individuals may be symptomatic for 1 month. Physical examination shows lower abdominal tenderness with normal or increased bowel sounds. Dehydration may occur in some cases, but peritoneal findings are rare and should suggest other diagnoses.

Infection with *Shigella* species may be associated with extragastrointestinal complications. Bacteremia occurs primarily in malnourished children and carries a 20% mortality as a result of renal failure, hemolysis, thrombocytopenia, gastrointestinal hemorrhage, and shock. Reiter's syndrome, a triad of arthritis, urethritis, and conjunctivitis, occurs most commonly in men between the ages of 20 and 40 years, and follows 2 to 4 weeks after infection with *Shigella* species (or certain strains of *Salmonella*, *Yersinia*, or *Campylobacter*). The syndrome, which has predilection for persons with the HLA-B27 phenotype, has a variable clinical presentation; limited forms are common, with little or no urethritis. The arthritic manifestations, which are distributed asymmetrically, are often chronic and relapsing. They may be associated with periostitis, tendonitis, heel spurs, and plantar fasciitis. They are managed with NSAIDs. Hemolytic-uremic syndrome may complicate infections with *Shigella* and *Escherichia coli*, with a mortality rate of >50%. It is characterized by acute hemolysis, renal failure, uremia, and disseminated intravascular coagulation. It has been postulated that hemolytic-uremic syndrome results from systemic effects of endotoxin.

Findings on Diagnostic Testing

Laboratory studies may reveal mild elevations in hematocrit, sodium, and urea nitrogen levels, indicative of volume depletion, although leukocytosis is rare. Stool examination reveals fecal leukocytes and erythrocytes. The laboratory diagnosis of infection with *Shigella* species is made by culture of a fresh fecal specimen.

Management and Course

Antibiotics reduce the duration and severity of symptoms in shigellosis and shorten the period of fecal excretion of the organism; they are therefore recommended for all patients with diarrhea, except those with mild symptoms (Table 46-1). Because antibiotic-resistant organisms are prevalent, the choice of an antibiotic to treat shigellosis ideally should be based on in vitro sensitivity testing. However, there is not always time for such testing with acute and severe disease. Ciprofloxacin (500 mg twice daily,) tetracycline (500 mg four times daily), ampicillin (500 mg four times daily), and trimethoprim-sulfamethoxazole (twice daily for 5 days) are effective against the dysentery. In addition, oral or intravenous rehydration should be given. Antidiarrheal agents are contraindicated because they may prolong symptoms and delay clearance of the organism. Oral vaccines against infection with *Shigella* organisms are being developed.

TABLE 46-1
Effectiveness of Antibiotic Therapy in Enteric Infections

DEGREE OF EFFECTIVENESS	INFECTION
Very effective	Typhoid fever
Effective	Shigellosis
	Cholera
	Clostridium difficile
	Traveler's diarrhea
	Giardiasis
	Amebiasis
Ineffective or minimally effective	Diarrhea caused by *Campylobacter* spp.
	Intestinal salmonellosis
	Cryptosporidiosis
	Enterohemorrhagic *Escherichia coli*

INFECTION WITH *CAMPYLOBACTER* SPECIES

Incidence and Epidemiology

Campylobacter jejuni (and *Campylobacter coli*) cause up to 20% of cases of bacterial dysentery in the United States. The organism is transmitted by ingestion of contaminated poultry, eggs, raw milk, and water, and exposure to sick pets.

Etiology and Pathogenesis

Campylobacter species are motile, gram-negative rods that possess oxidase and catalase activity. The histopathologic course of acute infection suggests that *C jejuni* invades and destroys epithelial cells, much like *Shigella* species. Some strains produce a cytotoxin and a heat-labile enterotoxin that stimulates secretion. Acute infection with *Campylobacter* species appears to confer short-term immunity against subsequent infection.

Clinical Features

Children younger than 5 years are most susceptible to infections caused by *Campylobacter* organisms, followed by young adults. The spectrum of disease ranges from asymptomatic carriage to life-threatening colitis with toxic megacolon. Fatigue and myalgia develop 1 to 6 days after exposure. This is followed by abdominal cramps, nausea, anorexia, tenesmus, and diarrhea, which may be watery or bloody. Although the disease usually resolves within 1 week, some patients experience a relapsing course similar to ulcerative colitis. Physical examination may reveal localized tenderness suggestive of appendicitis. Complications of infections with *Campylobacter* species include bacteremia, toxic megacolon, Reiter's syndrome, and hemolytic-uremic syndrome. Recurrent infection in patients with acquired immunodeficiency syndrome (AIDS) may stem from persistence of the organism in the gallbladder.

Findings on Diagnostic Testing

Laboratory studies show evidence of volume depletion and leukocytosis in some patients infected with *Campylobacter* species. Stool examination reveals leukocytes and erythrocytes. The diagnosis is confirmed by positive stool cultures.

Management and Course

The mainstay of therapy for infections with *Campylobacter* species is fluid and electrolyte replacement. Erythromycin (250 mg four times daily for 5 days) is often given for severe dysentery or relapsing infection, but there is no evidence that the antibiotic reduces the duration or severity of symptoms. Ciprofloxacin is an alternate choice, but quinolone-resistant strains have been described.

COLITIS INDUCED BY *ESCHERICHIA COLI*

Enteroinvasive Escherichia coli

Etiology and Pathogenesis

Enteroinvasive *E coli* (EIEC) is an important cause of traveler's diarrhea, foodborne gastroenteritis, and diarrhea in children in developing countries. This strain of *E coli* invades and proliferates within colonocytes, causing cell death, because of the presence of virulence plasmids. The roles of cytotoxins and enterotoxins elaborated by EIEC are unknown.

Clinical Features, Diagnosis, and Management

Patients with EIEC report fever, malaise, anorexia, abdominal cramps, and watery diarrhea followed by passage of blood-tinged stool or mucus. The disease is usually self-limited and uncomplicated. Fecal blood and leukocytes are present in many but not all patients. Laboratory confirmation of EIEC in clinical practice requires serotyping of *E coli* O and H antigens. The role of antibiotic therapy in EIEC infection is undefined, but it is reasonable to give trimethoprim-sulfamethoxazole, ampicillin, or ciprofloxacin to patients with dysentery.

Enterohemorrhagic Escherichia coli

Etiology and Pathogenesis

Infection with enterohemorrhagic *E coli* (EHEC) is caused by the O157:H7 strain, which can be found in poorly cooked ground beef, unpasteurized dairy products, and fecally contaminated water. Outbreaks are clustered in schools, day care centers, and nursing homes. EHEC does not invade colonic epithelium, but produces two Shiga-like toxins that are enterotoxic and cytotoxic by inhibiting the synthesis of cellular protein.

Clinical Features, Diagnosis, and Management

The typical manifestations of infections with EHEC are watery diarrhea and cramps, followed by bloody diarrhea 12 to 24 hours later. The severity of blood loss ranges from blood-tinged mucus to passage of large clots. Fever and vomiting occur in <25% of cases. Complications of infection with EHEC include hemolytic-uremic syndrome and thrombotic thrombocytopenic purpura, which occur most commonly in children or in those with severe bleeding and leukocytosis (white blood cell count of more than 20,000 per µl). Fecal examination reveals leukocytes and erythrocytes. *E coli* O157:H7 can be cultured on sorbitol-MacConkey medium. Recovery without sequelae is the usual outcome, although patients with hemolytic-uremic syndrome or thrombotic thrombocytopenic purpura may have long-term renal failure or neurologic deficits. Antibiotics are not recommended for this infection, because they may increase toxin production.

ENTEROCOLITIS INDUCED BY *CLOSTRIDIUM DIFFICILE*

Incidence and Epidemiology

Diarrhea and colitis caused by *Clostridium difficile* result most commonly from hospital-acquired infection and less commonly from oral antibiotic regimens administered at home. The incidence of *C difficile* carriage in patients ranges from 7% to 21%; however, diarrhea develops in only one-third of these patients. The organism can be cultured from bathrooms, toilets, scales, mops, and hands and shoes of hospital personnel. *C difficile* is also prevalent in chronic care facilities, nursing homes, newborn nurseries, and neonatal intensive care units. To reduce transmission of *C difficile*, hospital personnel should wear disposable gloves when handling stool or linen, and they should wash their hands after patient contact. Incontinent patients with diarrhea caused by *C difficile* should be placed in isolation. Bleach solutions may be effective against environmental contamination.

Etiology and Pathogenesis

C difficile is a gram-positive, obligate anaerobic rod that does not colonize the gastrointestinal tract unless the endogenous microflora has been altered by antibiotics, cancer chemotherapy, or the presence of another pathogen (e.g., *Salmonella* or *Shigella* species). The organism produces colonic damage by releasing two potent exotoxins. Toxin B possesses cytopathic activity against fibroblasts and other cells in culture, but it is not believed to be primarily responsible for colonic damage. Toxin A, the enterotoxin of *C difficile*, possesses lethal properties for laboratory animals and is cytotoxic for cultured fibroblasts. Toxin A produces inflammation of the lamina propria and elicits secretion of an inflammatory exudate containing neutrophils, lymphocytes, erythrocytes, proteins, and mucus.

TABLE 46-2
Tests for *Clostridium difficile* and Its Cytotoxin in Patients with Various Manifestations of Infection with *C difficile*

CONDITION	*C DIFFICILE* CULTURE (% POSITIVE)	*C DIFFICILE* CYTOTOXIN (% POSITIVE)
Pseudomembranous colitis	95–100	95–100
Colitis without pseudomembranes	75–90	60–75
Antibiotic-associated diarrhea	20–40	15–30
Hospitalized adults, asymptomatic	10–15	2
Healthy adults	0–3	0
Healthy neonates and children	30–80	25–50

Clinical Features

In addition to existing in a symptomatic carrier state, *C difficile* produces a spectrum of disease ranging from, in order of decreasing severity, pseudomembranous colitis, antibiotic-associated colitis without pseudomembranes, to antibiotic-associated diarrhea. With pseudomembranous colitis, diarrhea and cramps usually begin during the first week of antibiotic therapy, although symptom onset as late as 6 weeks is reported. Other symptoms include nausea, vomiting, tenesmus, fever, and dehydration. Occult fecal blood loss is common but hematochezia is rare. In severe cases, pseudomembranous colitis may progress to toxic megacolon, perforation, and peritonitis. Findings suggestive of a fulminant course include fever, tachycardia, localized tenderness, guarding, ascites, decreased bowel sounds, and signs of toxemia.

The clinical presentation of antibiotic-associated colitis without pseudomembranes is milder, with insidious development of fecal urgency, cramps, watery diarrhea, malaise, fever, and abdominal tenderness. Antibiotic-associated diarrhea without colitis is characterized by the absence of systemic findings, and by diarrhea that resolves when antibiotics are stopped. Infection with *C difficile* can also complicate the course of inflammatory bowel disease. Therefore, stool toxin assay should be performed on patients with Crohn's disease or ulcerative colitis who have unexplained relapses, especially after recent exposure to antibiotics.

Findings on Diagnostic Testing

Stool examination reveals leukocytes in 50% of patients with pseudomembranous colitis, but fecal leukocytes are less common with milder infections caused by *C difficile*. The diagnostic test of choice for *C difficile* is the stool cytotoxin assay. If stools are positive for toxin, cellular rounding or detachment of cultured human fibroblasts is observed after an incubation of 24 to 48 hours. The cytotoxin assay is positive in 95% to 100% of patients with pseudomembranous colitis and in 60% to 75% of patients with colitis without pseudomembranes. Positive assays are less frequent with milder disease (Table 46-2). Latex bead agglutination assays and rapid enzyme immunoassays have been introduced to expedite the diagnosis, and in some cases may be performed in lieu of the tissue culture assay. Although sensitive for detection of infection with *C difficile*, positive stool cultures do not differentiate asymptomatic carriers from patients with colitis; thus, their utility is limited.

Sigmoidoscopy is not required to diagnose infection with *C difficile*, but the finding of pseudomembranes on sigmoidoscopy can provide the impetus to initiate appropriate therapy while awaiting results of the stool toxin assay. This can be important for very ill hospitalized patients in whom diagnostic delay may have adverse consequences. Pseudomembranes appear as yellow-white raised plaques 2 to 5 mm in diameter, which may become confluent with severe disease. Although rectal sparing occurs in 30% of patients, colonoscopy is only rarely needed for diagnosis. Examination of a biopsy specimen of a pseudomembrane reveals a summit lesion, an exudate of fibrin, mucus, and inflammatory cells erupting from an epithelial microulceration.

Management and Course

Because of the significant morbidity of colitis associated with *C difficile*, most patients are given antibiotics to eradicate the organism from stools. Oral vancomycin (125 mg four times daily) can effectively eradicate *C difficile* after 1 week of therapy. Although resistant organisms have not been described, vancomycin is not the initial drug of choice because of its cost. For this reason, metronidazole (250 mg four times daily for 10 days) is the recommended initial course for treating pseudomembranous colitis. In patients with ileus, intravenous metronidazole is an alternate therapy. Other antibiotics with efficacy against *C difficile* include bacitracin and teicoplanin. Opiate antidiarrheals (e.g., loperamide, diphenoxylate with atropine) are not recommended in the treatment of severe colitis, but may be useful in mild cases.

Fifteen percent to 20% of patients with pseudomembranous colitis relapse after successful antibiotic treatment, usually 1 to 5 weeks after completion of therapy. The mechanisms for this phenomenon are poorly understood, although antibiotic resistance is not a factor. Possible causes include persistence of spores or vegetative forms of the organism, or reinfection from environmental sources. Mild relapses usually do not require a second course of antibiotics. Regimens proposed for recurrent pseudomembranous colitis include prolonged courses (4 to 6 weeks) of oral vancomycin, oral vancomycin plus rifampicin, or vancomycin and an anion exchange resin (e.g., cholestyramine, colestipol) that binds the *C difficile* toxins. Because resins also bind vancomycin and metronidazole, they should be administered hours before or after the antibiotic. In refractory cases, oral administration of nonpathogenic organisms (e.g., *Saccharomyces boulardii*) that inhibit growth of *C difficile* has been successful in pathogen eradication.

SEXUALLY TRANSMITTED COLORECTAL PATHOGENS

Gonorrheal Proctitis

Asymptomatic rectal carriage of *Neisseria gonorrhoeae* is common in promiscuous gay men. The symptoms of acute rectal gonorrhea include a creamy rectal discharge, hematochezia, constipation or obstipation, and anal dyspareunia. It may be complicated by perirectal abscesses, fistulae, strictures, and sepsis. Sigmoidoscopy reveals rectal erythema and friability. The diagnosis of gonococcal proctitis is based on positive results of cultures obtained from rectal swabs. A second swab study can be performed using Gram's stain, but this technique misses the diagnosis in 50% of cases. Therapies for rectal gonorrhea that produce cures in 95% of cases include intramuscular procaine penicillin G (4.8 million units) with oral probenecid (1.0 g) or intramuscular spectinomycin (2.0 g). Third-generation cephalosporins are effective against penicillin-resistant strains.

Proctitis Caused by Chlamydia trachomatis

Infection with *Chlamydia trachomatis*, the causative agent of lymphogranuloma venereum, accounts for 20% of proctitis in gay men. Asymptomatic carriage of the organism occurs in 2% to 5% of gay men. Patients with acute chlamydial proctitis present with bloody diarrhea, mucopurulent discharge, and, less commonly, rectal pain, tenesmus, constipation, and fistulae. Physical examination may reveal tender, enlarged inguinal lymph nodes (buboes). Biopsy specimens of the rectum show granulomatous inflammation with giant cells, inflammation with neutrophils, eosinophils, and crypt abscesses, and visible organisms on Giemsa staining. The diagnosis of proctitis caused by *C trachomatis* is confirmed by culture of rectal swabs. The treatment of choice is tetracycline, 500 mg four times daily for 2 to 3 weeks.

Proctitis Caused by Herpes Simplex Virus

Proctitis cased by herpes simplex virus (HSV) presents with intense anal pain, tenderness, tenesmus, discharge, constipation, urinary symptoms (retention, weak stream), pain (in the abdomen, buttocks, and thighs), impotence, and sacral paresthesias. Sigmoidoscopy during acute infection may reveal focal ulcers and vesicles. Biopsy specimens show acute and chronic inflammation, microabscesses, and superficial ulcerations. The diagnosis of proctitis caused by HSV depends on viral isolation from rectal swabs or biopsy specimens. Acyclovir appears to hasten clinical recovery in this condition.

Anorectal Syphilis

Proctitis caused by *Treponema pallidum* is characterized by rectal pain, discharge, and tenesmus. Primary syphilis may produce anal chancres, the exudate of which may reveal spirochetes on dark-field microscopic examination. Secondary syphilis produces flat, wartlike perianal and penile lesions called condylomata lata. The diagnosis of syphilis is confirmed by serologic testing, although false-negative tests are common in early disease. Therapy for anorectal syphilis includes intramuscular benzathine penicillin, 2.4 million units (single dose), or tetracycline, 500 mg four times daily for 15 days.

Anal Warts

Anal warts or condyloma acuminata are verrucous, skin-colored or pink papilliform skin lesions resulting from infection with human papilloma virus. Warts occur on the glans penis in men and on the labia, vulva, and cervix in women. Anal warts in men are frequently but not always associated with receptive anal intercourse. They may cause strictures, discharge, and bleeding. Therapies for anal warts include podophyllin, cryotherapy, and surgical fulguration, but recurrences and post-therapy anal strictures are common.

CHAPTER 47

Inflammatory Bowel Disease

INCIDENCE AND EPIDEMIOLOGY

The chronic inflammatory bowel diseases (IBDs) include ulcerative colitis, a disorder in which inflammation affects the mucosa and submucosa of the colon, and Crohn's disease, in which inflammation is transmural and may involve any or all segments of the gastrointestinal tract. The incidence of ulcerative colitis is 2 to 10 per 100,000 population in the United States, whereas the incidence of Crohn's disease is 1 to 6 per 100,000. There is an increased incidence of IBD in relatives of patients with IBD, indicative of a genetic predisposition. Both ulcerative colitis and Crohn's disease are more prevalent in Jews (especially Ashkenazi Jews) and less common in persons of black American heritage. The peak age of onset of both diseases is between 15 and 25 years, with a second peak sometimes set between 55 and 65 years of age. Women are affected as often or more often than men, depending on the series. Ulcerative colitis is more common than Crohn's disease in children younger than 10 years of age. Among patients with ulcerative colitis, there is a lower incidence of tobacco smoking than in the general population, whereas the incidence of smoking in patients with Crohn's disease patients is as high or higher than in the general population.

ETIOLOGY AND PATHOGENESIS

Potential Causes

There is clear evidence of immune system activation in IBD, with infiltration of the lamina propria with lymphocytes, macrophages, and other cells, although the antigenic trigger is unknown. Various viruses and bacteria (e.g., measles virus, *Mycobacterium paratuberculosis*) have been proposed as triggers, but there is little support for any specific infectious cause of IBD. A second hypothesis is that some dietary antigen or normally nonpathogenic microbial agent activates an abnormal immune response. As a result of failure of normal suppressor mechanisms, immune activation in IBD may be an inappropriately vigorous and prolonged response to a normal lumenal antigen. In healthy persons, lumenal antigens are exposed only to M cells overlying lymphoid tissue, whereas in those with IBD, because of epithelial destruction, lumenal antigens have access to the immune cells of the lamina propria, thus triggering aberrant immune responses. A third hypothesis is that the trigger in IBD is an autoantigen expressed on the patient's intestinal epithelium. In this theory, the patient mounts an initial immune response against a lumenal antigen, which then persists and may be amplified because of antigenic similarity between the lumenal antigen and host proteins. This autoimmune hypothesis involves the destruction of the epithelial cells by antibody-dependent cellular cytotoxicity or direct cell-mediated cytotoxicity. The presence of autoantibodies (e.g., antineutrophil cytoplasmic antibodies) in some patients with IBD is supportive of this hypothesis, but these antibodies are found in patients who have conditions with no intestinal involvement.

The Immune Response

Various immune system mechanisms are altered in IBD. Cell-mediated immune responses may be involved in the pathogenesis of IBD, but alterations in blood lymphocyte populations usually result from medication therapy or malnutrition, not the diseases themselves. There is increased antibody secretion by intestinal mononuclear cells in IBD, especially of the IgM and IgG classes, in contrast to the IgA secreted by normal mucosa. Ulcerative colitis is associated with increased production of IgG1 and IgG3, subtypes that commonly respond to proteins and T-cell–dependent antigens, whereas Crohn's disease is associated with increased IgG2 production, which normally responds to carbohydrates and bacterial antigens. There is also increased production of proinflammatory cytokines (IL-1, IL-6, IL-8) by macrophages in the lamina propria. Cytokines, particularly IL-1, tumor necrosis factor (TNF), and interferon-γ, stimulate epithelial, endothelial, mesenchymal, and immune cells. They are also involved in wound healing and fibrosis. IBD is associated with migration of neutrophils from the bloodstream to the mucosa and submucosa, which may be dependent on inflammatory cytokines (IL-8, TNF), platelet activating factor, and leukotriene B_4 (LTB$_4$). Supporting this hypothesis is the demonstration that LTB$_4$ concentrations are much higher in the mucosa of patients with IBD than in healthy controls. Activation of neutrophils results in activation of protease and production of superoxide and reactive oxygen species, which then participate in destruction of the epithelium.

Role of Genetic Factors

The incidence of IBD among first-degree relatives of patients with IBD is 15%, which is 30 to 100 times that of the general population. The incidence of ulcerative colitis, as well as that of Crohn's disease, is increased in relatives of patients with Crohn's disease; similarly, the predisposition to develop either disease is

---

TABLE 47-1
Classification of Ulcerative Colitis

Severe
    Diarrhea: six or more bowel movements per day, with blood
    Fever: mean evening temperature >37.5°C or >37.5°C on at
        least 2 of 4 days at any time of day
    Tachycardia: mean pulse rate higher than 90 beats/min
    Anemia: hemoglobin of <7.5 g/dl, allowing for recent transfusions
    Sedimentation rate: >30 mm/hr
Mild
    Mild diarrhea: fewer than four bowel movements per day, with only small amounts
        of blood
    No fever
    No tachycardia
    Mild anemia
    Sedimentation rate: <30 mm/hr
Moderately severe
    Intermediate between mild and severe

---

increased in relatives of patients with ulcerative colitis, suggesting that ulcerative colitis and Crohn's disease are related diseases. Monozygotic twins have a higher concordance rate than dizygotic twins. There is no increase in IBD in spouses of affected patients, indicating that genetic factors, not environmental factors, determine the incidence of IBD in families. The HLA-DR1/DQw5 haplotype is associated with Crohn's disease, and HLA-DR2 is associated with ulcerative colitis. Increases in intestinal permeability have been demonstrated in asymptomatic first-degree relatives of patients with Crohn's disease. Similarly, clinically healthy relatives of patients with ulcerative colitis have an increased incidence of antineutrophil cytoplasmic antibody positivity, suggesting that the autoantibody is more than just a marker of colonic inflammation.

CLINICAL FEATURES

Ulcerative Colitis

The dominant symptom in ulcerative colitis is diarrhea, which is often bloody. Bowel movements may be frequent but of low volume as a result of rectal inflammation. Abdominal pain (usually lower quadrant), fever, and weight loss in general result from pancolonic involvement. Localized rectal involvement may be characterized only by bloody diarrhea, with or without urgency, tenesmus, or pain. Rarely, elderly patients report constipation as a result of rectal spasm. Patients with ulcerative colitis can be classified according to disease severity, which helps direct disease management (Table 47-1). Diarrhea and rectal bleeding are the only complaints of mild disease, which is often associated with a normal finding on physical examination. Most patients with ulcerative proctitis have mild disease. Moderate disease, which occurs in 27% of patients, is characterized by five or six bloody stools per day, abdominal pain, abdominal tenderness, low-grade fever, and fatigue. Patients with severe ulcerative colitis represent 19% of cases. The clinical features of severe disease are frequent episodes of bloody diarrhea (>6 stools per day), profound weakness, weight loss, fever, tachycardia, postural hypotension, significant abdominal tenderness, hypoactive bowel sounds, and laboratory findings of anemia and hypoalbuminemia. Abdominal distention with severe disease raises the possibility of toxic megacolon.

Most cases of ulcerative colitis begin indolently and gradually worsen over the course of several weeks, but some cases exhibit fulminant disease in the beginning. At initial presentation, colitis extending to the cecum is present in 20% of patients, whereas 75% have no disease proximal to the sigmoid colon. More than 90% of patients with mild disease go into remission after the first attack. Patients with initially severe disease often require colectomy. In most patients, the disease follows a chronic intermittent course, with long quiescent periods interspersed with acute attacks lasting weeks to months. In some, however, the disease is continuously active. Older patients are more likely to report long periods of disease quiescence, but they may be more resistant to treatment-induced remission. For those with severe disease at initial presentation, 50% will need colectomy within 2 years, whereas <10% of patients with mild disease or proctitis require surgery after 10 years.

Severe ulcerative colitis can result in life-threatening complications. If the inflammatory process extends beyond the submucosa into the muscularis, the colon dilates, producing toxic megacolon. Clinical criteria suggestive of toxic megacolon include a fever of >38.6°C, a heart rate of >120 beats per minute, a neutrophil count of >10,500 cells per μl, dehydration, mental status changes, electrolyte disturbances, hypotension, abdominal distention, tenderness (with or without rebound), and hypoactive or absent bowel sounds. Toxic megacolon usually occurs in patients with pancolitis, often early in the course of their disease. Perforation of the colon may complicate toxic megacolon or may occur in cases of severe ulcerative colitis without megacolon. Strictures are uncommon, but lumenal narrowing may occur in 12% of patients after 5 to 25 years of disease, usually in the sigmoid colon and rectum. Strictures may occur with increased diarrhea or fecal incontinence and may mimic malignancy on endoscopic or radiographic evaluation. These patients require careful assessment.

Crohn's Disease

There are three main patterns of disease distribution in Crohn's disease: (1) involvement of the ileum and cecum (40% of patients); (2) disease confined to the small intestine (30%); and (3) disease of only the colon (25%), which is pancolonic in two-thirds and segmental in one-third. Less commonly, the disease affects the proximal gastrointestinal tract. Predominant symptoms in Crohn's disease include diarrhea, abdominal pain, and weight loss. They may exist for months to years before a diagnosis is made (Table 47-2). With colonic disease, diarrhea may be of small volume and associated with urgency and tenesmus, whereas involvement of the small intestine produces larger stool volumes that may be steatorrheic if disease is extensive. Diarrhea in Crohn's disease involving the small intestine may result from loss of mucosal absorption producing either bile salt–induced or osmotic diarrhea, bacterial overgrowth from stricturing, and enteroenteric or enterocolonic fistulae that bypass the absorptive surface. Pain results from intermittent partial obstruction or serosal inflammation. Commonly, pain and distention are reported in the right lower quadrant, accompanied by

---

TABLE 47-2
Frequency of Clinical Features in Crohn's Disease

	DISEASE LOCATION		
FEATURE	Ileitis (%)	Ileocolitis (%)	Colitis (%)
Diarrhea	~100	~100	~100
Abdominal pain	65	62	55
Bleeding	22	10	46
Weight loss	12	19	22
Perianal disease	14	38	36
Internal fistulae	17	34	16
Intestinal obstruction	35	44	17
Megacolon	0	2	11
Arthritis	4	4	16
Spondylitis	1	2	5

---

nausea and vomiting caused by the involvement of the terminal ileum. Weight loss occurs in most Crohn's patients because of malabsorption and reduced oral intake; 10% to 20% of patients lose >20% of their body weight. Gastroduodenal involvement in Crohn's disease may produce epigastric pain, nausea, and vomiting secondary to stricture or obstruction. When the disease is active, the patient may appear chronically ill, exhibiting pallor; temporal and interosseous wasting; abdominal tenderness; and a sensation of abdominal fullness or a mass secondary to thickened bowel loops, mesenteric thickening, or an abscess. Several attempts have been made to establish scoring systems of disease severity for research studies. The most widely accepted of these, the Crohn's Disease Activity Index, assigns numerical scores to stool frequency, abdominal pain, sense of well-being, systemic manifestations, use of antidiarrheal agents, abdominal mass, hematocrit, and body weight.

Crohn's disease is a relapsing and remitting disease that spontaneously improves without treatment in 30% of cases. Patients in remission can expect to remain in remission for 2 years in 50% of cases. However, 60% of patients require surgery within 10 years of diagnosis. Of patients who undergo surgical resection, 45% will eventually require reoperation. Crohn's disease can produce significant disability, and 50% of patients make significant changes in employment to accommodate decreased working hours and leaves of absence.

Crohn's disease often is associated with gastrointestinal complications. Abscesses and fistulae result from extension of a mucosal breach through the intestinal wall into the extraintestinal tissue. Abscesses occur in 15% to 20% of patients, most commonly arising from the terminal ileum, but they may occur in iliopsoas, retroperitoneal, hepatic, and splenic regions, and at anastomotic sites. Patients with abscesses present with fever, localized tenderness, and a palpable mass. Infection usually is polymicrobial (e.g., *Escherichia coli*, *Bacteroides fragilis*, enterococcus, and α-hemolytic *Streptococcus* species). Patients with Crohn's disease have a 20% to 40% prevalence of fistulae. Fistulae may be enteroenteric, enterocutaneous, enterovesical, or enterovaginal. They develop when disease is active and may persist after remission. Large enteroenteric fistulae produce diarrhea, malabsorption, and weight loss. Enterocutaneous fistulae produce persistent drainage that usually is refractory to medical therapy. Rectovaginal fistulae lead to foul-smelling vaginal discharge, and enterovesical fistulae produce pneumaturia and recurrent urinary infection. Obstruction, especially of the small intestine, is a common complication caused by mucosal thickening, muscular hyperplasia and scarring from prior inflammation, or adhesions. Perianal disease, including anal ulcers, abscesses, and fistulae, can also affect the groin, vulva, or scrotum. It is a complication of Crohn's disease that often is difficult to treat. Fistulae drain serous or mucous material, whereas perianal abscesses cause fever; redness; induration; and pain that is exacerbated by defecation, sitting, and walking.

Extraintestinal Features

Extraintestinal manifestations of ulcerative colitis and Crohn's disease are divided into two groups: those in which clinical activity follows the activity of the bowel disease, and those in which clinical activity is unrelated to the activity of the bowel disease. Ulcerative colitis and Crohn's colitis are associated with extraintestinal disease more often than is Crohn's disease of the small intestine. Colitic arthritis is a migratory arthritis of the knees, hips, ankles, wrists, and elbows that usually lasts a few weeks and rarely produces joint deformity. Successful treatment of bowel inflammation often results in improvement in the arthritis. In contrast, the activity of sacroiliitis and ankylosing spondylitis does not follow the course of the bowel disease and does not respond to the therapy for intestinal inflammation. Sacroiliitis often is asymptomatic and is found incidentally on radiography. The prevalence of ankylosing spondylitis, which is characterized by morning stiffness, low back pain, and stooped posture, is increased 30-fold with ulcerative colitis. It is associated with the HLA-B27 phenotype. Unlike colitic arthritis, ankylosing spondylitis can be relentlessly progressive and unresponsive to medications.

Hepatobiliary complications of IBD include steatosis, pericholangitis, chronic active hepatitis, cirrhosis, sclerosing cholangitis, and gallstones. Pericholangitis, histologically defined by lymphocytic and eosinophilic inflammation of the portal tract and degeneration of the bile ductules, produces asymptomatic elevations of alkaline phosphatase levels. Sclerosing cholangitis is a chronic cholestatic disease marked by fibrosing inflammation of the intrahepatic and extrahepatic bile ducts; it occurs in 1% to 4% of patients with ulcerative colitis and in lesser numbers of patients with Crohn's disease. Conversely, the prevalence of IBD is so high in patients with sclerosing cholangitis that colonoscopy should be performed even on those without intestinal symptoms. Early in the course of sclerosing cholangitis, liver biopsy specimens show portal tract enlargement, edema, and bile duct proliferation, which progress to fibrosis and cirrhosis in advanced disease. Patients may be asymptomatic at first, but as the disease progresses, fever, right upper quadrant pain, jaundice, or even death may occur. Cholangiocarcinoma develops in 10% to 15% of patients with IBD who have long-standing sclerosing cholangitis. Cholesterol gallstones develop in patients with Crohn's disease because of the bile salt depletion that occurs with ileal disease or resection.

Complications of IBD may involve other organ systems. Urinary tract complications include the formation of oxalate renal stones with ileal Crohn's disease because of intralumenal calcium binding by malabsorbed fatty acids, urinary tract infection resulting from fistulae, and ureteral obstruction caused by localized inflammation. Pyoderma gangrenosum, a discrete ulcer with a necrotic base usually found on the lower extremities, occurs in 1% to 5% of patients with ulcerative colitis and less frequently in patients with Crohn's disease. Lesions almost always develop after a bout of acute colitis. Erythema nodosum is a condition in which raised, tender nodules are found usually over the anterior surface of the tibia. This complication is associated with Crohn's disease in children. The lesions respond well to treatment of the intestinal disease. Uveitis is an inflammation of the anterior chamber resulting in blurred vision, headache, eye pain, photophobia, and conjunctival irritation. Episcleritis is characterized by scleral injection and burning eyes. Amyloidosis may produce end-stage renal disease; it does not improve with treatment of the bowel disease. Deep vein thrombosis, pulmonary emboli, and intracranial and intraocular thromboembolic events may result from clotting factor activation and thrombocytosis.

FINDINGS ON DIAGNOSTIC TESTING

Laboratory Studies

Laboratory studies most likely to reflect disease activity in ulcerative colitis are hemoglobin level, leukocyte count, levels of serum albumin and serum electrolytes, and erythrocyte sedimentation rate. Laboratory values usually are normal in mild to moderate disease, although mild anemia and elevations in the sedimentation rate may be seen. In contrast, if disease is severe, anemia, hypoalbuminemia, hypokalemia, and metabolic alkalosis may be prominent. At the initial evaluation, it is important to consider differential diagnoses, in particular, infectious colitis. Therefore, stool should be examined for leukocytes and cultures should be obtained for *Campylobacter*, *Shigella*, *Salmonella*, *Yersinia*, and other organisms. For watery diarrhea, examination of stool for ova and parasites of agents such as *Giardia lamblia* should be performed. If antibiotics have been taken recently, stool should be examined for *Clostridium difficile* toxin, and a specimen should also be cultured. Once the diagnosis of ulcerative colitis is established, symptom exacerbations do not mandate repeat stool cultures unless there is a risk of infection. In immunosuppressed patients, consideration should be given to the possibility of cytomegalovirus colitis, which can have a clinical presentation similar to that of ulcerative colitis.

Laboratory findings in Crohn's disease may be nonspecific. Anemia may result from chronic disease; blood loss; and iron, folate, and vitamin B_{12} deficiency. Active Crohn's disease is often associated with leukocytosis and sedimentation rate elevations, but marked increases suggest formation of an abscess. Hypoalbuminemia may be an indicator of malnutrition or protein-losing enteropathy. In patients with diarrhea, testing of stools for infectious agents is indicated as for ulcerative colitis. Measurement of fecal fat levels, either qualitatively (Sudan stain) or quantitatively, will provide evidence of ileal disease.

Complications and extraintestinal manifestations of IBD may be suggested by findings of laboratory studies. Profound leukocytosis with a neutrophil predominance in patients with ulcerative colitis is suggestive of perforation or toxic megacolon. Hepatobiliary manifestations such as pericholangitis and sclerosing cholangitis may produce striking liver chemistry abnormalities, especially with marked elevations of alkaline phosphatase levels. In a patient with Crohn's disease, urinalysis may reveal pyuria, suggesting an enterovesical fistula, or it may show hematuria, raising the possibility of renal stones.

TABLE 47-3
Colonoscopic Findings in Inflammatory Bowel Disease

FEATURE	ULCERATIVE COLITIS	CROHN'S DISEASE
Inflammation		
Distribution		
Colon		
Contiguous	+++	+
Symmetric	+++	+
Rectum	+++	+
Friability	+++	+
Topography		
Granularity	+++	+
Cobblestoned	+	+++
Ulceration		
Location		
Colitis	+++	+
Ileum	0	++++
Discrete lesion	+	+++
Features		
Size >1 cm	+	+++
Deep	+	++
Linear	+	+++
Aphthoid	0	++++
Bridging	+	++

Specificity index range: 0 (not seen) to ++++ (diagnostic).

Endoscopic Studies

Colonoscopic examination of a patient with possible IBD is often indicated at the initial presentation to help establish a diagnosis and define the extent of disease. However, with severe disease, the risks of perforation may preclude an evaluation of the entire colon. In these cases, sigmoidoscopy or proctoscopy may provide enough information to initiate therapy. The presence of deep ulceration or suspected toxic megacolon is a contraindication to endoscopy. In ulcerative colitis, the inflammation begins in the rectum and extends proximally to the point where visible disease ends without skipping any areas (Table 47-3). In mild disease, there are superficial erosions, loss of vascularity, granularity, exudation, and friability. In severe disease, large ulcers and areas of denuded mucosa may dominate. In chronic disease, the mucosa flattens, and inflammatory polyps (pseudopolyps) may develop. Pseudopolyps are not premalignant and do not need to be resected. Crohn's colitis in many but not all cases will exhibit a different endoscopic appearance. In early or mild disease, aphthous ulcers may predominate, whereas severe disease is characterized by cobblestoning and large, deep, linear or serpiginous ulcers. Similarly, with gastroduodenal Crohn's disease, antral aphthous and linear ulcers may be seen on upper gastrointestinal endoscopy. Unlike ulcerative colitis, mucosal involvement in Crohn's disease is not contiguous; patches of colon are often relatively disease free (areas skipped), and the rectum may or may not be involved. Strictures are more common with Crohn's disease, as is perianal involvement. Strictures and mass lesions seen in a patient with long-standing ulcerative colitis (>10 years) strongly suggest malignancy. In addition to its diagnostic capability, colonoscopy has therapeutic potential (e.g., pneumatic dilation) in patients with colonic strictures.

Specialized endoscopic studies may be of value in assessing the extraintestinal manifestations of IBD. Endoscopic retrograde cholangiopancreatography (ERCP) is the procedure of choice for diagnosing sclerosing cholangitis and cholangiocarcinoma. ERCP also can be used to dilate or stent the extrahepatic strictures that occur in sclerosing cholangitis, possibly reducing pruritus and other manifestations of obstructive jaundice.

Histologic Studies

Histologic evaluation of colonic biopsy specimens may help to distinguish ulcerative colitis from Crohn's disease and both forms of IBD from acute self-limited colitis. Distortion and atrophy of the crypts, acute and chronic inflammation of the lamina propria, and a villous mucosal surface are more common with ulcerative colitis than with acute self-limited colitis. The presence of granulomas provides the best histologic distinction between the two diseases. In one series, granulomas were found in 60% of patients with Crohn's disease and in 6% of patients with ulcerative colitis. Crypt atrophy, neutrophilic infiltration, and surface erosions are more common in ulcerative colitis than in Crohn's disease. Despite these variations, a histologic distinction between the two forms of chronic IBD cannot be made in 15% to 25% of cases.

Histologic evaluation also can assist in the diagnosis of extrahepatic manifestations of IBD. Liver biopsy specimens may show the characteristic findings of pericholangitis described above. However, liver biopsy findings in sclerosing cholangitis may be indistinguishable from those in pericholangitis; in appropriate clinical settings, ERCP findings can help make the distinction. A skin biopsy may be necessary to diagnose pyoderma gangrenosum.

Radiographic Studies

Radiography is complementary to endoscopy in evaluating a patient with IBD. Abdominal radiography findings may be normal or demonstrate dilation of the colon in toxic megacolon, air-fluid levels characteristic of intestinal obstruction in Crohn's disease, or pneumoperitoneum seen with perforation. Barium enema radiographs may appear normal early in the course of ulcerative colitis, but in more advanced or severe disease, a narrowed, shortened, and tubular form of the lumen is revealed. The haustra disappear and the colon appears straightened. The mucosa may be granular with mild ulcerative colitis but nodular with severe disease. Rectal inflammation may increase the presacral space (i.e., the distance from the sacrum to the rectal lumen) to >2 cm. Fifteen percent to 20% of patients with ulcerative colitis exhibit a dilated and irregular terminal ileum, consistent with backwash ileitis. Mild Crohn's disease exhibits multiple aphthous ulcers, which enlarge, deepen, and interconnect to form the characteristic cobblestone appearance of more severe disease. Barium enema radiography is far more likely to detect fistulae and strictures than is endoscopy. On barium radiography of the small intestine, strictures as well as mucosal changes and fixation of bowel loops may be observed. These features usually are most prominent in the ileum. In contrast to the radiographic findings of backwash ileitis in ulcerative colitis, the terminal ileum in Crohn's disease is often narrowed and ulcerated, with wall thickening and fistula formation. Antral and duodenal erosions revealed on upper gastrointestinal barium radiography indicate proximal involvement in Crohn's disease.

Other diagnostic modalities may be useful in select cases. Computed tomographic and ultrasound studies are useful in detecting abscesses (including those that are perianal) and fluid collections and may assist in their percutaneous drainage. Nuclear scans with labeled white blood cells have been used to localize areas of intestinal inflammation and quantitate their severity.

Imaging studies are useful in characterizing the complications and extraintestinal manifestations of IBD. Gallium scintiscans may reveal sites of abscess formation in patients with Crohn's disease. Intravenous pyelography and other imaging studies of the urinary tract may show enterovesical fistulae or renal stones. Radiography of the spine may show squaring of the vertebrae, straightening of the spine, and lateral and anterior syndesmophytes in ankylosing spondylitis. Radiographs of the pelvis in sacroiliitis reveal blurring of the margins of the sacroiliac joints, with patchy sclerosis. Ultrasound may detect cholesterol gallstones; in patients with cholecystitis, biliary scintigraphy may suggest the diagnosis. Percutaneous transhepatic cholangiography may detect sclerosing cholangitis or cholangiocarcinoma in some patients when ERCP is not possible.

Gross Pathology in Inflammatory Bowel Disease

Ulcerative colitis and Crohn's disease exhibit characteristic findings in gross specimens removed at the time of surgery. Pathologic findings in ulcerative colitis are generally limited to the mucosa and submucosa; the muscularis propria is involved only in fulminant disease. In contrast, the bowel wall is thickened and stiff with Crohn's disease because of transmural involvement. The mesentery is thickened and edematous and may be contracted. Adipose tissue creeps over the serosal surface, and intestinal loops may be matted together. Lymphoid aggregates may be observed on histologic examination involving the submucosa and occasionally the muscularis propria. Granulomas are found in many intestines surgically resected because of Crohn's disease and may also be discovered in lymph nodes, mesentery, peritoneum, and liver.

MANAGEMENT AND COURSE

Nutritional Management

Library Resource Center
Renton Technical College
3000 N.E. 4th St.
Renton, WA 98056

For most patients with IBD, the only nutritional therapy required is a well-balanced diet. Some patients with Crohn's disease of the small intestine are secondarily lactase deficient and should reduce lactose in their diet or use supplemental lactase. Oral iron supplements may be necessary if there is significant blood loss. Specific supplements of calcium, magnesium, zinc, vitamin B_{12}, vitamin D, and vitamin K may be required for clinical or biochemical evidence of deficiency caused by disease of the small intestine. Extensive terminal ileal resections (>100 cm) may lead to malabsorption of vitamin B_{12} as well as malabsorption of fat and bile salts. Fat-induced diarrhea can be managed by decreasing dietary fat. Bile salt–binding resins (e.g., cholestyramine) can reduce bile salt diarrhea. In some cases, medium-chain triglycerides, which are absorbed in the proximal intestine, can be substituted for conventional long-chain triglycerides. For patients whose oral intake is inadequate, enteral feedings may be provided by nasogastric, gastrostomy, or jejunostomy infusion. Elemental enteral feedings may reduce the antigenic load to the distal intestine, but there has been no convincing demonstration that these feedings alone alter the course of disease. Patients with severe exacerbations of IBD or with extensive resection of the small intestine as a result of Crohn's disease may be candidates for total parenteral nutrition. Parenteral nutrition is especially helpful in improving the nutritional status of patients with ulcerative colitis before colectomy.

Medications Used in Inflammatory Bowel Disease

5-Aminosalicylate Preparations

Drugs containing 5-aminosalicylate (5-ASA) are a mainstay of therapy for mild to moderate ulcerative colitis and Crohn's disease. The most commonly used drug in this class, sulfasalazine, is composed of sulfapyridine and 5-ASA joined by an azo bond. Seventy-five percent of ingested sulfasalazine reaches the colon, where the azo bond is cleaved by colonic bacteria, releasing the active 5-ASA molecule and the inert sulfapyridine moiety. With this drug, the colonic lumenal surface is exposed to high levels of 5-ASA, whereas the bloodstream absorbs little. The mechanism of action of 5-ASA in the treatment of IBD is unknown, although inhibition of local lipoxygenase pathways and free radical scavenging are current hypotheses. Sulfasalazine is the drug of choice for patients with mild to moderate flares of ulcerative colitis. Initially, 500 mg is taken twice daily with meals. The dose is slowly increased to 1 g four times daily over the course of 1 to 2 weeks. Responses can be expected in 2 to 4 weeks. After remission is achieved, doses can be tapered to 2 g per day for long-term maintenance therapy. This regimen has been shown to reduce relapses from 75% to 20% at 1 year. Sulfasalazine is also useful for Crohn's colitis with or without involvement of the small intestine; however, it is ineffective for disease confined to the small bowel. Demonstrations that long-term sulfasalazine therapy prevents relapses of Crohn's disease have not been convincing. Most of the side effects of sulfasalazine stem from the sulfapyridine component: Dose-related effects include nausea, vomiting, headache, abdominal discomfort, and hemolysis; hypersensitivity reactions include rash, fever, aplastic anemia, agranulocytosis, and autoimmune hemolysis. Abdominal discomfort may be reduced by use of enteric coated sulfasalazine. Sulfasalazine also causes reduced sperm counts (which recover 3 months after the patient stops taking the drug), folate deficiency (caused by inhibition of intestinal folate conjugase; many patients require folate supplements), and rarely, bloody diarrhea (caused by the 5-ASA component). Sulfasalazine can interfere with digoxin bioavailability, reducing serum levels of this drug.

Other 5-ASA preparations have recently become available in the United States. Enemas containing 4 g 5-ASA are effective in treatment of flares of distal ulcerative colitis, inducing remission in 93% of patients. 5-ASA suppositories (500 mg) have been released for treatment of disease that affects only the rectum. 5-ASA has also been formulated in coated granules that release the drug slowly in a pH-dependent fashion. Mesalamine (Asacol) is coated with a methacrylic acid copolymer (Eudragit-S) that releases 5-ASA in the terminal ileum and colon at pH 7 or above. A different form of mesalamine (Pentasa) uses a semipermeable membrane that releases significant amounts of 5-ASA at pH 6 and above in the small intestine and therefore may be more useful in treating small bowel involvement. Both drugs are as effective as sulfasalazine in treating acute ulcerative colitis. Pentasa has been shown to maintain remission in ulcerative colitis, whereas Asacol is effective in maintaining remission in Crohn's disease, especially with ileitis. Olsalazine is composed of two 5-ASA molecules covalently bound by an azo bond, which is cleaved by colonic bacteria. Olsalazine is effective in treating acute ulcerative colitis and in maintaining remission, but in 5% to 10% of patients it may cause watery diarrhea.

Corticosteroids

Corticosteroids block both the early and late manifestations of inflammation. They also have significant immunosuppressive effects. Oral steroids (e.g., prednisone, 40 mg every morning) are effective in most patients with moderate ulcerative colitis; improvement is seen within 3 weeks. If administered in hospital, intravenous steroids (e.g., methylprednisolone, 48 to 60 mg daily) are useful in patients with more severe ulcerative colitis. In Crohn's disease, corticosteroids produce remission in 60% to 92% of cases within 7 to 17 weeks. However, the clinician may need to ascertain whether an abscess is present before starting therapy to minimize the risk of uncontrolled sepsis. Maintenance steroid therapy has been demonstrated to be ineffective in preventing recurrences in both ulcerative colitis and Crohn's disease. Corticosteroid enemas are effective in treating left-sided ulcerative colitis reliably, up to the level of the middle of the descending colon. However, systemic absorption of active drug is significant; therefore, long-term use may lead to significant sequelae. Eighty percent of patients with ulcerative proctitis achieve remission within 2 to 3 weeks after nightly enemas. Steroid foams are also available for distal ulcerative colitis. Corticosteroids that have minimal systemic effects include beclomethasone enemas, and oral and enema forms of budesonide, but these are not yet available in the United States.

The side effects of corticosteroids may limit their use in the treatment of IBD. Patients taking 10 mg or more of prednisone for >3 weeks may have a suppressed hypothalamic-pituitary-adrenal axis for 1 year after therapy is discontinued and should receive supplemental steroids for surgery or severe illness. Common side effects include increased appetite, centripetal obesity, moon facies, acne, insomnia, depression, psychosis, growth retardation (in children), increased infections, hypertension, and glucose intolerance. Avascular necrosis of the femoral head may produce permanent disability. Osteoporosis is a devastating side effect of steroid therapy that can occur with prednisone doses as low as 8 to 10 mg per day. Patients on long-term steroid therapy should receive supplemental calcium and vitamin D. They should also have their calcium stores monitored through bone densitometry studies. Estrogen therapy may reduce bone loss in amenorrheic or postmenopausal women. Ocular complications of steroid use include cataracts, irreversible glaucoma, and, in rare cases, blindness.

Immunosuppressive Drugs

Azathioprine and 6-mercaptopurine (6-MP) at 2 to 2.5 mg per day have shown efficacy in the treatment of Crohn's disease, but a therapeutic response usually is not seen until after 3 or more months of therapy. Candidates for azathioprine or 6-MP include patients with disease refractory to steroid therapy and those who develop significant side effects to steroid therapy. Immunosuppressants may be of some benefit in healing fistulae in Crohn's disease. Azathioprine and 6-MP play a smaller role in ulcerative colitis because of the curative effects of colectomy, but, as with Crohn's disease, these drugs can achieve similar steroid-sparing effects. Initially, doses of 50 mg per day are given. If the patient tolerates the drug, the dose is gradually increased. Blood counts are monitored frequently because of the marrow-suppressive effects of these agents. Side effects of azathioprine and 6-MP include leukopenia, pancreatitis (3.3%), bone marrow depression (2%), infections (7%), and allergic reactions (2%). The risk of the development of malignancy with these agents is undefined.

Intravenous cyclosporine (4 mg per kg per day for 1 to 2 weeks) has been shown to be effective in treating severe ulcerative colitis refractory to steroid therapy, but it is not clear that long-term oral cyclosporine therapy ultimately prevents the need for colectomy in the majority of these patients. Oral cyclosporine at low doses (5.0 to 7.5 mg per kg per day) has shown only limited efficacy in Crohn's disease. Higher doses have been proposed, but these levels produce a number of side effects, the most significant being renal insufficiency. Methotrexate has been used to treat some patients with Crohn's disease, but the therapeutic response may be delayed. A potential side effect of methotrexate therapy is the development of cirrhosis.

Antibiotics

Broad-spectrum antibiotics play an important role in treating suppurative complications of Crohn's disease, including abscesses and perianal disease. They may also reduce diarrhea in patients with bacterial overgrowth secondary to involvement of the small intestine. Metronidazole has efficacy in Crohn's patients, especially those with perianal disease and possibly those with colitis. However, its mechanism of action is uncertain—it may not be related to its antimicrobial properties. For perianal involvement, many clinicians recommend high doses of metronidazole (10 to 20 mg per kg per day). Significant side effects include peripheral neuropathy, a bad taste in the mouth, and disulfiram-like reactions.

Miscellaneous Agents

Antidiarrheal agents (e.g., loperamide, diphenoxylate with atropine) may reduce defecation frequency and fecal urgency in patients with mild IBD. Similarly, anticholinergic drugs can reduce pain, cramps, and fecal urgency, especially after meals. These drugs, as well as opiate analgesics, should be avoided in severe disease because of the risk of toxic megacolon.

Medical Management of Ulcerative Colitis

The medical management of ulcerative colitis depends on the extent and severity of disease. Steroid or 5-ASA enemas are given nightly for 2 to 3 weeks for mild disease extending to 60 cm of the distal colon. If the patient responds, the frequency of enemas can be tapered to alternate nights, then to every third night to minimize disease recurrences. 5-ASA suppositories or corticosteroid foam may be used for proctitis. Oral sulfasalazine, Asacol, or Pentasa may also be used for mild distal ulcerative colitis; however, therapeutic responses are slower with these agents than with rectal therapy. Patients with refractory disease or severe distal colitis may respond to corticosteroids or 6-MP therapy, whereas those with very mild disease may need only antidiarrheal agents. Maintenance therapy for proctitis may include sulfasalazine (2 to 4 g per day) or 5-ASA enemas every other night.

In cases of pancolitis, mild disease is usually treated with sulfasalazine or an oral 5-ASA compound. Patients who have more than five to six bowel movements per day or those in whom a therapeutic response is desired in less than 3 to 4 weeks should receive oral prednisone, which will produce a response in a few days to 3 weeks. Patients with severe diarrhea, bleeding, or systemic symptoms are initially given 40 mg per day, whereas those with lesser symptoms may receive lower doses. After symptoms are controlled, the dose is reduced by 5 mg every 1 to 2 weeks while the patient is switched to sulfasalazine or 5-ASA preparations for maintenance. If steroids cannot be withdrawn and the patient remains on >15 mg prednisone per day for 6 months, consideration should be given to 6-MP or azathioprine therapy or colectomy.

The mainstays of treatment for severe ulcerative colitis are bed rest, intravenous hydration, blood transfusions as needed, parenteral antibiotics for signs of infection, and intravenous steroids (methylprednisolone, 48 to 60 mg per day; prednisolone, 60 to 80 mg per day; or hydrocortisone, 300 mg per day). The patient is given nothing by mouth, and nasogastric suction is performed if ileus is present. Total parenteral nutrition is provided if oral nutrition is to be withheld for a prolonged period. If there is no response within 7 days, continuous intravenous cyclosporine is given for 7 days, with doses aimed at obtaining serum levels of 100 to 400 ng per ml. Patients who respond to cyclosporine are switched to oral cyclosporine (8 mg per kg per day), whereas those who do not improve are considered for colectomy.

Medical Management of Crohn's Disease

It is difficult to provide generally applicable guidelines for management of Crohn's disease because of the varied clinical presentations. For mild to moderate colonic or ileocolonic disease, sulfasalazine or an oral 5-ASA preparation is reasonable initial therapy. Because of its preferential release in the small intestine, Pentasa may be a better choice for treating disease that is proximal to the terminal ileum. Oral prednisone is used as first-line therapy for ileal disease, for more active colonic or ileocolonic disease, and for patients who have failed to respond to 5-ASA compounds. The approach to severe Crohn's disease is similar to the approach to severe ulcerative colitis. Immunosuppressive agents are indicated for patients with prolonged disease or disease refractory to steroids and for patients who have side effects from steroid therapy. If tolerated, corticosteroids are continued with the immunosuppressant until a therapeutic response is observed or for 4 to 6 months, before tapering the steroid dose. If effective, immunosuppressants are usually continued for 1 to 3 years. The role of maintenance therapy for Crohn's disease requires further definition, but some trials have suggested efficacy for Asacol and Pentasa as well as for immunosuppressants.

Surgical Management of Inflammatory Bowel Disease

Ulcerative Colitis

Twenty percent to 25% of patients with ulcerative colitis eventually undergo colectomy, which is curative of the colonic disease and many but not all of the extraintestinal manifestations. Urgent indications for colectomy in ulcerative colitis include toxic megacolon, perforation, refractory fulminant colitis in the absence of dilation, and severe hemorrhage. Nonurgent indications include failure of medical therapy, severe drug side effects that prevent adequate medication regimens, dysplasia, and carcinoma. Uveitis, pyoderma gangrenosum, and colitic arthritis usually respond to colectomy, whereas ankylosing spondylitis and sclerosing cholangitis do not.

The ileal pouch–anal canal anastomosis has become the procedure of choice for young patients with uncomplicated ulcerative colitis undergoing colectomy because it preserves the normal continence. In this operation, the colon is completely removed, and the mucosa and submucosa are dissected from the rectum. A pouch is constructed from the distal 30 cm of ileum and sewn to the anal canal. A temporary diverting ileostomy may be needed until this anastomosis heals. Postoperatively, defecation frequency gradually decreases to five to six bowel movements per day after 1 year. Complications such as incontinence, intractable diarrhea, infection, or anastomotic breakdown occur but are uncommon. In older or severely ill patients, a Brooke's ileostomy may be performed with proctocolectomy in a one-stage or two-stage (colectomy and ileostomy followed by proctectomy) procedure. The disadvantage of this procedure is the need to wear an appliance to collect the ileal discharge. Complications of Brooke's ileostomy are rare but include stomal prolapse, retraction, herniation, and stenosis. The Kock continent ileostomy involves construction of an ileal valve that can be periodically drained with a rubber catheter, thus removing the need to wear an external bag. However, this operation has largely been replaced by the ileal pouch–anal canal anastomosis.

Crohn's Disease

In contrast to ulcerative colitis, surgery is not curative in Crohn's disease; therefore, the extent and frequency of resections should be minimized. Indications for surgery in Crohn's disease include disease intractability, failure of medical therapy, obstruction, fistulae, and abscess formation. Approximately 60% of patients with Crohn's disease require surgery within 10 years of diagnosis; of these, 50% will need a repeat operation within 10 years. Even in those who do not require reoperation, disease recurrences are frequent (>70%) postoperatively. For extensive colitis with rectal involvement, total proctocolectomy with Brooke's ileostomy is the procedure of choice. The ileal pouch–anal canal anastomosis is contraindicated because of the likelihood of recurrent ileal disease and the possibility of anastomotic breakdown and infection.

Management of Complications and Extraintestinal Manifestations of Inflammatory Bowel Disease

As described above, many complications of IBD are managed surgically, but there is also a role for medical management. In toxic megacolon, medical therapy may lead to improvement, obviating the need for surgery. Nasogastric suction is initiated to decompress the abdomen. Broad-spectrum antibiotics often are administered in anticipation of peritonitis. Fluid and electrolyte replacement should be aggressive, as electrolyte disturbances may contribute to impaired colonic motility in this setting. A successful medical response is defined by improvement in signs of toxicity and reduction in colonic diameter on abdominal radiography within 24 to 48 hours. If there is no improvement within 48 hours, colectomy should be performed because of the high risk of perforation. Broad-spectrum antibiotics are indicated for abscesses in Crohn's disease, in addition to percutaneous or surgical drainage. After the abscess has been drained and the inflammation subsided, resection of the affected bowel usually is required. Fistulae may respond to azathioprine or 6-MP, but they often recur when the immunosuppressive agents are discontinued. Surgical excision of the fistula is then required, especially if it is proximal to a stricture.

Many extraintestinal manifestations of IBD respond to medical treatment. Colitic arthritis usually responds to corticosteroid therapy, whereas ankylosing spondylitis often progresses despite medical intervention. NSAIDs may reduce pain in these conditions, but they may also exacerbate the underlying IBD. Pruritus secondary to sclerosing cholangitis may respond to cholestyramine. Pyoderma gangrenosum and erythema nodosum usually abate if the intestinal disease is controlled with corticosteroids. Pyoderma gangrenosum has also been reported to respond to cyproheptadine (Periactin), dapsone, cyclosporin, azathioprine, and direct local corticosteroid injection.

Surveillance for Colonic Neoplasia in Inflammatory Bowel Disease

Patients with ulcerative colitis have an increased likelihood of developing colon carcinoma, with a lifetime risk of 3% to 5%. For patients with pancolitis, the risk is appreciable 8 to 10 years after diagnosis. Patients with left-sided disease are at less risk. Disease severity is a lesser factor; colon cancer has been reported in patients with ulcerative colitis whose disease has been quiescent for >10 years. In contrast to the normal population, the development of colon cancer in patients with ulcerative colitis does not follow the standard progression of adenoma to carcinoma. Moreover, multicentric tumors, which are rare in the general population (2% to 3%), occur in up to 26% of patients with ulcerative colitis who have cancer. Therefore, surveillance programs must be designed to detect premalignant dysplastic tissue in areas of mucosa that appear no different from surrounding regions. Dysplasia is defined by nuclear stratification, loss of nuclear polarity, and nuclear and cellular pleomorphism. Areas of special concern are dysplasia-associated lesions or masses, which are visibly nodular or raised colonic regions; there is a 40% chance that these lesions will be carcinomas.

The usual approach to surveillance of a patient with pancolitis is to perform colonoscopy every 1 to 2 years beginning 8 to 10 years after diagnosis, taking one to two biopsy specimens every 10 cm of colon. If high-grade dysplasia is found, colonoscopy with biopsy is repeated. If high-grade dysplasia is confirmed, colectomy is performed. If the biopsy specimen shows low-grade dysplasia, colonoscopy is repeated at 3 months. The management of persistent low-grade dysplasia is controversial; some clinicians advocate colectomy. For left-sided colitis, surveillance can be delayed until 15 to 20 years after diagnosis.

The incidence of colon cancer in patients with Crohn's colitis is significantly less than in patients with ulcerative colitis, but it is higher than in the general population. There are currently no data to support a role for colonoscopic surveillance of these patients. There is an increased risk of development of adenocarcinoma of the small intestine in patients with ileal Crohn's disease.

Inflammatory Bowel Disease in Special Patient Populations

Pregnancy and Inflammatory Bowel Disease

Most pregnant women with IBD produce healthy babies, although the incidence of spontaneous abortion is slightly higher than in the general population. Active disease may lead to a slight increase in rates of prematurity. Sulfasalazine use has not been shown to increase spontaneous abortion, prematurity, or fetal abnormalities or to impair fetal growth; therefore, there is no need to discontinue the drug during pregnancy. Folate supplements should be given to prevent fetal deficiencies. Similarly, the risk of fetal complications is not increased by corticosteroid use. If possible, women should use the minimal dose or delay pregnancy until the disease is quiescent and medications can be withdrawn. Azathioprine, 6-MP, and metronidazole are potentially teratogenic and should be withdrawn unless required for control of the disease.

In general, inactive IBD at the time of conception will remain inactive throughout pregnancy, but active ulcerative colitis may worsen during pregnancy. The course of active Crohn's disease is less consistent during pregnancy. Fertility in women with IBD is normal or only minimally impaired.

Inflammatory Bowel Disease in Childhood and Adolescence

For the most part, IBD in childhood has a clinical presentation similar to IBD in adulthood, although extraintestinal manifestations may be more prevalent in the pediatric population. Growth failure, retarded bone development, and delayed sexual maturation may complicate Crohn's disease. Corticosteroids can also contribute to growth failure. Nutritional supplementation is important in children with IBD and should provide more calories (50 to 93 kcal per kg per day) than would normally be required. The principles of medication therapy for children with IBD are similar to those for adults, with dose adjustments for body weight. The indications for surgery are the same for children and adults. The success of surgical resection in reversing growth retardation is disappointing, however.

CHAPTER 48

Miscellaneous Inflammatory and Structural Disorders of the Colon

COLLAGENOUS AND LYMPHOCYTIC COLITIS

Etiology and Pathogenesis

Collagenous colitis and lymphocytic colitis are syndromes characterized by chronic watery diarrhea with histologic evidence of mucosal inflammation but normal endoscopic and radiographic appearances. Both disorders exhibit infiltration of the mucosal lamina propria with mononuclear cells (e.g., lymphocytes, plasma cells, macrophages, eosinophils, and mast cells), epithelial cell damage, preserved crypt architecture without cryptitis, and increased numbers of intraepithelial lymphocytes. Collagenous colitis is distinguished from lymphocytic colitis by the presence of a subepithelial band of collagen that is 10 to 100 μm thick (normal is <4 μm). This thickened collagen layer is most prominent beneath the surface epithelium between the crypts, preferentially involving the cecum (82% of cases) and transverse colon (83% of cases) and often sparing the rectum (27% of cases). The mean age at presentation is 60 to 65 years old, and most patients are women.

These disorders appear to be immunologically mediated. Many of the histologic features resemble those of celiac sprue, which is associated with collagenous and lymphocytic colitis, as are arthritis and other autoimmune disorders. However, colonic inflammation does not respond to a gluten-free diet, and the two colitides are not associated with HLA-B8 and HLA-DR3, as is celiac sprue. NSAIDs are used more frequently by patients with the two disorders than by control populations, suggesting an etiologic role for these medications. Other proposed causes include a genetic predisposition, bile salt malabsorption, and the ingestion of injurious agents. Diarrhea in lymphocytic colitis is caused by defective sodium and chloride absorption and defective chloride/bicarbonate exchange. Active colonic net chloride secretion has also been reported.

Clinical Features, Diagnosis, and Management

Symptoms of collagenous and lymphocytic colitis include the insidious onset of chronic nonbloody diarrhea (300 to 1700 g per day) associated with nocturnal stools, fecal incontinence, cramping, nausea, weight loss, and abdominal distention. Diarrhea usually abates somewhat with fasting. Laboratory abnormalities are unusual, although anemia, hypoalbuminemia, elevations in sedimentation rate, and, rarely, steatorrhea may occur. The diagnosis of these disorders is made with colonoscopy with biopsy. Several specimens must be taken from different colonic regions. The results of the biopsy studies will be positive in 82% of patients in a single sampling, if specimens from the rectum, sigmoid, and descending colon are pooled. Careful histologic analysis should exclude other causes of diarrhea, including acute infectious colitis, inflammatory bowel disease, radiation colitis, ischemia, amyloidosis, and eosinophilic gastroenteritis. Clinical symptoms of collagenous and lymphocytic colitis may spontaneously remit, sometimes after NSAIDs are discontinued. Drugs that have shown efficacy in treating these conditions include 5-aminosalicylate (5-ASA), sulfasalazine, and prednisone. Celiac sprue should be excluded in patients refractory to anti-inflammatory drugs, and antihistamines should be considered for patients with large numbers of mast cells in biopsy specimens.

DIVERSION COLITIS

Etiology and Pathogenesis

Inflammation may develop in bypassed colonic segments within Hartmann's pouches or mucous fistulae. Histologic findings include diffuse follicular lymphoid hyperplasia with germinal centers. Early inflammatory changes include the infiltration of lymphocytes, plasma cells, and neutrophils, with aphthous ulcers and reactive epithelial cells. More advanced lesions include crypt abscesses, mild crypt distortion, Paneth's cell metaplasia, and, rarely, mucin granulomas. Severe involvement produces diffuse nodularity and minute ulcerations. The pathogenesis of diversion colitis is incompletely defined, although it has been postulated that fecal diversion abolishes the supply of short-chain fatty acids that provide fuel to the colonocytes. This is supported by the observation that short-chain fatty acid enemas improve clinical, endoscopic, and histologic variables in some patients with diversion colitis. However, other factors are likely involved—for example, lumenal growth factors, dietary constituents, and bacterial metabolic products. The incidence of the disorder is higher if surgery was performed for inflammatory bowel disease (89%) than for carcinoma (23%), suggesting that pre-existing disease may play an important role in the development of diversion colitis.

Clinical Features, Diagnosis, and Management

One-third of patients with bypassed colonic segments develop mucoid discharges that progress to rectal bleeding and pain 1 to 9 months after diversion.

Endoscopic findings include erythema, granularity, friability, aphthous ulcers, and exudate. Biopsy specimens show lymphoid follicular hyperplasia, neutrophilic infiltration, and crypt inflammation. The clinical, endoscopic, and histologic manifestations of diversion colitis resolve on restoration of the fecal stream. Therapy is not needed for most mild cases. In severe cases, short-chain fatty acid enemas (acetate, 60 mmol per liter; propionate, 30 mmol per liter; and butyrate, 40 mmol per liter) induce remission in some patients, but using them is unpleasant. 5-ASA enemas may be useful; however, corticosteroid enemas usually are ineffective.

ENDOMETRIOSIS

Etiology and Pathogenesis

Endometriosis, defined as the presence of endometrial glands and stroma outside the uterus, occurs in 15% of menstruating women (usually 32 to 41 years of age), 37% of whom have intestinal implants. Postmenopausal women may experience symptomatic endometriosis if they are taking estrogen replacements. Most (95%) patients have rectosigmoid involvement; appendiceal (10%), ileal (5%), and other locations are less common. Bluish-gray peritoneal or serosal implants, 0.2 to 2.0 cm in diameter, may invade the bowel wall, causing localized muscular hypertrophy and fibrosis, rarely involving the mucosa. Mucosal biopsy specimens infrequently show crypt distortion, crypt abscesses, or ulceration.

The cause of endometriosis is unknown. Retrograde menstruation with ectopic implantation of viable uterine tissues has been proposed as the mechanism for peritoneal seeding. Hematogenous and lymphatic spread may account for remote implants such as rarely occur in pleural, pericardial, and lymph node endometriosis. Others have suggested that peritoneal cells undergo metaplastic transformation to endometrial epithelial cells. Some have hypothesized that shed endometrium in the abdomen and pelvis induces endometrial metaplasia of peritoneal cells.

Clinical Features, Diagnosis, and Management

Gastrointestinal manifestations of endometriosis include symptoms of partial obstruction (including abdominal pain and constipation), diarrhea, rectal bleeding, localized abdominal tenderness, palpable nodules on rectal examination, and, very rarely, appendicitis. Pelvic symptoms (dysmenorrhea, dyspareunia, infertility, dysfunctional uterine bleeding) occur in 80% of cases. Less than 50% of patients report a temporal association of their intestinal symptoms with their menstrual cycle. Barium enema radiography and colonoscopy findings may be normal in the presence of noninvasive serosal implants. Obstructing lesions can produce extrinsic compression or smooth strictures with overlying normal mucosa. Endoscopic evaluation with biopsy may be diagnostic in patients with rectal bleeding caused by mucosal invasion. Endoscopic ultrasound may detect colonic wall invasion. Computed tomographic (CT) and magnetic resonance imaging scans rarely are useful. Definitive diagnosis often requires laparoscopy or laparotomy.

Superficial serosal implants can be treated by hormonal therapy or nonresective surgery. Danazol, medroxyprogesterone, and gonadotropin-releasing hormone analogs (e.g., leuprolide) reduce pain and diminish the size of pelvic endometrial nodules. Anterior rectal and rectovaginal septal implants may be ablated with a laser during laparoscopy. Partial colonic obstructions often do not respond to medication, which may indicate the presence of malignancy. Segmental colectomy is usually required to treat this condition.

CHEMICAL-INDUCED COLONIC INJURY

Etiology and Pathogenesis

Chemicals delivered in enema form may cause damage to the colonic epithelium. Diarrhea produced by soap-associated colitis can be mild and watery or severe and bloody. Corresponding endoscopic appearances range from mucosal edema with loss of vascularity to mucosal sloughing and ulceration as deep as the muscularis propria. Histologically, the disorder resembles the liquefaction necrosis seen with the ingestion of caustic substances: an acute necrotic phase (days 1 to 4), an ulceration/granulation phase (days 3 to 5), and a cicatrization phase (weeks 3 to 4). Hyperosmolar water-soluble contrast medium (e.g., Gastrografin, Hypaque, and Renografin-76) can induce colitis, ranging from minimal inflammation to severe colitis with necrosis and perforation. This response generally occurs proximal to obstructing lesions, mainly in the cecum and ascending colon. Lumenal distention may be an important factor in contrast medium–induced colitis. Hydrogen peroxide enemas, historically used in the treatment of fecal impaction and meconium ileus and in the removal of intestinal gas, can cause ischemic damage to the mucosa, submucosa, and muscularis as a result of the penetration of gas into the bowel vasculature, which reduces blood flow. Colitis has also been reported after ethanol, hydrofluoric acid, calcium carbonate, and vinegar enemas.

Clinical Features, Diagnosis, and Management

Patients with colitis secondary to irritant enemas present with abdominal pain, bloody or nonbloody diarrhea, tenesmus, fever, rectal and abdominal tenderness, and possible peritoneal signs. Leukocytosis is frequently present. Colonoscopic findings are nonspecific. Perianal excoriations may suggest the diagnosis. Treatment involves intravenous fluids, bowel rest, and possibly intravenous antibiotics or surgery.

MEDICATION-INDUCED COLONIC INJURY

Medications can cause colonic injury by a variety of mechanisms (Table 48-1).

Laxative Effects on the Colon

Etiology and Pathogenesis

Melanosis coli is a dark pigmentation of the colonic mucosa that appears as a reticulated pattern of striations and spots. It results from the use of anthraquinone

TABLE 48-1
Therapeutic Agents That Induce Colonic Injury

Enemas
   Soap
   Water-soluble contrast media (e.g., Gastrografin)
   Hydrogen peroxide
Agents that induce ischemia
   Oral contraceptives
   Vasopressin
   Ergotamine
   Cocaine
   Dextroamphetamine
   Neuroleptics
   Digitalis
Laxatives
   Anthraquinones (e.g., cascara sagrada, aloe, rhubarb, senna, frangula)
Miscellaneous
   NSAIDs
   Gold
   Isotretinoin
   Antibiotics
   Chemotherapy
   Methyldopa
   Flucytosine

laxatives (cascara, aloe, rhubarb, senna, frangula). Melanosis usually develops 9 months after the initiation of anthraquinone laxatives and disappears 9 months after their withdrawal. The condition mainly affects the cecum and rectum, although the entire colon may be involved. It is associated with increases in brown pigment-laden macrophages in the lamina propria. The source of the pigment is unknown.

Cathartic colon is a well-recognized entity resulting from chronic use (>15 years) of irritant laxatives (usually anthraquinones). It leads to muscularis mucosae hypertrophy, thinning of the muscularis propria, submucosal fat deposition, loss of myenteric plexus neurons, and replacement of ganglia by Schwann cells. Toxic effects of anthraquinones on colonic myenteric nerves are the likely cause of the cathartic colon syndrome.

Clinical Features, Diagnosis, and Management

Melanosis coli is a benign condition without symptoms. Its presence implies chronic anthraquinone use; therefore, the physician should question any such patient concerning the use of these potentially harmful laxatives. Patients with cathartic colon complain of bloating, fullness, pain, and incomplete fecal evacuation, although some surreptitious users may present with chronic unexplained diarrhea or protein-losing enteropathy. Patients may increase laxative doses gradually until spontaneous defecation is impossible without laxative intake. Therapy for cathartic colon centers on the withdrawal of irritant laxatives, which is accomplished with bulking agents, a high-fiber diet, and a bowel retraining program (using osmotic laxatives or Fleet's enemas). Subtotal colectomy may be necessary in severe cases, but this option should be a last resort, as many cases of cathartic colon are reversible.

Medications that Produce Colonic Ischemia

Etiology and Pathogenesis

Oral contraceptive use (10 days to 11 years) is associated with mesenteric arterial and venous thromboses, typically presenting as ischemic colitis. Estrogen produces hypercoagulability, mesenteric vasospasm, and endothelial proliferation with subendothelial fibrosis. Vasopressin causes colonic ischemia by reducing blood flow, whereas cocaine and dextroamphetamine evoke intense mesenteric vasospasm. Ergot preparations produce colonic vasospasm, whereas ergotamine suppositories can cause rectal ulcers with obliteration of small blood vessels, endothelial proliferation, and thickening of the vascular wall. Ischemic colitis has been reported after the use of neuroleptics and tricyclic antidepressants. Digitalis preparations are associated with colonic ischemia, in part because of the underlying low-flow states (e.g., congestive heart failure) that produce colonic hypoperfusion. These agents produce mesenteric vasoconstriction in animal models, however, and may directly contribute to consequent ischemia.

Clinical Features, Diagnosis, and Management

Patients with medication-induced colonic ischemia present with abdominal pain (possibly with rebound tenderness and guarding), bloody or nonbloody diarrhea, tenesmus, nausea, vomiting, and fever. Leukocytosis may be present, and abdominal radiography may show thumbprinting. Colonoscopy may reveal friability, edema, erythema, granularity, ulceration with or without pseudomembranes, and necrosis.

Miscellaneous Medication-Induced Colitides

Etiology and Pathogenesis

It is estimated that 10% of newly diagnosed cases of colitis are related to the use of NSAIDs, including mefenamic and flufenamic acid, diclofenac, indomethacin, enteric-coated aspirin, ibuprofen, phenylbutazone, naproxen, and piroxicam. NSAID-associated colitis typically affects the elderly. It usually resolves with NSAID withdrawal. Relapse of quiescent inflammatory bowel disease, especially ulcerative colitis, has also been associated with NSAID use. NSAIDs have been reported to cause segmental colonic ischemia, colonic perforation (including diverticular perforation), colonic hemorrhage, proctitis, eosinophilic colitis, and diaphragm-like strictures of the colon.

Several other drugs produce colonic injury. Gold salts, used in treatment of rheumatoid arthritis, produce colitis, probably because of their local toxic effects. Isotretinoin, a vitamin A analog used in treating acne, causes acute colitis and may reactivate quiescent inflammatory bowel disease. Hemorrhagic colitis of unknown cause has been reported after ampicillin, amoxicillin, and erythromycin use; testing for *Clostridium difficile* produced negative results in these cases. Chemotherapeutic agents used to treat cancer (e.g., cytosine arabinoside, methotrexate, cyclophosphamide, and 5-fluorouracil) may induce colonic injury. Methyldopa has been associated with colitis, and the antifungal agent, flucytosine, produces colonic inflammation resembling ulcerative colitis.

Clinical Features, Diagnosis, and Management

Patients with NSAID-induced colonic injury present with diarrhea, occult or gross gastrointestinal bleeding, weight loss, and fever. Laboratory studies may show anemia, leukocytosis, or an elevation in the sedimentation rate. Colonoscopy reveals variable findings, including mild proctitis, patchy inflammation, thin strictures or membranes, focal ulcerations, and severe ulcerative pancolitis. Gold salt–induced colitis presents with bloody diarrhea, pain, tenesmus, fever, and leukocytosis. Colonoscopic findings in this condition include ulceration and friability. Lesions are most often in the rectosigmoid, although colitis may be diffuse. In most instances, withdrawal of the offending medication leads to improvement in the drug-induced colitis. Some patients with gold salt–induced colitis have required medical therapy with steroids, sulfasalazine, British anti-Lewisite, or oral cromolyn. Rarely, patients have undergone surgical resection for this condition.

COLONIC ULCERS

Isolated Nonspecific Colonic Ulcer

Etiology and Pathogenesis

Isolated nonspecific colonic ulcers most often are found in the cecum (67%). The patient population exhibits a slight female predominance and a mean age at presentation of 45 years. Most ulcers are round or oval and solitary (0.5 to 6.5 cm in diameter), located on the antimesenteric side of the lumen and on histologic examination exhibit nonspecific inflammatory changes (Table 48-2). The etiology of nonspecific ulcers is uncertain, although vascular factors, changes in local acid-base balance, foreign body trauma, infection, neurologic stress, toxins, and medications (NSAIDs, corticosteroids, oral contraceptives) have been reported as possible causative factors.

Clinical Features, Diagnosis, and Management

Clinical presentations of nonspecific colonic ulcers include right lower quadrant abdominal pain, hematochezia, occult blood loss, perforation, abdominal mass, obstruction, fever, and leukocytosis. Colonoscopy is the diagnostic procedure of choice; barium enema radiography studies may appear falsely normal in one-third of cases. CT scanning is useful for detecting perforation or abscess complications, whereas angiography may be needed for evaluation of brisk bleeding that obscures endoscopic visualization. Surgery (ulcer oversew, ulcer excision, or right hemicolectomy) is recommended for ulcer perforation, significant hemorrhage, or abscess formation. If biopsy specimens appear unremarkable and the course is uncomplicated, the patient with nonspecific colonic ulcer can be managed conservatively. Follow-up colonoscopy is recommended after to 4 to 6 weeks to document healing.

TABLE 48-2
Clinical Characteristics of Colonic Ulcers

TYPE OF ULCER	PRIMARY LOCATION	SIZE	FEATURES
Nonspecific ulcer	Cecum	0.5–6.5 cm	Antimesenteric location, oval to round
Dieulafoy's ulcer	Variable	<2 mm	Erosion into large submucosal artery
Stercoral ulcer	Sigmoid, rectosigmoid	1–4 cm	Associated with fecal impaction, antimesenteric location
Solitary rectal ulcer	Anterior rectum	≤1 cm	Associated with rectal prolapse, motor disturbances of the pelvic floor
Crohn's disease	Right colon	0.2–2.0 cm	Multiple ulcers, nodularity, strictures
Ischemic ulcer	Splenic flexure, descending colon	1–10 cm	Circumferential, shallow, diffuse, dusky mucosa
Malignant ulcer	Variable	Variable	Associated with mass, stricture

Dieulafoy's-Type Colonic Ulcer

Etiology and Pathogenesis

All patients with Dieulafoy's-type colonic ulcers have been men ages 20 to 74 years. The colonic lesions exhibit a pathologic picture similar to that of Dieulafoy's ulcers in the stomach (a solitary mucosal defect extending into the upper submucosa, with erosion of a submucosal large-caliber artery without inflammation, aneurysm, or vasculitis). The cause of this disorder is unknown.

Clinical Features, Diagnosis, and Management

Patients usually present with massive hematochezia and no other symptoms. Mesenteric angiography is usually necessary for diagnosis, as the magnitude of hemorrhage precludes endoscopic visualization. The definitive therapy is surgical resection in most cases.

Stercoral Ulcer

Etiology and Pathogenesis

Colonic ulceration may result from ischemic pressure necrosis from a large stercoral (or fecal) mass. Risk factors for stercoral ulceration include chronic constipation, confinement to a chronic care facility or nursing home, renal failure or transplantation, hypothyroidism, colonic strictures, foreign bodies, and use of constipating medications (aluminum antacids, opiates, phenothiazines). Stercoral ulceration may lead to perforation, usually on the antimesenteric side of the lumen of the sigmoid or rectosigmoid colon, and peritonitis.

Clinical Features, Diagnosis, and Management

Affected patients have abdominal pain with or without peritoneal signs, a palpable abdominal or rectal mass, rectal bleeding, and leukocytosis. Abdominal radiography may reveal pneumoperitoneum, marked fecal retention, and calcific fecaliths. Surgical resection is the definitive therapy for perforated and nonperforated stercoral ulcers. Resection of the perforation with an end colostomy and Hartmann's pouch or mucous fistula has the lowest mortality rate of the surgical options.

Solitary Rectal Ulcer Syndrome

Etiology and Pathogenesis

Solitary rectal ulcer syndrome has variable appearances. There may only be a single ulcer of <5 cm in diameter on the anterior rectal wall, 6 to 10 cm proximal to the anal verge, or there may be multiple ulcers, polypoid lesions, or a flat region of rectal erythema. Histologic criteria for diagnosis include replacement of the lamina propria by fibroblasts, smooth muscle, and collagen, hypertrophy and disorganization of the muscularis mucosae, erosion of the mucosa, displacement of the mucosal glands, and the presence of submucosal cystic glands. Proposed causes of solitary rectal ulcers include self-digitation, congenital rectal wall abnormalities, localized inflammatory bowel disease, and infection, but the most likely cause is rectal prolapse–induced mucosal trauma or ischemia.

Clinical Features, Diagnosis, and Management

Patients present with constipation, tenesmus, incomplete evacuation, straining on defecation, lower abdominal pain, rectal bleeding, passage of mucus, fecal incontinence, and rectal prolapse. Patients with polypoid lesions may respond to bowel retraining, the use of bulk laxatives, and reassurance. Surgery (i.e., abdominal rectopexy) is advised for patients with rectal prolapse who respond poorly to medical therapy. Rarely, more extensive resection or a diverting colostomy is needed.

Typhlitis

Etiology and Pathogenesis

Typhlitis, an acute necrotizing colitis primarily of the cecum, occurs mainly in immunosuppressed patients with leukemia. It has also been seen in patients with immunosuppression caused by cancer chemotherapy, drug-induced granulocytopenia, aplastic anemia, periodic neutropenia, immunosuppressive medication therapy for renal transplants and autologous bone marrow transplants, and possibly with acquired immunodeficiency syndrome. Involved segments of the intestinal tract may exhibit ulcers, wall thickening, edema, hemorrhagic necrosis, and lumenal dilation. Histologic findings include submucosal edema, mucosal necrosis without inflammation, the presence of fungal organisms in some cases, and bacterial infiltration of small blood vessels. It has been proposed that typhlitis results from sequential destruction of the colon wall beginning with failure to maintain an intact epithelial barrier, followed by bacterial invasion and intramural proliferation, production of bacterial endotoxins, necrosis, hemorrhage, perforation, and, finally, sepsis.

Clinical Features, Diagnosis, and Management

Typhlitis must be considered in a febrile, neutropenic patient with abdominal pain (usually localized to the right lower quadrant), nausea, vomiting, distention, diarrhea (which may be bloody), and associated stomatitis and pharyngitis. Peritoneal signs suggest perforation. Blood cultures positive for *Pseudomonas*, *Candida*, or other enteric organisms suggest sepsis. Abdominal radiographs may show a fluid-filled cecum, a dilated small intestine, diminished colonic gas, thumbprinting, a soft tissue mass, or cecal pneumatosis. CT scans reveal cecal thickening with pericecal fluid or a soft tissue mass. Ultrasound may show the target or halo sign of a solid mass with an echogenic center. Barium enema radiography and colonoscopy are relatively contraindicated because of the risk of perforation, but gentle sigmoidoscopy may be performed to exclude other forms of colitis. Medical therapy includes nasogastric suction, intravenous hydration and antibiotics to treat *Pseudomonas* organisms, and avoidance of antimotility drugs. Amphotericin B is added to the regimen if fever persists for >72 hours. Indications for surgery include perforation, severe hemorrhage, uncontrolled sepsis, and refractory disease. Regardless of therapy, typhlitis has a high mortality rate (40% to 50%).

COLITIS CYSTICA PROFUNDA

Etiology and Pathogenesis

Colitis cystica profunda is a benign disease characterized by the presence of large, submucosal, mucus-filled cysts, usually in the rectum. The lesions can be solitary or multiple in a localized, segmental, or diffuse distribution. The pathogenesis is not known, but the condition is associated with local trauma of the bowel wall, and symptoms regress after diverting colostomy. Colitis cystica profunda may be one manifestation of a spectrum of disease states, including solitary rectal ulcer syndrome and rectal prolapse. Localized disease is probably caused by ischemia secondary to trauma induced by rectal prolapse.

Clinical Features, Diagnosis, and Management

Patients present at a mean age of 30 years with bloody or mucous rectal discharge, diarrhea, abdominal or rectal pain, tenesmus, or obstruction. Rectal examination may reveal palpable smooth masses, rectal wall thickening, and stenosis. Endoscopic findings include obvious cysts with overlying mucosa that may be normal, or they may show erythema, edema, friability, ulceration, mass effect, prolapse, or stricture, usually on the anterior rectal wall within 12 cm of the anal verge. Barium enema radiography may reveal thickened valves of Houston, an increased presacral space, filling defects, stricture, and prolapse. Definitive diagnosis is based on histologic findings obtained by surgical excision. The findings include enlargement of the submucosa with benign cysts; replacement of the lamina propria with collagen and smooth muscle cells; and adjacent mucosal edema, ulceration, inflammation, pseudomembranes, and crypt distortion. Most cases follow a chronic, stable course, although adenocarcinoma may be adjacent to areas of colitis cystica profunda. Patients with minimal symptoms can be managed with reassurance and dietary fiber supplementation. Local surgical procedures (cyst excision, posterior proctectomy, electrocautery, injection sclerosis) are needed to treat more symptomatic patients (i.e., those with hemorrhage, obstruction, pain, stenosis). Despite therapy, recurrence is common. Diverting colostomy is reserved for the most disabled patients.

PNEUMATOSIS CYSTOIDES INTESTINALIS

Etiology and Pathogenesis

Pneumatosis cystoides intestinalis is characterized by multiple, thin-walled, gas-filled cysts ranging in size from a few millimeters to several centimeters with no epithelial lining in the wall of the small intestine or colon. The condition is associated with chronic obstructive pulmonary disease, intestinal obstruction, rheumatologic disease (scleroderma), bowel infarction, pseudomembranous colitis, and necrotizing enterocolitis. It may occur after surgery or endoscopy. The cysts contain hydrogen gas and are located in the submucosa or subserosa, near the mesenteric border. Inflammation with neutrophils, eosinophils, plasma cells, lymphocytes, and epithelioid granulomas may be observed. Theories of pathogenesis include mechanical introduction of gas into the bowel wall, invasion of bowel wall by gas-producing bacteria, and trapping of excess intralumenal gas produced by bacterial carbohydrate fermentation within the bowel wall.

Clinical Features, Diagnosis, and Management

Patients may be asymptomatic (with discovery of the condition on routine radiography or endoscopy), or they may present with diarrhea, abdominal discomfort, distention, hematochezia, mucus discharge, and weight loss. Complications include volvulus, pneumoperitoneum, obstruction, intussusception, tension pneumoperitoneum, hemorrhage, and perforation. Abdominal radiography may reveal linear or cystic bowel wall lucencies, pneumoperitoneum, or retroperitoneal air. A CT scan is more sensitive than barium radiography in detecting intramural gas and portal or mesenteric gas. On endoscopy, pneumatosis cystoides intestinalis appears as multiple, pale, blue, rounded, soft masses. Cysts usually resolve with treatment of the underlying medical condition, but some patients benefit from high-flow oxygen or even hyperbaric oxygen therapy. Antibiotics (metronidazole, ampicillin) and elemental diets have been used to resolve cysts in some patients. Surgery is reserved for severe refractory symptoms or complications, but postoperative cyst recurrence is common.

MALAKOPLAKIA

Etiology and Pathogenesis

Malakoplakia is characterized by yellow soft plaques or nodules (1 to 20 mm) appearing on the mucosal surface anywhere in the gastrointestinal tract, with the rectum, sigmoid, and descending colon being the most common sites. Other organs that can be affected are the urinary tract, genitals, skin, lung, bone, and brain. Predisposing conditions include chronic coliform infection, sarcoidosis, tuberculosis, immunosuppression, and colorectal carcinoma. The pathogenesis may relate to a defect in the phagocytic or digestive activity of macrophages.

Clinical Features, Diagnosis, and Management

Patients may be asymptomatic, or they may have diarrhea, abdominal pain, rectal bleeding, obstruction, an intestinal mass, or a fistula. The diagnosis is confirmed by histologic demonstration of a diffuse histiocytic infiltrate with periodic acid–Schiff (PAS)-positive eosinophilic cytoplasm (von Hansemann's cell) containing basophilic, laminated cytoplasmic calculospherules (Michaelis-Gutmann bodies). When the disorder is found, a thorough evaluation for associated malignancy or infection is indicated. Localized disease can be excised or fulgurated, whereas diffuse involvement can be treated with antituberculosis medications, antibiotics (e.g., trimethoprim-sulfamethoxazole, ciprofloxacin), or cholinergic agonists (bethanechol).

CHAPTER 49

Colonic Polyps and Polyposis Syndromes

The term *polyp* is a morphologic description of any lesion that is an elevation or lumenal protrusion of a mucosal surface. Although several histopathologic types of colonic polyps exist, >80% are adenomatous or hyperplastic (Table 49-1).

ADENOMATOUS POLYPS

Incidence and Epidemiology

Wide regional variation in the prevalence of colonic adenomas exists. In some areas of South America, <5% of the middle-aged population have polyps, whereas >50% of age-matched persons in Hawaii have polyps. The prevalence of adenomatous polyps parallels the risk of development of colon cancer, which is consistent with the presumed pathologic progression of adenomas to carcinoma. There is no difference in the frequency of adenomatous polyps between the sexes, but the prevalence increases to 30% to 40% in persons older than 60 years.

Etiology and Pathogenesis

Histopathology

Adenomatous polyps are benign neoplasms that result from disordered cell proliferation and differentiation. In normal colonic crypts, only colonocytes in the lower third of the crypts proliferate. In adenomas, cell proliferation extends into the upper portion of the crypt. All adenomas exhibit varying degrees of dysplasia, characterized by enlarged hyperchromatic nuclei, decreased cellular mucin, and increased mitotic forms. These features differentiate adenomas from hyperplastic polyps. Proliferation of stromal tissue also contributes to adenoma formation and architecture. In tubular adenomas, restricted mesenchymal proliferation hinders epithelial proliferation, leading to the branching tubular pattern characteristic of these tumors. With increased mesenchymal proliferation, epithelial proliferation is unimpeded, resulting in long glandular projections characteristic of villous adenomas.

TABLE 49-1
Histologic Classification of Colonic Polyps

TYPE	SIZE (cm)	HISTOLOGIC FEATURES	PERCENTAGE MALIGNANT
Tubular adenoma	<2	Epithelial tubules	5
Tubulovillous adenoma	0.5–5.0	Tubules and villi	20
Villous adenoma	>2	Villous projections	40
Hyperplastic	<0.5	Elongated crypts, serrated surface	0
Inflammatory	<1	Regenerative epithelium	0
Lymphoid	<0.5	Lymphoid follicles	0
Juvenile	<2	Mucus-filled glands	0
Peutz-Jeghers	<2	Normal glands surrounded by smooth muscle	0

Adenoma-to-Carcinoma Sequence

The cellular events responsible for the loss of growth regulation are still being elucidated. Analyses of polyps in various stages in the progression to malignancy have uncovered a sequence of genetic alterations that appear to be vital to neoplastic transformation and carcinogenesis. Mutations in the adenomatous polyposis coli (*APC*) gene and DNA methylation appear to be early events that cause epithelial cells to become hyperproliferative. Subsequently, the accumulation of mutations in the K-*ras* oncogene and deletions of the *p53* and *DCC* (deleted in colon cancer) tumor suppressor genes result in an increase in cellular atypia and eventually in development of malignancy. In general, the level of polyp dysplasia correlates with the number of these genetic alterations. These findings provide a genetic model for the progression of colonic adenomas to carcinoma.

Morphologic studies of adenomatous polyps support the putative adenoma-to-carcinoma sequence. Large adenomas frequently have small foci of adenocarcinomas. The chance of finding adenocarcinoma in a polyp increases with an increase in polyp size, a greater degree of cellular atypia, and a higher percentage of villous architecture. The predilection of polyps to occur on the left side of the colon parallels the higher incidence of colon cancers in the left colon. Studies confirm that removal of adenomatous polyps reduces the risk of colon cancer.

Risk Factors

The causes of these cellular and genetic changes are probably multifactorial. Hereditary factors play a primary role in adenoma formation in patients with familial adenomatous polyposis (FAP) and hereditary nonpolyposis colon cancer (HNPCC), but these disorders account for a small minority of adenomas and colon cancers. Other less well-defined genetic factors play a role in up to 20% to 30% of patients with colonic adenomas. Epidemiologic surveys suggest that a diet high in fat and low in fiber increases the risk for development of colonic adenomas and carcinoma, indicating the importance of environmental factors. Dietary fats increase the synthesis and delivery of bile acids to the colon, some of which have cancer-promoting properties. The impact of other dietary factors (e.g., antioxidants) remains unclear.

Development of colonic adenomas has been linked to several extraintestinal disorders. Patients with ureterosigmoidostomies with a colonic conduit exhibit an increased incidence of adenoma formation, which develops months to several years postoperatively. Patients with acromegaly have a 2- to 6-fold increased risk of developing colonic adenomas. The risk is particularly high in those patients with skin tags. Other diseases that have inconsistently been associated with colonic adenomas include breast cancer, prior cholecystectomy, atherosclerosis, diverticular disease, and hyperplastic polyps. The high risk of adenomatous polyps in patients with ureterosigmoidostomy or acromegaly have prompted recommendations for colonoscopic screening of these populations. No such broadbased recommendations can be made for the disorders less clearly linked to colonic adenomas.

Clinical Features

Adenomatous polyps remain asymptomatic until they are 1 cm or larger. The majority are detected during screening examinations or during evaluation of symptoms unrelated to the polyps themselves. If patients are symptomatic, overt bleeding or pallor and fatigue secondary to iron deficiency anemia are the common presentations. Polyps smaller than 1.5 cm rarely bleed. Occasionally, pedunculated adenomas will spontaneously slough, resulting in acute lower gastrointestinal hemorrhage. Large bulky polyps may interfere with stool passage and produce constipation or abdominal discomfort. In rare instances, large villous adenomas, usually in the rectum, may cause secretory diarrhea and volume depletion. The physical examination of a patient with colonic adenoma is often unrevealing. Digital rectal examination may detect polyps in the distal 7 to 10 cm of the rectum. Large polyps may intermittently bleed enough to produce a positive fecal occult blood test.

Findings on Diagnostic Testing

Laboratory Studies

Laboratory studies usually are normal in patients with colonic adenomas. Patients with large adenomas may exhibit iron deficiency anemia, which is a finding that also suggests colonic adenocarcinoma. Large secreting villous adenomas may cause electrolyte abnormalities.

Endoscopic Studies

Colonoscopy is the procedure of choice if the clinical presentation suggests that a patient has a colonic polyp; it has a sensitivity of 95% for detecting adenomatous polyps and a specificity approaching 100%. The performance characteristics of polypectomy and biopsy are superior to any other diagnostic modality. Because the endoscopic appearance of a polyp is an unreliable means of differentiating adenomatous polyps from non-neoplastic polyps, biopsy or polypectomy is essential to confirm the diagnosis. Endoscopically, tubular adenomas appear as smooth erythematous polyps. In contrast, villous adenomas have a lobular appearance, and they are larger and often friable.

Histologic Evaluation

Approximately 80% of adenomatous polyps are primarily tubular in architecture, and 5% are primarily villous. The residual 15% are mixed tubulovillous adenomas. The cellular atypia of any adenoma can be graded as mild, moderate, or severe. Severe focal atypia implies that a carcinomatous focus is present that does not interrupt the basement membrane. When malignant cells invade the basement membrane but do not penetrate the muscularis mucosae, the lesion is termed *intramucosal carcinoma*. In general, the risk of an adenoma harboring a high-grade lesion or invasive adenocarcinoma correlates with the size of the polyp and the fraction of the surface that exhibits villous architecture.

Radiographic Studies

When performed by an experienced radiologist, double-contrast barium enema radiography detects 90% of colonic polyps with a specificity of 85%. Single-contrast barium enema radiography is inferior and should not be used as the sole means of detection. Air insufflation enhances mucosal detail and exposes polyps, which appear as intralumenal protrusions coated with barium or as discrete rings with barium collected at their bases or along the stalks of pedunculated polyps. Not uncommonly, residual fecal material is misinterpreted to be a polyp. Even for experts, the rectosigmoid region is often difficult to visualize. Therefore, flexible or rigid sigmoidoscopy is necessary for a complete evaluation of the colon. Because barium enema radiography does not afford the capability to obtain histologic specimens, colonoscopy is required when a barium study suggests the presence of a colonic polyp.

Management and Course

Natural History

Colonic adenomas are premalignant lesions, but the percentage of adenomatous polyps that progress to adenocarcinoma remains unknown. Longitudinal follow-up of patients who have unresected polyps suggests that the risks of developing adenocarcinoma at the site of a 1-cm polyp are 3% at 5 years, 8% at 10 years, and 24% at 20 years after diagnosis. The growth rate and malignant potential of individual polyps vary significantly. Serial follow-up over several years shows that some polyps remain stable or even regress. Based on the average patient ages at the times of diagnosis of colonic adenomas and adenocarcinoma, the mean time of progression from adenoma to colorectal cancer is estimated to be 7 years. Other epidemiologic studies suggest that adenomatous polyps manifesting severe atypia progress to cancer in 4 years, whereas those manifesting mild atypia take 11 years on average.

Endoscopic and Surgical Therapy

Most adenomatous polyps can be removed by endoscopic polypectomy. Diminutive (<5 mm) polyps can be excised with cautery biopsy or bipolar electrocoagulation. Cautery biopsy enhances hemostasis and facilitates polyp obliteration, but residual adenomatous tissue may be left behind in up to 20% of polyps. Occasionally, numerous diminutive polyps are encountered, particularly in the rectum, rendering endoscopic differentiation of adenomatous and hyperplastic polyps impossible. In this setting, several polyps should be sampled for histologic examination, and polypectomy performed later if any of the polyps are adenomatous. Polyps of >5 mm and all pedunculated polyps are excised with snare electrocautery. Most polyps can be completely removed in a single resection, and the intact polyp can be examined histologically to confirm the absence of adenomatous tissue at the resection margin. Large, broad-based, sessile polyps may require piecemeal snare resection performed in one or more sessions. Because the results of histologic studies of the tissue margins are unreliable after piecemeal resections, patients should have a repeat colonoscopy several months after the resection to exclude the presence of residual adenoma.

Although all colonic adenomas have malignant potential, the decision to proceed with polypectomy is based on the patient's clinical status. As a general rule, patients with a life expectancy of at least several years should have adenomatous polyps removed. The risk of a diminutive polyp progressing to malignancy over a 3-year interval is small. Therefore, if patients have severe life-limiting illnesses or if endoscopic obliteration poses an extreme risk, endoscopic removal of asymptomatic polyps can be deferred. Contraindications to colonoscopic polypectomy include severe coagulopathy, recent myocardial infarction, uncontrolled cardiopulmonary symptoms, pregnancy, abdominal perforation, and recent colonic surgery. In general, polypectomy is safe; the complication rate is <3%.

If large or multiple polyps cannot be removed by endoscopic polypectomy, laser ablation or surgical resection may be necessary. Nd:YAG laser ablation is particularly useful for removing clusters of diminutive adenomatous polyps. However, the technique carries a 5% rate of hemorrhage or stenosis. Retrieval of the intact polyp for histologic examination is not possible. Controlled surgical resection is often necessary for the safe removal of large, sessile polyps.

Principles of Surveillance Programs

Because synchronous polyps are common (50%) in patients with adenomatous polyps, patients with a documented colonic adenoma should undergo a colonoscopic examination of the entire colon. Similarly, the prevalence of recurrent (metachronous) polyps warrants a surveillance program of follow-up colonoscopies to detect the development of new polyps before they progress to adenocarcinoma. The data from the National Polyp Study suggest that the recurrence rate for metachronous polyps is approximately 10% per year. Polyps with high-grade atypia and multiple polyps have a slightly higher recurrence rate. Based on this study, it has been recommended that patients undergo surveillance colonoscopy every 3 years once the colon is completely cleared of adenomatous polyps. Subsequent studies suggest that for average-risk patients, a 5-year interval may be suitable. When there is doubt about the adequacy of the polyp resection, if the polyps removed contain high-grade dysplasia, or if the patient has multiple neoplasms, more frequent surveillance is advised.

Malignant Polyps

Colonic adenomas with severe atypia or noninvasive carcinoma do not metastasize because there are no lymphatic channels above the muscularis mucosae. These lesions are cured by colonoscopic polypectomy. The distinction between noninvasive and invasive carcinoma requires meticulous histologic examination by an experienced pathologist. When malignant cells penetrate the muscularis mucosae, the polyp is considered to have invasive carcinoma. In this case, the decision to perform colonoscopic resection only or surgical resection

TABLE 49-2
Poor Prognostic Features of Malignant Polyps in Decreasing Order of Importance

Incomplete endoscopic resection
Venous or lymphatic invasion
Sessile or very short stalk
Poorly differentiated carcinoma
Involvement of or within 2 mm of polypectomy margins
Cancer larger than one-half of polyp volume
Polyp size of >2 cm

is based on the characteristics of the malignant polyp. Poor prognostic features include the presence of incomplete endoscopic resection, venous or lymphatic invasion, sessile morphology, extension through the base of the polyp stalk, poorly differentiated carcinoma, and carcinoma within 2 mm of the resection margin (Table 49-2). The presence of any of these features favors surgical resection of the underlying bowel. Pedunculated polyps that can be completely resected and that lack all of these high-risk features may be treated with polypectomy alone. All patients with malignant polyps managed with polypectomy alone should have surveillance colonoscopy within 1 to 3 months and at 1 year.

NONADENOMATOUS POLYPS

Hyperplastic Polyps

Hyperplastic polyps account for >50% of all diminutive polyps and >15% of all polyps reported in colonoscopic surveys. Hyperplastic polyps rarely exceed 1 cm and are almost universally asymptomatic. Endoscopically, they appear as small, sessile protrusions of pale epithelium, found predominantly in the rectum. Histologically, they are composed of elongated glands with epithelial infoldings, which produce a serrated pattern. Cellular proliferation and differentiation are normal; hyperplastic polyps are nonneoplastic and have no malignant potential. Some studies have suggested that patients with hyperplastic polyps have a higher incidence of adenomatous polyps, but this association remains controversial. No treatment or surveillance is recommended for hyperplastic polyps, but they are often resected because it is difficult to visually distinguish them from adenomatous polyps.

Inflammatory Polyps

Any chronic inflammatory process in the colon can produce two types of mucosal polyps. Pseudopolyps represent islands of residual colonic mucosa surrounded by excavated or denuded mucosa. Inflammatory polyps represent areas of regenerating mucosa and granulation tissue that develop in response to chronic inflammation. These polyps are commonly seen in inflammatory bowel disease, but they can occur in any chronic inflammatory disorder of the colon and are frequently found in association with surgical anastomoses and the solitary rectal ulcer syndrome. Inflammatory polyps may become large and pedunculated, and occasionally they may produce symptoms of hemorrhage or obstruction. The major clinical challenge in diagnosing inflammatory polyps is differentiating them from adenomatous polyps. This is particularly important in inflammatory bowel disease, given the high risk of colonic adenocarcinoma with long-standing ulcerative colitis. If numerous apparent pseudopolyps are found in a patient with ulcerative colitis, biopsy specimens of several polyps should be obtained to exclude adenomatous changes.

Juvenile Polyps

Juvenile polyps are most commonly found in children between the ages of 1 and 10 years, but occasionally they are observed in adulthood. They are present in 2% of asymptomatic children but account for >95% of polyps found in children younger than 15 years of age. The most common presenting symptom is rectal bleeding, which results from spontaneous sloughing of the polyp. Prolapse of the polyp through the rectum and constipation may rarely occur. On colonoscopy, juvenile polyps appear as pedunculated, smooth, cherry-red polyps. They are often friable or ulcerated. Histologic examination reveals mucin-filled cystic glands and abundant lamina propria. The appearance of retained mucin prompted use of the term *retention polyp* to describe these polyps. Juvenile polyps are hamartomas with no malignant potential, but a low incidence of adenomatous changes suggests that they should be resected.

SUBMUCOSAL MASSES

Because polyps represent intralumenal projections of mucosa, any submucosal mass may mimic a mucosal polyp. Lymphoid hyperplasia in the lamina propria is characterized by discrete, white polypoid lesions smaller than 5 mm. Diffuse nodular lymphoid hyperplasia (submucosal lymphoid follicles) appears as diffuse polyposis, but biopsy specimens reveal normal mucosa or focal submucosal lymphocyte collections. Diffuse nodular lymphoid hyperplasia may occur in association with Gardner's syndrome, intestinal lymphoma, human immunodeficiency virus infection, and common variable immunodeficiency. In most cases, lymphoid hyperplasia is found incidentally, and no specific treatment is necessary.

Colitis cystica profunda is a submucosal mass that is frequently mistaken for a sessile neoplastic polyp. Usually found in the rectum, these polyps consist of dilated mucus-filled cysts within the muscularis mucosae and may be associated with inflammatory colitis or recent colonic surgery. They are presumed to represent normal colonic glands that are displaced in the healing process. Colitis cystic profunda is usually asymptomatic and requires no treatment.

Lipomas may appear as submucosal masses, most commonly near the ileocecal valve. Superficial lipomas have a distinctive yellow appearance. Other less common benign lesions include fibromas, neurofibromas, leiomyomas, and endometriosis. The colon is rarely the site of metastasis for melanoma, lymphoma, Kaposi's sarcoma, adenocarcinomas, and malignant carcinoids.

FAMILIAL ADENOMATOUS POLYPOSIS

Incidence and Epidemiology

Familial adenomatous polyposis (FAP), also known as adenomatous polyposis coli (APC) or familial polyposis coli, is an autosomal dominant disease characterized by the early onset of hundreds or thousands of intestinal polyps and the inevitable progression to colon cancer. Thirty percent of cases probably result from a new, spontaneous mutation of the *APC* gene. Three adenomatous polyposis syndromes are variants of FAP. Gardner's syndrome is characterized by polyposis and extraintestinal benign tumors, including osteomas, desmoids, and epidermoid cysts. Attenuated FAP is a less aggressive form of FAP. Turcot's syndrome is polyposis and central nervous system malignancies. Recent evidence suggests that some forms of Turcot's syndrome may be more closely related to HNPCC, which is reviewed in Chapter 50.

Approximately 0.5% of all colon carcinomas arise from FAP. Worldwide, the frequency of FAP ranges from 1 in 7000 to 1 in 30,000 persons. Gardner's syndrome is less common than FAP. Adenomatous polyps develop in adolescence or young adulthood and colonic adenocarcinoma develops at a mean age of 39 years (Table 49-3). In attenuated FAP, the age of presentation is approximately 10 years later.

Etiology and Pathogenesis

The colonic polyps in FAP are primarily tubular adenomas, which may become so numerous that they carpet the entire colon. Histologically, adenomas are indistinguishable from sporadic tubular adenomas. Microadenomas—that is, foci of adenomatous epithelium within a single crypt—are a distinctive feature of FAP.

FAP results from a germline mutation of the *APC* gene, which has been localized to chromosome 5. Mutations that lead to FAP almost invariably result in truncation of the APC protein, which has an unknown function. The truncated protein appears to inactivate the normal APC protein generated from the normal *APC* allele. This dominant negative inhibition helps explain the autosomal dominant pattern of inheritance. The entire colonic epithelium in FAP patients is characterized by increased proliferation along the crypts, leading to the hypothesis that inactivation of the *APC* gene causes hyperproliferation. This hyperproliferative epithelium is susceptible to subsequent mutations or deletions of genes such as K-*ras*, *p53*, and *DCC*, which appear to be critical in neoplastic transformation and carcinogenesis.

The germline mutations in Gardner's syndrome are identical to those in FAP, although other genetic alterations may be responsible for development of mesenchymal tumors in this syndrome. Although patients with attenuated FAP tend to have mutations close to the 5' end of the *APC* gene, the mechanisms by which mutations in specific regions of the *APC* gene generate altered phenotypic expression are unknown. Most patients with Turcot's syndrome also have truncating mutations of the *APC* gene. This syndrome appears to be genetically het-

TABLE 49-3
Characteristics of the Polyposis Syndromes

SYNDROME	POLYP TYPE	POLYP DISTRIBUTION (%)	RISK OF COLON CANCER	ASSOCIATED LESIONS
Familial adenomatous polyposis and Gardner's syndrome	Adenoma	Colon (100) Stomach (30–100) Duodenum (46–93) Small intestine (20–40)	100%	CHRPE, Gardner's syndrome (desmoids, osteomas, dental abnormalities)
Peutz-Jeghers syndrome	Peutz-Jeghers hamartomas	Colon (60) Stomach (24–49) Small intestine (64–96)	Slightly increased	Orocutaneous pigmented lesions
Familial juvenile polyposis	Juvenile hamartomas	Colon (nearly 100) Stomach (may occur) Small intestine (may occur)	At least 9%	

CHRPE = congenital hypertrophy of the retinal pigment epithelium.

erogeneous, however, as some patients have mutations in the genes responsible for HNPCC as their primary germline defect.

Clinical Features

Gastrointestinal Polyposis

Patients with FAP usually develop adenomatous polyps in adolescence or young adulthood, but colonic adenomas have been reported to occur as early as age 4 years and as late as age 40 years. Polyps often carpet the colon and number in the hundreds to thousands, but they rarely produce symptoms until late in the course of disease. Patients typically present with rectal bleeding, diarrhea, and abdominal pain in the third and fourth decades. At the time symptoms occur, nearly 70% of patients have colon cancer. Patients with attenuated FAP often have fewer polyps, and the onset of adenomas and progression to adenocarcinoma is delayed by 10 years. Differentiating these patients from patients with HNPCC may be difficult, but the presence of duodenal polyps or extraintestinal features of FAP may be helpful clues.

Thirty percent to 100% of patients have gastric polyps, which are usually numerous, asymptomatic, occur in the proximal fundus or body, and exhibit a hyperplastic histologic appearance. Duodenal polyps occur in 4% to 90% of patients with FAP, but they are usually adenomatous. These polyps tend to be multiple, developing in the periampullary region, where they may rarely cause biliary obstruction or pancreatitis. Polyps have also been observed in the jejunum and ileum, but malignant transformation is rare.

Extraintestinal Manifestations

Sixty percent to 85% of patients with FAP exhibit a characteristic retinal abnormality known as congenital hypertrophy of the retinal pigment epithelium, consisting of hamartomas of retinal epithelium and appearing as multiple discrete round or oval areas of hyperpigmentation. Pupillary dilation may be necessary to visualize the lesions. Although the pathogenesis remains unknown, the presence of multiple lesions in both eyes is essentially pathognomonic for FAP.

Gardner's syndrome is a clinical variant of FAP with distinctive extraintestinal manifestations. Desmoid tumors are benign mesenchymal neoplasms that occur throughout the body but frequently in the mesentery and other intra-abdominal regions. These masses may infiltrate adjacent structures or compress adjacent visceral organs or blood vessels, producing abdominal pain. Abdominal examination may demonstrate a mass lesion. Osteomas are benign bony growths that occur throughout the skeletal system but most commonly involve the skull and mandible. Detection of osteomas may predate the diagnosis of Gardner's syndrome, but isolated osteomas may also occur in normal individuals. Osteomas have no malignant potential, and symptoms are related to their mass effect. Other abnormalities associated with Gardner's syndrome include dental cysts, unerupted teeth, supernumerary teeth, numerous cutaneous fibromas, and epidermoid cysts. These lesions are benign and generally cause no symptoms.

Turcot's syndrome is characterized by adenomatous polyposis in association with a 90-fold increased risk for development of central nervous system malignancies (e.g., medulloblastoma, glioblastoma), which usually occur in the first two decades of life. Neurologic surveillance may be indicated for persons at risk for the development of FAP, especially in families with Turcot's syndrome.

Findings on Diagnostic Testing

Genetic Testing and Endoscopic Studies

The universal progression to malignancy and the long asymptomatic premalignant polyposis phase mandate screening of children and young siblings of FAP patients. Genetic testing is now recommended for FAP screening in affected families. One currently available database, Helix, provides information about which laboratories offer clinical genetic testing (http://healthlinks.washington.edu/helix). Screening should begin with in vitro protein truncation for the proband, and if successful (80%), be extended to all family members. If not successful, linkage testing can be done if two other members have FAP. Children found to be carriers should then be screened endoscopically. Because polyps are distributed throughout the colon in FAP, flexible sigmoidoscopy is considered an adequate screening procedure. Screening should begin at age 10 to 12 years and continue every 1 to 2 years until age 35 years, after which the examination interval can be increased to 3 years. Relatives of patients with attenuated FAP require colonoscopy as a screening procedure because this syndrome produces far fewer polyps. Screening for these persons should be initiated at an age 10 years younger than the earliest age of diagnosis of colon cancer within the family. Screening can also be accomplished by DNA linkage analysis if two other affected family members are available for testing. Because this test is not 100% accurate, patients with negative test results should still undergo an endoscopic screening program until age 40 years. If genetic testing is unsuccessful or unavailable, all relatives should be screened endoscopically. Once the diagnosis of FAP is established, patients should be screened every 1 to 3 years for concurrent duodenal adenomatous polyps using a side-viewing duodenoscope that can assess the periampullary region.

Radiographic Studies

The diagnosis of Gardner's syndrome often requires bone radiography to document the sclerotic lesions characteristic of osteomas. Patients with abdominal pain or a palpable mass are examined with computed tomographic (CT) scanning. Abdominal CT scans can define the extent of intra-abdominal desmoid tumors in patients with Gardner's syndrome. CT or magnetic resonance imaging scans of the head can identify malignancies in the central nervous system of patients with Turcot's syndrome.

Management and Course

Therapy for Colonic Polyposis

Initially, patients with FAP may have only a few polyps, but the number and size of adenomas gradually increase over the course of several years. Left untreated, the disease invariably progresses to colon adenocarcinoma—most patients develop cancer by age 40 years, and by age 50 years >90% have developed cancer. When the diagnosis of FAP is established, elective surgery to remove the colon is recommended. Colectomy can be delayed in young children until adolescence or early adulthood, but these patients should have surveillance colonoscopy every 6 to 12 months. Sulindac causes polyp regression in a subset of patients and may be useful if surgery is delayed. Adults, on the other hand, should have surgery promptly. Before surgery, all patients should undergo colonoscopy to survey the colon for gross evidence of malignancy. In addition, upper gastrointestinal endoscopy with a side-viewing duodenoscope and barium radiography of the small intestine should be performed to exclude concurrent malignancy in the small intestine and to treat small polyps.

The surgical options for FAP include total proctocolectomy with ileostomy, total colectomy with ileal pouch–anal canal anastomosis, and subtotal colectomy with ileorectal anastomosis. In the last procedure, the rectal stump remains at risk for adenomatous polyp formation, and surveillance sigmoidoscopy is required every 3 to 6 months. Sulindac may slow the progression of adenomatous polyps in the retained rectal mucosal segment but does not obviate the need for surveillance and endoscopic ablation of incident rectal adenomas. Even with this aggressive approach, up to 30% of patients will eventually require completion of the rectal resection because of the inability to control polyps or to prevent progression to cancer. This has prompted many clinicians to consider the continence-sparing colectomy with ileal pouch–anal canal anastomosis as the procedure of choice.

Therapy for Duodenal Neoplasms

Progression of duodenal adenoma to adenocarcinoma, particularly periampullary cancer, occurs in up to 5% to 10% of patients with FAP, usually at a later age than colonic malignancy (mean age at diagnosis is 46 years). The optimal treatment of adenomatous duodenal polyps is undefined. Large villous adenomas should be considered for surgical resection given the high risk of coexisting malignancy. Smaller tubular adenomas can be safely treated with endoscopic ablation if they do not involve the papilla. It is not known if sulindac alters the natural course of duodenal adenomas.

Therapy for Extraintestinal Manifestations

Occasionally, extraintestinal tumors are a source of symptoms in patients with FAP. Desmoid tumors in Gardner's syndrome invade or compress blood vessels, nerves, and hollow viscera, accounting for 10% of deaths in FAP. Patients with small, asymptomatic lesions should be observed, but patients with enlarging or symptomatic desmoids should be given tamoxifen or sulindac. If this conservative treatment fails, chemotherapy, radiation therapy, or surgery may be necessary.

HAMARTOMATOUS POLYPOSIS SYNDROMES

Peutz-Jeghers Syndrome

Etiology and Pathogenesis

Peutz-Jeghers syndrome is a rare autosomal dominant disorder characterized by intestinal hamartomatous polyposis and mucocutaneous melanin spots. It is one-tenth as common as FAP. Unlike the latter disorder, a genetic locus has not yet been identified. The mucocutaneous manifestations are distinctive brown to black melanin spots 1 to 5 mm in diameter that are common in the perioral area (including the lips and buccal mucosa). They also occur on the face, palms, soles, and digits, and rarely on the colonic mucosa. The spots often appear in infancy, but those in the perioral region may fade in adulthood. Patients with Peutz-Jeghers syndrome are at increased risk for gastrointestinal and extraintestinal malignancies, including breast, cervical, and ovarian tumors in females; testicular tumors in males; and pancreatic tumors in males and females. Benign ovarian tumors are present in almost all female patients who have this syndrome.

Clinical Features, Diagnosis, and Management

Unlike FAP, polyps in Peutz-Jeghers syndrome are hamartomatous and fewer in number (10 to 20). Polyps occur in the stomach, small intestine, and colon and usually appear in the first decade of life (see Table 49-3). Symptoms usually do not manifest until young adulthood, when large polyps may cause hemorrhage or intestinal obstruction. Peutz-Jeghers polyps have a distinctive histologic pattern characterized by arborizing glands of normal epithelium surrounded by smooth muscle. Adenomatous changes occur in a small percentage of these polyps, and there appears to be an increased risk of gastrointestinal malignancies, particularly in the stomach and duodenum.

Because of the increased risk for development of gastrointestinal malignancy, all persons at risk for Peutz-Jeghers syndrome should undergo screening sigmoidoscopy every 3 years in conjunction with annual fecal occult blood testing beginning in early adolescence. When the diagnosis is suggested, the patient should undergo colonoscopy, upper gastrointestinal endoscopy, and barium radiography of the small intestine. All gastric, duodenal, and colonic polyps should be removed endoscopically. Polyps in the small intestine that are not endoscopically accessible are observed until they are symptomatic or >1.5 cm, at which point, they are surgically removed. The increased incidence of extraintestinal malignancies requires vigilant surveillance. Breast and testicular examinations should be performed routinely. Mammography and gynecologic screening should also be considered, although formal guidelines are not available.

Familial Juvenile Polyposis Coli

Etiology and Pathogenesis

Familial juvenile polyposis coli is a rare autosomal dominant disorder characterized by the presence of >10 juvenile polyps. The syndrome accounts for only a small portion of patients with juvenile polyps; up to two-thirds of patients with multiple juvenile polyps do not have the familial form of the disease.

Clinical Features, Diagnosis, and Management

The juvenile polyps in familial juvenile polyposis coli usually produce rectal bleeding during childhood, although some children present with abdominal pain, malnutrition, failure to thrive, or intussusception. Despite the hamartomatous nature of juvenile polyps, there does appear to be an increased risk for development of colon cancer, particularly in patients with the familial form of juvenile polyposis coli. The incidence of colonic adenocarcinoma is 10% to 20%, and the median age at diagnosis is 34 years. Unaffected relatives of patients with familial juvenile polyposis coli are also at increased risk of developing colon cancer, prompting recommendations to screen these persons.

The screening program should include a fecal occult blood test annually and flexible sigmoidoscopy every 3 to 5 years. When juvenile polyposis is found, patients should undergo complete evaluation with colonoscopy, upper gastrointestinal endoscopy, and barium radiography of the small intestine. Colonoscopic polypectomy can remove a small number of polyps, but unlike sporadic juvenile polyps, the polyps in familial juvenile polyposis coli often recur. When the number of polyps is more than 10 to 20, colectomy should be considered. The increased awareness of the risk of cancer in patients with this syndrome has made prophylactic colectomy a popular alternative to long-term endoscopic surveillance.

Cowden's Disease

Cowden's disease is an autosomal dominant disorder characterized by diffuse hamartomas of the skin and mucous membranes. The cardinal feature of the syndrome is facial keratotic papules that appear in adolescence. Most patients develop pinpoint red and verrucous papules of the oral cavity later in the course of the disease. One-third of patients exhibit gastrointestinal hamartomas, which may occur anywhere in the gastrointestinal tract, including the esophagus. Unlike other polyposis syndromes, these polyps rarely cause symptoms and do not increase the risk of gastrointestinal malignancy. The incidence of breast and thyroid malignancies is dramatically increased in patients with Cowden's disease, however. Breast cancer, in particular, may occur in as many as 50% of patients; the median age at diagnosis is 41 years.

ACQUIRED POLYPOSIS SYNDROMES

Cronkhite-Canada Syndrome

Etiology and Pathogenesis

Cronkhite-Canada syndrome is a rare disorder of unknown etiology. It is characterized by generalized gastrointestinal polyposis of the juvenile type throughout the stomach, small intestine, and colon. Adenomatous changes and colon cancer may occur in these polyps. Therefore, periodic colonoscopy with biopsies of polyps is recommended in long-term survivors.

Clinical Features, Diagnosis, and Management

Patients typically present at a median age of 59 years with cutaneous hyperpigmentation, hair loss, onychodystrophy, diarrhea, gastrointestinal hemorrhage, anorexia, weight loss, and skin changes. The prognosis of Cronkhite-Canada syndrome is variable. Some patients progress rapidly to death, usually because of complications of malnutrition, whereas others undergo spontaneous remission. Anecdotal reports have suggested that clinical improvement may result from corticosteroids, antibiotics, and total parenteral nutrition. Aggressive nutritional support is usually the initial therapy. Corticosteroids and antibiotics are reserved for patients who continue to deteriorate.

Miscellaneous Acquired Polyposis Syndromes

There are case reports of patients with hundreds of hyperplastic polyps throughout the colon, a condition that mimics FAP. These patients can be treated conservatively with periodic colonoscopy to exclude adenomas and to remove larger lesions.

CHAPTER 50

Malignant Tumors of the Colon

ADENOCARCINOMA

Incidence and Epidemiology

The majority of malignant neoplasms of the colon and rectum are adenocarcinomas, which represent a leading cause of cancer death in the United States. The United States and Eastern and Northern Europe have a high incidence of colon adenocarcinoma. Most developing countries have one-tenth the incidence of industrialized nations, which probably is attributable to environmental factors. When people migrate from a low-risk area to a high-risk area, they assume the higher risk of their new location. Approximately 150,000 patients are diagnosed with colorectal cancer annually in the United States, resulting in nearly 60,000 deaths per year. Urban populations and persons of higher socioeconomic status may have slightly higher risks, but the difference is not significant.

Etiology and Pathogenesis

Environmental Factors

Animal fats, particularly from red meat sources, have been associated with an increased risk for development of colon cancer. The per capita consumption of animal fats has a positive correlation with the incidence of colorectal cancer. Societies in which the dietary intake of marine fish is high have strikingly lower rates of colonic malignancy. Animal models suggest that high fat intake increases colonocyte proliferation and tumor formation, activities that may be mediated by increased colonic concentrations of bile acids, which are known cancer promoters. Several reports have observed an increased incidence of colon cancer in populations with low fiber intake. Because Western diets are often high in fat and low in fiber, it remains unclear whether these dietary factors are independent risk factors for development of colorectal cancer. Other dietary factors may alter the risk of colon cancer. Frequent ethanol use may produce a twofold to threefold increase in

445

colon cancer. Ingestion of the antioxidant vitamins E, A, and C has been postulated to lower the risk of malignancy, but currently there is no convincing evidence that supplements of these vitamins prevent colorectal cancer. Studies have demonstrated a higher incidence of colonic adenocarcinoma in patients infected with *Schistosoma japonicum*, a protozoan endemic to regions of China. This organism appears to be responsible for the high rate of colon cancer within these regions, despite an overall low incidence throughout most of the country.

Genetic Factors

Several inherited disorders are associated with the development of colonic adenocarcinoma at a young age, including the polyposis syndromes reviewed in Chapter 49. Whereas the polyposis syndromes account for <1% of all colorectal cancers, hereditary nonpolyposis colorectal cancer (HNPCC) may account for 3% to 5% of colorectal cancers. HNPCC is an autosomal dominant disorder that results from mutations in mismatch repair genes, which serve a housekeeping function for DNA replication. Protein products of mismatch repair genes recognize and repair DNA replication errors in postmitotic cells. Cells without mismatch repair activity accumulate random mutations and therefore are more likely to acquire mutations responsible for carcinogenesis. Because all colonic cells of affected persons have one intact copy of the gene, a second somatic mutation of this gene is required before mismatch repair function is lost. This "second hit" mechanism explains the absence of polyposis in HNPCC, as only a small portion of colonic cells will have damage to both alleles. To date, five mismatch repair genes have been identified (*hMSH2*, *hMLH1*, *hPMS1*, *hPMS2*, and *hMSH6*). A mutation in one of these genes is present in most but not all relatives of patients with HNPCC. Future research will probably define other mismatch repair genes. HNPCC is distinguished by the early onset of colorectal cancer (mean age at diagnosis is 40 years), a higher risk of synchronous tumors (18% versus 6%), right-sided tumors (65% versus 25%), and more frequent mucinous tumors (35% versus 20%) compared with sporadic colorectal cancer. HNPCC is often divided into two variants: Lynch syndromes I and II. Lynch syndrome I is an isolated, early-onset colorectal cancer, whereas Lynch syndrome II manifests as the early occurrence of carcinoma at other sites as well (e.g., endometrium, ovaries, genitourinary tract, stomach, small intestine).

There are familial factors that increase the susceptibility to colorectal cancer that are not transmitted in a standard mendelian pattern. A history of colorectal cancer in a first-degree relative increases the risk of colorectal cancer threefold, an observation that is supported primarily if the affected relative is younger than 55 years of age or if there are multiple affected family members. Identification of the genetic factors responsible for this familial risk may further clarify the molecular mechanisms of carcinogenesis.

Other Risk Factors

Several clinical disorders have been associated with an increased risk of colonic adenocarcinoma. Inflammatory bowel disease, particularly ulcerative colitis, is associated with an increased frequency of colorectal cancer. This increased risk becomes evident 8 to 10 years after diagnosis of ulcerative pancolitis; 10% of patients develop this complication every decade thereafter. The manifestation of colon adenocarcinoma in patients with long-standing inflammatory bowel disease may be confounded by symptoms of the underlying disease. The risk of development of colorectal malignancy is much lower in patients with left-sided ulcerative colitis or Crohn's disease. Patients with histories of pelvic irradiation for cervical cancer or ureterosigmoidostomy for bladder cancer have increased risks for development of colon adenocarcinoma, although the onset may be delayed by decades. Other clinical entities associated with colon cancer include group D *Streptococcus* bacteremia, acromegaly, skin tags, and alcoholism. Although tobacco use has been associated with an increased risk for development of colonic adenomas, there is no evidence to suggest that it increases the risk of colorectal cancer.

Adenoma-to-Carcinoma Sequence

Investigations have provided overwhelming evidence in favor of the adenoma-to-carcinoma sequence. On average, patients diagnosed with adenomatous polyps are 7 years younger than those diagnosed with colonic adenocarcinoma. In addition, the prevalence of colorectal cancer within a population correlates well with the prevalence of adenomatous colon polyps. Pathologic analyses of surgically excised colorectal carcinomas often reveal adjacent adenomatous tissue, whereas larger colorectal adenomas often exhibit cellular atypia with microscopic foci of invasive carcinoma. The most convincing evidence that adenocarcinomas arise from adenomas came from the report of the National Polyp Study Group, indicating that removal of adenomatous polyps lowered the rate of development of colorectal malignancy.

The progression from normal colonocytes to adenomatous tissue and finally to colon carcinoma involves a stepwise accumulation of mutations, each of which provides a growth advantage to involved cells. The initial events appear to involve somatic mutations of the adenomatous polyposis coli (*APC*) gene, providing the normal cell with increased proliferative capacity, which may be the critical step in the transition from the normal colonocyte to adenomatous tissue. Subsequent mutations in the K-*ras* oncogene, which occur in most large colonic adenomas, lead to further growth dysregulation. Perhaps the most important step in colorectal carcinogenesis is mutation of the tumor suppressor gene *p53*. The protein product of the *p53* gene normally serves to halt cellular proliferation in cells with damaged DNA. *p53* mutations lead to uninhibited replication of cells with damaged DNA, permitting these cells to accumulate even more severe genetic damage. Replication of these defective cells can result in losses of chromosomal segments containing several alleles, a phenomenon termed *loss of heterozygosity*, which can lead to deletions of other tumor suppressor genes, including *DCC* (deleted in colon cancer), which appears to be a late event in the transformation to malignancy. Not all colonic malignancies contain all of these mutations, and there are likely to be other genetic alterations vital to carcinogenesis that have not been discovered. However, this sequential mutation model of carcinogenesis does provide a conceptual framework for understanding the final common pathway leading to colorectal cancer. Successive waves of clonal expansion occur as cells accumulate mutations that provide incremental growth advantages. When sufficient damage to growth regulatory genes occurs, the clonal expansion transforms into a neoplasm. Eventually, the cells acquire the capability to invade, or metastasize, at which point the neoplasm is considered to be malignant.

Clinical Features

Most colorectal cancers develop after age 50 years, and most patients are diagnosed after age 60 years. In its early stages, colonic adenocarcinoma may be asymptomatic or produce only subtle changes in bowel habits. As the tumor grows, relative or complete colonic obstruction may develop, most commonly in the transverse, descending, and sigmoid colons, where lumenal diameters are lower. Incomplete colonic obstruction may be perceived initially as intermittent abdominal pain. As obstruction becomes complete, however, nausea, vomiting, distention, and obstipation supervene.

Colorectal adenocarcinomas are prone to bleeding as a result of tumor friability and ulceration. Most patients with tumor-related blood loss have occult bleeding, but hematochezia is the presenting feature in a small percentage of patients. Depending on the type of assay employed and the location and stage of the tumor, 50% to 90% of colorectal cancers give rise to positive fecal occult blood tests (FOBTs). Patients with tumors in the distal colon are more likely to have hematochezia or a positive result on FOBT as the presenting feature, whereas patients with right-sided colonic lesions are more likely to present with iron deficiency anemia.

Tumor invasion into adjacent structures may produce organ-specific symptoms. Invasion of the perirectal fat may cause tenesmus. Bladder involvement can lead to recurrent urinary infections because of the development of colovesical fistulae. Fistulae may also develop between the colon and stomach or small intestine. Malignant ascites results from local tumor extension through the serosa, with peritoneal dissemination. Metastatic disease to the liver is often asymptomatic initially, but advanced disease may be characterized by abdominal pain, jaundice, and portal hypertension. Some patients with colonic adenocarcinomas present with profound weight loss despite a small tumor burden. The cause of this metabolic disorder may stem from the systemic effects of mediators such as tumor necrosis factor.

Findings on Diagnostic Testing

Laboratory Studies

Laboratory studies may produce normal results or exhibit iron deficiency anemia. Liver chemistry abnormalities raise the possibility of hepatic metastases. The serum level of carcinoembryonic antigen (CEA) is elevated in most but not all cases of colorectal adenocarcinomas. A baseline CEA level should be obtained in a patient diagnosed with colorectal cancer. This value can serve as a reference and be compared with levels obtained after treatment to assess for incomplete tumor resection or recurrence. Because nonspecific elevations are caused by many other conditions, measurement of CEA is not used as a screening test in patients without a prior history of colonic adenocarcinoma.

Endoscopic Studies

Patients with symptoms suggestive of colonic obstruction or invasion and those older than 40 years with occult gastrointestinal bleeding should undergo diagnostic evaluation to exclude colorectal cancer. Colonoscopy is the procedure of choice because of its superior accuracy in detecting colonic neoplasms and because biopsies and endoscopic polypectomy can also be performed. The sensitivity of colonoscopy for detecting small malignancies is superior to barium enema radiography, and its sensitivity for neoplasms larger than 1 cm approaches 100%. If colorectal cancer is diagnosed in the distal colon, it is imperative that the entire colon be visualized, given the 5% incidence of synchronous malignancies. The entire colon can be visualized in 90% to 95% of studies. If a complete colonoscopy cannot be performed, barium enema radiography should be performed to image the remainder of the colon.

Radiographic Studies

When performed and interpreted well, double-contrast barium enema radiography detects the majority of colon cancers. Technical limitations may preclude adequate imaging of the rectosigmoid region; therefore, if barium enema radiography is chosen to evaluate a patient with suspected colonic adenocarcinoma, flexible sigmoidoscopy should be performed to exclude a neoplasm in this region. The sensitivity of barium enema radiography is highly dependent on the skill of the radiologist; diagnostic misinterpretation is common in inexperienced hands. In addition, many patients cannot comply with the body position changes necessary for an adequate examination. When colorectal malignancy is diagnosed, an abdominal computed tomographic scan is performed to exclude hepatic metastases. Similarly, chest radiography is required to exclude pulmonary dissemination.

Management and Course

Prognosis

The prognosis of patients with colorectal cancer is directly related to the stage of the tumor. The most widely used staging classification is the modified Dukes' classification (Table 50-1). Malignant mucosa that does not penetrate the muscularis mucosae is considered intramucosal carcinoma and is cured with adequate endoscopic or surgical resection. Dukes' stage A refers to invasive cancer confined to the submucosa. Stage B is subdivided into stage B1, which includes tumors invading the muscularis propria, and stage B2, which includes tumors extending into the surrounding serosa. Stage C is defined by the presence of regional lymph node involvement, which can be subdivided into stages C1 (one to four nodes involved) and C2 (more than four nodes involved). Stage D disease is defined by the presence of any distant metastatic disease. The age-adjusted 5-year survival rates for colorectal adenocarcinoma are 99%, 85%, 67%, and 14% for Dukes' stages A, B, C, and D, respectively.

Other features correlate with the prognosis for patients with colonic adenocarcinoma. Poorly differentiated or mucinous tumors are associated with a poor 5-year survival rate. Aneuploid malignancies, characterized by cell populations with irregular DNA content as a result of genetic instability, are also associated with a poor prognosis. Despite the predictive value of tumor stage, there is no evidence that the size of the tumor mass is an independent predictor of survival.

Surgical Therapy

Except for colonoscopic removal of malignant polyps with favorable prognostic features (see Chapter 49), the only reliable method of curing colorectal adenocarcinoma is surgical resection. Tumors in the cecum, ascending colon, and transverse colon require a right hemicolectomy; lesions in the splenic flexure and descending colon are treated with a left hemicolectomy. Rectosigmoid malignancies located >6 cm from the anal verge can be removed with a low anterior resection. Localization and staging of rectal tumors is critical because

TABLE 50-1
Dukes' Classification of Colorectal Tumors

STAGE	DEPTH OF INVASION	FREQUENCY (%)	AGE-ADJUSTED 5-YEAR SURVIVAL (%)
A	Submucosa	15	95–100
B1 B2	Muscularis propria Serosa	31	80–85
C1 C2	1–4 lymph nodes >4 lymph nodes	23	50–70
D	Distant metastases	30	5–15

lesions that invade the muscularis propria in the distal 6 cm require an extensive abdominoperineal resection with colostomy, whereas lesions confined to the submucosa may be amenable to a sphincter-sparing transanal resection. Transrectal ultrasound can be used to determine the depth of invasion. Some patients have a solitary hepatic metastasis or a small number of lesions localized to one hepatic lobe. Aggressive surgical resection can result in a 25% long-term survival rate. It is not known if resection of a solitary pulmonary metastasis improves survival.

Adjuvant Therapy

One-third of patients undergoing a surgical resection with curative intent will develop recurrent disease. Several trials have evaluated adjuvant chemotherapy for reducing postoperative recurrence of colorectal cancers. Patients with Dukes' stage A cancer rarely develop recurrent disease; therefore, most studies have targeted patients with Dukes' stage B or C tumors. For patients with Dukes' stage C colon cancer, 1 year of adjuvant therapy with levamisole and 5-fluorouracil results in a significant improvement in the disease-free interval and overall survival rate. This benefit has not been observed in patients with stage B disease, but improved selection of patients on the basis of other poor prognostic indicators may identify a subgroup of patients with Dukes' stage B tumors that may benefit from adjuvant therapy.

Patients with rectal cancer are often evaluated as a separate group in adjuvant therapy trials. Several studies have reported decreased pelvic recurrences and improved survival with adjuvant therapy for rectal carcinoma. In contrast to more proximal tumors, both Dukes' stage B2 and Dukes' stage C rectal tumors benefit from this therapy. Also in contrast to more proximal colon cancers, the adjuvant regimens for rectal cancer combine postoperative radiation therapy and chemotherapy (5-fluorouracil and methyl-CCNU). Preoperative radiation therapy for patients with unresectable rectal tumors may sufficiently decrease the tumor size to make resection possible. Such treatment of resectable tumors probably improves outcome and is an underused therapeutic option.

Management of Unresectable Disease

Although distant metastatic disease can preclude curative resection, palliative resection should be considered for patients with colonic lesions. Untreated colonic adenocarcinomas have a high incidence of obstruction. If resection is deferred until symptoms of obstruction develop, operative morbidity and mortality can be excessive. Nd:YAG laser photocoagulation may palliate rectal cancer in patients who are not operative candidates, but a high risk of perforation precludes laser palliation of lesions located above the peritoneal reflection.

Therapy for patients with extensive metastatic disease in the liver and other sites is limited. No systemic chemotherapy regimen has been demonstrated to improve survival rates. Most regimens include 5-fluorouracil and produce response rates of 15% to 20%. Delivery of 5-fluorouracil into the hepatic artery has been associated with 80% response rates. Surgery is required for catheter placement, however. This therapy has not been demonstrated to improve survival. Moreover, 80% of patients develop ischemic gastroduodenal ulcers and biliary strictures.

Principles of Screening Programs

Because effective therapy for colorectal cancer relies on early detection, attempts have been made to identify colonic neoplasia in a presymptomatic phase through population-based screening programs. The most widely available screening test is the FOBT. There are several assays to detect occult blood, but the guaiac-based Hemoccult II is most widely used. Colorless guaiac is converted to a pigmented quinone in the presence of peroxidase activity and hydrogen peroxide. Because hemoglobin contains peroxidase activity, the addition of hydrogen peroxide to the guaiac reagent transforms the slide to a blue color. The sensitivity of Hemoccult II for detecting colorectal malignancy ranges from 50% for a single test to 70% for six tests performed over 3 days. Although the false-positive rate is <1%, the low prevalence of colonic adenocarcinoma in healthy populations reduces the positive predictive value to <10%. Therefore, <10% of asymptomatic individuals with a positive Hemoccult test actually have colorectal cancer. Prolonged storage and delay in developing the slides can result in hemoglobin degradation, which decreases the sensitivity of the test. Using water to rehydrate slides that have dried out improves the sensitivity to approximately 90%, but this practice lowers the positive predictive value of FOBT to <5% and produces a higher false-positive rate. This translates into a larger number of unnecessary diagnostic evaluations, which dramatically increases the cost of screening.

These performance characteristics can be modified by dietary factors. Ingestion of red meats or peroxidase-containing legumes may increase the false-positive rate, particularly with rehydrated slides. Although iron supplements do not result in activation of the color indicator, the dark color of the stool may be misinterpreted as a positive test by an inexperienced processor. High doses of antioxidants (e.g., vitamin C) may interfere with guaiac oxidation to quinone. For these reasons, patients should be counseled to avoid ingesting red meats, peroxidase-containing legumes, and vitamin C several days before testing.

New assays have been developed in an attempt to improve the accuracy of FOBTs. HemeSelect relies on antibody detection of human hemoglobin and is performed in a laboratory setting. This test exhibits a sensitivity for detection of colonic adenocarcinoma of 94% to 97%, but it also has a high false-positive rate. HemeSelect and HemoccultSENSA seem to provide improved detection of adenomas of >1 cm in size. The sensitivities of Hemoccult II, HemoccultSENSA, and HemeSelect, are

42%, 60%, and 75%, respectively. HemoQuant provides a quantitative measure of fecal hemoglobin. The HemeSelect and HemoQuant assays avoid the confounding of dietary factors by measuring fecal hemoglobin, but both tests are cumbersome and cannot be performed at the bedside. Furthermore, the sensitivity and false-positive rate of the HemoQuant assay appear to be similar to those of Hemoccult II. The role of these newer FOBTs in colorectal cancer screening programs will likely be clarified by ongoing population-based studies.

Several reports have confirmed the efficacy of annual FOBT in reducing colorectal adenocarcinoma mortality. A diagnosis of Dukes' stage A cancer is made in 60% of screened persons compared with 10% to 15% of unscreened persons, which translates into a 33% reduction in colon cancer mortality. Because of these findings, it is recommended that FOBTs be performed every year in persons older than age 50 years. Unfortunately, patient compliance with screening programs using FOBTs may be as low as 38%.

Two-thirds of colonic adenocarcinomas are accessible for diagnosis with a flexible sigmoidoscope that reaches 65 cm. Case-control studies have documented 70% to 80% reductions in colorectal cancer deaths in patients screened with flexible sigmoidoscopy. Unlike FOBT, negative findings on sigmoidoscopic examination reduce the risk of cancer for up to 10 years. The magnitude of this benefit has prompted the American Cancer Society, the National Cancer Institute, and the U.S. Preventive Service Task Force to recommend screening sigmoidoscopy every 3 to 5 years for colorectal cancer in average-risk persons 50 years of age and older.

Principles of Surveillance Programs

Whereas screening programs are used for average-risk populations, persons at high risk for development of colonic adenocarcinoma undergo vigilant surveillance. The guidelines for surveillance in patients with adenomatous polyps and persons at risk for polyposis syndromes are discussed in Chapter 49. If HNPCC is identified, first-degree relatives should be considered for surveillance. The clinical criteria for HNPCC (Amsterdam criteria) are that at least three relatives develop colorectal cancer, that cancer occurs in at least two generations with one person being a first-degree relative of the other two, and that at least one individual is diagnosed before age 50 years. Although the test is not widely available, many patients are diagnosed with HNPCC by the detection of mutations of the mismatch repair genes *hMSH2*, *hMLH1*, *hPMS1*, *hPMS2*, or *hMSH6* in circulating lymphocytes or in tumor cells. Therefore, even if the Amsterdam criteria are not fulfilled, the detection of the familiar clustering of colon cancers or other Lynch syndrome II malignancies should prompt consideration of molecular genetic testing of the affected patient in order to identify relatives who should undergo surveillance colonoscopy. The initial colonoscopy in such relatives should be performed at an age that is 5 years younger than the youngest age at which colorectal cancer developed in a family member. If no polyps are found, colonoscopy should be repeated every 2 years; if polyps are found, the surveillance interval should be reduced to 1 year. If a cancer is found, subtotal colectomy with ileorectal anastomosis is the appropriate therapy, followed by annual surveillance of the rectal stump. The role of genetic testing for detection of mismatch repair gene mutations in relatives of affected patients is undefined.

Thirty percent of the population reports a history of at least one family member with colon cancer that does not adhere to any mendelian pattern of inheritance. There is no consensus on the appropriate surveillance program for this population. Persons with multiple first-degree relatives or with one first-degree relative younger than 55 years of age with colon cancer are at higher risk and should be considered for surveillance colonoscopy 5 years earlier than the earliest age at onset of colon cancer in the family. The subsequent surveillance procedures and intervals are then tailored according to the extent of the family history. Patients with only one affected member may be relegated to the same screening program as for average-risk populations, whereas patients with a family history that suggests HNPCC or attenuated FAP may require annual or biennial colonoscopy.

Surveillance of patients with prior colorectal adenocarcinoma can be divided into two stages. In the first postoperative year, colonoscopy is performed at 3 to 6 months and again at 12 months to evaluate for anastomotic recurrence. Subsequently, the surveillance program is no different than for individuals with prior adenoma (i.e., colonoscopy every 3 years).

The high risk of colon cancer development in patients with long-standing ulcerative colitis has prompted the suggestion that patients with pancolitic involvement of more than 8 to 10 years' duration should undergo surveillance colonoscopy every 1 to 2 years. Multiple biopsy specimens should be obtained randomly from all segments of the colon and from any polypoid, plaquelike, or masslike lesion. The implications of findings of morphologic dysplasia are discussed in Chapter 47.

COLONIC LYMPHOMA

Etiology and Pathogenesis

Primary colonic lymphoma accounts for <0.5% of all colonic malignancies, although increases in incidence are reported with Sjögren's syndrome, Wegener's granulomatosis, rheumatoid arthritis, systemic lupus erythematosus, and acquired immunodeficiency syndrome.

Clinical Features, Diagnosis, and Management

Patients usually present with nonspecific abdominal pain, weight loss, constipation, and gastrointestinal hemorrhage. On colonoscopy, tumors appear as discrete masses or, less commonly, as diffuse infiltrative lesions. One-half of colonic lymphomas occur in the ileocecal region, and 50% have associated malignant adenopathy. Most lesions can be diagnosed by colonoscopic biopsy. Although the optimal treatment has not been defined, most regimens include chemotherapy. Surgery may be effective for localized disease, but the overall 2-year survival rate is only 40%.

CARCINOID TUMORS

Carcinoids are part of the amine precursor uptake and decarboxylation family of tumors and are most common in the appendix, where they usually are diagnosed incidentally. Carcinoids are occasionally detected as asymptomatic rectal polyps, but up to 25% of rectal carcinoids present with hemorrhage. Neither appendiceal nor rectal carcinoids commonly metastasize (Table 50-2). Carcinoid tumors are extremely rare in other regions of the colon; however, tumors in these sites produce obstruction and hemorrhage and often metastasize, which is a course that may be associated with development of the carcinoid syndrome. Because of the malignant potential of colonic carcinoids, surgical resection is the treatment of choice.

TABLE 50-2
Distribution of Gastrointestinal Carcinoid Tumors

ORGAN	PERCENTAGE OF TOTAL	PERCENTAGE WITH METASTASIS
Stomach	3	18
Duodenum	1	16
Jejunum	2	35
Ileum	28	35
Appendix	47	3
Colon	2	60
Rectum	17	12

CHAPTER 51

Anorectal Diseases

HEMORRHOIDS

Etiology and Pathogenesis

Hemorrhoids occur in up to 50% of adults in the United States and result from dilation of the superior and inferior hemorrhoidal veins, which form the physiologic hemorrhoidal cushion. Internal hemorrhoids arise above the dentate line in three locations—right anterior, right posterior, and left lateral—and are covered by columnar epithelium. External hemorrhoids arise below the mucocutaneous junction and are covered by squamous epithelium. Skin tags are redundant folds of skin arising from the anal verge. They may be residua of resolved thrombosed external hemorrhoids. The pathogenesis of hemorrhoids is believed to involve deterioration of the supporting connective tissue of the hemorrhoidal cushion, causing hemorrhoidal bulging and descent. Internal hemorrhoids are similar to arteriovenous malformations, exhibiting high levels of oxygen saturation. Some investigators have suggested that anal sphincter hypertrophy may predispose an individual to hemorrhoidal enlargement. There is an increased incidence of hemorrhoids among those with constipation, diarrhea, and pelvic tumors and among pregnant women.

Clinical Features, Diagnosis, and Management

Patients with internal hemorrhoids may exhibit gross but not occult bleeding (rarely requiring transfusion), discomfort, pruritus ani, fecal soiling, and prolapse. First-degree hemorrhoids do not protrude from the anus. Second-degree hemorrhoids prolapse with defecation but spontaneously reduce. Third-degree hemorrhoids prolapse and require digital reduction, and fourth-degree hemorrhoids cannot be reduced and are at risk of strangulation. Most patients with new-onset bleeding should be evaluated with sigmoidoscopy (or colonoscopy) to confirm that the source of hemorrhage is hemorrhoidal. Most first- and second-degree hemorrhoids can be managed with a high-fiber diet, adequate fluid intake, possible use of bulking agents, sitz baths twice daily, and good anal hygiene. Suppositories, ointments, and witch hazel may relieve discomfort in some cases. Rubber band ligation, injection sclerotherapy with sodium morrhuate or 5% phenol, liquid nitrogen cryoprobes, electrocoagulation, or photocoagulation with lasers or infrared light are effective in treating selected patients with bleeding or other symptoms caused by first- and second-degree internal hemorrhoids. Surgical hemorrhoidectomy is the treatment of choice for most third-degree hemorrhoids, all fourth-degree hemorrhoids, and other hemorrhoids refractory to nonsurgical therapy. In patients with high resting anal sphincter pressures, lateral internal sphincterotomy may achieve results comparable with those of rubber band ligation.

Thrombosis of an external hemorrhoid can produce severe pain and bleeding. Most thrombosed external hemorrhoids can be managed with sitz baths, bulking agents, stool softeners, and topical anesthetics; resolution occurs after 48 to 72 hours. If surgical evacuation or excision is required, it should be performed within 48 hours of symptom onset. Symptoms of skin tags include sensation of a growth and difficulty with anal hygiene. Treatment is conservative, and surgical resection is rarely needed.

ANORECTAL VARICES

Etiology and Pathogenesis

Anorectal varices are unrelated to hemorrhoids and are found in patients with other manifestations of portal hypertension. Anorectal varices are discrete, serpentine, submucosal veins that compress easily, extending from the squamous portion of the anal canal into the rectum.

Clinical Features, Diagnosis, and Management

Massive, life-threatening bleeding may occur from the anal or rectal portion of the varix. Injection sclerotherapy, cryotherapy, rubber band ligation, and hemorrhoidectomy can all produce torrential hemorrhage. Treatment by underrunning the variceal columns with an absorbable suture controls bleeding in most cases, but portosystemic shunting may be required.

ANAL FISSURE

Etiology and Pathogenesis

Anal fissure is a painful linear ulcer in the anal canal, usually located in the posterior midline (90%) and occasionally in the anterior midline. Lateral fissures suggest a predisposing illness such as inflammatory bowel disease (usually Crohn's disease), proctitis, leukemia, carcinoma, syphilis, or tuberculosis. Fissures are caused by traumatic tearing of the posterior anal canal during passage of hard stool. They may become chronic in the setting of high resting anal sphincter tone. Patients have an abnormal overshoot anal contraction after the normal relaxation, which may cause pain and spasm.

Clinical Features, Diagnosis, and Management

Patients typically present with anal pain and bright red rectal bleeding. The fissure is best identified by simple inspection after spreading the buttocks. An anal fissure is a small, linear tear perpendicular to the dentate line. Chronic anal fissures appear as the triad of a fissure, a proximal hypertrophic papilla, and a sentinel pile at the anal verge. Patients usually respond to a high-fiber diet, the addition of bulking agents, stool softeners, topical anesthetics (e.g., benzocaine, pramoxine), and warm sitz baths. Lateral subcutaneous internal anal sphincterotomy may be necessary for some patients with a chronic fissure. Midline sphincterotomy with fissurectomy or manual dilation may also be curative, but complications such as fecal incontinence may occur.

ANORECTAL ABSCESS AND FISTULA

Etiology and Pathogenesis

Anorectal abscess, the acute manifestation of suppurative infection, is an undrained collection of perianal pus, whereas anorectal fistula, the chronic manifestation of infection, is an abnormal communication between the anorectal canal and the perianal skin. Diseases associated with these disorders include hypertension, diabetes, heart disease, inflammatory bowel disease, and leukemia. Infection, most commonly with *Escherichia coli*, *Enterococcus* species, or *Bacteroides fragilis*, results from obstruction of anal glands as a result of trauma, anal eroticism, diarrhea, hard stools, or foreign bodies. Abscess and fistula formation may occur without primary glandular infection in patients with Crohn's disease, anorectal malignancy, tuberculosis, actinomycosis, lymphogranuloma venereum, radiation proctitis, leukemia, and lymphoma.

Clinical Features, Diagnosis, and Management

Swelling and acute pain, which are exacerbated by sitting, movement, and defecation, are the presenting symptoms of anorectal abscess. Malaise and fever are common. The presence of a foul-smelling discharge suggests that the abscess is spontaneously draining through the primary anal orifice. Physical examination reveals erythema, warmth, swelling, and tenderness, although intersphincteric abscesses may produce only localized tenderness. Anorectal abscesses require surgical drainage to prevent necrotizing infection, which carries a 50% mortality rate. Superficial perineal or ischiorectal abscesses may be drained under local anesthesia, but abscesses in other sites require more extensive drainage procedures in an operating room setting. Antibiotics usually are not necessary and may mask signs of underlying suppurative infection. However, second- or third-generation cephalosporins are indicated for patients with diabetes, leukemia, valvular heart disease, or extensive soft tissue infection. Warm sitz baths, stool-softening agents, and analgesics can minimize disease recurrence postoperatively.

Anorectal fistulae produce chronic, purulent drainage, pain on defecation, and pruritus ani. Examination may reveal a red, granular papule that exudes pus. Patients who are neutropenic may exhibit point tenderness and poorly demarcated induration. These patients have high mortality rates from disseminated infection. Multiple perineal openings suggest the possibility of Crohn's disease or hidradenitis suppurativa. Anoscopy and sigmoidoscopy are performed to locate the primary orifice at the level of the dentate line and to exclude proctitis. The presence of an anorectal fistula is an indication for surgery, which involves removal of the primary orifice and opening of the fistulous tract but conservation of the external sphincter. Patients with Crohn's disease who have chronic fistulae may benefit from immunosuppressive therapy or use of metronidazole or from conservative surgical techniques, such as seton placement. Postoperative care is the same as for anorectal abscess.

RECTAL PROLAPSE

Etiology and Pathogenesis

Rectal prolapse is protrusion of the rectum through the anal orifice. The prolapse may be complete (all layers visibly descend), occult (internal intussusception without visible protrusion), or mucosal (protrusion of distal rectal tissue but not the entire circumference). Rectal prolapse in children may be idiopathic or secondary to spina bifida, meningomyelocele, or cystic fibrosis. In adults, the condition is associated with poor pelvic tone, chronic straining, fecal incontinence, pelvic trauma, and neurologic disease. Defects that may result from rectal prolapse include weakened endopelvic fascia, levator ani diastasis, loss of the normal horizontal rectal position, an abnormally deep pouch of Douglas, a redundant rectosigmoid colon, a weak anal sphincter, denervation of the striated muscle, and loss of the anocutaneous reflex. Disturbed sphincter function and innervation may explain the frequent reports of fecal incontinence after surgical correction of rectal prolapse.

Clinical Features, Diagnosis, and Management

Patients report prolapse of tissue as well as defecatory straining, incomplete evacuation, tenesmus, and incontinence. On examination, the prolapse may be obvious when the patient is asked to sit and strain. Endoscopy or barium enema radiography is performed to exclude malignancy; it may reveal concomitant solitary rectal ulcer. Defecography is the best test to demonstrate occult prolapse. Persistently prolapsed tissue must be promptly reduced manually with or without intravenous sedation to avoid strangulation, ulceration, bleeding, or perforation. Complete rectal prolapse should be treated surgically (anterior sling rectopexy or Ripstein procedure, abdominal proctopexy with or without sigmoid resection). Perineal exercises or buttock strapping can be suggested to patients who refuse or who cannot undergo surgery. Perineal or extra-abdominal rectosigmoidectomy or diverting colostomy may be performed for elderly or debilitated patients. Occult prolapse is treated surgically if incontinence or solitary rectal ulcer is present; otherwise, conservative therapy is recommended.

ANAL STENOSIS

Etiology and Pathogenesis

Anal stenosis may result from malignancy (anal carcinoma, rectal carcinoma, invasion by urogenital malignancy) or benign conditions (prior rectal surgery, trauma, inflammatory bowel disease, laxative abuse, chronic diarrhea, radiation injury, lymphogranuloma venereum, congenital causes).

Clinical Features, Diagnosis, and Management

Symptoms of anal stenosis include small caliber stools, painful or resistant defecation, and bleeding. Mild strictures may respond to periodic dilation and dietary fiber supplementation; severe stenosis may require surgical anoplasty with or without lateral internal sphincterotomy.

FECAL INCONTINENCE

Etiology and Pathogenesis

Fecal incontinence is the loss of rectal contents against one's wishes. Women, the elderly, and institutionalized persons are affected most often. Traumatic obstetric and surgical injuries, rectal or hemorrhoidal prolapse, and neuropathic disease may impair anal sphincter function and lead to incontinence (Table 51-1). Traumatic or neuropathic injury that leads to abnormal straightening of the anorectal angle can also cause incontinence. Pudendal nerve injury may result from chronic defecatory straining and vaginal childbirth (especially with multiparity, high birth weight, forceps delivery, and third-degree perineal tears). Other factors that predispose to fecal incontinence include loss of anal or rectal sensation secondary to neuropathy and large-volume diarrhea. Hypersensitivity to distention and abnormal rectal motility probably account for the incontinence often seen in patients with irritable bowel syndrome.

Clinical Features, Diagnosis, and Management

Partial incontinence is defined as minor soiling and poor flatus control. The elderly and those with internal anal sphincter deficiency, fecal impaction, and rectal prolapse are prone to partial incontinence. Major incontinence refers to frequent loss of large amounts of stool. It is caused by neurologic disease, traumatic

TABLE 51-1
Causes of Fecal Incontinence

Diarrhea
Fecal impaction
Irritable bowel syndrome
Anal diseases
    Anal carcinoma
    Congenital abnormalities
    Protruding internal hemorrhoids
    Rectal prolapse
    Perianal infections
    Fistulae
    Injury (e.g., surgical, obstetric, accidental)
Rectal diseases
    Rectal carcinoma
    Rectal ischemia
    Proctitis (e.g., inflammatory bowel disease, radiation therapy, infection)
Neurologic diseases
    Central nervous system (e.g., cerebrovascular accident, dementia, toxic or metabolic
        disorders, spinal cord injury or tumors, multiple sclerosis, tabes dorsalis)
    Peripheral nervous system (e.g., diabetes, cauda equina lesions)
Miscellaneous
    Chronic constipation
    Descending perineum
    Advanced age

injury, and surgical damage. Rectal examination may reveal anal deformity, tumors, infections, fistulae, prolapsing hemorrhoids, loss of anal tone, and absence of the anal wink. A rough estimate of the anorectal angle and puborectalis function can be made by palpation of this muscle in the posterior midline during rest and voluntary squeeze.

Several tools are available for assessing the mechanisms of continence. Flexible sigmoidoscopy is used to exclude malignancy or rectal inflammation. Anorectal manometry can be used to define resting and maximal anal pressures, rectal compliance, and the sensitivity of the rectum to distention. Miniature probes are used to measure thermal and electrical sensitivity of the anal canal. Electromyographic tests are used to assess external sphincter and puborectalis muscle activity. Anorectal ultrasound is used to measure sphincteric muscle thickness and detects muscular defects with traumatic or surgical injury. Defecography radiographically demonstrates the evacuation of a simulated barium stool and provides static and dynamic measurements of the anorectal angle, pelvic floor, and puborectalis function. Continence can be tested by measuring leakage of rectally infused saline or resistance to passage of a solid object.

Treatment of fecal incontinence depends partially on its cause. Fiber therapy or opiate antidiarrheals are indicated for treatment of diarrhea. Fecal impactions are removed with enemas or by manual disimpaction. Anal biofeedback may be attempted in motivated individuals; therapeutic success rates of about 70% have been documented. This technique involves the use of a manometry catheter to record anal contractions. The patient learns to associate external anal contractions with the visual manometric recording by repetition and trial and error. Then, sphincter contraction in response to rectal balloon distention is taught. Conditions that respond poorly to biofeedback therapy include severe organic disease with reduced rectal sensation, irritable bowel syndrome, anterior rectal resection, and prior posterior anal sphincterotomy. Surgery is generally reserved for patients with major incontinence. Prior anal injury may be reparable with external anal sphincter repair; posterior proctopexy may be performed for complex sphincter injury, pelvic neuropathy, and loss of the normal anorectal angle. Anterior reefing procedures may be useful for women with anterior sphincter defects. Gracilis muscle transposition with or without electrical stimulation may benefit patients with a destroyed sphincter or a congenital pelvic floor abnormality. An artificial sling may be constructed for nonreconstructable sphincters or primary neurogenic disease. As a last resort, placement of a colostomy should be considered.

PRURITUS ANI

Etiology and Pathogenesis

Pruritus ani is an itchy sensation of the anus and perianal skin that may result from perianal disease or from residual fecal material. Anorectal diseases that produce pruritus ani include fissures, fistulae, hemorrhoids, and anal malignancies. *Candida albicans* and dermatophyte infections may appear as localized erythematous rashes, but may also be present on apparently normal skin. Pinworm (*Enterobius vermicularis*) causes nocturnal pruritus ani in children and in adults exposed to infected children. Scabies (*Sarcoptes scabiei*) and pubic lice produce pruritus ani that may be associated with genital itching. Sexually transmitted diseases associated with the condition include herpes simplex, gonorrhea, syphilis, condyloma acuminatum, and molluscum contagiosum. Generalized skin conditions (e.g., psoriasis) as well as local irritants, allergens, and chemicals may produce perianal itching. Clinical experience suggests that certain dietary products such as coffee, cola, beer, tomatoes, chocolate, tea, and citrus fruits may be causative. Idiopathic pruritus ani results from a combination of perianal fecal contamination and trauma.

Clinical Features, Diagnosis, and Management

Most cases of pruritus ani are successfully managed. If identified, dermatologic, infectious, and anorectal disorders should receive specific treatment (Table 51-2). A diagnosis of pinworms can be confirmed by detection of eggs on adhesive cellophane tape applied to the perianal skin early in the morning. Foods that predispose to diarrhea or pruritus should be eliminated. The key to management in most cases rests on keeping the anal area clean and dry while minimizing trauma induced by wiping and scratching. Patients should cleanse the perianal skin with a moistened pad after defecation. Witch hazel or lanolin preparations can soothe irritated tissues. The area should be dried with a blow dryer or with a soft tissue using a blotting motion. Thin cotton pledgets may be needed for those with fecal discharge. Excess perspiration can be controlled with baby powder and loose cotton clothing. Healing can be facilitated by application of 1% hydrocor-

Table 51-2
Causes of Pruritus Ani

Anorectal diseases
  Diarrhea
  Fecal incontinence
  Hemorrhoids
  Anal fissures
  Fistulae
  Rectal prolapse
  Anal malignancy
Infections
  Fungal (e.g., candidiasis, dermatophytes)
  Parasitic (e.g., pinworms, scabies)
  Bacterial (e.g., *Staphylococcus aureus*)
  Venereal (e.g., herpes, gonorrhea, syphilis, condyloma acuminatum)
Local irritants
  Moisture, obesity, perspiration
  Soaps, hygiene products
  Toilet paper (e.g., perfumed, dyed)
  Underwear (e.g., irritating fabric, detergent)
  Anal creams and suppositories
  Dietary (e.g., coffee, beer, acidic foods)
  Medications (e.g., mineral oil, ascorbic acid, quinidine, colchicine)
Dermatologic diseases
  Psoriasis
  Atopic dermatitis
  Seborrheic dermatitis

Source: Adapted from R Hanno, P Murphy. Pruritus ani: classification and management. Dermatol Clin 1987;5:81.

tisone cream twice daily for no more than 2 weeks (because of atrophic effects on the skin) and zinc oxide ointment. Nocturnal pruritus may benefit from oral antihistamines (e.g., diphenhydramine). Intractable symptoms may respond to intracutaneous injections of methylene blue.

RECTAL FOREIGN BODIES AND TRAUMA

Etiology and Pathogenesis

A number of foreign bodies can become lodged in the rectum after insertion for medical treatment, concealment, assault, and eroticism. Foreign bodies are classified as low-lying if they are in the rectal ampulla and high-lying if they are at or proximal to the rectosigmoid junction. Rectal trauma may result from penetrating injury (e.g., gunshot), blunt trauma (e.g., motor vehicle collisions), impalement (e.g., assault), sexual activities (e.g., fist fornication), and iatrogenic injury (e.g., endoscopy, enemas, surgery).

Clinical Features, Diagnosis, and Management

Patients may be reluctant to divulge the existence of a rectal foreign body or trauma. Therefore, a careful history and physical examination is important. Anteroposterior and lateral radiographs may define the location of a foreign body. Small, low-lying objects can be removed through an anoscope, whereas larger objects (e.g., vibrators) may require regional anesthesia, anal dilation, and a grasping forceps. Large, bulky items may be removed by inflating Foley catheters in the colon proximal to the object, followed by gentle traction on the catheters for careful extraction. High-lying foreign bodies are removed using spinal anesthesia and the lithotomy position. Gentle pressure on the abdomen pushes the object to within the reach of forceps directed through a rigid sigmoidoscope. Laparotomy is indicated if objects cannot be delivered distally, if abdominal distress develops, or if broken glass is present. Surgical procedures required for some cases of major rectal trauma include a diverting colostomy, presacral drain placement, rectal irrigation, and sphincter preservation.

ANAL MALIGNANCIES

Etiology and Pathogenesis

Anal malignancies include a variety of histologic types: squamous cell (70% to 80%), basaloid or cloacogenic (20% to 30%), mucoepidermoid (1% to 5%), and small-cell anaplastic (<5%) types. Patients present at a mean age of 60 years. Risk factors for anal malignancy include receptive anal intercourse in men; genital or anal warts in both sexes; smoking; prior venereal disease (e.g., gonorrhea, herpes simplex, infection with *Chlamydia trachomatis*); a history of positive results on a Papanicolaou smear; genital tumors in women; renal transplantation; chronic anal inflammation and scarring; and Crohn's disease. Adenocarcinoma of the anal canal may arise in anorectal fistulae. Extramammary Paget's disease is a perianal glandular tumor that appears in the seventh decade as an erythematous, well-demarcated eczematoid plaque. Anal melanoma typically are large (>4 cm), nonpigmented in one-third of cases, and tend to metastasize early. Survival rates are poor. Basal cell carcinoma of the anus is characterized by rolled skin edges with central ulceration. Bowen's disease is a slow-growing, squamous cell carcinoma in situ that manifests as red-brown scaly or crusted plaques. This disease is associated with metachronous neoplasms of the lung, gastrointestinal tract, and urogenital system.

Clinical Features, Diagnosis, and Management

Bleeding, pain, pruritus, or palpable lymphadenopathy may be the presenting symptoms of anal cancer, although many patients are asymptomatic and the diagnosis is not suspected until routine physical examination is performed. At presentation, 15% to 30% of patients have lymph node involvement, and 10% have liver or lung metastases. The diagnosis is made by biopsy. Lesions arising from the anal canal are more aggressive, whereas those originating from the anal margin are more differentiated and less malignant. Findings that confer a poor prognosis include squamous cell tumors of >2 cm in size, basaloid or anaplastic carcinomas, sphincteric invasion, and nodal spread. Radiation therapy plus chemotherapy with

5-fluorouracil and mitomycin C cause complete tumor regression in most cases of small, noninfiltrating anal cancers, with a 5-year survival rate of 70% and preservation of sphincter function. Wide local excision remains a therapeutic option for some patients, although anal canal adenocarcinoma typically recurs despite resection. Surgical treatment of extramammary Paget's disease includes wide local excision or radical abdominoperitoneal resection with ipsilateral groin dissection for advanced disease with nodal involvement. Surgery is rarely curative for anal melanoma. Resection or radiation therapy provides excellent results in treatment of basal cell carcinoma. Resection is curative of Bowen's disease.

HIDRADENITIS SUPPURATIVA

Etiology and Pathogenesis

Hidradenitis suppurativa is a suppurative condition of apocrine glands in the axilla and inguinoperineal regions that manifests in adolescence and young adulthood. Risk factors include obesity, acne, perspiration, and mechanical trauma. Apocrine duct occlusion, inflammation, and bacterial infection lead to formation of glandular abscesses that enlarge and spread. Repeated inflammation and healing produce fibrosis and draining sinus tracts, including anal and rectal fistulae. Bacteria associated with disease activity include *Streptococcus milleri*, *Staphylococcus aureus*, and gram-negative bacilli.

Clinical Features, Diagnosis, and Management

Patients present with tender anogenital abscesses with or without axillary disease; sinuses; fistulae; scarring; and, rarely, anemia, inflammatory arthritis, and squamous cell carcinoma. Warm, wet compresses are applied, and antibiotics are administered topically and systemically, but surgery is usually necessary. Draining nodules are exteriorized, and the base is curetted and cauterized to destroy the infected tissue. Total excision and skin grafting are needed in severe cases, and a diverting colostomy may be performed to prevent fecal soiling.

PILONIDAL DISEASE

Etiology and Pathogenesis

Pilonidal disease is an acquired condition of the midline coccygeal skin in which small skin pits precede development of a draining sinus or abscess. In contrast to anorectal fistula or hidradenitis suppurativa, there is no communication with the anorectum.

Clinical Features, Diagnosis, and Management

Patients, usually young men, present with a painful swelling and drainage. Acute pilonidal abscess requires incision, drainage, and hair removal; chronic pilonidal disease is managed by excision with or without marsupialization or primary closure. Squamous cell carcinoma may complicate the course of pilonidal disease.

This malignancy is more aggressive than other tumors arising from chronically irritated skin lesions.

PROCTALGIA FUGAX AND LEVATOR ANI SYNDROME

Etiology and Pathogenesis

Proctalgia fugax is characterized by sudden, brief episodes of severe rectal pain and is associated with irritable bowel syndrome and psychogenic disorders. In most cases the cause is unknown. A familial internal anal sphincter myopathy has been described, however, that causes proctalgia fugax and difficulty with defecation. Patients with the levator ani syndrome present with aching rectal pain caused by tenderness and spasm of the levator ani muscle group (ileococcygeus, pubococcygeus, puborectalis).

Clinical Features, Diagnosis, and Management

Attacks of proctalgia fugax are described as intense stabbing or aching midline pain above the anus, lasting seconds to minutes, associated with an urge to expel flatus, a desire to lie on one side with hips flexed, cold sweats, syncope, and priapism. Often the attacks occur at night. No clear precipitating cause can be identified. Local therapies, none of which have been subjected to trial, include rectal massage, firm perineal pressure, and warm soaks or baths. Anecdotal reports claim that various medications reduce symptoms, including amyl nitrate, nitroglycerin, salbutamol, clonidine, and diltiazem.

The pain of the levator ani syndrome is more chronic, aching, and pressure-like and than that of proctalgia fugax. Defecation and prolonged sitting can precipitate the pain. On examination, palpable tenderness and spasm of the levator muscles may be elicited. Treatment includes reassurance, local heat, rectal massage, diazepam, and electrogalvanic stimulation.

OTHER CAUSES OF ANORECTAL PAIN

Coccygodynia refers to a sharp or aching pain in the coccyx that may radiate to the rectal region or buttocks. It can be caused by traumatic arthritis, dislocation or fracture, difficult childbirth, or prolonged sitting. Manipulation of the coccyx on examination reproduces the pain. Therapies include warm soaks, analgesics, local corticosteroid injection, and, rarely, coccygectomy.

Other causes of anorectal pain include a familial disorder of proctalgia, high resting anal sphincter tone, cauda equina tumors, pelvic tumors, perianal endometriosis, intermittent enteroceles, and retrorectal tumors and cysts.

CHAPTER 52

Structural Anomalies and Hereditary Diseases of the Pancreas

EMBRYOLOGY AND ANATOMY OF THE PANCREAS

The pancreas begins as two separate outpouchings of the digestive tract. The ventral pancreas forms at the base of the hepatobiliary diverticulum and is drained by the duct of Wirsung, which usually shares a common channel with the distal common bile duct before emptying into the duodenum. The dorsal pancreas is an elongated structure that is drained by the duct of Santorini directly into the duodenum. In the second month of gestation, the ventral pancreas rotates to the left of the duodenum and migrates with the distal common bile duct to lie below the dorsal pancreas. Fusion of the duct of Wirsung and the distal portion of the duct of Santorini forms the main pancreatic duct. Most pancreatic secretions drain out the duct of Wirsung through the ampulla of Vater. The duct of Santorini usually drains only a small proportion of the pancreatic secretions. It is an accessory duct that drains into the duodenum through the minor papilla. It often regresses or ends blindly in the duodenal wall.

The adult pancreas is a 12 to 20 cm long, flattened, transversely oriented gland without a fibrous capsule that lies behind the peritoneum of the posterior abdominal wall. The pancreatic head is adjacent to the duodenal sweep. The pancreatic neck, a constricted part of the gland 3 to 4 cm wide, extends from the head of the pancreas to the left. In front of the aorta in the midline, the pancreatic body continues to the left, posterior to the gastric antrum and body. The pancreas terminates in the tail, which is adjacent to the hilum of the spleen. The sphincter of Oddi consists of circular smooth muscle that surrounds the common channel of the common bile duct and the main pancreatic duct.

The arterial blood supply to the pancreas originates from the celiac and superior mesenteric arteries. The pancreatic head and the duodenum have a common blood supply from the anterior and posterior pancreaticoduodenal arteries. The body and tail of the pancreas derive their blood supply from branches of the splenic artery. The general pattern of venous drainage of the pancreas is the same as that of the arterial supply; blood from the pancreas ultimately drains into the portal vein. The duodenum and pancreatic head have a common lymphatic drainage. Lymph eventually flows into the celiac and superior mesenteric groups of the para-aortic lymph nodes. The lymphatics of the pancreatic tail pass to the splenic nodes, and those of the body pass upward to the pancreaticosplenic nodes. The sympathetic efferent innervation of the pancreas derives from the greater, lesser, and least splanchnic nerves, whereas the parasympathetic innervation derives from the vagus nerves. Intrapancreatic ganglion cells are observed within the pancreatic interlobular tissues, with unmyelinated fibers passing to exocrine and endocrine cells.

The pancreas is a lobulated organ with lobular subunits consisting of acini. The acini are rounded or tubular and are lined by single rows of epithelial cells. The acinar lumen connects with intralobular ducts to form the interlobular ducts, which ultimately coalesce to form the main pancreatic duct. Ductules are lined by columnar, goblet, and argentaffin cells. Acinar cells contain highly basophilic cytoplasm reflective of the numerous ribosomes that are involved in protein production. The endocrine portion of the pancreas consists of 1 million islets of Langerhans. The islets are diffusely distributed throughout the gland, except in the tail, where they are relatively concentrated. Seventy-five percent to 80% of cells in the islets are B cells, which secrete insulin. The remainder are A, D, EC, and PP cells, which produce glucagon, somatostatin, 5-hydroxytryptamine, and pancreatic polypeptide, respectively.

PANCREAS DIVISUM

Incidence and Epidemiology

Pancreas divisum is the most common congenital structural anomaly of the pancreas. It is caused by the failure of the primordial ducts of Santorini and Wirsung to fuse during embryologic development. Autopsy series suggest a prevalence of 5% to 10%, but endoscopic series report a prevalence of 2% to 4%. Pancreas divisum is found in up to 25% of patients with idiopathic pancreatitis (in some series), which suggests that the condition may be an important cause of pancreatitis. Although pancreas divisum is a congenital anomaly, it usually is not detected until adulthood.

Etiology and Pathogenesis

Pancreas divisum results from failure of the ventral (Wirsung) and dorsal (Santorini) pancreatic ducts to fuse during the second month of embryonic development. In some cases there is a thin ductal stricture joining the two large ducts, an anomaly termed *incomplete pancreas divisum*. In pancreas divisum, most of the pancreas is drained by the accessory duct rather than by the proximal main pancreatic duct. It is postulated that increased resistance and ductal hypertension caused by the smaller caliber of the accessory duct and the minor papilla may induce pancreatitis.

Clinical Features

Most patients with pancreas divisum are asymptomatic and experience no significant clinical sequelae from the condition. It is not uncommon for the diagnosis to be made incidentally on endoscopic retrograde cholangiopancreatography.

In some patients, however, pancreas divisum is believed to be the cause of recurrent attacks of acute pancreatitis. As with pancreatitis induced by other causes, steady, severe epigastric pain, often radiating to the back, nausea, vomiting, and ileus are the dominant symptoms. Some patients report complete resolution of symptoms between attacks, whereas others have chronic abdominal pain and steatorrhea as a result of the chronic pancreatitis. Some patients experience only subtle episodic abdominal discomfort, which may represent a mild episode of pancreatitis. Patients with pancreatitis associated with pancreas divisum may experience any of the sequelae and complications found with acute or chronic pancreatitis secondary to other causes.

Findings on Diagnostic Testing

Laboratory Studies

Laboratory findings in patients with pancreatitis associated with pancreas divisum are similar to findings in patients with pancreatitis associated with other causes.

Structural Studies

Endoscopic retrograde pancreatography (ERP) is the definitive means of diagnosing pancreas divisum. Injection of contrast medium into the pancreatic duct through the major papilla reveals a short, narrow, arborizing duct in the pancreatic head that tapers to a blind end; the neck, body, and tail of the pancreas do not fill with contrast. In some patients, cannulation of the duct of Wirsung is not possible because of its small size. The diagnosis is confirmed by dye injection of the minor papilla, which demonstrates filling of a separate duct of Santorini all the way to the tail of the pancreas. In patients with recurrent acute pancreatitis, this duct may appear normal or slightly dilated. Patients with chronic pancreatitis usually have other ductal changes: ductal dilation and ectasia, dilated and blunted secondary radicals, intraductal stones, and possibly pseudocysts.

Management and Course

Patients with recurrent attacks of acute pancreatitis attributable to pancreas divisum may benefit from endoscopic sphincterotomy of the minor papilla, after which a pancreatic stent may be placed across the papilla to protect the duct from edema and inflammation. Although this therapy seems to decrease the episodes of acute pancreatitis, minor sphincterotomy is not effective for patients with chronic pancreatitis. Medical therapy with enzyme supplements and analgesics should always be the initial treatment of patients with chronic pancreatitis. Patients with refractory pain or pseudocysts may require surgical intervention.

ANNULAR PANCREAS

Etiology and Pathogenesis

Annular pancreas is characterized by a band of pancreatic tissue encircling the second portion of the duodenum. The annulus probably results from the tethering of a portion of the ventral pancreas as the ventral and dorsal pancreas rotate around the duodenum in the first 2 months of embryologic development. Annular pancreas is associated with other congenital defects, including Down's syndrome, Meckel's diverticulum, intestinal malrotation, tracheoesophageal fistulae, imperforate anus, and cardiac abnormalities.

Clinical Features, Diagnosis, and Management

Most patients present in the first year of life with vomiting and failure to thrive as a result of duodenal obstruction. Occasionally, annular pancreas is diagnosed in adulthood when patients complain of postprandial fullness or bloating and some develop gastrointestinal hemorrhage and acute pancreatitis. In infants, abdominal radiography may show the double bubble sign resulting from duodenal obstruction. Upper gastrointestinal barium radiography demonstrates a concentric narrowing, 0.5 to 5.0 cm in length, of the second portion of the duodenum. Symptomatic patients require surgical bypass of the obstructed segment. Division of the annulus is not recommended because of the high rate of development of postoperative pancreatic fistulae.

HETEROTOPIC PANCREAS

Etiology and Pathogenesis

Aberrant rests of pancreatic tissue can occur anywhere in the gastrointestinal tract, and rarely in extra-abdominal sites such as the lung. The probable cause is abnormal differentiation of pluripotent endodermal stem cells. The incidence is 0.6% to 15%, but most cases are subclinical.

Clinical Features, Diagnosis, and Management

Seventy-five percent of pancreatic rests occur in the submucosa of the stomach and small intestine. Upper gastrointestinal endoscopy or upper gastrointestinal barium radiography demonstrates a 2- to 4-cm submucosal nodule that often has a central depression. These lesions occasionally ulcerate, producing gastrointestinal hemorrhage. Because pancreatic rests contain the full histologic complement of normal pancreatic tissue, there is an extremely small risk of adenocarcinoma, islet cell tumors, or pseudocysts developing within these rests. Asymptomatic rests need no treatment, but symptomatic pancreatic rests should be surgically excised.

AGENESIS OR HYPOPLASIA OF THE PANCREAS

Agenesis of the pancreas is a rare congenital anomaly that results in absolute endocrine and exocrine insufficiency. In hypoplasia of the pancreas, also known as *lipomatous pseudohypertrophy of the pancreas*, the islets of Langerhans are intact but the acinar cells are replaced by fatty tissue. Although the mechanisms for development remain unclear, an intrauterine infection may be the primary insult that disrupts embryologic development of the exocrine gland.

CONGENITAL CYSTS

Congenital pancreatic cysts are usually solitary and sporadic, but some hereditary disorders such as polycystic kidney disease, cystic fibrosis, and von Hippel–Lindau syndrome manifest multiple pancreatic cysts. Most congenital cysts are diagnosed in infancy as an abdominal mass, which may cause symptoms related to gastroduodenal or biliary obstruction. Some congenital cysts are not detected until adulthood, and in this setting they must be differentiated from pseudocysts, cystadenomas, and cystadenocarcinomas. Asymptomatic lesions require no therapy, but surgical enucleation is the treatment of choice for symptomatic cysts.

CYSTIC FIBROSIS

Incidence and Epidemiology

Cystic fibrosis, an autosomal-recessive disease with an incidence of 40 in every 100,000 live births in white populations, is the most common hereditary disease of the exocrine pancreas. The gene frequency may be as high as 5% among persons of Northern European ancestry, but the disease may occur in any social or ethnic group. In the United States, there are >7 million asymptomatic heterozygotes and 30,000 affected homozygotes.

Etiology and Pathogenesis

The cystic fibrosis gene encodes a chloride channel termed the *cystic fibrosis transmembrane conductance regulator* (CFTR). The mutation of this gene results in the loss of a single amino acid, accounting for 70% of mutant alleles in patients with cystic fibrosis and preventing transport of the CFTR protein to the cell surface. Under normal conditions, chloride secretion through the CFTR activates a chloride-bicarbonate exchange and promotes transcellular movement of sodium and water. A defect of CFTR function impairs apical bicarbonate secretion as well as transcellular sodium and water secretion. This defective dilution and alkalinization leads to inspissation of protein-rich pancreatic secretions and ultimately to ductal obstruction and acinar disruption. As the disease progresses, pancreatic autodigestion contributes to the pancreatic injury, which culminates in diffuse fibrosis and cystic degeneration. Although islet cells are spared in the early stages of the disease, insulin production may be compromised in the late stages. Defective CFTR function is also responsible for obstructive secretions in the lungs, genital tract, and biliary tract, where focal biliary cirrhosis may result.

Clinical Features

The pancreatic manifestations of cystic fibrosis are apparent at 2 years of age in 80% of patients. The earliest complication is meconium ileus, which occurs in 15% of cases, and presents in the first week of life as abdominal distention, bilious vomiting, and delayed passage of meconium. The inspissated meconium becomes impacted in the small intestine. Some patients may have associated atresia of the small intestine or volvulus, which may be complicated by peritonitis.

The most common clinical presentation of pancreatic insufficiency is poor weight gain and growth retardation despite adequate caloric intake. In the first few months of life, stools are watery, but later in the first year, the stools are bulky and greasy, characteristic of steatorrhea. Frequent passage of bulky stools, chronic coughing, and decreased muscle mass contribute to the development of rectal prolapse in 20% of patients. Older children and adults may present with bowel obstruction or intussusception caused by inspissated stool or partially digested food. Deficiencies of fat-soluble vitamins A, D, E, and K may occur at any age with significant steatorrhea. Rarely, a patient with cystic fibrosis who does not have exocrine insufficiency may present with acute pancreatitis. In addition to exocrine insufficiency, 10% to 15% of young adults with cystic fibrosis develop diabetes mellitus.

Hepatobiliary disorders (e.g., gallbladder cysts and gallstones) are common in patients with cystic fibrosis, but the most clinically significant disease is focal biliary cirrhosis, which occurs in 5% of young children and adults. Inspissation of bile in intrahepatic bile ducts leads to periportal inflammation and fibrosis and bile duct proliferation. Patients may present with asymptomatic alkaline phosphatase elevations, jaundice, splenomegaly, and complications of portal hypertension.

Findings on Diagnostic Testing

Laboratory Studies

Patients with cystic fibrosis exhibit several laboratory abnormalities. Hypoproteinemia may result from chronic catabolism and malabsorption. Minimal elevations in serum amylase and lipase levels may reflect low-grade pancreatitis, whereas a rare patient with acute pancreatitis may have marked enzyme elevations. Hepatic involvement is characterized by nonspecific elevations in liver chemistry values, with a disproportionate increase in alkaline phosphatase levels. Deficiencies in vitamin K or vitamin B_{12} may manifest as a prolongation of prothrombin time or macrocytic anemia. Chronic pulmonary infections and malnutrition cause other nonspecific abnormalities, including anemia, leukocytosis, and low serum nitrogen levels.

Evaluation of Exocrine Function

Patients with pancreatic exocrine insufficiency usually have steatorrhea, which is best assessed by a quantitative 72-hour fecal fat assay. Testing of pancreatic exocrine function with administration of secretin or cholecystokinin, followed by measurement of pancreatic bicarbonate or enzyme output, frequently reveals diminished secretory capacity before clinically significant maldigestion is detected. ERP is rarely necessary, but if performed, the ductal structures may display a range of nonspecific changes similar to those in chronic pancreatitis.

Sweat Testing

The gold standard for confirming the diagnosis of cystic fibrosis is the sweat test. When performed in an experienced laboratory, analyses of sodium and chloride concentrations in sweat are 99% sensitive for detecting affected homozygotes. The sweat in patients with cystic fibrosis typically has sodium and chloride concentrations of >77 and >74 mEq per liter, respectively, because of the diminished water content of sweat. False-positive assays may occur with dehydration, edema, congestive heart failure, malnutrition, adrenal insufficiency, and diabetes insipidus.

Genetic Testing

When the sweat test result is equivocal or prenatal screening is desired, genetic analysis may be useful if the patient has one of the common CFTR mutations. A mutation in a single amino acid at a nucleotide binding site accounts for 70% of the mutant alleles. However, the sensitivity of genetic screening is limited; the remaining 30% of mutant alleles are the result of >60 diverse mutations not easily detected by current methods.

Management and Course

The natural course of cystic fibrosis is dominated by recurrent pulmonary infections, impaired growth, and malnutrition. Improvement in the median survival time to approximately 30 years is the result of recent therapeutic advances. The clinical severity of cystic fibrosis varies widely; some patients have relatively uncomplicated courses of disease and live into their fourth and fifth decades. This variability may be caused by different CFTR mutations and the corresponding defects in chloride channel function.

Although the pulmonary complications of cystic fibrosis are the most common cause of hospitalization and mortality, gastrointestinal complications may contribute significantly to morbidity, and specific therapeutic intervention is often warranted. Pancreatic enzyme replacement improves steatorrhea and corrects nutritional deficiencies. Large enzyme doses and acid suppression with H_2-receptor antagonists ensure adequate delivery of intact enzymes to the small intestine. Patients deficient in vitamin A, D, E, and K should receive supplements. If severe protein and calorie malnutrition persist despite these measures, enteral or parenteral nutrition may be necessary.

Obstruction of the small intestine by meconium or an impacted, partially digested food bolus may be confirmed with a meglumine (Gastrografin) enema. The high osmolarity of this water-soluble contrast stimulates lumenal water secretion, which may disrupt the impaction. The mucolytic agent, *N*-acetylcysteine, given orally or rectally, is also helpful for relieving the obstruction. If conservative therapy fails or signs of peritonitis develop, surgical exploration is necessary.

HEREDITARY PANCREATITIS

Hereditary pancreatitis is an autosomal dominant syndrome characterized by recurrent attacks of pancreatitis that often progresses to chronic pancreatitis. The mean age at onset is 10 years. The genetic alterations and pathophysiologic mechanisms of this syndrome remain poorly defined; however, investigators have identified a potentially pathogenic mutation in the cationic trypsinogen gene. With long-standing disease, the pancreas becomes calcified, and large calcium stones in the pancreatic ducts are common. Patients with hereditary pancreatitis develop maldigestion, chronic pain, pancreatic pseudocysts, splenic vein thrombosis, and distal bile duct strictures. Adenocarcinoma of the pancreas develops in 5% of patients. It is not clear if this increased risk of malignant transformation warrants surveillance with computed tomography or ultrasound.

SHWACHMAN SYNDROME

Shwachman syndrome is an autosomal recessive disorder characterized by pancreatic exocrine insufficiency, neutropenia, metaphyseal dysostosis, and eczema. With an incidence of 5 in every 100,000 live births, it is the second most common cause of pancreatic insufficiency in children, after cystic fibrosis. Neutropenia is classically cyclical and may be associated with anemia and thrombocytopenia. Infectious complications resulting from neutropenia are the most common cause of death. Remarkably, patients surviving into adulthood often experience improvement in pancreatic exocrine function.

CHAPTER 53

Acute Pancreatitis

INCIDENCE AND EPIDEMIOLOGY

Acute pancreatitis is a clinical syndrome of sudden-onset abdominal pain and elevations in the levels of serum pancreatic enzymes caused by an acute necroinflammatory response in the pancreas. The hospitalization rates for acute pancreatitis vary between communities because of the demographic differences in the cause of acute pancreatitis (Table 53-1). In the United States, >80% of cases of acute pancreatitis are caused by binge drinking of ethanol or by biliary stones. In urban settings, the majority of cases are associated with alcohol use, whereas in suburban or rural settings, gallstones tend to be the predominant cause. In contrast, infection with *Ascaris lumbricoides* may be the cause of pancreatitis in 10% to 20% of patients in Asian populations.

ETIOLOGY AND PATHOGENESIS

Pathogenic Mechanisms

Although the mechanisms responsible for pancreatitis are not well defined, the fundamental defects appear to be breakdowns in the normal exocrine function

TABLE 53-1
Differential Diagnosis of Acute Pancreatitis

Ethanol
Gallstones
   Choledocholithiasis
   Biliary sludge
   Microlithiasis
Mechanical/structural injury
   Sphincter of Oddi dysfunction
   Pancreas divisum
   Trauma
   Post–endoscopic retrograde cholangiopancreatography
   Pancreatic malignancy
   Peptic ulcer disease
   Inflammatory bowel disease
Medications
   Azathioprine/6-mercaptopurine
   Dideoxyinosine
   Pentamidine
   Sulfonamides
   L-Asparaginase
   Thiazide diuretics
Metabolic
   Hyperlipidemia
   Hypercalcemia
Infectious
   Viral
   Bacterial
   Parasitic
Vascular
   Vasculitis
   Atherosclerosis
Miscellaneous
   Scorpion bite
   Hereditary pancreatitis
   Idiopathic pancreatitis
   Cystic fibrosis
   Coronary bypass
   Tropical pancreatitis

and cellular defenses of the pancreas. Premature activation of intrapancreatic zymogens by trypsinogen autoactivation or the lysosomal enzyme cathepsin B appears to be the pivotal derangement and may result from intracellular retention and impaired cellular transport of zymogen granules. The normal zymogen granule has protective levels of pancreatic trypsin inhibitor, which may be quantitatively reduced or functionally defective in acute pancreatitis. Excessive cholinergic stimulation may also contribute to pancreatic injury. Once intrapancreatic zymogen activation is initiated, a cascade of inflammatory cells and chemical mediators potentiates cellular destruction, increases vascular permeability, and promotes local ischemia. Although the causes of acute pancreatitis are diverse, intracellular zymogen activation followed by a necroinflammatory response of variable severity appears to be the final common pathway.

Risk Factors

Gallstones and biliary sludge appear to induce pancreatitis by producing transient obstruction of the main pancreatic duct. Patients with gallstones have a 20-fold increased risk of pancreatitis, but the incidence of pancreatitis is <0.2% per year in this patient population. Microlithiasis, microscopic crystals of cholesterol monohydrate or calcium bilirubinate, as well as ultrasonographically visible biliary sludge, also increase the risk of pancreatitis, presumably by mechanisms similar to those for gallstones. Microlithiasis and biliary sludge may account for up to two-thirds of cases of idiopathic pancreatitis.

Ethanol induces pancreatitis by several mechanisms: main pancreatic duct obstruction resulting from altered sphincter of Oddi function, small ductule obstruction by concretions of secreted protein, altered fluidity of the pancreatic cell membrane, and ethanol-induced hypertriglyceridemia. Pancreatitis usually occurs in the setting of long-standing alcohol abuse or binge drinking, but only 5% of heavy drinkers develop clinical pancreatitis. Most patients with ethanol-induced acute pancreatitis have underlying chronic pancreatitis, a finding that is consistent with the observation that initial pancreatitis attacks almost always present after years of significant alcohol intake.

Obstruction of pancreatic secretion is a less common cause of acute pancreatitis. Sphincter of Oddi dysfunction occurs mostly in patients who have had a cholecystectomy. It is associated with increases in sphincter pressure caused by increased smooth muscle tone or fibrotic stricturing. Pancreas divisum results from failure of the ventral and dorsal ducts to join during fetal development. The small accessory duct of Santorini and minor papilla may produce a relatively high outflow resistance. Sphincter of Oddi dysfunction or pancreas divisum is observed in >25% of patients with idiopathic pancreatitis in some series. Whether this represents a causal or coincidental association in any individual patient is difficult to discern.

Other disease processes are associated with pancreatitis. Ten percent of patients with pancreatic adenocarcinoma manifest acute pancreatitis. Penetrating duodenal ulcers may extend into the pancreas and produce a focal pancreatitis. Two metabolic disturbances that can trigger acute pancreatitis are hypercalcemia and hyperlipidemia. Hyperlipidemia also may be a consequence of the fat necrosis in acute pancreatitis resulting from any cause, but levels of serum triglycerides of more than 1000 mg per dl have been reliably defined as a precipitant of pancreatitis. Pancreatic infarction resulting from atherosclerotic disease or vasculitis is a rare cause of acute pancreatitis. Infections with mumps, coxsackie B virus, and cytomegalovirus may be complicated by pancreatitis. A *lumbricoides* infection causes up to 20% of cases of acute pancreatitis in Asia. Other infectious causes of pancreatitis are common in patients with acquired immunodeficiency syndrome. A rare familial form of pancreatitis, hereditary pancreatitis, frequently evolves into chronic pancreatitis and is associated with a high risk for development of pancreatic cancer.

Trauma or manipulation of the pancreatic duct can cause pancreatitis. Endoscopic retrograde cholangiopancreatography (ERCP) is the most common iatrogenic cause of pancreatitis; up to 5% of patients develop the complication. Sphincterotomy, underlying sphincter of Oddi dysfunction, excessive dye injection of the pancreas (acinarization), and hyperosmolar contrast all increase the risk of pancreatitis. Blunt abdominal trauma can cause pancreatitis, usually by disruption of the main pancreatic duct as it crosses over the vertebral body. Postoperative pancreatitis occurs most often after upper abdominal procedures. Other surgical procedures, especially coronary bypass surgery, have been associated with hyper-amylasemia, but clinical pancreatitis is unusual. Percutaneous biopsy of the pancreas and lithotripsy have been reported to induce pancreatitis.

Medications are common causes of pancreatitis (see Table 53-1). Of the patients taking azathioprine or 6-mercaptopurine, 3% develop acute pancreatitis, almost always in the first month of therapy. Pentamidine, even in aerosol form, produces pancreatitis. The onset of pancreatitis associated with 2',3'-dideoxyinosine (ddI) may be several months after drug initiation. Medications that have been less convincingly associated with pancreatitis include sulfonamides, 5-aminosalicylates, furosemide, thiazides, estrogens, tetracyclines, and cimetidine. The etiologic role of corticosteroids remains uncertain. With the exception of estrogens, which may produce pancreatitis by induction of hypertriglyceridemia, the mechanism of drug-induced pancreatitis is unknown.

CLINICAL FEATURES

The initial symptom of acute pancreatitis is almost always abdominal pain, which is described as a boring visceral-type epigastric pain that develops over several hours. It persists for hours to days and radiates to the middle to lower back. Patients frequently are restless and cannot remain still. Increased pain when supine prompts many patients to sit leaning forward in an effort to minimize discomfort. However, 5% of patients with acute pancreatitis present without abdominal pain.

Nausea and vomiting are present in most patients. Low-grade fever is commonly observed in uncomplicated pancreatitis, but high fever and rigors suggest coexisting infection. In some cases of severe pancreatitis, the diagnosis is overlooked because of the patient's inability to report pain in the setting of delirium, hemodynamic instability, or extreme respiratory distress.

Physical examination of a patient with pancreatitis may reveal several findings. Abdominal tenderness with guarding is common and usually most pronounced in the epigastric region. Bowel sounds are diminished as a result of superimposed ileus. Tachycardia may be secondary to severe pain, but hypovolemia is common, and severe cases may be complicated by hypotension resulting from extravasation of fluids or hemorrhage in the retroperitoneum. Rare patients present with peri-umbilical (Cullen's sign) or flank (Grey Turner's sign) ecchymoses. Ethanol-induced pancreatitis is occasionally accompanied by signs or symptoms of alcoholic liver disease, including jaundice, hepatomegaly, ascites, and encephalopathy. It is estimated that 1% of alcoholics will have pancreatitis and liver disease. Gallstone pancreatitis may be accompanied by jaundice caused by a retained common bile duct stone, although any severe cause of pancreatitis may be associated with jaundice that is caused by biliary obstruction from an edematous pancreas or associated fluid collection.

FINDINGS ON DIAGNOSTIC TESTING

Laboratory Studies

Elevated serum amylase and lipase levels are the most common abnormalities seen in laboratory studies of patients with acute pancreatitis and result from increased release and decreased renal clearance of the enzymes. Elevations greater than fivefold are virtually diagnostic of pancreatitis, but disease severity does not correlate with the degree of enzyme elevation. Total serum amylase is composed of pancreatic and salivary isoforms. Salivary amylase levels increase with salivary gland disease, chronic alcoholism without pancreatitis, cigarette smoking, anorexia nervosa, esophageal perforation, and several malignancies. The pancreatic amylase isoform may also be elevated in cholecystitis, intestinal perforation, and intestinal ischemia. Five percent to 10% of episodes of acute pancreatitis produce no increases in serum amylase and lipase, which is most common in the setting of underlying chronic alcoholic pancreatitis and long-term glandular destruction and fibrosis with loss of functional acinar tissue. Macroamylasemia is characterized by persistent elevation of serum amylase levels because of decreased renal excretion of a high-molecular-weight macroamylase. The disorder is benign. Differentiation from pathologic hyperamylasemia relies on calculation of the amylase-to-creatinine clearance ratio (ACCR), which equals

(serum creatinine × urine amylase)/(urine creatinine × serum amylase) × 100.

An ACCR of <1% suggests macroamylasemia.

Serum lipase has been reported to be a more specific marker of pancreatitis, but mild elevations are observed in other conditions (e.g., renal failure and intestinal perforation). In pancreatitis, lipase levels may remain elevated for several days after amylase levels have normalized. Therefore, if there is a delay in diagnosis, hyperlipasemia may be the only abnormal laboratory finding. A lipase-to-amylase ratio of >2 has been reported to be specific for alcoholic pancreatitis; however, this should not replace the history and physical examination as the primary means of discerning the cause of pancreatitis.

Patients often have other laboratory abnormalities. Leukocytosis can result from inflammation or infection. An increased hematocrit may signal decreased plasma volume caused by extravasation of fluid; a decreased hematocrit may be caused by retroperitoneal hemorrhage. Electrolyte disorders are common, particularly hypocalcemia, which in part is caused by sequestration of calcium salts as saponified fats in the peripancreatic bed. Patients with underlying liver disease or choledocholithiasis may have abnormal liver chemistry values.

Structural Studies

Ultrasound is the most sensitive noninvasive means of detecting gallstones, biliary tract dilation, and gallbladder sludge. Intralumenal gas may obscure images of the pancreas, however, rendering ultrasound an insensitive technique for detecting the changes associated with pancreatitis. Computed tomographic (CT) scanning is superior to ultrasound for imaging the peripancreatic bed. In mild cases, the pancreas may appear edematous or enlarged. More severe inflammation may extend into surrounding fat planes, producing a pattern of peripancreatic fat streaking. CT scanning also is optimal for defining inhomogeneous pancreatic phlegmons with ill-defined margins or well-defined pseudocysts. A dynamic arterial phase CT scan can identify areas of tissue necrosis, which are at significant risk of subsequent infection. The magnitude of pancreatic necrosis is predictive of overall prognosis. Given its high cost and the limited yield in evaluating mild disease, CT scanning should be reserved for patients with severe disease. Once pancreatitis has resolved, CT scanning

TABLE 53-2
Prognostic Criteria for Acute Pancreatitis

RANSON CRITERIA	SIMPLIFIED GLASGOW CRITERIA
On admission	Within 48 hrs of admission
Age >55 yrs	Age >55 yrs
Leukocyte count >16,000/μl	Leukocyte count >15,000/μl
Lactate dehydrogenase >350 IU/liter	Lactate dehydrogenase >600 IU/liter
Glucose >200 mg/dl	Glucose >180 mg/dl
Aspartate aminotransferase >250 IU/liter	Albumin <3.2 g/dl
48 hrs after admission	Calcium <8 mg/dl
Hematocrit decrease by >10%	Arterial Po_2 <60 mm Hg
Serum urea nitrogen increase by >5 mg/dl	Serum urea nitrogen >45 mg/dl
Calcium <8 mg/dl	
Arterial Po_2 <60 mm Hg	
Base deficit >4 mEq/liter	
Estimated fluid sequestration >6 liter	

Sources: Adapted from N Agarwa, CS Pitchumoni. Assessment of serverity in acute pancreatitis. Am J Gastroenterol 1990;85:356; and JB Marshall. Acute pancreatitis: a review with an emphasis on new developments. Arch Intern Med 1993;153:1185.

may have a role in excluding pancreatic cancer as a cause of pancreatitis in older patients.

ERCP is primarily a therapeutic tool in acute biliary pancreatitis; it has no role in diagnosing acute pancreatitis. Once acute pancreatitis has been resolved, ERCP should be considered if the cause of the pancreatitis is unclear.

MANAGEMENT AND COURSE

Prognosis

The most common prognostic criteria used to assess acute pancreatitis are the Ranson criteria, which are observations made at admission and at 48 hours after admission, and the simplified Glasgow criteria, which are variables measured at any time during the first 48 hours (Table 53-2). The prognostic accuracy of the two scales is similar. Although the Ranson criteria were developed to assess alcoholic pancreatitis, they are frequently applied to pancreatitis of other causes. If two signs or fewer are present, mortality is <1%; three to five signs predict a mortality rate of 5%; and six or more signs increase the mortality rate to 20%. Other factors associated with a poor prognosis include obesity and extensive pancreatic necrosis.

Complications

Patients with severe pancreatitis may develop peripancreatic fluid collections or pancreatic necrosis, either of which can become infected. The role of prophylactic antibiotics in patients with severe pancreatitis is controversial. If administered, the combination of a quinolone and metronidazole provides resistance against the gram-negative and anaerobic organisms most frequently encountered. Infections occurring in the first 1 to 2 weeks usually involve peripancreatic fluid collections or pancreatic necrosis and are characterized by florid symptoms. More indolent courses are characteristic of pancreatic abscesses, which can arise several weeks after a bout of pancreatitis in well-defined pseudocysts or areas of resolving pancreatic necrosis. Gram's stain and culture of fluid obtained by CT-guided aspiration is mandatory if infection is suspected. Infected necrotic tissue and pancreatic abscesses require immediate surgical debridement, although some well-defined abscesses may be drained percutaneously.

Pseudocysts develop in 10% of patients with acute pancreatitis. Pseudocysts can persist for several weeks, causing pain, compressing adjacent organs, and eroding into the mediastinum. Cysts more than 5 to 6 cm in diameter are associated with a 30% to 50% risk of complications, including rupture, hemorrhage, and infection. Although many pseudocysts spontaneously resolve or decrease in size, persistent (>6 weeks) large cysts or rapidly expanding cysts should be drained using surgical, endoscopic, or percutaneous procedures. Percutaneous drainage may be complicated by formation of a pancreaticocutaneous fistula. Administration of the somatostatin analog octreotide may lower the risk of fistula formation by decreasing pancreatic secretions. Endoscopic drainage may be achieved by transpapillary stent placement or transgastric placement of a cystenterostomy.

Pancreatitis may be complicated by several pulmonary processes. Mild hypoxemia is present in most patients with pancreatitis. Chest radiography may demonstrate increased interstitial markings or pleural effusions, which usually are left-sided and small but occasionally are large enough to compromise respiration. The interstitial edema occurs in the setting of normal cardiac function; the etiology is unclear. Severe adult respiratory distress syndrome requires artificial respiratory support. Multisystem organ failure may accompany this syndrome.

Other systemic complications of severe pancreatitis include stress gastritis, renal failure, hypocalcemia, delirium, and disseminated fat necrosis (involving bones, joints, and skin). Extension of the inflammatory process into the peripancreatic bed may produce splenic vein thrombosis, which may be complicated by development of gastric varices and gastrointestinal hemorrhage.

Therapy

Therapy for most cases of acute pancreatitis is supportive, although severe cases may require massive volume repletion with crystalloids and colloids. Patients should receive nutrition and electrolytes intravenously, not enterally. If symptoms are expected to persist more than 2 to 3 days, total parenteral nutrition should be considered. Parenteral meperidine is preferred over morphine as an analgesic because of the risk of morphine-induced sphincter of Oddi spasm. Nasogastric suctioning is primarily useful for intractable vomiting, but it is not needed in all cases. There is no evidence to support the routine use of antibiotics or somatostatin. The decision to reinitiate feeding should not be based on serum enzyme levels but rather on the clinical status of the patient. Resolution of pain and emergence of hunger reliably indicate that the patient is ready to eat.

Gallstone pancreatitis is managed differently from acute pancreatitis of other causes. Emergency ERCP with sphincterotomy and stone extraction reduces the complication rate and shortens the hospital stay for patients with severe gallstone pancreatitis. These procedures should be reserved for patients with severe disease or for those who fail to improve with conservative treatment. It is important to note that ERCP does not appear to significantly worsen pancreatitis. Patients with mild gallstone pancreatitis should be treated conservatively; ERCP is performed after recovery to assess for retained bile duct stones. The risk of recurrent gallstone pancreatitis is up to 33%; therefore, all patients should undergo expeditious and definitive surgical therapy. For patients who are poor operative risks, endoscopic sphincterotomy without cholecystectomy is an acceptable therapeutic option.

CHAPTER 54

Chronic Pancreatitis

INCIDENCE AND EPIDEMIOLOGY

Chronic pancreatitis causes irreversible morphologic and functional damage to the pancreas. In many cases, there are intermittent flares of acute pancreatitis. The clinical distinction between acute recurrent pancreatitis, with restoration of normal pancreatic function and structure between attacks, and chronic pancreatitis may be difficult. Ethanol use accounts for most cases of chronic pancreatitis in the United States, whereas in Asia and Africa, malnutrition is the major cause (Table 54-1). The prevalence of chronic pancreatitis in autopsy series is 0.04% to 5.0%, although it may be as high as 45% in alcoholics. Most cases are probably subclinical; only 5% to 10% of heavy ethanol users develop clinical pancreatitis.

ETIOLOGY AND PATHOGENESIS

Ethanol Use

Alcohol is responsible for up to 80% of cases of chronic pancreatitis in Western societies. Alterations in pancreatic secretion appear to play a pathogenic role in ethanol-induced chronic pancreatitis. Alcohol consumption increases the sensitivity of the pancreas to cholecystokinin (CCK), resulting in increased enzyme secretion. The resultant high-protein, high-viscosity output of the pancreas provides the substrate for protein plug formation in secondary ductules. Ethanol may fur-

---

TABLE 54-1
Causes of Chronic Pancreatitis

Ethanol (70–80%)
Idiopathic (including tropical) (10–20%)
Other (10%)
    Hereditary
    Hyperparathyroidism
    Hypertriglyceridemia
    Obstruction
    Trauma
    Cystic fibrosis

---

ther promote ductal precipitates by decreasing the production of lithostatin, a pancreatic protein that inhibits the formation of calcium stones. The main cause of pancreatic injury and dysfunction is the blockage of small ductules and eventually the main pancreatic duct by protein plugs and stones.

There does not seem to be a threshold level of alcohol consumption below which there is no risk of pancreatitis. Persons who consume as little as one ethanol-containing beverage per day have a higher risk for development of chronic pancreatitis than persons who abstain. The risk increases with increased mean daily consumption and duration of ethanol use, but the type of alcohol and pattern of drinking do not influence the risk. Alcohol consumption alone does not appear to be sufficient to induce pancreatitis, given the small percentage of alcoholics who manifest clinical disease. Other factors such as diet composition and genetic susceptibility probably interact with ethanol to produce chronic pancreatitis.

Malnutrition

Malnutrition-induced (or tropical) pancreatitis is the most prevalent form of chronic pancreatitis in developing Asian and African countries. Consumption of cassava, a plant indigenous to these regions, may contribute to pancreatic injury by increasing serum thiocyanate levels, which subsequently increases cellular free radical production. Ingestion of a diet deficient in micronutrients and antioxidants then exposes the pancreas to injury by unopposed free radicals. Pancreatic calculi and ductular obstruction also contribute to ongoing injury, as seen with alcoholic pancreatitis.

Other Causes

Disorders that produce long-standing obstruction of the main pancreatic duct are associated with chronic pancreatitis, including tumors, traumatic strictures, and pancreas divisum. The association of sphincter of Oddi dysfunction with chronic pancreatitis remains controversial. A small percentage of patients with hyperparathyroidism develop pancreatic duct stones and calcific pancreatitis as a result of increased pancreatic calcium secretion. Genetics plays a role in the rare syndrome of hereditary pancreatitis. This disease appears in childhood or young adulthood and is transmitted in autosomal dominant fashion. In Western countries, idiopathic chronic pancreatitis is the second most common form of the disease. A bimodal age distribution in adolescents and the elderly suggests that there may be two distinct pathophysiologic causes. Cystic fibrosis is a common cause of chronic pancreatic insufficiency in pediatric practices.

CLINICAL FEATURES

Abdominal pain and malabsorption are the most common clinical features of chronic pancreatitis. Pain, which is present in 85% of patients, is probably caused by noxious stimulation of peripancreatic afferent nerves or increased intraductal pressure. Typically felt in the upper quadrants, the pain may radiate to the back. It often is less intense while sitting forward. Patients may report several days of pain with pain-free intervals. Some patients have steady, unremitting pain. Food ingestion increases the intensity of pain, leading to a fear of eating (sitophobia), which is the main cause of weight loss in chronic pancreatitis.

Malabsorption in chronic pancreatitis results from inadequate pancreatic enzyme secretion. Maldigestion is the physiologic defect that occurs when exocrine function is <10% of normal. Steatorrhea is the initial manifestation of malabsorption, but in more advanced disease, azotorrhea occurs. Because mucosal absorptive capacity is intact, voluminous diarrhea is unusual; most patients complain of bulky or greasy stools. A pattern of steatorrhea, weight loss, and fat-soluble vitamin deficiencies in the absence of abdominal pain is common in idiopathic chronic pancreatitis.

Most patients eventually develop symptomatic hyperglycemia. Although insulin is frequently necessary to control symptoms, most patients are not prone to ketosis. Patients with ethanol-induced chronic pancreatitis may have symptoms of liver disease, including ascites, encephalopathy, variceal bleeding, and jaundice. Jaundice can also result from compression or stricturing of the intrapancreatic portion of the common bile duct.

Physical examination findings may be normal or there may be marked abdominal tenderness. Patients may have stigmata of chronic alcoholism including gonadal atrophy, gynecomastia, and palmar erythema. A midline mass suggests the presence of a pseudocyst or complicating neoplasm. Rarely, patients have pancreatic ascites or clinical evidence of fat-soluble vitamin (A, D, E, and K) deficiency.

FINDINGS ON DIAGNOSTIC TESTING

Laboratory Studies

The findings of laboratory evaluation are often normal in chronic pancreatitis. Rarely, patients exhibit hyperbilirubinemia and abnormal liver chemistry values as a result of concurrent alcoholic liver disease or common bile duct stricture. Acute flares of pancreatitis may be accompanied by leukocytosis. Macrocytic anemia occurs in a rare patient with vitamin B_{12} deficiency. Coagulopathy may result from vitamin K malabsorption or alcoholic liver disease. Because azotorrhea occurs only in advanced disease, serum albumin levels usually are normal despite profound weight loss. Serum amylase and lipase levels may be slightly elevated, but marked elevations, as observed in acute pancreatitis, are unusual. If exocrine function is severely impaired, serum lipase levels may be low, whereas serum amylase levels usually are normal in this setting because salivary amylase production is normal.

Assessment of Pancreatic Exocrine Function

Numerous methods of assessing pancreatic enzyme output are available. The simplest tests to perform are those that detect increased fat in the stool, which develops if exocrine secretion is reduced by >90%. Steatorrhea may be detected by qualitative fecal fat tests (Sudan stain) or quantitative 72-hour fecal fat measurements. In severe cases, the amount of fat excreted in the feces may approach the amount of fat ingested, indicative of profound reductions in pancreatic enzyme output. Such high degrees of steatorrhea are rarely observed with mucosal disease of the small intestine.

Pancreatic exocrine function is more accurately assessed by pancreatic stimulation tests after injection of secretin or CCK, or after ingestion of a high protein meal, with simultaneous collection of pancreatic secretions through a catheter positioned in the distal duodenum. The collected fluid is assayed for bicarbonate (for secretin stimulation) or lipase and trypsin (for CCK stimulation). Chronic pancreatitis is characterized by decreased secretory output in response to these stimulants. False-positive pancreatic stimulation tests may occur in diabetes mellitus, cirrhosis, and after Billroth II gastrojejunostomy. Incomplete duodenal recovery of pancreatic juice or gastric acid inactivation of enzymes may lead to an underestimation of pancreatic function. The sensitivity of pancreatic function tests for detecting chronic pancreatitis is 70% to 95%, including most patients with only mild to moderate pancreatic insufficiency.

The bentiromide test in an indirect measure of pancreatic function. Patients ingest a tripeptide that is cleaved by pancreatic chymotrypsin, releasing para-aminobenzoic acid (PABA). PABA is absorbed in the intestine and is measured in the urine, providing an index of chymotrypsin activity. The sensitivity of bentiromide testing is only 50% in early chronic pancreatitis, suggesting that the diagnostic value of this test is limited. The findings on Schilling's test are abnormal in chronic pancreatitis because of impaired cleavage of R protein, which prevents the binding of vitamin B_{12} to intrinsic factor. Expanding this test to include vitamin B_{12} bound to intrinsic factor can differentiate the maldigestion of R protein from malabsorption of the vitamin B_{12}–intrinsic factor complex. Ingestion of the triglyceride ^{14}C-olein with subsequent measurement of breath $^{14}CO_2$ excretion provides an assessment of triglyceride digestion and absorption. As with the bentiromide test, these studies exhibit low sensitivities in the detection of early chronic pancreatitis.

Structural Studies

Confirming the diagnosis of chronic pancreatitis usually requires imaging studies of the pancreas. Abdominal radiography demonstrates the diagnostic finding of pancreatic calcifications in 30% to 40% of patients with chronic pancreatitis, obviating the need for more expensive imaging procedures. Ultrasound has a sensitivity of 70% and a specificity of 90% in the detection of chronic pancreatitis. Findings include pseudocysts, dilation of the main pancreatic duct, and discrete, echogenic foci in the parenchyma. Ultrasound is also useful in excluding biliary dilation caused by a distal common bile duct stricture as the cause of hyperbilirubinemia. Although intralumenal gas may preclude adequate examination of the pancreas, confirming the diagnosis with ultrasound spares the patient from invasive testing.

If abdominal radiography and ultrasound fail to confirm the diagnosis, a computed tomographic (CT) scan demonstrates the architectural changes of chronic pancreatitis, with a sensitivity of 80% and a specificity of 90%. Chronic pancreatitis can also be differentiated from pancreatic carcinoma on a CT scan, and a CT scan can reveal splenomegaly and venous collaterals resulting from splenic vein thrombosis. Endoscopic retrograde pancreatography (ERP) provides the most detailed anatomic assessment of the pancreatic ducts. In the absence of a histologic specimen, ERP is the gold standard for the diagnosis of chronic pancreatitis. The main pancreatic duct is normal in early pancreatitis, but the side branches may be dilated. Patients at this stage often have normal secretory function, but occasionally exocrine function is reduced out of proportion to the ERP findings. With more advanced disease, dilation and an irregular contour of the main pancreatic duct may be observed. Although pancreatic cancer may produce a discrete stricture of the main pancreatic duct, chronic pancreatitis often leads to multiple ductal strictures and filling defects as a result of stone formation. Brush cytology specimens obtained under fluoroscopic guidance may be used to distinguish benign strictures from malignant strictures. Endoscopic ultrasound (EUS) has emerged as a means of obtaining detailed images of the pancreas. Several reports suggest that this technique is equivalent to ERP; both tests exhibit sensitivities and specificities of >90%. Unlike ERP, EUS has no risk for inducing pancreatitis. EUS-guided fine-needle aspiration can differentiate chronic pancreatitis from malignancy. ERP and EUS are costly, invasive procedures that should be used only when less invasive procedures fail to substantiate the diagnosis of chronic pancreatitis or if a diagnostic finding such as a stricture, ductal dilation, or intraductal calculus will alter management.

MANAGEMENT AND COURSE

Medical Therapy

Medical therapy for chronic pancreatitis focuses on relief of pain and repletion of digestive enzymes. If the patient has symptoms of maldigestion, pancreatic enzyme supplements should be taken before all meals. Although some preparations are specifically designed to release enzymes into the duodenum (Table 54-2), there is little evidence to suggest that encapsulated preparations are superior to standard supplements. It is usually more difficult to treat steatorrhea than azotorrhea. At least 25,000 to 30,000 units of lipase per meal are necessary to provide adequate lipolysis; therefore, patients will need to take 2 to 10 pills with each meal, depending on the preparation. Gastric acid can destroy pancreatic enzymes, necessitating the administration of enteric-coated preparations or acid suppressants (e.g., H_2-receptor antagonists or proton pump inhibitors) for some patients.

Enzyme replacement therapy may also decrease the pain associated with chronic pancreatitis. A decrease in enzyme secretion increases CCK levels, which in turn produce pancreatic hyperstimulation. By interrupting the feedback upregulation of CCK release, enzyme replacements reduce hormonal stimulation of the pancreas, thereby decreasing intraductal pressures. Non–enteric-coated preparations are the only supplements that reliably deliver enzymes to the proximal duodenum where feedback regulation begins. Similarly, only non–enteric-coated preparations have been shown in clinical trials to reduce pan-

TABLE 54-2
Pancreatic Enzyme Preparations

		CONTENTS (UNITS)		
PREPARATION	DELIVERY*	Lipase	Amylase	Protease
Cotazyme	Capsule	8,000	30,000	30,000
Cotazyme-S	Enteric-coated microsphere	5,000	20,000	20,000
Creon 10	Enteric-coated microsphere	10,000	33,200	37,500
Ilozyme	Uncoated tablet	11,000	30,000	30,000
Ku-Zyme HP	Enteric-coated microsphere	8,000	30,000	30,000
Pancrease MT-4	Enteric-coated microtablet	4,000	12,000	12,000
Pancrease MT-10	Enteric-coated microtablet	10,000	30,000	30,000
Pancrease MT-16	Enteric-coated microtablet	16,000	48,000	48,000
Protilase	Enteric-coated microsphere	4,000	20,000	25,000
Viokase	Uncoated tablet	8,000	30,000	30,000
Viokase	Powder	16,800	70,000	70,000
Zymase	Enteric-coated microsphere	12,000	24,000	24,000

*Enteric-coated microspheres and microtablets are encased in a cellulose capsule.

Source: Adapted from RR Berardi, VA Dunn-Kucharski. Pancreatitis and Cholelithiasis. In DiPiro JT, Talbert RL, Hayes PE, et al. (eds), Pharmacotherapy: A Pathophysiologic Approach. Norwalk, CT: Appleton & Lange, 1993;614.

creatic pain. For reasons that remain unclear, patients with advanced or alcohol-induced chronic pancreatitis appear to respond less often to enzyme supplements than do patients with idiopathic chronic pancreatitis.

Analgesics remain the primary means of controlling the pain of chronic pancreatitis. An initial trial of acetaminophen or NSAIDs is preferable. Patients should be cautioned about excessive doses of acetaminophen. Severe cases require administration of opiate analgesics. Concerns over addiction should not interfere with the goal of pain relief; a strong patient-physician relationship may prevent abuse of prescribed narcotics.

The somatostatin analog octreotide inhibits pancreatic secretion and has visceral analgesic effects; thus, it might be expected to decrease pain in chronic pancreatitis. Clinical trials are under way to ascertain the utility of this drug in patients with painful chronic pancreatitis. Octreotide may also have a role in management of refractory pancreatic fistulae or pseudocysts.

Nonmedical Therapy

A small percentage of patients are refractory to medical measures and require more invasive procedures to control pain. Although celiac plexus neurolysis has been effective for pain control in patients with pancreatic adenocarcinoma, results in patients with chronic pancreatitis have been disappointing. Most patients experience only transient relief. Endoscopic pancreatic stone extraction, occasionally performed in conjunction with extracorporeal shock wave lithotripsy, reduces pain in 50% to 80% of cases. Patients with tight strictures may obtain pain relief after endoscopic balloon dilation and stent placement. Controlled trials evaluating these techniques are not available.

For severe debilitating pain unresponsive to medical therapy, surgical therapy is a legitimate means of restoring quality of life to a patient with chronic pancreatitis. Patients with dilation of the main pancreatic duct are optimal candidates for pancreaticojejunostomy (modified Puestow procedure), a procedure with initial success rates of 80%. Unfortunately, many patients develop recurrent pain several years postoperatively. Patients without significant ductal dilation may require partial or subtotal pancreatectomy according to the extent of parenchymal disease. One-half of patients experience pain relief. Ketosis-prone diabetes invariably complicates subtotal pancreatectomy. Pancreatic islet cell autotransplantation at the time of the operation may prevent postoperative diabetes.

Complications

Patients with chronic pancreatitis who report severe refractory pain or worsening of pain should be evaluated for the development of a pseudocyst. Ultrasound detects many pseudocysts, but a CT scan is the definitive diagnostic procedure. Pseudocysts in chronic pancreatitis usually are found in the body of the gland. They may rupture, bleed, or become infected; the risk of these complications is much lower than the corresponding risk of complications associated with acute pseudocysts. Cysts larger than 6 cm rarely resolve and require internal drainage through surgical or endoscopic techniques. Percutaneous CT-guided catheter drainage has proved successful in some cases, although a persistent pancreaticocutaneous fistula may develop.

CHAPTER 55

Pancreatic Adenocarcinoma

DUCTAL ADENOCARCINOMA

Incidence and Epidemiology

With 27,000 deaths yearly, pancreatic adenocarcinoma is the fifth leading cause of cancer death in the United States. More than 80% of patients present after the age of 60 years. The incidence of this cancer has more than doubled since 1930, with especially prominent increases in women. The annual incidence of pancreatic adenocarcinoma is 12 per 100,000 in men and slightly less in women. Populations living in urban settings have a higher incidence than age-matched rural populations. Advanced age and the presence of other severe diseases contribute to the poor outcome for patients with pancreatic adenocarcinoma.

Etiology and Pathogenesis

Pathogenic Mechanisms

Although the events responsible for pancreatic carcinogenesis remain poorly defined, several genetic alterations occur in most pancreatic tumors. Point mutations in the oncogene Ki-*ras* are present in 90% of adenocarcinomas. Similarly, 50% to 70% of tumors harbor a defect in the tumor suppressor gene, *p53*, and another 50% have defective expression of *DCC*, the tumor suppressor gene frequently deleted in advanced colorectal polyps or cancer. Unlike the situation in colorectal neoplasia, there are no reliable means to detect premalignant pancreatic lesions; therefore, it is unclear if there is the stepwise accumulation of genetic instabilities that characterize the pathogenesis of pancreatic cancer, as there is with colorectal cancer.

Risk Factors

Several environmental exposures increase the risk for development of pancreatic adenocarcinoma (Table 55-1). Cigarette smoking is associated with a twofold

TABLE 55-1
Risk Factors for Pancreatic Adenocarcinoma

Advanced age
Men >40 years
Urban location
Diabetes mellitus
Hereditary pancreatitis
Tobacco smoking
High-fat diet
Occupational exposure to carcinogens (chemical, petroleum industries)

increase in the rate of pancreatic cancer; it manifests at least 10 years before similar neoplasia in nonsmokers. The dietary content of fat also correlates with the incidence of pancreatic carcinoma. Canada and the United States, with mean dietary fat intakes of >120 g per day, have twice the rates of pancreatic cancer of Japan and Italy, where mean fat intakes range from 40 to 80 g per day. Exposure to industrial chemicals and petroleum derivatives such as aminobenzene, methylnitrosourethane, and β-naphthylamine coal tar derivatives have been associated with pancreatic adenocarcinoma, but the magnitude of this risk is unclear. Preliminary reports have linked pancreatic cancer with excessive coffee and alcohol consumption, but further analyses have refuted these claims.

Pancreatic adenocarcinoma may develop in patients who have other pancreatic disease. Although pancreatic cancer induces glucose intolerance in up to 60% of affected patients, pre-existing diabetes mellitus has been postulated to predispose to pancreatic cancer. Twenty percent of patients with diabetes have had their disease for >2 years before being diagnosed with pancreatic carcinoma, suggesting that the biochemical or pathologic consequences of diabetes may promote tumor formation in small numbers of persons. Patients with chronic pancreatitis also are at increased risk for development of pancreatic adenocarcinoma. The risk increases with the duration of pancreatitis; it is 2% at 10 years and 4% at 20 years of disease. The risk is particularly high in patients with hereditary pancreatitis. Despite these increased cancer rates, the mechanism of tumor promotion in long-standing diabetes and chronic pancreatitis remains unclear.

Clinical Features

Most patients experience abdominal pain that often radiates to the back. The indolent onset of the pain contrasts with the acute severe pain of acute pancreatitis and cholangitis. Careful questioning of the patient often reveals that pain developed up to 3 months before the onset of jaundice. The pain of pancreatic cancer results from ductal obstruction or malignant perineural invasion. It usually is poorly localized and constant. As with other forms of pancreatic pain, the severity may be increased by lying supine and decreased by leaning forward while sitting.

Seventy percent of pancreatic adenocarcinomas occur in the head of the pancreas, and virtually all of these lesions produce obstructive jaundice. Cancers in the body or tail of the gland only rarely manifest jaundice because of the anatomic spacing between the tumors and the common bile duct that courses posterior to the head of the pancreas. Jaundice in patients with tumors in the pancreatic body or tail usually results from adenopathy in the porta hepatis or extensive liver metastasis. Pruritus and pale-colored stools are common with jaundice owing to impaired bile excretion in the setting of extrahepatic biliary obstruction.

Loss of >10% of body weight almost invariably occurs with pancreatic cancer. Weight loss usually results from anorexia and inadequate caloric intake. Sixty percent of patients with pancreatic adenocarcinoma have delayed gastric emptying, most often in the absence of mechanical gastroduodenal obstruction. Gastroparesis may be secondary to infiltration of the local splanchnic neural network and disruption of the neurohumoral mechanisms responsible for coordinated gastroduodenal motility. Reduced secretion of pancreatic enzymes with consequent maldigestion can also contribute to weight loss. Maldigestion is particularly prominent with tumors of the pancreatic head, as obstruction of the pancreatic duct in this location results in near total loss of pancreatic enzyme secretion.

Diabetes mellitus is present in >60% of patients with pancreatic adenocarcinoma. Most patients first experience glucose intolerance within 2 years of the diagnosis of pancreatic cancer, which suggests that the malignancy causes diabetes. Enhanced secretion of islet amyloid peptide from the islets of Langerhans adjacent to the tumor is the probable cause. Elevated serum levels of this peptide produce marked insulin resistance and relative glucose intolerance. Despite the frequent coexistence of diabetes mellitus, hyperglycemia rarely leads to significant morbidity in patients with pancreatic carcinoma.

Acute pancreatitis may be the initial manifestation in up to 5% of pancreatic tumors. Adenocarcinoma of the pancreas should be considered in any older adult with acute pancreatitis unrelated to gallstones or ethanol. Duodenal obstruction caused by local invasion of the pancreatic mass occurs in 10% of patients. Obstruction is rarely a presenting feature, and it is almost always a preterminal event. Other uncommon complications include gastric variceal hemorrhage resulting from splenic vein thrombosis, major depression, and migratory superficial thrombophlebitis (Trousseau's syndrome).

The physical examination of patients with pancreatic adenocarcinoma frequently reveals jaundice and evidence of significant weight loss. The chest and extremities may have extensive excoriations and lichenification as the result of constant scratching because of the effects of jaundice. Tumors in the body and tail may be detected as a palpable mass because they grow to an enormous size before causing symptoms. With long-standing biliary obstruction, the gallbladder may become markedly distended and palpable, defining the classic Courvoisier's sign.

Findings on Diagnostic Testing

Laboratory Studies

At the time of clinical presentation, patients often have several laboratory abnormalities, but none are specific for the diagnosis of pancreatic adenocarcinoma. Serum amylase and lipase levels may be mildly elevated, but this finding is not universal, and normal levels should not preclude further testing. There may be mild elevations of liver chemistry values and disproportionate increases in alkaline phosphatase levels. Hematologic abnormalities include anemia caused by nutritional deficiencies or blood loss and thrombocytopenia caused by splenomegaly associated with splenic vein thrombosis. The tumor markers carcinoembryonic antigen (CEA) and CA19-9 are elevated in 75% to 85% of patients with pancreatic adenocarcinoma. Assays of these serum markers lack the specificity necessary for a reliable diagnosis, however.

Imaging Studies

Ultrasound may identify pancreatic cancer, but overlying intralumenal gas and excess adipose tissue often compromise image quality. Even if examination of the pancreas is incomplete, ultrasound may demonstrate ancillary findings of pancreatic cancer, including dilation of the biliary tract and enlargement of the gallbladder. Computed tomography (CT) is superior to ultrasound, providing a sensitivity of 80% for detecting pancreatic masses. CT also has the capability to define the tumor stage using dynamic contrast-enhanced imaging. Spiral CT, also termed *helical CT*, represents an advance in tomographic technology; image resolution is improved and imaging during the arterial and venous phases of contrast enhancement is possible. Ongoing studies should clarify whether spiral CT is superior to standard dynamic CT for detecting and staging pancreatic masses. Ultrasound and CT guide needle biopsy of pancreatic masses; however, anecdotal reports of tumor seeding along the needle track have prompted concern about performing these procedures in patients with potentially resectable tumors.

Endoscopic retrograde cholangiopancreatography (ERCP) has a sensitivity and specificity of 90% for the diagnosis of pancreatic malignancy. Abrupt obstruction of both a dilated common bile duct and a dilated pancreatic duct is termed the *double-duct sign*. This finding is virtually diagnostic of pancreatic cancer and is usually indicative of an advanced tumor in the pancreatic head. Less advanced lesions and cancers in the body or tail more often produce discrete pancreatic duct strictures. Cytologic samples of a pancreatic stricture can be obtained at the time of ERCP, but the yield is limited and the sensitivity is only 30% to 40%.

Endoscopic ultrasound (EUS) has a sensitivity of >90% for the detection of pancreatic tumors. It is more sensitive than CT or ultrasound for the detection of tumors smaller than 2 cm. EUS is the most accurate imaging test for staging the local extent of pancreatic tumors and is particularly useful for detecting invasion of the major splanchnic vessels. EUS-guided fine needle aspiration of the mass can establish a histologic diagnosis of adenocarcinoma, with a sensitivity of 80% to 90%. Because the needle track is confined to the area of surgical resection, there is no concern of tumor seeding outside the field of resection.

Management and Course

Staging

Curative surgical resection provides the only chance for long-term survival to patients with pancreatic adenocarcinoma. Unfortunately, at the time of presentation, >85% of patients have unresectable disease. Preoperative staging is essential to establish the prognosis and to plan the optimal treatment strategy. As with many other cancers of the gastrointestinal tract, pancreatic tumors are classified on the basis of the TNM staging system (Table 55-2). Tumors invading the major splanchnic vessels (T3), except the splenic vein, or involving distant sites (M1) cannot be resected for cure. Because splenectomy, and hence splenic vein resection, is often performed at the time of pancreatic cancer resection, invasion of the

TABLE 55-2
TNM Staging of Pancreatic Cancer

Primary tumor (T)
   T1   Tumor <2 cm, confined to pancreas
   T2   Tumor >2 cm, confined to pancreas
   T3   Tumor invades adjacent major blood vessels or organs other than duodenum
Lymph nodes (N)
   N0   No regional lymph node metastasis
   N1   Regional lymph node metastasis
Distant metastasis (M)
   M0   No distant metastasis
   M1   Distant metastasis

splenic vein does not preclude complete excision of the tumor. Although metastasis to regional lymph nodes (N1) does not preclude complete surgical excision, patients with these tumors have an unfavorable prognosis relative to patients without lymph node metastasis. Several complementary procedures are used to define the stage of pancreatic cancer. Contrast-enhanced CT scanning is the best noninvasive means of detecting liver metastasis. Invasion of the large splanchnic vessels can be detected with a sensitivity of 30% to 50%. Angiography detects vascular invasion with a sensitivity of 75%. EUS has emerged as the most accurate means of detecting vascular invasion, with a sensitivity and specificity approaching 90%. As with angiography, EUS is not a reliable method of detecting distant metastatic disease, hence the optimal staging strategy combines CT and EUS studies. Magnetic resonance imaging has been refined to improve the definition of the vascular anatomy of the peripancreatic bed. Ongoing studies will define the staging role of this imaging modality.

Surgical Therapy

Surgical exploration with the intent of performing curative resection should be attempted in all patients who have apparently resectable disease. An initial staging laparoscopy should be performed as part of the planned resection to inspect the peritoneum and liver for evidence of distant metastases not detected on CT scans. Even when all staging procedures, including laparoscopy, indicate a resectable tumor, unresectable disease is found in 10% to 20% of patients after surgical dissection. Cancers localized to the pancreatic head require a pancreaticoduodenectomy—the Whipple procedure. Lesions in the body or tail can be treated with a distal pancreatectomy. Alternative procedures, including total pancreatectomy and the pylorus-sparing Whipple procedure, have no proven advantage relative to the standard operations. In the past, operative mortality rates for curative resection averaged 10% to 20%, but specialized centers are reporting mortality rates of 2% to 5%. The poor overall prognosis of pancreatic cancer is underscored by five-year survival rates of 10% to 25% for patients who undergo surgical resection. The long-term survival of patients with T1 cancers is only 35% to 40%; most deaths result from recurrent disease. Unfortunately, survival for 5 years does not guarantee a cure from this disease; 40% of these persons eventually die of recurrent pancreatic adenocarcinoma.

Palliative Therapy

Because most patients with pancreatic cancer have unresectable disease at the time of presentation and have an expected survival of 6 months, palliation of symptoms is the primary goal. Correction of nutritional deficiencies and control of pain can be achieved with supportive measures. Malabsorptive symptoms can be alleviated with adequate pancreatic enzyme supplementation. Adequate protein and caloric intake may require enteral nutrition, given the high rate of malnutrition in these patients. NSAIDs and acetaminophen may be adequate for pain control, but if pain is severe, narcotics should be administered. Narcotics may have constipating effects, necessitating the concomitant use of osmotic or stimulant laxatives. For relief of tumor-associated refractory pain, surgical or radiologically guided percutaneous injection of alcohol into the celiac ganglion is 90% effective.

Obstructive jaundice and pruritus may be treated by surgical biliary bypass or by endoscopic or percutaneous placement of a biliary stent. Endoscopic stent placement and surgical bypass are >90% successful in relieving biliary obstruction, but surgical therapy is associated with longer hospitalizations, higher morbidities, and higher periprocedural mortality rates. Percutaneous stent placement for distal common bile duct malignant strictures has a higher morbidity and mortality relative to endoscopic stent placement because of the hemorrhage and bile leaks associated with transhepatic puncture. Therefore, endoscopic placement is preferred. Unfortunately, 40% of biliary stents become obstructed with debris and sludge 5 to 6 months after placement. As a prophylactic measure, plastic stents often are replaced every 3 to 6 months to prevent cholangitis secondary to stent occlusion. Expandable metallic biliary stents have been associated with lower occlusion rates, but high cost precludes routine use. Further studies are needed to define the optimal roles of metallic versus plastic stents in patients with pancreatic adenocarcinoma.

In contrast to biliary obstruction, symptomatic duodenal obstruction is best managed surgically. This complication occurs in 10% of patients with pancreatic cancer. Gastrojejunostomy is the procedure of choice. Unfortunately, duodenal obstruction is often a preterminal event and surgical intervention may be contraindicated because of the overall poor clinical status of the patient.

The role of chemotherapy and radiation therapy for patients with pancreatic cancer is limited. Combined radiation and chemotherapy may prolong survival by 2 to 4 months, but there is often significant therapy-induced toxicity. Formal assessments of quality of life are lacking.

OTHER MALIGNANT AND PREMALIGNANT DISEASES OF THE PANCREAS

Cystic Neoplasms

Cystic neoplasms of the pancreas may be benign or malignant. These lesions must be differentiated from the pseudocysts that often complicate the course of acute and chronic pancreatitis. Cystadenomas are classified as mucinous, also termed *macrocystic adenomas,* and serous, also termed *microcystic adenomas.* The distinction is critical because serous cystadenomas have no malignant potential, whereas mucinous cystadenomas have a high incidence of progression to cystadenocarcinoma. Both lesions occur more commonly in women; serous lesions usually are diagnosed in elderly patients, and mucinous lesions usually are diagnosed in middle-aged patients. Because mucinous lesions are larger, abdominal pain, weight loss, and vomiting are common presenting symptoms. Serous lesions are usually less than 4 to 6 cm and contain many small cysts less than 1 to 2 cm in diameter. One-third of serous lesions exhibit a characteristic stellate "sunburst" calcification, sometimes evident on abdominal radiography. In contrast, mucinous cystadenomas contain a few large cysts, and a curvilinear calcification of the cyst capsule may occur. Despite these characteristic anatomic features, distinguishing the two neoplasms on the basis of imaging alone is unreliable. Although increases in cyst fluid viscosity and CEA levels may favor the diagnosis of a mucinous neoplasm, only surgical biopsy can confirm the diagnosis. Asymptomatic serous lesions require no further therapy, but all mucinous lesions and symptomatic serous lesions require surgical resection. In comparison with the poor survival rate associated with ductal adenocarcinoma, patients with mucinous cystadenomas and cystadenocarcinomas have a 5-year survival rate of 50% after surgical resection.

Solid and Papillary Epithelial Neoplasms

Solid and papillary epithelial neoplasms arise from the epithelium of ductules, usually in the tail of the pancreas. Most patients are women. Tumors are often larger than adenocarcinomas and frequently exhibit a cystic appearance on CT or ultrasound studies as a result of liquefaction necrosis. Despite their large size, many tumors remain localized. Resection is associated with long-term survival.

Mucinous Ductal Ectasia

Mucinous ductal ectasia, also referred to as a mucin-producing cystic tumor, is a premalignant lesion of the pancreatic duct. The etiology is unknown. Massive dilation of the pancreatic duct is characteristic. Patients present with abdominal pain, weight loss, and steatorrhea. On endoscopic examination, the ampulla of Vater may be seen to release copious amounts of viscous mucus into the duodenum. Papillary projections of dysplastic mucosa and intraductal collections of mucinous debris often produce diffuse filling defects on ERCP. At the time of presentation, patients often have coexisting adenocarcinoma, which suggests that mucinous ductal ectasia is a variant of mucinous cystadenocarcinoma. Surgical excision is curative if the lesion is detected before carcinoma develops. Because the lesion often involves the entire pancreatic duct, pancreatectomy is the procedure of choice.

CHAPTER 56

Endocrine Neoplasms of the Pancreas

INCIDENCE AND EPIDEMIOLOGY

Pancreatic endocrine neoplasms are rare, having an estimated prevalence of 10 per 1 million population. Insulinomas and gastrinomas are the most common, whereas tumors that secrete vasoactive intestinal polypeptide (VIPomas) or glucagon are much less common. Only a small number of cases of symptomatic somatostatinomas have been reported, and the incidence of tumors that secrete growth hormone releasing factor (GRFomas) is unknown. Tumors that secrete pancreatic polypeptide (PPomas) and nonfunctional tumors do not generally produce clinical syndromes related to excess circulating hormone, but may account for one-third of all pancreatic endocrine tumors.

ETIOLOGY AND PATHOGENESIS

Endocrine tumors of the pancreas are neoplastic proliferations of small round cells with immunohistochemical features characteristic of APUDomas (amine precursor uptake and decarboxylation [APUD]). Other members of this tumor family include medullary carcinoma of the thyroid, pheochromocytoma, melanoma, and carcinoids. Pancreatic endocrine tumors are subclassified on the basis of the clinical and pathophysiologic consequences of excess hormone production. Although immunohistochemical staining of these tumors often demonstrates the presence of more than one hormone, the clinical features are almost invariably defined by the hypersecretion of only one hormone. Up to 20% of pancreatic endocrine tumors do not secrete hormones. Symptoms from these nonfunctional tumors are caused by local mass effects. A variable percentage of each tumor subtype is associated with the autosomal dominant syndrome, multiple endocrine neoplasia (MEN) type I. Eighty percent of patients with MEN I syndrome have pancreatic endocrine tumors, which are more often multicentric than are sporadic tumors. Pancreatic endocrine tumors are rare and cause significant morbidity, and, with the exception of insulinomas, a large percentage have malignant potential.

CLINICAL FEATURES

Insulinoma

Patients with insulinomas almost invariably present with symptoms of hypoglycemia. Symptoms of neuroglycopenia include confusion, lightheadedness, syncope, visual disturbances, and behavioral changes. In some patients, the reactive sympathetic response dominates the presentation, producing tremor, irritability, malaise, and palpitations. Symptoms may be present for years before a diagnosis is established, and patients may be incorrectly diagnosed with psychiatric disorders. Insulinomas usually are smaller than 2 cm, and only 10% are malignant. Five percent of patients with insulinoma have MEN I; 95% are sporadic. The average age of onset is between 40 and 50 years.

VIPoma

VIPoma, also termed *Verner-Morrison syndrome* or the *WDHA* (watery diarrhea, hypokalemia, and achlorhydria) *syndrome,* produces secretory diarrhea that results from activation of adenylate cyclase, leading to increased net sodium and chloride secretion. Diarrhea may be intermittent in the early phase, but eventually it is profuse and watery. Hypokalemia is the result of potassium losses in the stool, and achlorhydria or hypochlorhydria results from VIP inhibition of gastric acid secretion. Twenty percent of patients experience flushing because of VIP-induced vasodilation. Other metabolic changes include glucose intolerance, which is secondary to VIP-mediated glycogenolysis, and hypercalcemia, which develops by unknown pathways. Similar to insulinomas, VIPomas in adults are almost invariably localized to the pancreas. VIPomas often are larger than 5 cm and up to 60% are malignant. VIPoma is only rarely associated with the MEN I syndrome. The sporadic form can occur at any age.

Glucagonoma

Glucagonomas produce a syndrome of dermatitis, weight loss, anemia, and glucose intolerance, most often in persons 50 to 60 years of age. Many clinicians assume that all patients with glucagonoma are glucose intolerant, but up to 15% of patients are euglycemic. In fact, other catabolic effects of glucagon such as weight loss and hypoaminoacidemia are more consistently associated with these tumors. The classic cutaneous finding is necrolytic migratory erythema, which begins as erythematous patches in the intertriginous and perioral regions. As lesions expand, they become confluent, raised, and bullous. Necrolytic migratory erythema typically waxes and wanes. Chronic lesions become hyperpigmented. Correction of hypoaminoacidemia may improve the rash. The anemia is normochromic and normocytic and develops by unknown mechanisms. Other less common features of glucagonoma include thromboembolic phenomena, diarrhea, and steatorrhea. Tumors are large and located almost exclusively in the pancreas; 50% are malignant.

Somatostatinoma

Most symptoms of the somatostatinoma syndrome result from the inhibitory effects of somatostatin on the secretion of other gastrointestinal hormones. Inhibition of cholecystokinin (CCK) and gastrin release results in decreased pancreatic enzyme and gastric acid secretion. The decrease in pancreatic exocrine function may be sufficient to cause maldigestion and steatorrhea. Somatostatin also decreases the intestinal transit time and inhibits intestinal absorption. Therefore, development of diarrhea and steatorrhea is probably multifactorial. A decrease in circulating CCK leads to gallbladder stasis, which fosters sludge and gallstone formation. Inhibition of insulin release results in glucose intolerance or overt diabetes mellitus. The net catabolism and malabsorption caused by the somatostatin-secreting tumor leads to weight loss in most patients. Tumors usually are large, and most are malignant. Forty percent to 50% of somatostatinomas originate in the intestine. Diabetes, weight loss, diarrhea, and gallbladder disease are less common in patients with intestinal somatostatinomas.

GRFoma

GRFomas stimulate excessive growth hormone secretion, producing the clinical manifestations of acromegaly. The incidence of these tumors is unknown. GRFomas usually are larger than 6 cm and most are extrapancreatic. In 30% of cases, the tumors are malignant. One-third of patients with a GRFoma have MEN I.

PPoma and Nonfunctional Tumors

Excess circulating pancreatic polypeptide does not produce significant symptoms; therefore, PPomas are clinically indistinguishable from nonfunctional tumors. Symptoms of PPomas and nonfunctioning endocrine tumors are caused by the local and regional effects of the mass. Patients may report abdominal pain, back pain, or weight loss. Tumors usually are larger than 5 cm, and most are metastatic at the time of diagnosis.

FINDINGS ON DIAGNOSTIC TESTING

Laboratory Studies

Confirming the diagnosis of pancreatic endocrine neoplasms rests on the demonstration of inappropriately elevated levels of the relative hormone as well as the localization of the tumor. Several provocative tests can establish unregulated insulin secretion, but the most accepted assay relies on documenting an increase in serum insulin concentration during fasting-induced hypoglycemia. Patients are fasted in an inpatient setting for up to 72 hours. Blood glucose and insulin levels are monitored every 2 to 4 hours, or more frequently if the blood sugar level decreases to <50 mg per dl. The test is terminated if blood glucose levels are persistently <40 mg per dl or if neuroglycopenic symptoms develop. In the setting of hypoglycemia, an insulin-to-glucose ratio of >0.3 or failure of

---

TABLE 56-1
Differential Diagnosis of Fasting Hypoglycemia

Endogenous mediators
    Insulinoma
    Spontaneous autoimmune anti-insulin antibody syndrome
    Autoantibodies to insulin receptor
    Noninsulin tumor–associated hypoglycemia
Reduced hepatic glucose output
    Deficient gluconeogenesis or glycogen storage
    Hormonal deficiencies (e.g., adrenal insufficiency)
    Enzyme defects (e.g., glucose-6-phosphatase deficiency)
    Ethanol consumption and poor nutrition
    Diffuse liver disease
Medication or other pharmacologic causes
    Sulfonylureas or biguanides
    Insulin administration
    Ingestion of ackee fruits (i.e., hypoglycin)
    Other medications (e.g., aspirin, pentamidine)

Sources: Modified from G Boden. Insulinomas and glucagonomas. Gastroenterol Clin North Am 1989;18:831; and R Comi, P Gordon, FL Doppman. Insulinoma. In Go VLW, Di Magno EP, Gardner JD, et al. (eds), The Pancreas: Biology, Pathobiology and Disease (2nd ed). New York: Raven Press, 1993;979.

serum insulin levels to decrease to <6 mU per ml is consistent with the diagnosis of insulinoma. More than 90% of insulinomas are detected with this assay, but alternative diagnoses such as surreptitious use of insulin or sulfonylureas should be considered (Table 56-1). Therefore, serum assays should also be performed to determine levels of C-peptide (elevated in insulinoma, decreased in surreptitious use of insulin), sulfonylureas, and antibodies to insulin.

With the exception of gastrinomas, the other pancreatic endocrine tumors do not require provocative testing to document unregulated hormone secretion. Glucagonoma is suggested by marked elevations of serum glucagon levels, which may also occur with severe stress, renal insufficiency, or hepatic dysfunction. Similarly, the diagnoses of VIPoma, somatostatinoma, GRFoma, and PPoma require documentation of elevated serum levels of the corresponding peptides.

Structural Studies

Imaging procedures are required to characterize nonfunctional tumors. Imaging studies also play a critical role in localizing and establishing the extent of symptomatic pancreatic endocrine neoplasms. The sensitivities of ultrasound, computed tomography (CT), and magnetic resonance imaging (MRI) depend on the size of the tumor. These tests detect up to 80% of tumors larger than 3 cm, but fail to identify 90% of tumors smaller than 1 cm. Glucagonomas, VIPomas, PPomas, and nonfunctional tumors usually are detected as large pancreatic masses, which renders these imaging modalities well suited to their identification. However, ultrasound and computed tomography identify only 10% to 40% of gastrinomas and insulinomas; specialized procedures usually are required to precisely localize small tumors.

Endocrine tumors are typically hypervascular. Selective angiography demonstrates a characteristic vascular mass in 60% to 70% of cases and may also identify hepatic metastases. Provocative angiographic studies may localize small insulinomas and gastrinomas. Selective portal vein sampling for insulin involves transhepatic placement of a catheter into the portal vein. Serum insulin measurements taken from various locations along the splenic, superior mesenteric, and portal veins permit successful localization of insulinomas in 77% to 90% of patients. One technique uses selective injection of calcium into arterial tributaries of the pancreas followed by measurement of serum insulin levels from the hepatic veins. This method of venous sampling for insulin avoids the risks of transhepatic puncture of the portal vein and accurately defines the pancreatic location of 90% to 100% of insulinomas. A similar technique of selective intra-arterial injection of secretin followed by hepatic vein measurement of gastrin levels successfully localizes 75% of gastrinomas.

Endoscopic ultrasonography (EUS) is particularly useful for defining insulinomas. Accuracy approaches 100% when performed in experienced centers. EUS is helpful in localizing pancreatic gastrinomas, but its sensitivity for detecting extrapancreatic gastrinomas is about 50%. With the exception of insulinomas, the majority of endocrine tumors contain somatostatin receptors. Nuclear scintigraphic techniques using radiolabeled analogs of somatostatin have been shown to detect a large subset of endocrine tumors and may be particularly useful in identifying distant metastatic disease. Intraoperative ultrasound, palpation of the pancreas, and examination of the small intestine are the most direct means of identifying endocrine tumors.

MANAGEMENT AND COURSE

Surgical Therapy

All patients with pancreatic endocrine neoplasia without evidence of metastatic disease on angiography, somatostatin scintigraphy, CT, or MRI studies should undergo exploratory laparotomy by a surgeon who has extensive experience in the evaluation and treatment of gastrointestinal endocrine tumors. If imaging studies fail to identify a tumor, exploratory surgery along with intraoperative ultrasound should be performed to search for the primary tumor. Complete surgical excision is curative for >90% of cases of insulinoma. It usually involves simple enucleation or a distal pancreatectomy. Multicentric or metastatic disease is present in the majority of the other endocrine tumors; complete surgical resection is possible in some patients. If complete resection is achieved, the 10-year survival rate is 90%, whereas the corresponding survival rate for unresectable tumors is 20%. The only reliable means of determining the malignant nature of an endocrine tumor is the presence of metastases; therefore, all localized tumors should be resected unless severe illness precludes surgical intervention. The role of tumor debulking in patients with unresectable disease has not been defined, although some patients experience improved survival and symptom control.

Medical Therapy

Patients awaiting surgical excision and patients with inoperable disease as a result of metastatic spread or other severe illness usually require medical therapy for tumor-associated symptoms. Nutritional deficits, hypovolemia, and

TABLE 56-2
Effects of Octreotide in Patients with Pancreatic Endocrine Tumors

| | TUMOR TYPE | | | |
	Insulinoma	*VIPoma*	*Glucagonoma*	*GRFoma*
Number of patients treated	48	29	16	8
Number of patients treated >1 month	10	26	14	8
Symptoms improved (%)	31	86	81	100
Marker hormone level reduced (%)	41	86	75	100
Dose range (μg/day)	50–1,500	100–450	100–2,250	100–1,500
Decrease in tumor size (% of patients)	22	0	0	16

GRFoma = tumor that secretes excess growth hormone releasing factor; VIPoma = tumor that secretes excess vasoactive intestinal polypeptide.

electrolyte disorders should be corrected. Although patients with symptomatic insulinomas should have expeditious surgery, control of hypoglycemia may be difficult in the preoperative period. Many patients avoid symptoms by eating frequent meals, but occasionally refractory hypoglycemia requires more aggressive therapy. Large amounts of parenteral glucose may produce hypokalemia as a result of intracellular sequestration of potassium. Diazoxide inhibits insulin release and stimulates glycogenolysis; it is useful in controlling refractory hypoglycemia in preoperative patients and in patients with unresectable disease.

The somatostatin analog octreotide is a potent inhibitor of hormone release from gastrinomas, VIPomas, glucagonomas, and GRFomas, but it is a less effective suppressor of insulin secretion (Table 56-2). Octreotide improves the skin rash, diarrhea, and weight loss in patients with glucagonoma, but it has little effect on glucose intolerance. The analog improves diarrhea in patients with gastrinoma by inhibiting gastric acid secretion. It corrects the diarrhea in patients with VIPoma by inhibiting VIP secretion. Initial doses range from 50 to 150 μg subcutaneously three times daily. Escalating doses, up to 750 μg three times daily, may be required if tachyphylaxis develops. Whether octreotide has tumoricidal effects is controversial, but a small percentage of patients experience reductions in tumor size. Side effects (e.g., steatorrhea, gallstones) are common with high doses. Glucose intolerance may develop or worsen, and a small percentage of patients experience nausea, vomiting, and crampy abdominal pain.

Several chemotherapy regimens have been evaluated in patients with metastatic pancreatic endocrine neoplasms. Streptozocin in combination with doxorubicin or 5-fluorouracil is associated with response rates of 50% to 70%. Streptozocin plus doxorubicin is the regimen of choice because it may also provide a survival advantage. Chlorozotocin, an analog of streptozocin that has fewer adverse effects, may prove to be superior to streptozocin. High-dose leukocyte interferon produces variable response rates, but most reports suggest it is minimally effective. Hepatic artery chemoembolization reduces the size of liver metastases and improves symptoms in most patients, but procedure-related morbidity is common.

CHAPTER 57

Abdominal Cavity: Structural Anomalies, Hernias, Intra-Abdominal Abscesses, and Fistulae

ABDOMINAL CAVITY EMBRYOLOGY AND ANATOMY

The abdominal (peritoneal) cavity appears early in embryonic development as the caudal part of the celomic cavity. It is covered by splanchnic mesoderm. During the migration of the abdominal organs, the mesodermic bands elongate and form the abdominal ligaments, the mesenterium, and the greater and lesser omenta. The dorsal mesogastrium of the foregut develops to a larger extent than its ventral counterpart, folding to the left. The space within the mesogastrial fold becomes the lesser sac. The greater omentum, a structure that hangs free to the pelvis, forms from enlargement of the dorsal mesogastrium, and extends from the greater gastric curvature to the transverse colon and mesocolon. The omentum receives arterial blood from the gastroepiploic arteries and becomes laden with fat. In an adult, the remnants of the ventral mesogastrium are the ligaments of the liver—the coronary, falciform, and teres—and the gastrohepatic ligament (lesser omentum). In the developing fetus, the umbilical vein follows the ligamentum teres hepatis and terminates in the portal vein. The mesentery is formed from elongation and folding of the dorsal mesodermic attachment. The mesenteries of the ascending and descending colon fuse with the posterior body wall, and the mesentery of the small intestine extends from the transverse mesocolon to the ileocecal junction.

The abdominal cavity is bounded superiorly by the diaphragm, laterally by the abdominal walls, and inferiorly by the pelvis. The peritoneum is a layer of endoderm that covers the walls and organs of the abdominal cavity. The pancreas, part of the duodenum, the right and left colon, and the rectum are retroperitoneal, whereas the intraperitoneal organs are supported by thickened peritoneal bands (gastrohepatic, gastrosplenic, gastrocolic, splenorenal, splenocolic, falciform, coronary, teres). The abdominal cavity has three compartments: lesser sac, supramesocolic, and inframesocolic. The lesser sac communicates with the rest of the abdominal cavity through the foramen of Winslow. The supramesocolic compartment (containing the stomach, duodenum, pancreas, liver, and spleen) and the inframesocolic compartment (containing the intestine) are separated by the transverse mesocolon, inserted in the anterior duodenum and pancreas. The area between the colon and the inferior margin of the liver is called Morison's pouch, a potential site for fluid accumulation. The most inferior part of the peritoneum between the rectum and urogenital organs is the pouch of Douglas. The inguinal region is bounded by the arch of the aponeurosis of the transversus abdominis muscle and by the upper ramus of the pubis and the psoas muscle. The inguinal canal contains the vas deferens, spermatic artery and vein, and cremasteric muscle. The omentum and mesentery are rich in lymphatics and blood vessels, providing macrophages and lymphocytes to aid in clearance of abdominal foreign bodies and infections.

The parietal peritoneum lines the abdominal cavity, diaphragm, and pelvis, and the visceral peritoneum covers the intraperitoneal organs and forms the mesenteries. The parietal peritoneum is innervated by somatic and visceral afferent nerves and responds to noxious stimuli with a sensation of localized, sharp pain, whereas the visceral peritoneum receives afferent information from the autonomic nervous system and responds to traction and pressure with poorly localized, dull pain. The peritoneum and mesentery are supplied by splanchnic blood vessels and branches of the lower intercostal, lumbar, and iliac arteries.

The retroperitoneum is the space behind the abdominal cavity from the diaphragm to the peritoneal reflection, where it continues as the extraperitoneal pelvic space. The anterior retroperitoneum contains the pancreas, duodenum, and ascending and descending colons. The posterior retroperitoneum contains the kidneys, adrenal glands, vessels, lymphatics, and nervous structures.

DEVELOPMENTAL ABNORMALITIES OF THE ABDOMINAL CAVITY

Omphalocele and Gastroschisis

Etiology and Pathogenesis

The embryonic celomic cavity is too small to accommodate the intestines until the tenth gestational week, when they re-enter the abdomen. Omphalocele occurs when the viscera herniate through the umbilical ring and persist outside the body, covered by a membranous sac. Gastroschisis is a condition in which the peritoneal sac has ruptured in utero and the viscera are in free contact with the exterior. Associated congenital abnormalities, including incomplete rotation and fixation of the midgut, intestinal atresia, trisomy 13, trisomy 18, vascular disruptions, and renal and gallbladder agenesis, are present in 30% to 50% of cases. Beckwith-Wiedemann syndrome, also known as *EMG syndrome* (exomphalos, macroglossia, gigantism), is characterized by somatic and visceral overgrowth and omphalocele.

Clinical Features, Diagnosis, and Management

The diagnosis of omphalocele or gastroschisis is obvious on examination at birth. It also can be diagnosed prenatally by ultrasound examination. Immediate treatment of these conditions is required to prevent dehydration, visceral desiccation, sepsis, and death. Antiseptic solutions are applied to the sac in infants with omphalocele. With gastroschisis, the viscera are wrapped in a silicone sheet, which is sutured to the abdominal wall until growth of the infant permits reduction of the hernia and closure of the defect. Amnion inversion is an alternate therapy for high-risk infants. Despite aggressive intervention, the mortality rate of these abnormalities is 40% to 50%. Of the infants who survive, many exhibit slow recovery of bowel function.

Diaphragmatic Hernias

Etiology and Pathogenesis

Congenital diaphragmatic hernias are common defects that occur in weak areas of the diaphragm. Anteromedial diaphragmatic hernias through the sternocostal area (i.e., hernia of Morgagni) contain the stomach, colon, or omentum. Posterolateral diaphragmatic hernias through the lumbocostal area (i.e., hernia of Bochdalek) are large and associated with hypoplasia of the ipsilateral lung.

Clinical Features, Diagnosis, and Management

Anterior diaphragmatic hernias are usually small and rarely cause significant symptoms. Chest radiographs show an air shadow lateral to the xiphoid. Surgical correction of anterior hernias is accomplished with minimal morbidity and mortality. Posterolateral diaphragmatic hernias produce respiratory distress, mediastinal displacement, and nausea and vomiting as a result of intestinal obstruction. Respiratory sounds may be absent on the affected side, heart sounds may be audible in the right side of the chest, and bowel sounds may be audible in the left hemithorax. The abdomen may be scaphoid. Chest radiographs show left thoracic air–fluid levels, mediastinal displacement, and loss of the diaphragmatic line. Upper gastrointestinal radiography using water-soluble contrast may reveal intestinal loops in the thorax. Mortality from congenital diaphragmatic hernias results from respiratory insufficiency, malnutrition, failure to thrive, and intestinal strangulation. Surgery is necessary for posterolateral hernias, but the mortality rate is as high as 50% in the first week of life. Extracorporeal membrane oxygenation may reduce the pulmonary consequences of this condition.

Umbilical Hernias

Etiology and Pathogenesis

Umbilical hernias are caused by congenitally large umbilical rings or by rings that are distended by high intra-abdominal pressures. Predisposing factors include prematurity, Down's syndrome, gargoylism, amaurotic family idiocy, cretinism, and Beckwith-Wiedemann syndrome.

Clinical Features, Diagnosis, and Management

Most umbilical hernias reduce and heal spontaneously; strangulation complicates only 5% of cases. Surgery before 3 years of age is indicated only for large, symptomatic hernias or in the event of incarceration or strangulation. If the hernia does not spontaneously improve by 3 to 4 years of age, elective surgery is performed.

HERNIAS IN ADULTS

Epigastric Hernias

Etiology and Pathogenesis

Epigastric hernias occur in the midline of the abdominal wall between the umbilicus and the xiphoid in a congenital weakness of the linea alba that is small and may contain incarcerated preperitoneal fat. Multiple hernias are reported in 20% of cases.

Clinical Features, Diagnosis, and Management

Epigastric hernias produce symptoms ranging from a small, painless nodule to acute obstruction of the small intestine. Pain that is exacerbated by exertion and relieved by reclining is characteristic. The diagnosis, which may be difficult in obese patients with small hernias, is made by palpation of a tender mass on physical examination. Pain may increase as the patient raises his or her head from the examining table. Surgery is indicated for epigastric hernias.

Umbilical Hernias

Etiology and Pathogenesis

Umbilical hernias in adults occur in multiparous and cirrhotic patients with ascites. Intestinal or omental incarceration and strangulation complicates 20% to 30% of cases, especially if the umbilical ring is small. Other complications in cirrhotic patients with ascites are hernia ulceration and perforation, which may be further complicated by peritonitis (often caused by *Staphylococcus aureus*) or renal failure.

Clinical Features, Diagnosis, and Management

Large umbilical hernias are obvious on physical examination. If the diagnosis is not self-evident, abdominal radiographs may demonstrate an intestinal loop outside the abdominal wall. Umbilical hernias are treated surgically. In cirrhotic patients, control of ascites with medications or shunting procedures is essential. If perforation occurs, the patient requires hospitalization,

TABLE 57-1
Epidemiology of Groin Hernias*

HERNIA TYPE	OCCURRENCE (%)
Inguinal	80
Indirect	(48)
Direct	(24)
Both	(8)
Femoral	5
Inguinal and femoral	2
With a sliding component	12
Sigmoid	(8)
Cecum	(4)
Other	2

*Groin hernias account for 85% of all hernias.

antibiotic treatment for gram-positive organisms, and fluid and electrolyte replacement.

Groin Hernias

Etiology and Pathogenesis

Groin hernias represent 85% of all hernias. There are three clinically relevant types: indirect inguinal hernias (through the internal inguinal ring into the inguinal canal), direct inguinal hernias (superior to the inguinal ligament but not through the inguinal canal), and femoral hernias (inferior to the inguinal ligament and medial to the epigastric vessels) (Table 57-1). Most groin hernias contain ileum, omentum, colon, or bladder. An indirect inguinal hernia containing a Meckel's diverticulum is known as a *Littre hernia.*

Clinical Features, Diagnosis, and Management

A patient with a groin hernia presents with an inguinal mass that appears with increased intra-abdominal pressure. Pain usually is mild. Constant pain suggests incarceration; colicky pain indicates strangulation. The diagnosis of hernias of the groin is made on physical examination by inserting the finger through the external inguinal ring into the inguinal canal to the internal ring. Indirect hernias are felt exiting the internal ring, whereas direct hernias are palpated laterally. Femoral hernias are felt below the inguinal ligament in the femoral region. Strangulation affects 5% of indirect hernias, and 20% to 30% of femoral hernias strangulate, whereas direct hernias rarely develop this complication. Laparoscopy may visualize the site of herniation and the area of bowel that is trapped. Surgery is indicated for groin hernias using local or general anesthesia.

Pelvic Hernias

Etiology and Pathogenesis

Pelvic hernias involve bowel herniation through the obturator foramen, the greater or lesser sciatic foramina, or the perineal muscles. Pelvic hernias are rare; obturator hernias are the most prevalent. Obturator hernias usually contain ileum and are more common in women.

Clinical Features, Diagnosis, and Management

Patients with obturator hernia often have a history of transient attacks of acute intestinal obstruction. Diagnosis usually is made at laparotomy because the obturator is not easily palpated in the thigh. On rectal or vaginal examination, however, a soft, tender, anterolateral, fluctuating mass may be palpated. The Howship-Romberg sign—medial thigh pain radiating to the knee or hip—is present in 50% of patients. An abnormal gas shadow in the intestine may be detected on radiographs of the obturator foramen. A computed tomographic (CT) scan may be diagnostic if there is hernia incarceration. Pelvic hernias are treated surgically.

Lumbar Hernias

Etiology and Pathogenesis

Lumbar hernias are congenital, or they are acquired through flank or rib trauma, through iliac crest fracture, or by removal of a fragment of the iliac crest for bone grafting. Lumbar herniation in the posterior abdominal wall may be superior (bounded by the twelfth rib, internal oblique, and sacrospinalis) or inferior (bounded by the iliac crest, latissimus dorsi, and external oblique).

Clinical Features, Diagnosis, and Management

Lumbar hernias can be asymptomatic, or they can produce lumbar pain referred to the back or pelvis. Surgery is indicated because these hernias generally increase in size.

Spigelian Hernias

Etiology and Pathogenesis

A spigelian hernia is a small protrusion through the external oblique fascia lateral to the rectus abdominus muscle, below the arcuate line of Douglas. Spigelian hernias are rare and usually occur in elderly persons.

Clinical Features, Diagnosis, and Management

Patients present with discomfort on straining or coughing. Sensation of a mass may be reported. A gas shadow may be seen on radiographs of the abdominal wall, whereas upper gastrointestinal contrast radiography may demonstrate bowel lumen outside the abdominal cavity. Surgery is mandatory.

Traumatic Diaphragmatic Hernias

Etiology and Pathogenesis

Penetrating or blunt trauma may produce diaphragmatic tears. The most common injury is a tear from the esophageal hiatus to the left costal attachment, with herniation of the stomach, spleen, colon, and left hepatic lobe into the thorax.

Clinical Features, Diagnosis, and Management

Diaphragmatic injury produces upper abdominal pain referred to the left shoulder and scapula. Visceral herniation causes nausea and vomiting, central abdominal pain and diaphoresis as a result of traction of the mesentery and blood vessels, and respiratory distress from lung compression and mediastinal deviation. In rare cases, symptoms are mild, and the hernia remains undiagnosed for years. Chest radiographs, upper gastrointestinal contrast radiographs, ultrasound, and CT scans may demonstrate abdominal viscera in the thorax. The disorder requires immediate surgical repair.

Internal Hernias

Etiology and Pathogenesis

An internal hernia is the protrusion of an intraperitoneal viscus into a compartment within the abdomen. Paraduodenal hernias originate from a defect in midgut rotation and may involve bowel herniation into the left fossa of Landzert or the right fossa of Waldeyer. Herniation through the foramen of Winslow into the lesser sac is facilitated by a large foramen and abnormal colonic mobility. The small intestine is involved in 70% of cases and the colon in 25%. Pericecal hernias are characterized by passage of the ileum through the ileocecal fossa into the right paracolic gutter. Loops of the small intestine rarely become incarcerated in the intersigmoid fossa, which is a pocket between the two sigmoid loops. Approximately 5% to 10% of internal hernias in adults occur through defects in the mesentery and omentum. These hernias are the most common type of internal hernia in infants and are often associated with an atretic segment of the intestine.

Clinical Features, Diagnosis, and Management

Internal hernias produce recurrent nausea, vomiting, and pain as a result of intermittent obstruction of the small intestine. The diagnosis relies on abdominal radiography or laparotomy. Arteriography is also useful for diagnosis because it can demonstrate blood vessel displacement or reversal of their course. Radiographs of left paraduodenal hernias show encapsulated small intestine with superior displacement of the stomach and inferomedial displacement of the left colon, whereas right paraduodenal hernias are shown to displace the right colon anteriorly. Radiographs of hernias through the foramen of Winslow reveal gas-distended bowel loops in the lesser sac and anterior displacement of the stomach and colon. Intersigmoid hernias produce retrograde ileal filling that can be seen on barium enema radiography. Therapy for internal hernias is surgical.

Iatrogenic Hernias

Etiology and Pathogenesis

Iatrogenic hernias result from surgical creation of weak areas and abnormal foramina in the abdominal cavity. A retroanastomotic hernia is the herniation of the intestine through a mesenteric space left open during construction of an anastomosis (e.g., Billroth II). Incisional hernias are caused by defective abdominal muscle suturing, defects at exteriorized drain sites, vertical laparotomies, multiple incisions, infraumbilical incisions, malnutrition, anemia, and wound hematomas or infections.

Clinical Features, Diagnosis, and Management

Retroanastomotic hernias are frequently acute and cause intestinal obstruction. Upper gastrointestinal barium radiography is diagnostic. Immediate surgical treatment is mandatory. Incisional hernias are detected on physical examination. Operative correction is generally required.

ABSCESSES

Etiology and Pathogenesis

Abscesses are fluid collections containing necrotic debris, leukocytes, and bacteria. The usual causes are operative complications, trauma, visceral perforation, pancreaticobiliary disease, and genitourinary infection. Sources of bacterial contamination include exogenous seeding from penetrating trauma, hematogenous spread from adjacent or distant sites, and local spread from gastrointestinal perforation. Peritoneal inflammation by any mechanism leads to host-protective responses, including transudation of protein-rich fluid, complement production, and leukocyte attraction and activation. These protective responses have both beneficial and undesirable effects. For example, fibrin formation, resulting from activation of tissue thromboplastin, traps bacteria; bacterial proliferation is promoted, lymphatic clearance of bacteria is impaired, and phagocytosis of bacteria by neutrophils is inhibited.

Most intra-abdominal abscesses are contaminated by multiple microbes, including gram-negative facultative organisms (*Escherichia coli* and *Klebsiella*, *Enterobacter*, *Proteus*, and *Pseudomonas* species) and anaerobes (e.g., *Bacteroides fragilis*). Aerobic bacteria promote anaerobe growth by consuming oxygen. Some anaerobes interfere with neutrophil phagocytosis, thereby promoting proliferation of aerobes and anaerobes. Abscesses can develop almost anywhere in the peritoneal cavity. Initially localized inflammatory processes such as appendicitis and diverticulitis may produce localized abscesses in the lower abdomen if perforation occurs after the inflammatory reaction is walled off. If perforation occurs before the development of a localized inflammatory process, generalized peritonitis may result. Abscess formation in dependent areas in the recumbent patient, such as the subdiaphragmatic, subhepatic, and pelvic spaces, is associated with generalized peritonitis.

Clinical Features, Diagnosis, and Management

Patients with intra-abdominal abscesses present with intermittent fever (usually >39°C), abdominal pain (localized to the site of inflammation or diffuse), anorexia, and malaise. Abscesses under the diaphragm may produce shoulder pain and hiccups. Abscesses adjacent to the bladder or rectum may produce urinary or fecal urgency, respectively. Physical findings are variable, ranging from point tenderness and a focal mass to advanced sepsis with obtundation and hypotension. Bowel sounds may be reduced or absent, and rectovaginal examination may reveal a localized mass or tenderness. Even if the physical examination is unrevealing, clinicians must maintain a high degree of suspicion with all patients at risk for abscess formation. Factors associated with poor outcome in patients with an intra-abdominal abscess include advanced age, associated organ failure, a recurrent or persistent abscess, and multiple abscesses. Complications of abscesses include sepsis, secondary abscesses caused by direct extension or hematogenous spread, bowel obstruction or fistula formation, and blood vessel erosion with massive hemorrhage.

Blood testing can suggest but not confirm the presence of an abscess. A complete blood count may show mild anemia or leukocytosis. Liver chemistry values may reveal hyperbilirubinemia secondary to the effects of bacteremia. Peripancreatic abscesses can produce hyperamylasemia. Blood cultures may be positive for one or more organisms, usually gram-negative bacilli or anaerobes.

A variety of imaging techniques can be helpful in diagnosing an intra-abdominal abscess. Chest radiographs may show pleural effusions, an elevated hemidiaphragm, and atelectasis. Abdominal radiographs may demonstrate air-fluid levels, increased bowel gas, extraintestinal gas bubbles, and visceral displacement. A CT scan is the imaging test of choice for most patients, being positive in 90% of cases. Abscesses on CT scans appear as well-defined fluid collections. Ultrasound may be useful in selected regions, including the right upper quadrant, retroperitoneum, and pelvis, but lumenal gas may obscure visualization of other intra-abdominal sites. Radionuclide scans with [67]Ga- or ^{111}In-labeled neutrophils demonstrate increased uptake in regions of white cell accumulation, such as abscesses, with accuracies ranging from 60% to 95%. However, the results of these scans are also positive with fresh surgical scars, recent fractures, and surgical drain sites. Indium has the advantage over gallium of not being excreted into the gut lumen or concentrated in the reticuloendothelial system, allowing visualization of these potential sites of infection. Conversely, areas of reduced radionuclide uptake visualized on liver-spleen scintigraphy or renal scintigraphy suggests abscesses in solid organs such as the liver, spleen, or kidneys.

The mainstay of treatment of intra-abdominal abscess is drainage. Percutaneous drainage may be performed for single abscesses containing thin fluid, whereas operative drainage is usually required for multiple abscesses, loculated abscesses, infected hematomas, or abscesses containing thick viscous fluid. Factors associated with failure of percutaneous drainage include age older than 60 years and pancreatic abscesses. Patients whose abscesses are drained by either method who do not respond within 4 days should be restudied with a CT scan or

---

TABLE 57-2
Etiologic Classification of Enteric Fistulae

Congenital
    Tracheoesophageal fistula
    Patent vitelline duct
Postoperative
    Inadvertent injury
    Failure of anastomosis
    Proximity of drain
Post-traumatic
    Direct injury
    Open abdominal wound
Inflammatory
    Crohn's disease
    Adjacent abscess
Postirradiation
    Spontaneous
    Postoperative
Malignant
    Adherence of tumor to adjacent bowel or abdominal wall with subsequent tumor
      necrosis

---

ultrasound, and repeat percutaneous drainage or surgery should be considered. Antibiotics are adjunctive therapy for intra-abdominal abscesses. Antibiotic therapy should be broad enough to treat gram-negative and gram-positive aerobes and anaerobes. The duration of antibiotic therapy should be determined by the patient's condition and the results of blood and tissue cultures. Recurrent infection is least likely in those patients who were afebrile and who had normal leukocyte counts.

FISTULAE

Etiology and Pathogenesis

Fistulae are abnormal communications from a hollow organ (gut, biliary tract, pancreatic duct, urinary tract) to another hollow organ or the skin. Fistulae develop in response to surgery, the use of prosthetic mesh to close abdominal wall defects, radiation therapy, inflammatory bowel disease, trauma, and malignancy (Table 57-2). Rarely, fistulae develop when abscesses erode into adjacent bowel.

Clinical Features, Diagnosis, and Management

The most common presentations of abdominal fistulae include enteric drainage through the skin and signs and symptoms of an intra-abdominal abscess. High-output fistulae (>500 ml per day) involving the proximal gut produce significant fluid and electrolyte abnormalities—for example, metabolic acidosis from duodenal fistulae, and hypochloremic, hypokalemic metabolic alkalosis from gastric fistulae. Fluid loss may be so severe as to cause dehydration, hypotension, and renal failure. Skin irritation may result from exposure to activated digestive enzymes. Malnutrition may result from protein and nutrient loss from the fistula, decreased oral intake, and the increased energy demands of the underlying illness. Malnutrition can significantly increase morbidity and mortality rates associated with fistulae. The presence of multiple, recurrent, or complex fistulae should suggest Crohn's disease. Recurrent urinary tract infection or pneumaturia should raise the possibility of an enterovesical fistula, whereas diarrhea and malnutrition may be the presenting symptoms of an enteroenteric fistulae that bypasses significant segments of gut.

Various studies may be needed to accurately diagnose the presence of a fistula. The course of enterocutaneous fistulae can be defined by careful injection of a radiographic contrast medium into the skin opening. Enterovesical fistulae may be suggested by persistently positive urine cultures for enteric organisms. Upper or lower gastrointestinal contrast radiography may demonstrate disease that leads to fistula formation, but rarely defines the fistula itself. Cystoscopy is the most helpful test for diagnosing enterovesical fistulae. Gastrointestinal contrast radiographs usually demonstrate enteroenteric fistulae, whereas endoscopy often is not helpful. CT scanning and ultrasound may rarely detect fistulae but can be helpful in defining predisposing factors such as intra-abdominal abscess cavities.

The goals of treatment of an abdominal fistula include correction of fluid and electrolyte abnormalities, drainage of associated abscesses, protection of the skin, nutrient repletion, reduction of fistula drainage, and treatment of the underlying disease. For high-output fistulae, daily adjustments in replacement fluids may require direct measurement of the electrolyte composition in the fistula fluid. Effective drainage of associated abscesses is achieved by placement of sump drains. Skin can be protected with stoma appliances, similar to those used for surgically placed ileostomies or colostomies. The choice of enteral versus parenteral nutrition in patients with gastrointestinal fistulae must be individualized. Enteral feedings may increase fluid output from proximal fistulae of the small intestine, rendering parenteral nutrition more useful. In contrast, patients with fistulae of the distal small intestine or colon may be adequately nourished by enteral feedings without increasing fistulous output. Somatostatin and its analog, octreotide, reduce pancreatic and intestinal secretion and have been proposed for use in patients with intestinal or pancreatic fistulae. Some studies have shown faster closure of fistulae with these agents; however, further controlled studies are required. Factors that predict an unfavorable response to conservative management of fistulae include malignancy, inflammatory bowel disease, foreign bodies, poorly drained abscesses, distal gut obstruction, disruption of >50% of the bowel wall, a fistula tract <2.5 cm from the skin, age older than 65 years, fistula output of >500 ml per day, chronicity, and localization to the distal small intestine and colon. Surgery is considered for fistulae that persist after 4 to 6 weeks.

CHAPTER 58

Diseases of the Mesentery, Peritoneum, and Retroperitoneum

DISEASES OF THE MESENTERY

The mesentery and omentum can be affected by various disease processes (Table 58-1).

Mesenteric Panniculitis and Retractile Mesenteritis

Etiology and Pathogenesis

Mesenteric panniculitis is a nonspecific inflammation of the adipose tissue of the mesentery. The cause may be trauma, infection, or ischemia, but it is often unknown. It can be part of the generalized Weber-Christian disease. Grossly, panniculitis exhibits a thickened mesentery, usually a solid mass, representing excess growth of fat with subsequent degeneration, fat necrosis, xanthogranulomatous inflammation (macrophages, histiocytes, lymphocytes, foreign body giant cells), fibrosis, and calcification. If mesenteric panniculitis progresses to retractile mesenteritis, the thickened mesentery becomes fibrotic. Fat necrosis may produce mesenteric pseudocysts.

Clinical Features, Diagnosis, and Management

Symptoms of mesenteric panniculitis include abdominal cramps, weight loss, nausea, vomiting, and low-grade fever. Sixty percent of the abdominal masses are palpable, and 40% are discovered at laparotomy. Radiographic findings include displacement and extrinsic compression of bowel, stretching of the vasa recta and vascular encasement on angiography, and an inhomogeneous mass on computed tomographic (CT) scans. Retractile mesenteritis produces similar symptoms as well as obstruction of the small intestine, mesenteric thrombosis, lymphatic obstruction with ascites, steatorrhea, or protein-losing enteropathy. The prognoses for these

TABLE 58-1
Classification of Mesenteric and Omental Diseases

Mesenteric diseases
  Primary mesenteric inflammatory diseases
      Mesenteric panniculitis
      Retractile mesenteritis
  Mesenteric cysts
      Embryonic and developmental cysts
      Traumatic or acquired cysts
      Neoplastic cysts
      Infective and degenerative cysts
  Mesenteric tumors
      Benign
          Lipoma
          Hemangioma
          Leiomyoma
          Ganglioneuroma
      Malignant
          Leiomyosarcoma
          Liposarcoma
          Rhabdomyosarcoma
          Metastatic disease
  Mesenteric fibromatosis
  Mesenteric vascular diseases
Omental diseases
  Mass lesions
      Primary tumors and cysts
      Metastatic disease
  Vascular lesions compromising blood flow
      Torsion
          Primary
          Secondary (e.g., hernia, adhesion, tumor)
      Infarction
          Primary
          Secondary (e.g., torsion, incarceration in hernia)
      Inflammatory lesions
          Adhesions and inflammation caused by peritonitis

conditions depend on the underlying disease. Therapy should rely on surgical bypass; resection usually is not possible. Some patients have been reported to respond to prednisone with azathioprine or cyclophosphamide, but further studies are needed to confirm the effectiveness of this therapy.

Mesenteric Fibromatosis

Etiology and Pathogenesis

Library Resource Center
Renton Technical College
3000 N.E. 4th St.
Renton, WA 98056

Mesenteric fibromatosis (or mesenteric desmoid) is a benign, noninflammatory fibromatous proliferation arising from the mesentery. The desmoid tumor has an ill-defined margin, lacks encapsulation, and infiltrates into surrounding muscle and fascial planes. The condition may occur spontaneously or in association with the familial polyposis coli syndromes (especially Gardner's syndrome). Other cases are associated with trauma, prior surgery, or estrogen use.

Clinical Features, Diagnosis, and Management

Patients with mesenteric fibromatosis may present with an asymptomatic abdominal mass or with intestinal obstruction or perforation resulting from involvement of mesenteric blood vessels. Ultrasound shows a solid mass, and CT scans show a nonenhancing mass with soft tissue density. Wide local excision is the treatment of choice but may be precluded by mesenteric root involvement. Some cases may require palliative intestinal bypass. There are anecdotal reports of successful treatment with prostaglandin synthesis inhibitors and antiestrogens (e.g., tamoxifen) alone or in combination. Cytotoxic chemotherapy and radiation therapy have not proved useful in the treatment of mesenteric fibromatosis.

Mesenteric and Omental Cysts and Solid Tumors

Etiology and Pathogenesis

Lymphangiomas are large cysts of the mesentery of the small intestine, the mesocolon, or the omentum. Lymphangiomas are characteristically found in children. Histologically, these are cystic structures lined with flattened lymphatic endothelium with smooth muscle and abundant lymphoid tissue made up of foam cells containing lipoid material in the cyst wall. Other mesenteric cysts (nonpancreatic pseudocysts, enteric cysts, mesothelial cysts) have cuboidal, columnar, or no epithelial lining. Cystic teratomas, cystic smooth muscle tumors, and cystic mesotheliomas are included in the differential diagnosis of lymphangiomas.

Most mesenteric malignancies arise from other sites and secondarily involve the mesentery through direct spread or metastasis. Primary solid tumors of the mesentery and omentum are rare. These solid tumors may be benign (leiomyoma, hemangiopericytoma, neurofibroma, lipoma, myxoma, xanthogranuloma) or malignant (leiomyosarcoma, fibrosarcoma, liposarcoma, rhabdomyosarcoma). Patients present with inflammatory fibrosarcomas at a mean age of 15 years. These tumors are locally aggressive and possibly metastatic, leading to death.

Clinical Features, Diagnosis, and Management

Lymphangiomas are often large, causing abdominal distention, nausea, and vomiting. Nonlymphangiomatous cysts occur in older persons and may not be symptomatic. Abdominal radiographs demonstrate bowel displacement and proximal bowel dilation. Ultrasound, CT, and magnetic resonance imaging (MRI) studies may show homogeneous or inhomogeneous cysts with uni- or multilocular characteristics. The definitive management of these lesions is surgical resection. Total excision may require resection of adjacent intestinal segments.

Mesenteric and omental tumors are often detected as a palpable abdominal mass. Patients usually present with pain and sometimes with ascites or vomiting. Abdominal radiographs may show bowel loop displacement. The mass can be localized to the mesentery or omentum from CT scans. Angiography may be able to determine if the mass is extrinsic or intrinsic to the mesentery. If possible, primary omental and mesenteric tumors should be surgically excised, as 50% of lipomatous, histiocytic, and leiomyomatous mesenteric tumors and 25% of omental tumors are malignant. Metastases to the mesentery produce mesenteric shortening, angulation, and fixation of the bowel, resulting in obstruction or infarction as a result of vascular occlusion. Curative resection usually is not possible in this setting, but surgery may have palliative value for patients with metastatic carcinoid because of the indolent nature of these tumors.

Omental Vascular Accidents

Etiology and Pathogenesis

Primary vascular accidents of the omentum, such as torsion, infarction, and hemorrhage, may occur as a complication of a hernia or as a result of bifid omentum, obesity, vascular anomalies, embolism from the heart or aorta, thrombosis, abdominal trauma, violent exercise, coughing, straining, and acute changes in body position.

Clinical Features, Diagnosis, and Management

Patients present with acute abdominal pain that may be generalized or localized to the right abdomen, nausea, vomiting, anorexia, low-grade fever, and mild leukocytosis. The physical examination may reveal a mobile, tender mass; guarding may or may not be detected. Most patients require surgical resection of the involved omentum.

Mesenteric and Omental Granulomatous Infections

Granulomatous diseases such as tuberculosis or mycoses may be clinically similar to metastatic malignancy, lymphoma, and inflammatory bowel disease. CT scans may show lymphadenopathy, involvement of the liver, spleen, and adrenals, and nodularity and thickening of the mesentery and omentum. Biopsy specimens stained and cultured for fungi and acid-fast bacillus are necessary for diagnosis.

DISEASES OF THE PERITONEUM

Peritonitis

Peritonitis is a localized or generalized inflammation of the parietal and visceral peritoneum. It may be the primary disease, or it may be secondary to diseases of or injury to the intra-abdominal organs.

Acute Suppurative Peritonitis

Etiology and Pathogenesis. Acute suppurative peritonitis results from primary intra-abdominal disease (e.g., perforated ulcer, appendicitis, diverticulitis), penetrating trauma, or iatrogenic perforation after endoscopy or radiographic procedures.

Clinical Features, Diagnosis, and Management. Patients present with pain that is exacerbated by movement and respirations, anorexia, nausea, vomiting, fever (38°C to 40°C), and signs of hypovolemia (e.g., tachycardia, dry mucous membranes, hypotension). Abdominal examination may reveal distention, hypoactive or absent bowel sounds, tenderness (point or diffuse), involuntary guarding, and rigidity. Laboratory studies are most remarkable for significant leukocytosis, often with increased bands. Abdominal radiographs may show dilation of the small intestine and colon and pneumoperitoneum.

Early diagnosis and prompt surgical intervention are essential to reduce morbidity and mortality from multiple organ failure that results from untreated peritonitis. Isotonic crystalloid fluids (e.g., Ringer's lactate) should be administered to correct hypovolemia and electrolyte imbalances. Response to fluid resuscitation should be monitored carefully, and vital signs and urine output should be assessed frequently. Nasogastric suction decompresses the stomach, and supplemental oxygen overcomes mild hypoxemia. Broad-spectrum antibiotics to treat aerobic and anaerobic organisms should be started before and continued during and after surgery. The mainstay of therapy for acute suppurative peritonitis is expeditious surgery, including copious irrigation of the peritoneum and repair of the ruptured viscus.

Granulomatous Peritonitis

Etiology and Pathogenesis. Granulomatous peritonitis is characterized by peritoneal inflammation with formation of granulomas and development of adhesions. The most common cause is tuberculosis. Tuberculous peritonitis usually is associated with a primary focus of tuberculosis elsewhere, most often the lung, despite normal chest radiographs in about two-thirds of cases. The omentum, intestine, liver, spleen, and female genital tract can also be involved. The organism gains entry into the peritoneal cavity transmurally from diseased bowel, from tuberculous salpingitis, or by hematogenous spread from a pulmonary focus. Granulomatous peritonitis may also be caused by infections (e.g., fungal organisms, such as *Candida* or *Histoplasma* species, and parasites, such as ameba or *strongyloides*), and iatrogenic sources (e.g., glove talc, or cellulose fibers from gauze, surgical drapes, or gowns).

Clinical Features, Diagnosis, and Management. Generally, the onset of tuberculous peritonitis is insidious; symptoms include fever, anorexia, weakness, malaise, weight loss, and abdominal distention due to ascites or partial intestinal obstruction. The abdominal examination may reveal tenderness and ascites; the classic doughy abdomen is rare. Laboratory studies usually show no leukocytosis and only a mild anemia. Tuberculin skin tests produce positive results in most cases, but results may be negative in anergic persons. Chest radiographs are abnormal in 80% of patients. Abdominal radiographs are rarely useful. CT scans may show thickened bowel and ascites. Ascitic fluid protein levels usually exceed 3.0 g per dl, and glucose levels are <30 mg per dl in >80% of cases. Most patients have ascitic fluid leukocyte counts of >250 cells per μl, which are predominantly lymphocytic. Centrifugation of >1 liter of ascitic fluid with subsequent acid-fast staining identifies the organism in some cases; ascitic cultures often need 4 to 6 weeks to incubate. Some laboratories are using polymerase chain reaction testing, which can detect 10 to 100 mycobacteria in an ascitic fluid sample. Laparoscopy and laparotomy are often diagnostic, revealing characteristic stalactite-like fibrinous masses and granulomatous peritoneal studding. Isoniazid plus two additional drugs for 18 to 24 months is the indicated medical therapy for tuberculous peritonitis. Corticosteroids for 2 to 3 months may prevent development of dense adhesions.

Chemical Peritonitis

Etiology and Pathogenesis.   Peritoneal irritation results from exposure to bile, urine, and chyle, which may occur secondary to injury or surgery. Barium spillage from contrast radiographic procedures produces a severe peritoneal reaction.

Clinical Features, Diagnosis, and Management.   Patients present with typical peritoneal findings. Therapy relies on adequate intravenous fluids, broad-spectrum antibiotics, and laparotomy to irrigate the abdomen and control the source of inflammation.

Peritonitis with Chronic Peritoneal Dialysis

Etiology and Pathogenesis.   Peritonitis is the most common complication of chronic ambulatory peritoneal dialysis (CAPD), occurring 1.4 times per patient-year of treatment. Most CAPD-related peritonitis involves a single organism, which usually is a gram-positive coccus such as *Staphylococcus epidermidis*, *Staphylococcus aureus*, or a *Streptococcus* or *Enterococcus* organism. One-fourth of cases result from infection with gram-negative bacteria (e.g., *Escherichia coli*, *Pseudomonas aeruginosa*). Fungal peritonitis is a rare but severe complication of CAPD.

Clinical Features, Diagnosis, and Management.   Most patients with CAPD-related peritonitis have less severe symptoms than patients with acute suppurative peritonitis. Diffuse abdominal pain, fever, hyperhydration, diarrhea, hypotension, and pain over the catheter tunnel are common presenting symptoms. Blood testing usually reveals leukocytosis. The diagnosis relies on the presence of two of three criteria: abdominal pain or tenderness, a turbid dialysate with a neutrophil count of >100 per μl, and a positive peritoneal fluid culture. Most patients are effectively treated by an outpatient course of intraperitoneal antibiotics determined by pathogen susceptibility (e.g., vancomycin, cephalosporins, aminoglycosides). Heparin is added to the dialysate to prevent postinfection adhesions. CAPD catheters should be removed in cases of persistent peritonitis after 4 to 5 days of treatment, fungal or tuberculous peritonitis, fecal peritonitis, or skin infection at the catheter site.

Peritonitis in the Acquired Immunodeficiency Syndrome

Peritonitis in patients with acquired immunodeficiency syndrome can be caused by perforation of the small intestine or colon secondary to cytomegalovirus enteritis and by infection with *Mycobacterium avium-intracellulare* complex, *Mycobacterium tuberculosis*, *Cryptococcus neoformans*, and *Strongyloides* organisms. Most patients present with severe abdominal pain. Principles of management include emergency laparotomy, intravenous fluids, and broad-spectrum antibiotics.

Primary Mesothelioma

Etiology and Pathogenesis

Twenty percent to 40% of mesotheliomas occur in the peritoneum; the majority originate in the pleura. The incidence of mesothelioma is linked to asbestos exposure, radiation exposure, and use of the angiographic contrast agent Thorotrast.

Clinical Features, Diagnosis, and Management

Patients with mesotheliomas present with epigastric or right upper quadrant pain, nausea, vomiting, malaise, fever, weight loss, diarrhea, and anemia. Ascites is present in 90% of patients. Primary mesotheliomas can produce and secrete various hormones such as antidiuretic hormone, growth hormone, and insulin-like factors, all of which can cause paraneoplastic syndromes, manifesting as hyponatremia, hypoglycemia, thrombocytosis, and increased production of fibrin-degradation products. Findings on ultrasound and CT scanning can suggest the diagnosis, demonstrate the extent of tumor, and aid in directed biopsy of suggestive lesions. In most cases, the diagnosis is confirmed by laparoscopy or laparotomy. Other neoplasms in the differential diagnosis include benign papillary and fibrous mesotheliomas, adenomatoid tumors, and multicystic peritoneal mesotheliomas. Therapy for mesothelioma rarely prolongs survival. Doxorubicin, alone or in combination with other antineoplastic agents, achieves the best response. Most patients survive <1 year after diagnosis.

Pseudomyxoma Peritonei

Etiology and Pathogenesis

Pseudomyxoma peritonei is characterized by the accumulation of large quantities of diffuse, gelatinous material in the peritoneum and omentum arising from mucinous neoplasms of the appendix or ovary.

Clinical Features, Diagnosis, and Management

Patients most commonly present with increased abdominal girth, secondary to mucinous ascites or intestinal obstruction. Ultrasound shows multiple intraperitoneal multilocular cysts and ascitic septation. A CT scan reveals scalloping of the hepatic and bowel margins as a result of compression by the gelatinous mass. Treatment involves aggressive surgical debulking of the tumor, along with appendectomy and bilateral oophorectomy. Pseudomyxoma peritonei is a low-grade malignancy; the 5-year survival rate is 54%. Repeat laparotomy is indicated for recurrent disease.

DISEASES OF THE RETROPERITONEUM

Retroperitoneal Fluid Collections

Etiology and Pathogenesis

Lymphoceles are cystic masses that contain lymph. They occur in the retroperitoneum after injuries, diseases, or operations (renal or pancreatic transplant) that interrupt the lymph channels traversing the posterior pelvis and abdomen. Duodenal succus results from duodenal injury secondary to injury, sphincterotomy, and ulcer or diverticular perforation. Pancreatic duct injury caused by acute and chronic pancreatitis, trauma, or pancreatic surgery can produce localized collections of pancreatic juice. Abdominal trauma and endoscopic or surgical manipulation can injure the distal common bile duct, causing bile leakage. Injury of the collecting system of the kidney can produce perinephric urine extravasation.

Clinical Features, Diagnosis, and Management

CT or ultrasound studies can be used to direct the aspiration of retroperitoneal fluid collections. A lymph collection can be readily distinguished from blood but not urine on CT scans. Duodenal perforations are diagnosed with upper gastrointestinal meglumine (Gastrografin)-enhanced radiography. A CT scan may differentiate a duodenal hematoma from a full-thickness perforation. Preoperative or intraoperative pancreatography can be used to assess pancreatic duct injury. Intravenous pyelography or a CT scan can be used to evaluate the function of an injured renal collecting system.

Surgical intervention is needed to treat many significant retroperitoneal fluid collections. Conservative management may be possible for early duodenal perforation, but retroperitoneal infection mandates operative therapy. Drainage procedures are performed for small pancreatic ductal injuries, but partial pancreatectomy is needed for major duct damage. Isolated bile duct injuries require primary repair or T-tube drainage with secondary repair. Complex injuries that involve the bile ducts, pancreas, and duodenum may need a Whipple procedure. Avulsion of the renal collecting system necessitates nephrectomy, whereas renal pelvis laceration and ureteropelvic junction avulsion can usually be repaired. Ureter injury may be managed by suture repair with or without stenting and nephrostomy.

Retroperitoneal Hemorrhage

Etiology and Pathogenesis

The major cause of retroperitoneal hemorrhage is traumatic vessel injury associated with pelvic or vertebral fracture or avulsion of a renal vascular pedicle. Other causes include anticoagulation therapy, spontaneous hemorrhage into an adrenal gland or retroperitoneal tumor, acute pancreatitis, ruptured aortic aneurysm, and ruptured utero-ovarian veins during pregnancy. Most abdominal aortic aneurysms are caused by atherosclerosis; aneurysms secondary to bacterial or fungal infection are less common.

Clinical Features, Diagnosis, and Management

The clinical course of most retroperitoneal hemorrhage depends on the intensity and cause of bleeding. Ruptures of atherosclerotic abdominal aortic aneurysms manifest as severe back pain and a tender, pulsatile mass on abdominal examination. Inflammatory aneurysms are characterized by discomfort, tenderness, and ureteral obstruction. Ultrasound may confirm the presence of aneurysmal rupture, but this test should not be performed on an unstable patient if doing so would create a delay in surgery. CT scanning and aortography are time-consuming procedures, which precludes their routine use in patients suspected of having aneurysm rupture. Emergency surgery is mandatory for ruptured aortic aneurysms, all cases of massive or persistent retroperitoneal hemorrhage, hemorrhage during pregnancy, and penetrating wounds. Postoperative complications of aortic aneurysm surgery include myocardial infarction, stroke, renal failure, bleeding, and ischemic colitis.

Retroperitoneal Fibrosis

Etiology and Pathogenesis

Retroperitoneal fibrosis is characterized by progressive fibrosis of connective and adipose tissue. It originates in the lower retroperitoneum and spreads bilaterally toward the renal hilus, encircling the vessels and ureters. The most common form of disease is idiopathic; however, fibrosis may result from paraneoplastic phenomena (e.g., carcinoid, Hodgkin's disease, sarcoma), drugs (e.g., methysergide), other fibrotic processes (e.g., mesenteric fibrosis, sclerosing cholangitis, orbital pseudotumor), radiation therapy, retroperitoneal infection or fluid collections, or inflammatory abdominal aortic aneurysms.

Clinical Features, Diagnosis, and Management

Patients present with abdominal or back pain, anorexia, fatigue, fever, jaundice, edema, protein-losing enteropathy, portal hypertension, peripheral thrombosis, intermittent claudication, hydronephrosis, pyelonephritis, and progressive renal failure with anuria. An abdominal mass is present in 15% of patients. Intravenous pyelography shows medial displacement and narrowing of the ureters. A CT scan demonstrates the extent of the fibrous plaque. Disease progression may be slowed by steroid therapy alone or in combination with surgery. The options for treating renal damage include ureterolysis, renal autotransplantation into the pelvis, ureteral catheter placement, or nephrostomy.

Retroperitoneal Inflammation and Necrosis

Noninfectious retroperitoneal inflammation is found with retroperitoneal fibrosis, inflammatory aortic aneurysms, fluid collections, acute pancreatitis, or tumors. In severe pancreatitis, serial CT scans may document retroperitoneal inflammation and necrosis that typically spread to the left and right pararenal spaces, the mesenteric roots, both paracolic gutters, and para-aortically into the lower retroperitoneum. The initial management is conservative, but major pancreatic necrosis mandates necrosectomy, lavage, and drainage.

Retroperitoneal Infections

Etiology and Pathogenesis

Retroperitoneal abscesses usually occur in the anterior compartment and result from appendicitis, pancreatitis, penetrating duodenal ulcer, perforating colonic carcinoma and diverticulitis, and Crohn's disease. Psoas abscesses may be primary (e.g., *S aureus* in children), or they may be secondary to extension of an intra-abdominal infection (Crohn's disease, appendicitis, diverticulitis, malignancy) or a vertebral infection. One-fourth of extrapulmonary tuberculosis infections affect the retroperitoneum, which is seeded at the time of initial dissemination. Renal tuberculosis originates in the cortex and spreads to the medulla, causing papillary necrosis and cavitation. The adrenal glands are susceptible to disseminated histoplasmosis, paracoccidioidomycosis, and blastomycosis. Renal and psoas abscesses may form in the setting of coccidioidomycosis.

Opportunistic fungi (e.g., *Candida*, *Aspergillus*, or *Cryptococcus* organisms) may disseminate in the retroperitoneum in patients with altered immune responses. Retroperitoneal actinomycosis may be caused by appendiceal or colonic perforation. It is characterized by chronic abscesses with multiple sinus tracts exuding "sulfur granules." Retroperitoneal infections caused by *Nocardia* organisms usually occur in the kidney and are the result of dissemination from a pulmonary focus. These infections usually affect immunosuppressed patients.

Clinical Features, Diagnosis, and Management

Patients with retroperitoneal abscesses present with fever; malaise; leukocytosis; a retroperitoneal mass; and pain in the flank, back, abdomen, or thigh. A CT scan is most accurate in evaluating retroperitoneal abscesses. It also facilitates needle aspiration of abscess fluid for culture. Operative drainage with broad antibiotic coverage is the treatment of choice. Percutaneous drainage is successful in selected patients with well-defined abscess cavities. The symptoms of retroperitoneal tuberculous infection include dysuria, urinary frequency, hematuria, flank pain, and sterile pyuria. Some symptoms are associated with characteristic findings on intravenous pyelography. Retroperitoneal tuberculous infection is treated with antituberculous chemotherapy. Spinal tuberculosis with a secondary psoas abscess may also require incision and drainage. Involvement of the adrenals in fungal infections may result in life-threatening Addison's disease. On CT scans, the findings with retroperitoneal fungal infections include bilateral adrenal enlargement with focal hemorrhage, necrosis, and cavitation. Retroperitoneal fungal infections are treated with amphotericin B; a total 1 to 4 g is administered in the course of the treatment. Actinomycosis is rarely diagnosed without laparotomy. It is treated with incision and drainage, combined with 0.5 to 20 million units of penicillin daily for 4 to 12 weeks. *Nocardia* infections are treated with a combination of trimethoprim and sulfamethoxazole for 3 to 4 months.

Retroperitoneal Neoplasms

Etiology and Pathogenesis

Primary retroperitoneal neoplasms derive from soft tissue, lymphoid tissue, or germ cells. Most are malignant sarcomas: liposarcomas, leiomyosarcomas, and fibrous histiocytomas. Lymphomas (usually non-Hodgkin's) result from lymphatic metastases of primary neoplasms. In children, rhabdomyosarcomas, neuroblastomas, ganglioneuroblastomas, and teratomas predominate. Neoplasms of the abdomen, lower extremities, and genitourinary systems can metastasize to the retroperitoneum.

Clinical Features, Diagnosis, and Management

Larger retroperitoneal neoplasms produce fatigue, abdominal pain, radiating pain to the back and thigh, and symptoms of lymphatic, venous, and urinary obstruction. CT or MRI studies may define the site of origin and gross morphology of a retroperitoneal neoplasm; however, angiographic demonstration of invasion of adjacent organs may be necessary to define the malignant nature of the tumor. Percutaneous needle biopsy can determine the histologic character of a retroperitoneal neoplasm in 80% of cases. The therapy of choice for retroperitoneal tumors is complete resection of the tumor and involved structures; this is possible in 50% of cases. Debulking may be of value with large, symptomatic sarcomas. Sarcomas respond poorly to adjuvant radiation therapy and chemotherapy. In contrast, lymphomas respond better to these modalities.

CHAPTER 59

Structural Anomalies, Tumors, and Diseases of the Biliary Tree

EMBRYOLOGY AND ANATOMY OF THE BILIARY TREE

The biliary tree and liver originate near the junction of the foregut and the midgut as a ventral diverticulum. Shortly after it develops, this diverticulum divides into the cranial bud, which develops into the liver and intrahepatic bile ducts, and the caudal bud, which develops into the gallbladder and cystic duct. The stalk of the diverticulum forms the extrahepatic bile ducts. These primordial buds are initially composed of solid cords of endodermal cells, which later vacuolize, forming the patent lumen of the biliary tree.

The gallbladder lies in a depression on the inferior surface of the liver at the boundary between the right and left lobes. The area of the gallbladder not attached to the liver is covered by the peritoneum and is in contact with the duodenum, pancreatic head, and hepatic flexure of the colon. The fundus is the rounded end of the gallbladder that projects beyond the liver. The body is the largest part of the gallbladder. It is connected to the liver on one side and covered by peritoneum on the free surface. The infundibulum is the transitional area between the body and neck of the gallbladder, an S-shaped structure in the deepest part of the cystic fossa. The arterial supply of the gallbladder is derived from the cystic artery. Venous drainage is by multiple small veins directly into the liver or toward the cystic duct. The lymphatic drainage parallels that of the venous drainage. Sympathetic innervation originates in the celiac plexus, whereas the parasympathetic supply is through branches of both vagal nerves. The gallbladder mucosa has many folds that increase the surface contact with bile. The well-developed muscularis is covered by an almost avascular connective tissue layer and the serosa.

The intrahepatic segmental bile ducts coalesce to form the right and left hepatic ducts, which merge to form the common hepatic duct. The lengths of the right and left hepatic ducts vary from 0.5 to 2.5 cm. They join outside the liver in 95% of cases. The cystic duct, which is 0.1 to 0.4 cm in diameter and 0.5 to 8.0 cm in length, connects the gallbladder neck to the common hepatic duct. The spiral valves of Heister are projections of the cystic duct mucosa that prevent excessive distention or collapse of the gallbladder. The common bile duct is 5 to 17 cm long, with a diameter of 0.3 to 1.1 cm. It consists of scanty circular muscle covered by a fibroareolar coat. The lumen is lined by columnar epithelium that is continuous with that of other biliary structures. The lumens of the common bile duct and main pancreatic duct usually join to form the ampulla of Vater, although these ducts drain separately in 30% of cases. A complex system of circular and longitudinal smooth muscle, known as the sphincter of Oddi, surrounds the intraduodenal segment of the common bile duct and the ampulla of Vater.

DEVELOPMENTAL ANOMALIES OF THE BILIARY TREE

Etiology and Pathogenesis

Failure of vacuolization of the primordial hepatic buds can result in intra- or extrahepatic biliary atresia or congenital absence of the gallbladder. Incomplete vacuolization can lead to a septated gallbladder or biliary hypoplasia with stenosis. Abnormal migration of the caudal bud into the cranial bud may produce an intrahepatic gallbladder. Inadequate caudal migration leads to a free-floating gallbladder.

Clinical Features, Diagnosis, and Management

Biliary atresia is the most frequent cause of death from liver disease in children and occurs in 1 in 10,000 live births. Infants with biliary atresia are jaundiced. Obliteration of the bile ducts is evident several weeks after birth. Treatment requires definitive surgical drainage (e.g., a Kasai procedure). Even after adequate drainage, 5-year survival is only 50%, and liver transplantation may be necessary.

BILIARY CYSTS

Incidence and Epidemiology

Cystic anomalies occur throughout the biliary system. The incidence of biliary cysts is highest in Japan and other Asian countries; they are far less common in Western countries, including the United States. With the exception of choledochoceles, which occur with equal frequency in males and females, biliary cysts are more common in females. Many patients (40% to 60%) are diagnosed before 10 years of age; up to one-third present after 20 years of age.

Etiology and Pathogenesis

Five types of biliary cysts are described by the Todani classification. Type I cysts are characterized by saccular dilation of the common bile duct and are the most common type, accounting for 75% to 85% of biliary cysts. Type II cysts are diverticula of the extrahepatic ducts and are rare, accounting for 2% to 3% of cases. Type III cysts (termed choledochoceles) represent a dilated, prolapsed segment of the intraduodenal portion of the common bile duct. Choledochoceles are further classified into type A, which are saccular dilations of the intraduodenal portion of the common bile duct, and type B, which are diverticula of the intraduodenal portion of the common bile duct. Type IV cysts are diffuse cystic dilations in the intra- and extrahepatic biliary tree. Type V cystic dilations are limited to the intrahepatic biliary system (also known as Caroli's disease).

Several mechanisms are probably involved in the formation of biliary cysts. Theories on their origins include abnormal embryogenesis with unequal proliferation of the endodermal cell cords. Other investigators suggest that biliary cysts are acquired because of the insertion of the pancreatic duct high into the common bile duct, which is an anomaly observed in many patients with biliary cysts. Long-term exposure to pancreatic juice may result in chronic inflammation, edema, fibrosis, and obstruction of the bile ducts, with subsequent dilation of the common bile duct. The presence of an abnormal distal muscle segment, similar to the colonic abnormalities of Hirschsprung's disease, has also been suggested as a possible cause.

Clinical Features

Patients with type I choledochal cysts typically present in infancy with jaundice and failure to thrive, although 20% of patients present after 2 years of age with intermittent abdominal pain and recurrent jaundice. Rarely, patients remain asymptomatic. Cirrhosis and portal hypertension are frequent complications, particularly when the cysts present in infancy. Patients with type II cysts classically present with obstruction of the common bile duct. Seventy-five percent of patients with choledochoceles (type III cysts) present after age 20 years with pain and obstructive jaundice. Pancreatitis is a complication in 30% to 70% of cases of choledochocele. Patients with type IV and type V cysts typically have recurrent cholangitis, liver abscesses, and portal hypertension. Caroli's disease may be associated with medullary spongy kidney, which should be distinguished from autosomal-dominant polycystic kidney disease. The latter disease is characterized by hepatic cysts, which are pathologically distinct from biliary cysts. Unlike biliary cysts, hepatic cysts do not communicate with the biliary tree.

Findings on Diagnostic Testing

Ultrasound and hepatobiliary scintigraphy are the primary noninvasive modalities used to diagnose type I, II, IV, and V biliary cysts. Characteristic ^{99m}Tc-labeled iminodiacetic acid scintigraphic findings include biliary dilation and tracer retention after 24 hours. The standard for diagnosis is direct visualization of the biliary system with endoscopic retrograde cholangiopancreatography (ERCP) or percutaneous transhepatic cholangiography (PTC). Definition of the anatomy is critical to surgical planning, especially because of

TABLE 59-1
Causes of Secondary Sclerosing Cholangitis

Operative trauma
Choledocholithiasis
Chronic pancreatitis
Ischemic cholangiopathy
    Liver allograft rejection
    Hepatic arterial infusion of chemotherapy
    Surgical trauma
Histiocytosis X
Cholangiocarcinoma

the high frequency of the anomalous union of the pancreatic duct and common bile duct.

Management and Course

Small intraduodenal choledochoceles are best treated with endoscopic sphincterotomy, but all other biliary cysts require surgical therapy. For extrahepatic cysts, excision and drainage is preferable to drainage alone because of the risks of recurrent cholangitis and malignant transformation. For localized intrahepatic cysts, resection is the preferred treatment. The patient with diffuse intrahepatic cysts may require hepatic transplantation if hepatic failure or portal hypertension develop. Chronic antibiotic therapy may reduce the risk of recurrent cholangitis, particularly in Caroli's disease.

In addition to cholangitis, pancreatitis (type III), biliary cirrhosis, and liver abscesses may complicate the course of disease in the patients with biliary cysts. Pregnant patients may develop cyst rupture during labor, prompting the recommendation that pregnant women with symptomatic cysts should deliver by cesarean section. The most feared complication is malignant degeneration. This risk is particularly high in adult patients; 15% develop carcinoma. Carcinoma may occur throughout the biliary and pancreatic tree, including the gallbladder and sites uninvolved by the cysts. The prognosis of these tumors is dismal. Almost all patients die soon after diagnosis.

SCLEROSING CHOLANGITIS

Incidence and Epidemiology

Bile duct injury characterized by inflammation, fibrosis, thickening, and stricture formation is termed *sclerosing cholangitis*. Primary sclerosing cholangitis (PSC) refers to bile duct injury not attributable to other causes, whereas secondary sclerosing cholangitis describes bile duct injury in the setting of a known cause (Table 59-1).

TABLE 59-2
Disorders Associated with Primary Sclerosing Cholangitis

DISORDER	FREQUENCY (%)
Inflammatory bowel disease	
Chronic ulcerative colitis	50–75
Crohn's disease	<5
Immunodeficiency syndromes	Rare
Angioimmunoblastic lymphadenopathy	
Acquired immunodeficiency syndrome	
Familial immunodeficiency syndromes	
Miscellaneous	
Recurrent pancreatitis	4–25
Antiphospholipid antibody syndrome	Rare
Sjögren's syndrome	Rare
Rheumatoid arthritis	Rare
Retroperitoneal fibrosis	Rare

PSC is a disease that mostly affects young men. Two-thirds of patients are diagnosed before age 45 years, and the male-to-female ratio is 2:1. It is associated with many disorders that involve immune dysregulation (Table 59-2). Fifty percent to 75% of patients with PSC have associated ulcerative colitis. Less than 5% have Crohn's disease. Conversely, only 3% to 5% of patients with chronic ulcerative colitis are diagnosed with PSC, and there is no relationship between the severity and duration of ulcerative colitis and the risk of developing PSC.

Etiology and Pathogenesis

The etiology of PSC remains unknown, but the distinctive pattern of disease associations has generated several theories. Most patients with PSC have circulating immune complexes and autoantibodies. The most prevalent autoantibodies are characterized by immunoreactivity in the perinuclear region of neutrophils and are called *perinuclear antineutrophil cytoplasmic antibodies* (pANCA). Although their etiologic role remains unclear, the presence of pANCA in 50% to 80% of patients with ulcerative colitis and 90% of patients with PSC raises the possibility of a common pathogenetic link for these disorders. Other putative pathogenetic mechanisms in PSC include portal venous bacteremia with subsequent periductal inflammation; occult infection with cytomegalovirus; and a genetic predisposition, suggested by the association of the disease with HLA-B8 and -DR3.

The mechanisms of injury in secondary sclerosing cholangitis are specific to the precipitating condition (see Table 59-2). Ischemia is the cause of bile duct injury in patients undergoing hepatic artery catheter–delivered chemotherapy and in patients with liver allograft rejection. Gallstone-induced biliary sclerosis results from direct traumatic damage to the bile duct.

Clinical Features

The onset of PSC is insidious. Most patients experience symptoms an average of 2 years before diagnosis. Patients present with progressive fatigue, pruritus, and jaundice. Cholangitis is uncommon and often indicates the presence of superimposed choledocholithiasis or bile duct carcinoma. Patients with associated inflammatory bowel disease are more likely to have both intrahepatic and extrahepatic ductal disease. Isolated involvement of the extrahepatic ducts is more common in patients without inflammatory bowel disease (38%) than in patients with inflammatory bowel disease (7%). A small percentage of patients with PSC have other associated immune disorders (e.g., Sjögren's syndrome, hereditary acquired immunodeficiency syndromes, or the antiphospholipid antibody syndrome) (see Table 59-1).

Findings on Diagnostic Testing

Most patients exhibit at least a twofold elevation of alkaline phosphatase levels, which is out of proportion to the elevations of serum bilirubin levels. Aminotransferase levels are only mildly increased. The standard for diagnosis is ERCP, which is preferred over PTC because of the technical difficulties of cannulating strictured intrahepatic ducts. The characteristic cholangiographic features include multifocal strictures, usually in the intrahepatic and extrahepatic ducts, with intervening normal or dilated ductal segments, producing a "string of beads" pattern. This pattern is not specific for PSC and may be seen in patients with metastatic cancer to the liver, primary biliary cirrhosis, allograft ischemic injury, and the diffuse form of cholangiocarcinoma. Differentiating cholangiocarcinoma from PSC can be difficult, especially because bile duct cancer is a potential complication of PSC.

Management and Course

The clinical course of PSC usually is slowly progressive. A small subset of patients have stable disease for decades, but over years, most patients with PSC progress to portal hypertension and death from liver failure. The 5-year survival rate is 60% to 70%. Cholangiocarcinoma complicates the course of 7% to 15% of patients with PSC; it can be difficult to diagnose in view of the cholangiographic abnormalities observed in PSC. The mean age at diagnosis of cholangiocarcinoma in these patients is 42 years, compared with the mean age of 66 years for the general population.

The treatment of PSC patients is primarily supportive. Orthotopic liver transplantation is reserved for patients with end-stage disease. No immunosuppressive regimen has been demonstrated to slow the progression of disease. Although ursodeoxycholic acid may relieve pruritus and improve biochemical profiles, it also fails to halt disease progression. Prophylactic colectomy in patients with ulcerative colitis does not alter the natural course of PSC nor does it prevent the complication of cholangiocarcinoma. Dominant symptomatic strictures may be treated with endoscopic balloon dilation and stenting. Surgical resection and biliary reconstruction may be necessary for selected patients with refractory strictures or for those who may have bile duct carcinoma.

CARCINOMA OF THE BILE DUCTS

Incidence and Epidemiology

Cholangiocarcinoma is a rare tumor that generally occurs in middle-aged persons. The relatively young median age of onset results in part from the association with PSC and biliary cysts. Unlike gallbladder tumors, there are minimal racial and geographic differences in the incidence of bile duct carcinoma.

Etiology and Pathogenesis

No specific causes have been identified for bile duct cancer, but there are several disease associations. The high incidence of these tumors in Southeast Asia may be the result of chronic infestation with the liver fluke, *Clonorchis sinensis*. However, this infection does not have a proven pathogenetic role. Other disease associations include PSC and biliary cysts. There have also been reports of an increased incidence of cholangiocarcinoma in patients and relatives of patients with hereditary nonpolyposis colon cancer. Cholangiocarcinoma has not been linked to cirrhosis, gallstone disease, carcinogens, or drug exposures.

Clinical Features

Nonspecific symptoms of anorexia and weight loss are common in patients with cholangiocarcinoma. Jaundice develops if the extrahepatic ducts become obstructed. Pain and cholangitis are not typical symptoms unless the patient has had prior surgery or superimposed choledocholithiasis. Fifty percent of extrahepatic tumors involve the hilum of the right and left hepatic ducts (i.e., Klatskin's tumor), and the other 50% involve the common hepatic duct or common bile duct. Ten percent of tumors spread diffusely throughout the biliary tree and may mimic PSC. Bile duct tumors tend to invade locally, and patients generally do not present with widely metastatic disease.

Findings on Diagnostic Testing

Initially, ultrasound should be used to evaluate patients suspected of having bile duct tumors. Intrahepatic bile duct dilation with no evidence of extrahepatic dilation is suggestive of an extrahepatic bile duct tumor. A CT scan is more accurate in defining distal common bile duct lesions and is more sensitive than ultrasound in detecting intrahepatic lesions. A contrast-enhanced CT scan also can detect invasion of surrounding vascular structures. The definitive imaging procedure is cholangiography by PTC or ERCP. If a CT scan or ultrasound suggest obstruction in the hilar region, PTC is the preferred procedure for further evaluation.

Histologic confirmation of malignancy can be obtained by transhepatic or endoscopic cytologic brushings. These tests have sensitivities of 30%. The addition of forceps biopsy to cytologic testing increases the diagnostic yield to 70%. Many tumors are well differentiated and occur in the setting of PSC, making diagnosis very difficult without surgical resection.

Management and Course

Surgical resection is the only option for long-term survival. At the time of diagnosis, 20% to 30% of proximal duct tumors and 60% to 70% of distal duct tumors are resectable. Involvement of both the right and left hepatic lobes or invasion of the portal vein or hepatic artery are indicators of unresectability. The median survival time for patients who successfully undergo resection with tumor-free margins is 3 years, compared with 1 year for patients who have unresectable tumors.

Jaundiced patients with unresectable tumors should be considered for palliative biliary-enteric anastomosis. If the patient is a poor operative candidate, placement of a biliary stent during ERCP or PTC usually provides adequate drainage. Radiation therapy may also palliate symptoms and improve survival. Hepatic transplantation prolongs survival, but the high incidence of recurrent disease in these patients suggests that transplantation should only be done in the setting of a research protocol.

CARCINOMA OF THE GALLBLADDER

Incidence and Epidemiology

Carcinoma of the gallbladder is a disease of the elderly. It is three times more common in women than in men. The female predominance has been attributed to a strong association with gallstones, which are present in 80% of patients with gallbladder tumors. There is a marked ethnic and geographic variation in the incidence of this tumor. It is the most common gastrointestinal malignancy in Native Americans. It is also prevalent in Latin American women, Japanese women, and Northern Europeans.

Etiology and Pathogenesis

The strong association of gallbladder carcinoma with gallstone disease has led to speculation that the bacterial and chemical microenvironment in association with cholelithiasis is carcinogenic, but the mechanisms involved are unknown. The duration of gallstone disease is important, as patients with cholelithiasis for >40 years have a higher incidence of gallbladder carcinoma than those with stones for a shorter period. Despite this increased risk, the very low incidence of gallbladder cancer does not warrant prophylactic cholecystectomy in patients with asymptomatic stones. Other factors associated with a high risk of gallbladder cancer include calcification of the gallbladder wall (porcelain gallbladder), biliary cysts, and *Salmonella typhi* carriage. Although the carcinogens are unknown, workers in the textile, rubber, and automotive industries have higher incidences of gallbladder malignancies.

Clinical Features

The signs and symptoms of gallbladder carcinoma are nonspecific. Only 10% to 20% of patients have the diagnosis established preoperatively. Pain is the most common complaint, but the pattern is variable. Jaundice occurs in 30% to 60% of patients and is a poor prognostic sign, usually indicative of an unresectable tumor. Other symptoms include nausea, vomiting, anorexia, and weight loss. Cholecystenteric fistulae are rare complications of gallbladder tumors.

Management and Course

Most patients with gallbladder tumors have stage IV or unresectable disease. The median survival time for these patients is 5 months. Patients with noninvasive stage I tumors limited to the gallbladder can be cured with simple cholecystectomy. Stage II and stage III tumors have a small chance of cure with a radical cholecystectomy, which involves wedge resection of the liver and regional lymphadenectomy. The role of chemotherapy and radiation therapy has not been defined for treatment of gallbladder tumors.

CHAPTER 60

Biliary Tract Stones and Postcholecystectomy Syndrome

GALLSTONES

Incidence and Epidemiology

Gallstone-related conditions are among the most common gastrointestinal disorders requiring hospitalization. Prevalence varies widely among ethnic groups. Pima Indians, Chileans, and whites in the United States manifest the highest rates. Asians in Singapore and Thailand have exceptionally low incidences of gallstone disease. The composition of stones also varies among cultures. Cholesterol stones account for 75% of gallstones in Western countries, whereas pigment or bilirubinate stones predominate in Africa and Asia.

Etiology and Pathogenesis

Biliary tract stones are divided into two general categories: cholesterol stones and pigment stones. This classification results from distinct pathophysiologic alterations in bile composition and the disparate clinical associations and risk factors (Table 60-1). Cholesterol stones are predominantly composed of cholesterol monohydrate with small amounts of calcium salts and glycoproteins. Cholesterol gallstones may form whenever there is a disturbance in the tightly regulated process of cholesterol secretion in bile. Bile may become supersaturated with cholesterol if bile acid secretion is decreased or if free cholesterol secretion is increased. Because phospholipids help solubilize cholesterol into micelles, any decrease in bile phospholipid content also promotes stone formation. Stone formation is also fostered by stasis within the gallbladder. Several nucleation factors, including gallbladder mucin, make the gallbladder a fertile environment for stone formation.

TABLE 60-1
Risk Factors and Conditions Associated with Gallstone Formation

Cholesterol stones
    Age
    Female sex
    Estrogens
    Pregnancy
    Diabetes mellitus
    Obesity
    Hypertriglyceridemia
    Prolonged fasting
    Rapid weight loss
    Ileal disease or resection
    Cystic fibrosis
Black pigment stones
    Chronic hemolysis
    Cirrhosis
    High-protein diet
Brown pigment stones
    Biliary infections
    Foreign bodies (e.g., sutures)
    Low-protein diet

Pigmented biliary tract stones are subclassified into black and brown stones based on differences in chemical composition and associated clinical features (see Table 60-1). Both are composed of calcium bilirubinate. Black stones contain polymers of bilirubinate, whereas brown stones contain monomers of bilirubinate as well as cholesterol and fatty acid salts. β-Glucuronidase from bacteria and, to a lesser extent, from biliary mucosal sources serve to deconjugate bilirubin glucuronides. In the setting of gallbladder stasis, the unconjugated bilirubin then precipitates as calcium bilirubinate crystals, which subsequently accumulate to form pigment stones.

Clinical Features

Gallbladder stones produce a wide spectrum of clinical presentations, including episodic biliary colic, acute cholecystitis, and chronic cholecystitis. Passage of a gallstone through the common bile duct may lead to acute cholangitis or acute pancreatitis. Despite the high incidences of these complications in the general population, more than two-thirds of patients with gallstones will never develop symptoms.

Biliary Colic

Most patients with symptomatic cholelithiasis present with biliary colic. This is a visceral pain that is caused by transient gallstone obstruction of the cystic duct. The pain typically is severe and episodic, lasting 30 minutes to several hours. The term *biliary colic* is a misnomer because the pain is steady and does not fluctuate in intensity. It is usually epigastric and is often referred to the right shoulder or interscapular region. During attacks, patients are restless and may have associated diaphoresis and vomiting. The interval between attacks is highly variable and may be days to years. There is no convincing evidence that ingesting fatty foods precipitates an attack of biliary colic.

Acute Cholecystitis

When a biliary colic attack lasts >3 hours or if localized right upper quadrant tenderness and fever develop, the diagnosis of acute cholecystitis should be entertained. The pain of acute cholecystitis may wane but the tenderness usually increases. Murphy's sign, the abrupt cessation in inspiration in response to pain on palpation of the right upper quadrant, is a classic finding observed in 60% to 70% of patients. High fever, hemodynamic instability, and peritoneal signs suggest gallbladder perforation, which is a complication in 10% of patients with acute cholecystitis. Ten percent to 15% of patients develop jaundice, which is a symptom that may be caused by gallstone obstruction of the common bile duct, or by Mirizzi's syndrome, which is an obstruction of the common hepatic duct caused by edema and inflammation at the origin of the cystic duct.

Acalculous Cholecystitis

In 5% to 10% of patients with acute cholecystitis, there is no evidence of cholelithiasis. Acalculous cholecystitis occurs in critically ill patients, often in the setting of multiorgan failure, extensive burn injuries, major surgery, and trauma. Perforation is more common and the course is more fulminant.

Findings on Diagnostic Testing

Laboratory Studies

Most patients with acute cholecystitis exhibit leukocytosis with a left shift. Some patients may have elevations in aminotransferases, alkaline phosphatase, bilirubin, or amylase caused by choledocholithiasis or cystic duct edema with resulting biliary obstruction. Patients with uncomplicated biliary colic usually have normal biochemical profiles.

Structural Studies

Ultrasound is highly sensitive and specific for the diagnosis of cholelithiasis. In uncomplicated biliary colic, gallstones may be the only finding. Thickening of the gallbladder wall is a nonspecific finding commonly observed in acute and chronic cholecystitis. Pericholecystic fluid and intramural gas are specific ultrasonographic features of acute cholecystitis. Dilation of the intrahepatic or extrahepatic ducts suggests choledocholithiasis; however, ultrasound is insensitive for the imaging of common bile duct stones. ^{99m}Tc-labeled iminodiacetic scintigraphy can confirm a diagnosis of acute cholecystitis. The tracer is injected intravenously and excreted in bile. Failure to image the gallbladder within 90 minutes suggests cystic duct obstruction. The gallbladder cannot be visualized in 85% of patients with acalculous cholecystitis. Endoscopic retrograde cholangiopancreatography (ERCP) is the procedure of choice for evaluating patients with suspected choledocholithiasis. It also provides therapeutic potential through endoscopic sphincterotomy and bile duct stone extraction.

Management and Course

Most patients with gallstones remain asymptomatic, but over a 20-year period, 15% to 20% of these asymptomatic patients develop symptoms. Once symptoms occur, there is a high risk of recurrent attacks of pain and complications such as cholecystitis, pancreatitis, and cholangitis.

Although there are many nonsurgical alternatives, cholecystectomy is the definitive treatment for symptomatic cholelithiasis. Laparoscopic cholecystectomy is favored because there are fewer wound-related complications, shorter hospital stays, and more rapid recoveries. The technique results in a 2% to 3% incidence of bile duct injuries, however, a higher incidence than with open cholecystectomy. Open cholecystectomy is preferred if acute cholecystitis is evident, if extensive scarring from prior abdominal surgery exists, if exploration of the common bile duct is planned, or if visualization at laparoscopy is inadequate.

Given the overall benefits of surgical therapy, dissolution therapy with chenodeoxycholic acid or ursodeoxycholic acid should be reserved for patients who are at high risk for surgery. Because of its superior side-effect profile, ursodeoxycholic acid is the preferred agent. Small (<1.5 cm in diameter) noncalcified stones that float on oral cholecystography are suitable for dissolution. Candidate patients should demonstrate adequate gallbladder filling and emptying on oral cholecystography. Dissolution often requires >6 months of therapy. Response rates range from 60% to 70%. There are frequent recurrences after therapy is discontinued. Direct contact dissolution therapy with mono-octanoin and methyl tertbutyl ether is often successful in days to weeks, but it is associated with a high rate of complications and thus remains experimental.

Extracorporeal shock wave lithotripsy is 90% successful in achieving stone fragmentation and clearance of solitary, small, radiolucent stones. Most patients also require dissolution therapy. Similar to dissolution therapy, it may take months of extracorporeal shock wave lithotripsy to clear the gallbladder of stones. Approximately 20% of patients experience biliary colic for several weeks after fragmentation.

CHOLEDOCHOLITHIASIS

Incidence and Epidemiology

In the United States, most bile duct stones are cholesterol stones that have migrated from the gallbladder. Ten percent to 15% of patients undergoing cholecystectomy have concomitant bile duct stones, and 1% to 4% exhibit residual postoperative choledocholithiasis, even after exploration of the common bile duct. Conversely, more than 80% to 90% of patients with choledocholithiasis have gallbladder stones. The incidence of choledocholithiasis increases with age; one-third of octogenarians undergoing cholecystectomy have coexistent bile duct stones. The prevalence of choledocholithiasis and intrahepatic stones is higher in Asian societies. These populations have higher incidences of pigment stones, which usually are formed de novo in the bile ducts.

Etiology and Pathogenesis

Although most bile duct stones originate in the gallbladder, some stones (especially brown pigment stones) form de novo in the bile ducts. The major component of these stones is calcium bilirubinate. Any process that increases the concentration of unconjugated bilirubin in bile or increases bile stasis will foster intraductal brown stone formation. Bacterial β-glucuronidase probably plays a major role in deconjugating bilirubin, as most common bile duct stones are culture positive. A diet low in fat and protein may also promote bile duct stone formation; the factors involved are increased deconjugation of excreted bilirubin and sphincter of Oddi (SO) hypertension with associated bile stasis. Other potential risk factors include periampullary diverticula, ampullary stenosis, and foreign material in the bile ducts.

Clinical Features

Unlike with gallbladder stones, most patients with bile duct stones develop symptoms. Some remain asymptomatic for decades, and others present suddenly with potentially life-threatening cholangitis or pancreatitis. Patients with choledocholithiasis often present with biliary colic indistinguishable from the pain of cystic duct obstruction. The pain is steady, lasts for 30 minutes to several hours, and is located in the epigastrium and right upper quadrant.

Cholangitis is the result of superimposed infection in the setting of a biliary obstruction. Charcot's classic triad of right upper quadrant pain, fever, and jaundice may be present only in 50% to 75% of patients with acute cholangitis. Ten percent of episodes are marked by a fulminant course with hemodynamic instability and encephalopathy. *Reynold's pentad* refers to the constellation of Charcot's triad plus hypotension and confusion.

Findings on Diagnostic Testing

Laboratory Studies

Immediately after an attack, levels of serum aminotransferases often are elevated as a result of hepatocellular injury. Alkaline phosphatase levels are often elevated, mildly in asymptomatic patients, and not more than five times higher than normal in symptomatic patients. Most symptomatic patients have hyperbilirubinemia, the bilirubin level being in the range of 2 to 14 mg per dl. Higher elevations in alkaline phosphatase or bilirubin levels suggest malignant obstruction of the biliary tree.

Structural Studies

In contrast to gallbladder stones, bile duct stones are not readily detected by ultrasound; the sensitivity is <20%. A computed tomographic (CT) scan is more sensitive, but it may only detect 50% of common bile duct stones. The technological advances of helical CT scanning may improve this accuracy. ERCP has a sensitivity of 90% for the diagnosis of choledocholithiasis and has the advantage of facilitating therapeutic sphincterotomy and stone extraction. Endoscopic ultrasound can detect 95% of common bile duct stones, but current instruments cannot be used to perform stone extraction.

There is no consensus on the optimal evaluation for choledocholithiasis in patients undergoing elective cholecystectomy for gallstone disease. If open cholecystectomy is planned, intraoperative cholangiography and common bile duct palpation can be used. If stones are found, common bile duct exploration and stone extraction should be performed. Several alternative strategies are available to patients undergoing planned laparoscopic cholecystectomy. One strategy involves minimal preoperative assessment, including ultrasound and CT scanning. An intraoperative cholangiogram is performed during the laparoscopic procedure. Those patients with documented intraductal stones undergo stone extraction laparoscopically or by open cholecystectomy. Alternatively, ERCP with endoscopic sphincterotomy could be performed postoperatively. A second strategy identifies patients preoperatively as being at high or low risk for coexisting choledocholithiasis on the basis of biochemical profile and the presence or absence of biliary tract dilation on ultrasound. Patients at high risk undergo preoperative endoscopic ultrasonography or ERCP; those with confirmed biliary stones undergo endoscopic stone extraction. When the stones are cleared from the bile duct, the patient then proceeds to laparoscopic cholecystectomy. Patients with a low risk of choledocholithiasis undergo laparoscopic cholecystectomy with intraoperative cholangiography as previously described. There are benefits and risks associated with each strategy; the approach is largely determined by the resources available at individual institutions.

Management and Course

Common bile duct stones, even if asymptomatic, require therapy because of the high complication rate (e.g., cholangitis and pancreatitis). Secondary biliary cirrhosis may develop in cases of persistent biliary obstruction. Definitive therapy involves common bile duct exploration and stone extraction, but this procedure increases the operative mortality rate of a cholecystectomy from 0.5% to 3% to 4%. The perioperative mortality rate for patients younger than 60 years of age is 1.5%, whereas the risk for patients older than 65 years is 5% to 10%. On the basis of this high mortality rate, endoscopic sphincterotomy and stone extraction is a favorable approach, especially in older patients. The risk of recurrent symptoms is high if patients have an intact gallbladder; therefore, cholecystectomy should be performed. In elderly patients with severe comorbid illness, however, the surgical risks may outweigh the risk of recurrent gallstone symptoms. Endoscopic sphincterotomy alone is an acceptable therapy for these patients. If bile duct stones cannot be extracted endoscopically, long-term internal stenting is also a therapeutic option for this high-risk group. Young, healthy patients who have minimal operative risk factors may be treated with primary cholecystectomy and common bile duct exploration with stone extraction. The choice of endoscopic versus surgical removal of bile duct stones in this group may be determined by local expertise and resources. It is worth noting that even after surgical common bile duct exploration, 1% to 4% of patients have retained common bile duct stones.

Patients presenting with cholangitis or pancreatitis are treated initially with conservative measures, including parenteral fluid repletion, bowel rest, and parenteral antibiotics (for cholangitis). In patients with severe pancreatitis that progresses or fails to improve within 48 hours and in patients with severe cholangitis, emergency ERCP with possible stone extraction has been shown to reduce morbidity and mortality. Patients who do not pass their stones on ERCP or who have superimposed cholecystitis require emergency surgical intervention.

POSTCHOLECYSTECTOMY SYNDROME

Incidence and Epidemiology

After cholecystectomy, 20% to 40% of patients experience abdominal discomfort, and 2% to 10% have debilitating pain. Patients who do not have gallstones confirmed on surgical pathologic examination are more likely to remain symptomatic after cholecystectomy. Most of these patients have functional abdominal pain, but a small percentage of patients with the postcholecystectomy syndrome have symptoms originating from the biliary tract. Possible causes include retained common bile duct stones, postoperative bile duct strictures, biliary tumors, and SO dysfunction. SO dysfunction is primarily a disease of women who have undergone prior cholecystectomy. The disorder is uncommon and accounts for only 5% to 10% of patients presenting with postcholecystectomy pain. SO dysfunction is also the putative cause in 10% to 20% of patients with idiopathic pancreatitis.

Etiology and Pathogenesis

The basic mechanism by which SO dysfunction produces symptoms involves impedance to bile flow at the level of the SO. This can result from an anatomic narrowing, termed *papillary stenosis*, or abnormal motility, termed *sphincter of Oddi dyskinesia*. Stenosis may result from fibrosis or muscle hypertrophy secondary to prior choledocholithiasis. The cause of dyskinesia remains undefined but probably involves dysregulation of neurohormonal influences on the sphincter.

Clinical Features

Patients with SO dysfunction may manifest idiopathic pancreatitis or recurrent abdominal pain after cholecystectomy. The pain is similar to biliary colic; it is localized to the epigastrium and right upper quadrant and often radiates to the scapula.

Findings on Diagnostic Testing

Given the confounding possibility that either small gallbladder stones or sludge is the cause of symptoms, SO dysfunction can be reliably diagnosed only in patients who have undergone prior cholecystectomy. Liver chemistry profiles are obtained during an attack of pain and ultrasound is performed to exclude biliary dilation. ERCP is necessary to exclude alternative diagnoses, such as retained common bile duct stones or postoperative biliary strictures. ERCP can also assess the drainage capability of the biliary tree. The results of laboratory testing, ultrasound, and ERCP can be used to classify patients into groups with distinct probabilities of the presence of physiologic SO dysfunction. Type I describes patients with biliary pain, liver chemistry values elevated to at least twice normal on two occasions, a dilated common bile duct, and delayed contrast drainage from the common bile duct during ERCP. Type II is defined by biliary pain with one or two of the above criteria, and type III includes patients with biliary-type pain but none of the other features described. The incidence of manometrically confirmed SO dysfunction is nearly 100% in type I, 50% in type II, and 25% in type III patients.

If ERCP demonstrates biliary dilation and delayed common bile duct contrast drainage (>45 minutes) in a patient with liver chemistry abnormalities during two previous episodes of pain, a presumptive diagnosis of SO dysfunction can be made and the patient can be treated at the time of ERCP with endoscopic sphincterotomy. Papillary stenosis rather than sphincter dyskinesia is the mechanism of dysfunction in most type I patients. SO manometry is indicated to confirm high sphincter pressures in type II and type III patients. It is performed by passing a three-channel, water-perfused catheter into the common bile duct through a duodenoscope. The catheter is slowly withdrawn across the sphincter as basal and phasic pressures are recorded. Although many manometric abnormalities have been observed in patients with SO dysfunction, an elevated basal sphincter pressure (>40 mm Hg) is the only criterion that predicts a therapeutic response to endoscopic sphincterotomy. A basal pressure of >40 mm Hg is essential, therefore, to making the diagnosis of SO dysfunction in type II and type III patients.

Management and Course

Pharmacologic therapy for SO dysfunction has been disappointing, mostly because of its inefficacy in treating the papillary stenosis variant of the abnormality and the high incidence of side effects. The mainstay of therapy is disruption of the sphincter mechanism. Surgical sphincterotomy has a high success rate, but this approach has been supplanted by endoscopic sphincterotomy, which has become the standard therapy for SO dysfunction. Sphincterotomy alleviates abdominal pain in 90% of patients with manometrically confirmed SO dysfunction. Although results of longer follow-up periods are required, 5% of patients develop restenosis.

Endoscopic sphincterotomy carries a significant complication rate, especially for patients with SO dysfunction. The incidence of post-ERCP pancreatitis in these patients is 10% to 20%. The incidence is higher in patients without common bile duct dilation. Hemorrhage and perforation are less common complications.

MISCELLANEOUS COMPLICATIONS OF BILIARY TRACT STONES

Bile Duct Strictures

Trauma and the chronic inflammatory response induced by biliary stones can result in benign strictures of the extrahepatic bile ducts. Other common causes of benign strictures include surgical trauma, chronic pancreatitis, parasitic infection, and sclerosing cholangitis. Patients may present with cholangitis, painless jaundice, or asymptomatic elevations of alkaline phosphatase levels. Diagnosis requires direct bile duct visualization by ERCP or percutaneous transhepatic cholangiography. Given the inadequate long-term efficacy of biliary stenting, surgical decompression is the treatment of choice for benign strictures. Failure to relieve the obstruction predisposes the patient to cholangitis, stone formation, and secondary biliary cirrhosis.

Biliary Fistula

The most common cause of biliary fistula formation is surgical trauma. Most spontaneous biliary-enteric fistulae are produced by gallstones; alternative causes include malignancy, peptic ulcer disease, and penetrating trauma. Patients with gallstone-induced fistulae can be asymptomatic or they may present with nonspecific symptoms of anorexia, weight loss, and malabsorption. Gallstone ileus results when a large gallstone (>3 cm) passes into the gut through a cholecystenteric fistula and produces lumenal obstruction in the distal ileum. Biliary fistulae can often be detected on abdominal radiographs or upper gastrointestinal barium radiographs as air or barium in the biliary tree. Treatment requires surgical excision of the fistula, cholecystectomy, and extraction of all bile duct stones.

Hematobilia

Hemorrhage from the biliary tract is a rare complication of gallstones. The more common causes are penetrating trauma or iatrogenic trauma from a liver biopsy. In the United States, hepatobiliary tumors and aneurysms are possible causes, whereas parasitic diseases are possible causes in Asian societies. Diagnosis requires upper gastrointestinal endoscopy to exclude other sources of upper gastrointestinal hemorrhage. Angiography can confirm the site of bleeding. Angiographic embolization is the preferred initial treatment of hepatic causes of hematobilia. Surgical intervention is preferred to treat hemorrhage originating from the extrahepatic biliary tree.

Oriental Cholangiohepatitis

In selected regions of Southeast Asia, the most common presentation of gallstone disease is a syndrome characterized by intrahepatic bile duct stones, ductal dilation and stricturing, and recurrent cholangitis known as oriental cholangiohepatitis. It occurs primarily in patients older than 50 years of age and is associated with malnutrition and low socioeconomic status. There are inconsistent associations with infections caused by *Clonorchis sinensis* and *Ascaris lumbricoides,* but the pathogenetic role of these parasites remains unclear.

The stones in this disease are pigmented calcium bilirubinate stones that preferentially involve the left intrahepatic ducts. Patients typically present with relapsing cholangitis and hepatic abscesses. Ultrasound is of limited value because echogenic material often fills the intrahepatic ducts. The diagnosis relies on cholangiography. The primary treatment is surgical and often requires hepatic resection and extensive biliary reconstruction to relieve any obstruction and clear the ductal system of stones. Most patients require reoperation, although long-term prophylactic antibiotics may reduce the frequency of infectious complications.

CHAPTER 61

Cholestatic Syndromes

Cholestasis is defined as a defect in bile excretion. It can be classified as intrahepatic or extrahepatic based on the anatomic site of the disturbance. Extrahepatic cholestasis is caused by a structural impairment in bile secretion and flow in the large bile ducts and is primarily caused by disease processes reviewed in Chapters 59 and 60. Intrahepatic cholestasis is caused by a functional defect in bile formation at the level of the hepatocyte and terminal bile ducts. This chapter reviews the common causes of intrahepatic cholestasis (Table 61-1).

PRIMARY BILIARY CIRRHOSIS

Incidence and Epidemiology

Primary biliary cirrhosis (PBC) is a chronic, progressive, cholestatic disease that mainly affects women in their sixth and seventh decades of life. Patients may present as early as 30 years of age or as late as 90 years of age. PBC has been observed in all races, but appears to be more common among whites. Worldwide, PBC accounts for 0.6% to 2.0% of the deaths from cirrhosis. Epidemiologic surveys have failed to identify specific environmental risk factors, but developed regions have higher incidences than undeveloped regions. It is not known whether this represents a true difference in disease incidence or a detection bias resulting from health screening.

Etiology and Pathogenesis

Although several disease associations and well-characterized disturbances in immune regulation suggest that PBC is an immune-mediated disease, the etiology remains unknown. Associated immunologic abnormalities include the presence of antimitochondrial autoantibodies, IgM hypergammaglobulinemia, circulating immune complexes, and decreases in the number and function of suppressor T-lymphocytes. Other autoimmune diseases associated with PBC include Sjögren's syndrome, scleroderma, autoimmune thyroiditis, and, possibly, rheumatoid arthritis. PBC has also been linked to the HLA-DRw8 antigen, suggesting that there may be a genetic component to the disease.

Liver injury results from nonsuppurative destruction of small bile ducts in the lobule. The obstruction of bile flow leads to cholestasis and toxic hepato-

TABLE 61-1
Differential Diagnosis of Intrahepatic Cholestasis

Primary biliary cirrhosis
Sclerosing cholangitis
Hepatocellular disease
    Viral hepatitis
    Alcoholic hepatitis
    Medications
Intrahepatic cholestasis of pregnancy
Systemic infection
Total parenteral nutrition–associated cholestasis
Postoperative cholestasis

cyte injury as a result of accumulation of bile acids and copper. The disease evolves through four histologically described stages. In stage I, the portal tracts are expanded by chronic inflammatory cells and noncaseating granulomas adjacent to the damaged bile ducts. Stage II is characterized by expansion of the inflammatory infiltrate into the hepatic parenchyma and proliferation of the bile ducts. In stage III, interlobular fibrous septa are present. Stage IV represents cirrhosis.

Clinical Features

Forty percent to 50% of patients diagnosed with PBC are asymptomatic at the time of presentation. The disease is detected in the majority of these patients on the basis of an elevated serum alkaline phosphatase level. The remaining 50% to 60% present with pruritus and fatigue, whereas 25% have jaundice. The pruritus may be relentless and profound, prompting the patient to seek advice from a dermatologist before it is recognized as a complication of cholestasis. The skin may become excoriated and hyperpigmented as a result of incessant scratching. Other physical findings include hepatomegaly, splenomegaly, palmar erythema, spider angiomata, and xanthelasma. The last finding correlates with the hyperlipidemia observed in PBC. The defect in bile acid secretion leads to impaired fat digestion with resultant steatorrhea, weight loss, and fat-soluble vitamin deficiencies. Long-standing cholestasis can also result in bone resorption and osteoporosis, which frequently lead to vertebral compression fractures and long bone fractures. A rare patient may have hepatic failure or a complication of portal hypertension (e.g., variceal bleeding) as the initial manifestation of PBC.

Most patients with PBC have associated autoimmune diseases. Sjögren's syndrome and scleroderma are the most common disorders, but the diseases are usually mild and survival is dictated by the severity of hepatic dysfunction. Autoimmune thyroiditis and hypothyroidism also are often seen in PBC patients and may predate the diagnosis of liver disease. Other diseases associated with PBC include rheumatoid arthritis, psoriatic arthritis, Raynaud's phenomenon, and distal renal tubular acidosis. Although the evidence is inconclusive, there may be a higher incidence of breast cancer in patients with PBC.

Findings on Diagnostic Testing

Laboratory Studies

All patients with PBC have elevated serum alkaline phosphatase levels. Similar elevations in levels of 5'-nucleotidase, α-glutamyl transpeptidase, and leucine aminopeptidase help confirm the hepatic origin of the elevated alkaline phosphatase level. Serum bilirubin levels usually are normal at the time of diagnosis. But, as the disease progresses, >50% of patients develop hyperbilirubinemia, which is a poor prognostic indicator. As with other cholestatic syndromes, levels of aminotransferases usually are only slightly elevated. Other nonspecific surrogate markers of cholestasis are increased, including serum bile acids, cholesterol, and triglycerides.

Serologic Testing

The immunologic abnormalities observed in PBC provide useful diagnostic information. Antimitochondrial antibodies (AMAs) are present in 95% of PBC patients. Although other autoantibodies are present in a large number of cholestatic syndromes, elevated titers of AMAs are relatively specific for PBC. Similarly, the finding of IgM hypergammaglobulinemia on serum protein electrophoresis has a high predictive value for PBC. Other serologic abnormalities include increased titers of antinuclear antibodies, anti–smooth muscle antibodies, antithyroid antibodies, and rheumatoid factor, but these findings are not specific to PBC and are of limited diagnostic value.

Liver Biopsy

Confirmation of PBC requires percutaneous liver biopsy. The pathognomonic lesion is characterized by patchy destruction of interlobular bile ducts with a mononuclear inflammatory infiltrate. Granulomas may be present in some portal tracts, but their presence is not required to confirm a diagnosis of PBC. The severity of histologic damage can be classified into stages I to IV.

Structural Studies

Several imaging procedures may be used to evaluate PBC. These procedures are used primarily to exclude extrahepatic causes of cholestasis. Ultrasound generally demonstrates normal-sized bile ducts. Gallstones are revealed in >30% of cases. Computed tomographic scanning also helps to exclude bile duct dilation and may demonstrate portosystemic collaterals suggestive of portal hypertension. In patients lacking the serologic markers of PBC, endoscopic retrograde cholangiopancreatography (ERCP) may be necessary. Although the terminal intrahepatic ducts may be irregular, the larger ducts appear to be normal in size and contour on ERCP.

Management and Course

PBC is an invariably progressive disease, but the rate of progression varies. One-half of the patients with PBC are asymptomatic on presentation, but most become symptomatic within 2 to 4 years. As the disease progresses from the asymptomatic to symptomatic stages, the serum alkaline phosphatase and α-globulin levels often dramatically increase and subsequently reach a plateau. Once symptoms appear, there is an indolent worsening of fatigue and pruritus, usually over the course of years. Patients eventually develop muscle wasting, progressive jaundice, and hepatic dysfunction. The final stage of PBC is marked by complications of portal hypertension, including ascites, variceal hemorrhage, and encephalopathy.

The chronic inflammatory response and immune dysfunction observed in PBC have prompted clinical trials of several immunosuppressive regimens. Corticosteroids fail to alter the biochemical, histologic, and clinical progression observed in PBC. Azathioprine, cyclosporine, colchicine, and D-penicillamine may result in biochemical improvements, but none of these agents has been shown to alter disease progression or survival. Early trials of methotrexate are promising, demonstrating improvement in biochemical and histologic abnormalities. Given the high incidence of treatment-associated toxicity, however, no immunosuppressive regimen can be recommended until there is evidence of improved symptoms and survival.

The secondary bile acid ursodeoxycholic acid represents a unique approach to the treatment of PBC. Ursodeoxycholic acid may serve to stabilize hepatocyte membranes and decrease the production of more toxic bile acids. Several reports describe a decrease in the severity of pruritus in 50% of cases. Most patients experience biochemical improvement, but effects on histologic improvement have been inconsistent in short-term trials. Long-term studies of ursodeoxycholic acid treatment have demonstrated improved survival and delay in time to transplantation.

The control of pruritus is the goal of symptomatic treatment of PBC. Oral antihistamines are rarely of benefit in cholestasis-associated pruritus. Cholestyramine administered in doses of 4 g before each meal is effective but often causes profound constipation and bloating. This ionic resin binds intralumenal bile acids and other pruritogens, thus preventing the absorption of these substances. Cholestyramine and other ion resins also interfere with the absorption of medications such as digoxin, thyroxine, and penicillins. Steatorrhea and fat-soluble vitamin deficiencies can be exacerbated. Patients intolerant of cholestyramine may respond to phenobarbital or rifampicin. Refractory pruritus may respond to plasmapheresis or therapy with ultraviolet B light.

Survival of patients with PBC depends largely on the clinical and histologic stage of disease. Patients with asymptomatic PBC have a median survival time of 10 years, which is shorter than for age-matched controls. Survival time for symptomatic patients is shorter than for asymptomatic patients. Several models have attempted to predict survival on the basis of clinical variables. The most powerful predictor is the serum bilirubin level. Patients with bilirubin levels higher than 10 mg per dl usually survive <2 years.

Prediction of survival is critical in enabling the clinician to select optimal candidates for liver transplantation. Transplantation should be considered for patients with complications of portal hypertension, severe symptomatic osteodystrophy, or a predicted survival of <2 years. In properly selected candidates, liver transplantation is highly successful in treating PBC; the 2-year survival rate is >80%.

HEPATOCELLULAR DISEASES

Several liver diseases that characteristically produce hepatocellular injury and a disproportionate increase in levels of aminotransferases may demonstrate biochemical and clinical features more consistent with cholestasis. Alcoholic hepatitis may produce profound increases in levels of serum bilirubin and alkaline phosphatase with normal to minimally elevated levels of aminotransferases, a pattern that often correlates with severe hepatocellular injury. Patients with alcoholic hepatitis often have a very poor prognosis. Atypical variants of acute viral hepatitis A, B, and E are characterized by a syndrome of prolonged cholestasis. Although patients with hepatitis C typically manifest acute hepatitis, liver allograft recipients with recurrent infection with hepatitis C virus may develop pericholangitis and cholestasis.

INTRAHEPATIC CHOLESTASIS OF PREGNANCY

Pregnancy may be associated with abnormal liver chemistry values attributable to numerous physiologic alterations and disease processes. Perhaps the most common finding is a mild increase in the serum alkaline phosphatase levels as a result of placental release of this enzyme. Women may also have coincident liver diseases unrelated to their pregnancy—for example, alcohol-, viral-, and immune-mediated liver diseases. The impact of pregnancy on the natural history of these disorders remains unclear. Pregnancy may be complicated by several disorders unique to pregnancy, for example, pre-eclampsia–associated liver injury and the rare but devastating syndrome of acute fatty liver of pregnancy. These two disorders may exhibit cholestasis and are often accompanied by systemic complications such as disseminated intravascular coagulation, renal failure, and hepatic failure. Acute fatty liver and pre-eclampsia–related liver injury require prompt termination of the pregnancy. Unless diagnosed early, they are associated with high maternal mortality rates.

The most common liver disease unique to pregnancy is intrahepatic cholestasis of pregnancy. It accounts for 30% to 50% of all causes of jaundice in pregnancy. It is distinguished from the other disorders by its benign course. The syndrome is similar to the cholestasis associated with estrogen supplements. Moreover, women with a prior history of intrahepatic cholestasis of pregnancy often manifest cholestasis when challenged with oral contraceptives in the nonpregnant state. The etiology remains unknown, but familial clusterings suggest the presence of a genetically acquired sensitivity to the cholestatic effects of estrogens. Patients usually present with pruritus and mild jaundice in the third trimester. Liver chemistry values demonstrate a cholestatic pattern. A biopsy specimen from the liver reveals bland cholestasis with no inflammatory reaction. A biopsy is occasionally needed to differentiate the syndrome from acute fatty liver of pregnancy or other more morbid disorders. Supportive treatment with cholestyramine or phenobarbital can be initiated to relieve pruritus; cholestasis resolves with delivery.

SYSTEMIC INFECTION

Systemic gram-negative bacterial infections are often accompanied by cholestasis. Endotoxemia decreases bile flow and may result in conjugated hyperbilirubinemia, with bilirubin levels in the range of 5 to 10 mg per dl. Levels of aminotransferases are usually near normal, and the alkaline phosphatase level is variably elevated. Clinical manifestations are dominated by the underlying infection. Cholestasis improves with successful treatment of the responsible micro-organisms.

CHOLESTASIS ASSOCIATED WITH
TOTAL PARENTERAL NUTRITION

Patients receiving long-term total parenteral nutrition (TPN) may manifest any of several distinct patterns of hepatic dysfunction, including cholestasis. TPN-induced intrahepatic cholestasis is common in newborn premature infants. The mechanism is undefined but probably results from alterations in serum bile acid pools caused by changes in intestinal bacteria. Patients receiving TPN are often subjected to bowel rest; the resulting bile stasis promotes biliary sludge and stone formation. Therefore, extrahepatic cholestasis also should be considered in the evaluation of patients on long-term TPN.

POSTOPERATIVE CHOLESTASIS

The postoperative state may be complicated by jaundice caused by cholestasis and impaired bile formation or alterations in the production or excretion of bilirubin. Increased bilirubin production, which may exceed the excretory capacity of the liver, can be caused by several factors in a patient undergoing surgery. Hemolysis caused by systemic infections, transfusion reactions, mechanical trauma caused by artificial valves or circulatory bypass, or pre-existing red blood cell defects and hemoglobinopathies all increase the production of bilirubin. Similarly, massive transfusions and resorption of large hematomas may overwhelm the ability of the liver to excrete bilirubin. Increased bilirubin loads lead to a predominantly unconjugated hyperbilirubinemia. Patients with Gilbert's syndrome, the common autosomal dominant defect of bilirubin conjugation, often develop unconjugated hyperbilirubinemia as a result of physiologic stress and fasting in the perioperative period.

Hepatocellular injury also may cause jaundice in postoperative patients. Hypoxia and hypotension in the perioperative period can produce ischemic hepatitis. Similarly, viral hepatitis acquired from transfusions may result in jaundice weeks after an operation. Drug-induced hepatotoxicity, especially from anesthetic agents, can cause jaundice. All of these insults usually produce a marked increase in levels of aminotransferases in addition to hyperbilirubinemia.

Cholestasis in the postoperative state can be extrahepatic or intrahepatic in origin. Patients undergoing biliary surgery are prone to extrahepatic cholestasis if there are retained bile duct stones and bile duct injuries. Systemic infection, medications, and TPN all can produce intrahepatic cholestasis. When all other causes of postoperative jaundice and cholestasis have been excluded, the probable diagnosis is benign postoperative intrahepatic cholestasis. This transient syndrome of unknown etiology usually causes conjugated hyperbilirubinemia and elevated serum alkaline phosphatase levels by the third postoperative day. It gradually resolves over 1 to 2 weeks.

CHAPTER 62

Drug-Induced Hepatic Injury

INCIDENCE AND EPIDEMIOLOGY

Among the many adverse effects of medications, hepatobiliary toxicity is one of the most common, accounting for 5% of all reported drug reactions. The clinical and biochemical patterns of injury can mimic any acute or chronic liver disease (Table 62-1). Medications that predictably produce hepatic injury in a dose-dependent manner are termed *intrinsic hepatotoxins*. Although the exact mechanism of hepatic injury remains poorly defined, intrinsic hepatotoxins and their metabolites generally injure hepatocytes by direct structural and functional alterations of vital subcellular elements. Intrinsic hepatotoxins often produce a zonal pattern of injury, which is the result of metabolic production or accumulation in a particular region of the hepatic lobule. In contrast, idiosyncratic hepatotoxins unpredictably produce hepatic injury in a small percentage of susceptible individuals. These agents often cause immune-mediated injury through a hypersensitivity response. Therefore, the onset of idiosyncratic hepatotoxicity typically is delayed several weeks and may be accompanied by a fever, rash, eosinophilia, and hepatic granulomas.

ETIOLOGY AND PATHOGENESIS

One of the principal physiologic functions of the liver is the biotransformation of lipophilic substances to polar compounds that are subsequently excreted in bile or urine. Several diverse and overlapping mechanisms have evolved to metabolize and dispose of the ubiquitous xenobiotic and endobiotic chemicals circulating in the human body. The handling of these substances requires transcellular transport as well as biotransformation. The enzymes that catalyze the biotransformation reactions are usually found in the endoplasmic reticulum and cytosol of hepatocytes. Many of the substrates for biotransformation are toxic, and in several instances, the products of biotransformation are even more toxic. Because the liver is often the primary site of exposure to these toxins, hepatic injury is a frequent consequence. An understanding of the basic

TABLE 62-1
Patterns of Drug-Induced Liver Disease

HISTOLOGIC FINDINGS	MEDICATIONS
Cholestasis	
Inflammatory	Chlorpromazine, erythromycin estolate, haloperidol, captopril, chlorpropamide, sulfonamides, ketoconazole
Bland	Estrogens, anabolic steroids
Zonal necrosis	
Centrilobular (zone III)	Acetaminophen, halothane, carbon tetrachloride
Mid-zonal (zone II)	Yellow phosphorus
Periportal (zone I)	Allyl alcohol
Hepatitis	
Nonspecific acute	Isoniazid, phenytoin, methyldopa, penicillin
Granulomatous	Quinidine, allopurinol, sulfonylureas
Chronic active	Isoniazid, methyldopa, nitrofurantoin, amiodarone, oxyphenisatin, sulfonamides, NSAIDs
Steatosis	
Microvesicular	Valproic acid, tetracycline, dideoxyinosine, tolmetin, piroxicam, salicylates
Macrovesicular	Amiodarone, methotrexate, corticosteroids
Steatohepatitis	Amiodarone, methotrexate
Fibrosis and cirrhosis	Methotrexate, vitamin A, vinyl chloride
Portal hypertension	
Budd-Chiari syndrome	Estrogens
Veno-occlusive disease	Mitomycin C, adriamycin, busulfan, 6-thioguanine, azathioprine
Hepatic tumors	
Adenoma	Estrogens, androgens
Hepatocellular carcinoma	Androgens, (?) estrogens
Angiosarcoma	Vinyl chloride, Thorotrast, anabolic steroids

mechanisms of biotransformation is essential to any discussion of drug-induced liver injury.

The biotransformation process is often divided into two phases. In phase 1, the compound undergoes a redox reaction to a more polar substance, usually using the cytochrome P-450 (CYP) superfamily of enzymes. The products are often volatile and may be extremely toxic, as in the case of acetaminophen metabolism. Phase 1 is often referred to as a *toxification*. Phase 2 reactions detoxify the metabolites by conjugation with glucuronic acid, glycine, sulfates, and glutathione. Patients with severe liver disease have impaired phase 1 capacity, but phase 2 activities usually are intact.

The CYP superfamily is a group of >30 different enzymes, mostly found in the endoplasmic reticulum. These enzymes have distinct substrate specificities, but there is often some overlap—that is, two CYPs can contribute to the metabolism of one xenobiotic. CYP3A4, CYP2D6, CYP2E1, and CYP1A1 are among the most important enzymes in the CYP superfamily. The activity of CYP enzymes varies tremendously between individuals. In addition, these enzymes are susceptible to induction and inhibition by numerous specific substrates. These are the primary mechanisms of drug interactions. For example, phenobarbital induces CYP3A4, leading to increased metabolism of cyclosporine. Alternatively, ketoconazole inhibits CYP3A4, leading to decreased clearance of cyclosporine and potentially severe systemic drug toxicity. This type of interaction can also increase the risk of drug-induced liver injury. For example, ethanol induces CYP2E1, which increases the conversion of acetaminophen to the toxic intermediate, NAPQI. Because of interindividual variations and the multitude of potential drug interactions, drugs metabolized by the CYP enzymes generally do not have a predictable pharmacodynamic profile.

Uridine diphosphate (UDP)-glucuronosyltransferases are a group of enzymes that catalyze the conjugation of glucuronide to many xenobiotics and endobiotics. As with the CYP enzymes, the substrate specificities of UDP-glucuronosyltransferase isoforms overlap, providing redundant pathways for xenobiotic elimination. The formation of glucuronides is important for the excretion of bilirubin, steroids, and many medications. Glucuronidation is primarily a means of detoxifying substances; however, the glucuronides of several compounds may produce hepatobiliary injury. For example, the glucuronide of estradiol is probably responsible for cholestasis caused by endogenous and exogenous estrogens. Conjugation with sulfate is an important mechanism in the biotransformation of several drugs to water-soluble compounds. Many of the substrates for UDP-glucuronosyltransferases are also substrates for sulfotransferases.

One of the most important defenses against hepatocellular toxicity is glutathione conjugation by glutathione S-transferases. Glutathione is a tripeptide of glutamine, glycine, and cysteine. Glutathione protects cellular enzymes and membranes from oxidative injury by volatile metabolites. The rate-limiting factor for glutathione synthesis is the intracellular concentration of cysteine. In acetaminophen toxicity, an increased concentration of the volatile intermediate NAPQI rapidly exhausts the supply of glutathione. Supplying cysteine, in the form of N-acetylcysteine, replenishes glutathione and prevents the accumulation of hepatotoxic levels of NAPQI. Conditions that deplete glutathione levels (e.g., fasting) increase susceptibility to toxicity from substances detoxified by glutathione S-transferase.

CLINICAL FEATURES, DIAGNOSIS, AND MANAGEMENT

Cholestasis

Several medications produce biochemical and clinical evidence of cholestasis through multiple structural alterations in hepatocellular membranes and functional alterations in the transport proteins responsible for bile formation (see Table 62-1). Although dozens of drugs have been associated with cholestasis, the most commonly incriminated drugs are estrogens, anabolic steroids, phenothiazines, and the estolate form of erythromycin. Estrogenic and androgenic steroids usually produce a bland cholestasis with minimal inflammation, which can be observed on a liver biopsy specimen. Phenothiazines, haloperidol, and erythromycin estolate can produce a cholangiodestructive cholestasis histologically similar to primary biliary cirrhosis. This inflammatory cholestasis is often accompanied by systemic signs and symptoms of hypersensitivity, including fever, rash, arthralgias, and eosinophilia.

Drug-induced cholestasis usually resolves with removal of the offending agent, but the chlorpromazine-induced syndrome that resembles primary biliary cirrhosis can persist for months to years and eventually lead to cirrhosis.

Hepatitis

The most common histologic pattern of drug injury is a nonspecific hepatitis. Hepatocellular necrosis is patchy and associated with a variable degree of mononuclear inflammation. Many drugs produce a more severe lesion that is indistinguishable from viral hepatitis. Common culprits include halothane, isoniazid, phenytoin, and methyldopa. In these acute reactions, the patient may develop fulminant or subfulminant hepatic failure. For unclear reasons, the prognosis for patients with drug-induced hepatic failure is generally worse than for patients with other causes of fulminant hepatic failure.

Some medications cause a granulomatous hepatitis. Hepatic injuries caused by quinidine, sulfonamides, and allopurinol often are accompanied by noncaseating granulomas. Prolonged use of isoniazid, methyldopa, oxyphenisatin, and nitrofurantoin can produce a form of chronic active hepatitis that is indistinguishable from chronic viral hepatitis or autoimmune hepatitis. The latter type of drug-induced injury may be associated with circulating autoantibodies. With the exception of fatal cases of fulminant hepatitis, cessation of the agent accountable for any variant of hepatitis always results in clinical and histologic improvement. Patients with chronic active hepatitis may progress to cirrhosis if the clinician does not recognize the iatrogenic nature of the illness and discontinue the responsible drug.

Steatosis and Steatohepatitis

Several drugs disturb the metabolism of fatty acids and triglycerides, leading to triglyceride accumulation in hepatocytes. There are two distinct patterns of bland steatosis. In macrovesicular steatosis, large globules of triglycerides fill the cytoplasm and displace the nucleus peripherally. In microvesicular steatosis, small fat globules are distributed uniformly throughout the cytoplasm and do not displace the nucleus. Microvesicular steatosis is most commonly associated with valproic acid and intravenous tetracycline. This histologic lesion is also seen in Reye's syndrome and fatty liver of pregnancy, and similar to the clinical course of these disorders, drug-induced microvesicular steatosis can cause marked elevations in aminotransferase levels, severe hepatic dysfunction, and, eventually, hepatic failure. Macrovesicular steatosis is characteristic of ethanol, corticosteroids, methotrexate, and amiodarone exposure. The injury associated with amiodarone exposure resembles alcoholic hepatitis; both are characterized by the presence of Mallory bodies and an inflammatory infiltrate. Characteristic lysosomal inclusions produced by amiodarone can be observed on electron microscopy, but their presence does not correlate with the magnitude of liver injury. If unrecognized, the steatohepatitis caused by amiodarone can evolve into cirrhosis.

Cirrhosis

Numerous drugs and toxins produce cirrhosis with minimal clinical evidence of antecedent injury. Although high-dose vitamin A, arsenics, and vinyl chloride can be associated with cirrhosis, methotrexate is the agent most often implicated as the cause of cirrhosis. The risk of methotrexate liver injury is poorly defined, but it appears to increase with daily dosing, obesity, ethanol use, and diabetes. Baseline and surveillance biopsies of the liver are often recommended, as liver chemistry values are often normal. Early methotrexate injury is characterized by steatosis with variable degrees of inflammation; drug withdrawal is not necessary. Significant steatohepatitis warrants continued biopsy surveillance. If the patient has fibrosis, bridging portal tracts, or established cirrhosis, methotrexate should be discontinued.

Hepatic Tumors

Estrogenic and androgenic steroids have been associated with the development of hepatic adenomas and, rarely, hepatocellular carcinomas. Adenomas can become quite large and may be complicated by hemorrhage and rupture. Cessation of estrogen contraceptives has been associated with regression. Large or hemorrhagic lesions may require surgical intervention. Although focal nodular hyperplasia has been reported to occur with oral contraceptive use, the validity of this association remains in question. The risk of hepatocellular carcinoma appears to be minimal; the majority of reports link the tumor to prolonged use of anabolic steroids. Highly malignant angiosarcomas have been associated with anabolic steroids, vinyl chloride, and the radiologic contrast agent Thorotrast.

Portal Hypertension

In addition to drug-induced cirrhosis, portal hypertension may develop secondary to Budd-Chiari syndrome, a disease associated with oral contraceptive use. Underlying myeloproliferative disorders have been noted in many patients with contraceptive-associated Budd-Chiari syndrome. Patients may present with an acute illness characterized by right upper quadrant pain, hepatomegaly, and sudden-onset ascites. Alternatively, portal hypertension may develop insidiously over a period of several months.

Patients receiving high-dose chemotherapy with mitomycin C, adriamycin, and 6-thioguanine may present with a clinical illness similar to Budd-Chiari syndrome called *veno-occlusive disease*. Histologically, veno-occlusive disease is characterized by necrosis and obliteration of the central veins. It is most often seen in the setting of bone marrow transplantation. Patients usually present in the first weeks to months after ablation chemotherapy and radiation therapy. Patients may have progressive portal hypertension, or they may return to normal. Azathioprine, a drug used in the management of renal transplantation, has also been associated with veno-occlusive disease.

Acetaminophen Hepatotoxicity

Acetaminophen is the most common cause of life-threatening hepatic injury. Inadvertent and suicidal ingestions of large doses predictably cause severe acute liver injury and account for up to 20% of liver transplantations performed for fulminant hepatic failure. At therapeutic doses, 90% of acetaminophen is conjugated with glucuronide or sulfate and subsequently excreted in urine. A small percentage of acetaminophen is oxidized by CYP2E1 to the toxic intermediate NAPQI. Under normal physiologic conditions, the highly volatile NAPQI is rapidly detoxified by conjugation with glutathione. Any condition that increases the formation of NAPQI or decreases the reserve of glutathione predisposes the patient to acetaminophen hepatotoxicity. The most common scenario is consumption of a supratherapeutic dose of acetaminophen, usually more than 10 to 15 g, which saturates the glucuronidation pathway and increases NAPQI formation. Alternatively, induction of CYP2E1 by chronic ethanol consumption may increase the proportion of acetaminophen metabolized to NAPQI, even at therapeutic doses. In either scenario, the increased NAPQI rapidly overwhelms the reserve of glutathione, and the subsequent accumulation of NAPQI produces hepatocellular injury. Chronic alcoholism and prolonged fasting also deplete glutathione stores, and the small amounts of NAPQI produced with therapeutic doses of acetaminophen cannot be completely detoxified. The residual NAPQI can cause significant hepatocellular injury. Because the centrilobular region is the site of highest CYP2E1 activity and lowest glutathione concentration, acetaminophen toxicity manifests as necrosis in this region.

Acetaminophen is a classic intrinsic hepatotoxin, and ingestion of high doses predictably produces hepatocellular injury. In the setting of a single ingestion of an excessive dose, a well-described nomogram, based on serum acetaminophen levels, accurately identifies persons likely to incur hepatotoxicity. The first several hours after overdose, patients may experience nausea and vomiting that rapidly resolves. Over the next 24 to 48 hours, patients may appear deceptively well, with normal aminotransferase levels, but biochemical evidence of acute hepatitis appears within 48 hours of ingestion. By the third to fifth day after ingestion, many patients develop symptoms of acute hepatitis: recurrent nausea, vomiting, jaundice, and abdominal pain. Serum aminotransferase levels usually peak in the thousands. Increase in the bilirubin level and prolongation of prothrombin time are proportional to the severity of injury. Severe cases may meet the criteria of fulminant hepatic failure, with progression to encephalopathy and other complications of hepatic failure.

All patients suspected of overdosing on acetaminophen should receive gastric lavage, especially if they present within several hours of the ingestion. A toxicology evaluation of serum and urine should be completed, as many patients overdose with multiple agents. Activated charcoal delivered orally or through a nasogastric tube serves to nonspecifically prevent further absorption of residual quantities of intralumenal acetaminophen as well as other medications ingested in an overdose. Charcoal therapy may need to be delayed several hours if acetaminophen is the sole medication ingested, because the only route of antidote administration is enteral.

Because acetaminophen toxicity results from depletion of hepatic glutathione and the subsequent accumulation of NAPQI, therapy has focused on repletion of glutathione stores. N-acetylcysteine delivered orally supplies the liver with a source of cysteine, which is the rate-limiting factor in glutathione synthesis. If given within 16 hours of acetaminophen ingestion, there is virtually no risk of developing hepatic failure. Several reports indicate that N-acetylcysteine may be beneficial even after the onset of hepatitis, although efficacy clearly declines the longer therapy is delayed.

The nomogram for acetaminophen toxicity predicts that any patient with postingestion serum acetaminophen levels of 150 mg per ml at 4 hours, 70 mg per ml at 8 hours, or 35 mg per ml at 12 hours may suffer severe hepatotoxicity. This nomogram is applicable to only one-time ingestions of large doses by healthy adults. Similarly, the temporal relationship of serum levels to actual ingestion time is often unreliable. Given these limitations and the benign nature of *N*-acetylcysteine therapy, any patient with suspected acute or chronic acetaminophen overdose should receive *N*-acetylcysteine therapy. Also given the increased susceptibility of alcoholics and fasting patients, any acute liver injury in these settings should prompt clinicians to consider therapy for acetaminophen toxicity.

Most patients with acute hepatic injury secondary to acetaminophen ingestion gradually improve with no long-term sequelae, but the progression to fulminant hepatic failure, which is heralded by the onset of encephalopathy, may be fatal. Any patient with this complication should be referred to a center specializing in liver transplantation. Patients should be monitored in a critical care setting for metabolic complications such as hypoglycemia, acidosis, and renal failure. Reversible causes of encephalopathy should be corrected, and intracranial pressure should be monitored in grade III or IV encephalopathy. Recovery is unlikely if patients have an arterial pH of <7.30 or if patients have grade III or IV encephalopathy associated with a prothrombin time international ratio of >6.5 and a serum creatinine level of >3.5 mg per dl. Patients with these poor prognostic indicators who are otherwise suitable for liver transplantation should be placed at the highest priority for transplantation. Post-transplant survival rates of 50% to 70% greatly exceed the chance of recovery in patients with these poor prognostic indicators.

CHAPTER 63

Hepatitis

Hepatitis is a nonspecific clinicopathologic term that encompasses all disorders characterized by hepatocellular injury accompanied by histologic evidence of a necroinflammatory response. Hepatitis is classified into acute hepatitis, which is defined as self-limited liver injury of <6 months' duration, and chronic hepatitis, in which the inflammatory response persists after 6 months. These two fundamental forms of hepatitis can be further subdivided on the basis of the underlying disease process or cause. Several diseases, such as drug-induced hepatitis and viral hepatitis B and C, may manifest as both acute and chronic hepatitis. Others, such as viral hepatitis A and E, are strictly acute in nature. Hemochromatosis invariably presents as chronic liver injury.

HEPATITIS A

Incidence and Epidemiology

Hepatitis A virus (HAV) causes 200,000 cases of acute hepatitis annually. It is transmitted primarily by fecal-oral routes. Epidemics can be traced to contaminated water or food. Rarely, HAV is acquired through parenteral exposure. Thirty percent of the population of the United States has serum IgG antibodies to HAV, suggesting prior exposure. In developing countries, essentially all children are exposed to the virus, which often produces subclinical illness in this age group. Risk factors for acquisition of HAV include male homosexuality, household contact with an infected person, travel to developing countries, contact with children in day care, and consumption of raw mollusks.

Etiology and Pathogenesis

HAV is an RNA virus that produces hepatocellular injury by mechanisms that remain poorly understood. Direct cytopathic or immunologically mediated injury seem probable, but neither has been proved. After exposure, there is a 2- to 6-week incubation period before symptom onset, although the virus may be detectable in the stool 1 week before clinically apparent illness. The immune response to HAV begins early and may contribute to hepatocellular injury. Immunologic clearance of HAV is the rule, and unlike the hepatitis viruses B and C, HAV never enters a chronic phase. By the time symptoms are manifest, patients invariably have IgM antibodies to HAV (anti-HAV IgM), which typically persist for 3 to 6 months. IgG antibodies to HAV (anti-HAV IgG) also develop, providing life-long immunity against reinfection.

Clinical Features

Many patients with HAV infection, especially young children, may be asymptomatic. Only 5% to 10% of patients with serologic evidence of prior HAV infection recall an episode of jaundice. As many as 80% to 90% of childhood HAV infections may be asymptomatic. Factors that contribute to subclinical versus clinical infection remain unclear.

The syndrome of acute hepatitis caused by HAV is clinically indistinguishable from other viral causes of acute hepatitis. Patients usually present with a non-specific prodrome of fatigue, anorexia, nausea, headache, myalgias, and arthralgias. This is followed by jaundice and right upper quadrant pain. Some patients may experience pruritus, but this rarely requires treatment. Vomiting is common and may become intractable, leading to fluid and electrolyte imbalance. Physical signs include icterus and tender hepatomegaly. The spleen is palpable in a minority of patients. Spider angiomata may be present in HAV hepatitis and in other forms of acute hepatitis. They are not specific to chronic liver disease.

Findings on Diagnostic Testing

Elevations in levels of aminotransferases usually occur 1 to 2 weeks before the onset of symptoms and persist for up to 4 to 6 weeks. The alanine aminotransferase (ALT) level usually is higher than the aspartate aminotransferase (AST) level; absolute values often exceed 1000 IU per liter. The level of enzyme elevation does not correlate with disease severity. Asymptomatic cases may have serum AST or ALT levels in the thousands. Serum bilirubin levels usually peak 1 to 2 weeks after symptoms appear, but they rarely exceed 15 to 20 mg per dl. HAV infection occasionally produces a cholestatic pattern of liver biochemical abnormalities, with a disproportionate elevation in the alkaline phosphatase level. Other laboratory abnormalities include a relative lymphocytosis with a normal total leukocyte count.

Diagnosis relies on the detection of anti-HAV IgM in the serum. Because this IgM component of the humoral immune response only lasts 3 to 6 months, its presence implies recent or ongoing infection. Liver biopsy is not necessary in the setting of positive findings on serologic testing and is performed only if the diagnosis is in doubt. Although there are no distinguishing features of any form of viral hepatitis, patchy necrosis and lobular lymphocytic infiltrates are typical findings.

Occasionally ultrasound or computed tomographic (CT) scanning may be necessary to exclude biliary obstruction, particularly in patients with the cholestatic variant of HAV. These tests may confirm hepatomegaly and reveal an inhomogeneous liver parenchyma, but findings usually are nonspecific.

Management and Course

HAV is self-limited, and symptoms resolve over the course of 2 to 4 weeks. There is no specific treatment, and patients should be encouraged to maintain fluid and nutritional intake. Ten percent of patients require hospitalization for intractable vomiting, worsening coagulopathy, or comorbid illnesses. The overall mortality rate for hospitalized patients is <1%. Deaths are mainly the result of the rare case of fulminant hepatitis, which is characterized by signs of hepatic failure, including encephalopathy. These patients should be referred to specialized centers for consideration of liver transplantation.

Infection with HAV can be prevented by either passive or active immunization. Patients exposed to feces of HAV-infected individuals should be given immune globulin (0.02 ml per kg) within 2 weeks of the exposure. Travelers to endemic areas may be given immune globulin, which lasts approximately 3 months, or the formalin-inactivated hepatitis A vaccine, which provides long-term immunity.

HEPATITIS B

Incidence and Epidemiology

Hepatitis B virus (HBV) is an important cause of acute and chronic hepatitis. In regions of Africa, Asia, and the Mediterranean basin where HBV is endemic, there are high rates of chronic HBV infection. Worldwide, there are 350 million HBV carriers. In the United States, HBV accounts for 250,000 cases of acute hepatitis annually, and 5% of these enter a chronic phase. Approximately 0.3% of the population in the United States suffers chronic infection with HBV.

Although 30% to 50% of infections with HBV have no identifiable source, the main route of transmission is parenteral. Before universal blood bank screening,

HBV accounted for 10% of transfusion-related hepatitis. Currently, the most common means of transmission are intravenous drug use, intimate or sexual contact, and vertical transmission from mother to child. Several epidemiologic surveys have emphasized the importance of contact transmission among individuals in the same household, even in the absence of intimate or sexual contact. The mechanism of this contact-associated transmission remains poorly defined.

Etiology and Pathogenesis

HBV is a DNA virus surrounded by an envelope that contains a protein called *hepatitis B surface antigen* (HBsAg). Inside the envelope is a nucleocapsid that contains the hepatitis B core antigen (HBcAg), which is not detectable in serum. During virus replication, a third antigen termed the *hepatitis B e antigen* (HBeAg) as well as HBV DNA and DNA polymerase are detectable in the serum. While in the replicative phase, HBV produces hepatocellular injury primarily by activating the cellular immune system in response to viral antigens on the surface of hepatocytes. Cytotoxic CD8+ lymphocytes recognize viral proteins in association with HLA class I markers and subsequently lyse the infected cell. The vigor of the immune response determines the severity of acute HBV hepatitis and the probability of the infection entering a chronic phase. An exuberant response can produce fulminant hepatic failure, whereas a lesser response may fail to clear the virus.

After exposure to HBV, there is an incubation period of several weeks to 6 months before the onset of symptoms. HBsAg appears in the serum, followed shortly by HBeAg late in the incubation period. Detectable levels of HBeAg correlate with active viral replication, as does the presence of HBV DNA and HBV DNA polymerase. The first detectable immune response is antibody to HBcAg (anti-HBc), which is usually present by the time symptoms occur. As with HAV, the initial antibody response is primarily IgM, which persists for 4 to 6 months and is superseded by a life-long IgG response. Antibodies to HBsAg (anti-HBs) develop in >90% of individuals with acute hepatitis. They usually appear several weeks after disappearance of HBsAg and resolution of symptoms. Anti-HBs provide life-long immunity to reinfection, although titers may decrease to undetectable levels over the course of years. Antibodies to HBeAg (anti-HBe) appear earlier than anti-HBs and usually signify the clearance of HBeAg and cessation of replication.

In chronic HBV infection, the virus may be in a replicative phase characterized by the presence of HBsAg, HBeAg, and HBV DNA, along with an immune-mediated chronic inflammatory response. Alternatively, HBV may enter a nonreplicative state, formerly referred to as the carrier state, in which HBV is maintained by insertion into the host genome. In this phase, HBsAg persists, but HBeAg and HBV DNA disappear and anti-HBe appears. The inflammatory response in this nonreplicative state is usually minimal.

Clinical Features

Most acute HBV infections are asymptomatic, especially if acquired at a young age when chronicity is more probable. Thirty percent of infections with HBV in adults result in acute hepatitis, which is indistinguishable from other forms of acute viral hepatitis. The illness usually has a 1- to 6-month incubation period. Hepatitis may be preceded by a serum sickness syndrome characterized by fever, urticaria, arthralgias, and, rarely, arthritis. This syndrome is probably caused by immune complexes of HBV antigens and antibodies, which may also produce glomerulonephritis and vasculitis in patients with chronic HBV infection.

Patients with chronic HBV infection may have a history of a distant bout of acute hepatitis, but a history of icterus is unusual. Most patients with chronic HBV infections remain asymptomatic for years. When symptoms develop, they usually are nonspecific, including malaise, fatigue, and anorexia. Some patients exhibit jaundice and complications of portal hypertension, such as ascites, variceal hemorrhage, or encephalopathy. Physical examination in the chronic phase may be normal, although hepatomegaly is common. Some patients may present with stigmata of cirrhosis and portal hypertension, including ascites, dilated abdominal veins, gynecomastia, and spider angiomata.

Findings on Diagnostic Testing

Diagnosis of acute hepatitis B is based on a typical serologic pattern in the setting of acute hepatitis. Serum aminotransferase elevations in the thousands and other liver biochemical abnormalities are indistinguishable from alternative causes of acute viral hepatitis. Acute infection is accompanied by IgM antibodies to HBcAg (anti-HBc IgM) and evidence of ongoing infection represented by HBsAg, HBeAg, and HBV DNA. In 5% to 10% of patients with acute hepatitis, the latter three markers may be cleared before clinical presentation, leaving anti-HBc IgM as the only indicator of recent infection. It is important to distinguish the IgM subtype, because the isolated presence of IgG antibodies to HBcAg (anti-HBc IgG) is a common serologic pattern in distant HBV infection that has been cleared. The timing of HBsAg disappearance is variable, but it is absent in 80% to 90% of cases by 4 months after infection. Persistence of HBsAg beyond 6 months indicates chronic infection. Several weeks after the disappearance of HBsAg, anti-HBs appears. This antibody provides life-long immunity, but titers may drop to undetectable levels over the course of years. As with acute HAV, liver biopsy for acute HBV is needed only when the diagnosis is not substantiated by serologic testing.

Chronic HBV may produce several serologic patterns based on the replicative state of the virus. The presence of HBsAg, HBeAg, and HBV DNA and the absence of anti-HBs and anti-HBe are characteristic of active virus replication. The presence of HBsAg and anti-HBe in the absence of HBeAg, HBV DNA, and anti-HBs is representative of the nonreplicative or chronic carrier state. All patients with chronic HBV have anti-HBc IgG. A small number of patients may have low titers of anti-HBc IgM, particularly when the virus is transitioning from the replicative phase to the nonreplicative phase.

The levels of serum aminotransferases usually are mildly elevated with chronic HBV infection. Biochemical variables and symptoms correlate poorly with the histologic severity of liver damage. Liver biopsy provides important prognostic information in patients with chronic hepatitis. Patients with active viral replication demonstrate a variable degree of chronic periportal inflammation. Extension of chronic inflammatory cells into the hepatic lobule is termed *piecemeal necrosis,* whereas inflammation and hepatocellular destruction extending from portal tract to portal tract is termed *bridging necrosis.* Patients in the nonreplicative phase or chronic carrier state usually have minimal to no inflammation. Variable stages of fibrosis or even cirrhosis can be present in any patient with chronic HBV. Determining the extent of inflammation and fibrosis is often critical in making therapeutic decisions for chronic HBV.

Management and Course

Acute HBV hepatitis usually resolves clinically and biochemically over several weeks to months. As with other forms of acute viral hepatitis, treatment is supportive. One percent of cases follow a fulminant course resulting in hepatic failure and encephalopathy. These patients should be referred to transplantation centers.

The risk of HBV infection establishing a chronic course seems to be associated with the patient's age at acquisition. Chronicity rates are 90% if the infection is acquired in utero or at birth. The rate is lower in older children and <5% in adults. The mechanism of this variability in the ability of HBV to enter a chronic phase is probably related to changes in immune tolerance with aging.

Once established, chronic HBV infection is usually life-long. Annually, 1% to 2% of chronic HBV carriers lose HBsAg and develop anti-HBs, suggesting complete viral eradication. Also each year, the replicative phase of the virus transforms into the nonreplicative phase in 5% to 20% of patients; HBeAg is lost, and anti-HBe is gained. An acute clinical and biochemical flare of the infection often accompanies this seroconversion. The transition to a nonreplicative state does not indicate complete clearance of HBV. Many patients exhibit reactivation of replication with reappearance of HBeAg at some point in the future.

Although cirrhosis may develop at any stage of chronic HBV infection, it usually requires many years of infection. The risk is greatest for patients with bridging necrosis and active viral replication. Because chronic HBV is indolent and produces minimal or no symptoms, complications of cirrhosis, including ascites, variceal hemorrhage, and encephalopathy, may be the initial manifestations of chronic HBV. Patients with chronic HBV infection also have up to a 200-fold increased risk of hepatocellular carcinoma; therefore, patients with HBV infection for >10 years should be screened every 6 months by serum α-fetoprotein measurements and ultrasound to facilitate early detection. The course of acute and chronic HBV infection can also be complicated by superinfection with hepatitis D virus.

Attempts to clear HBV with antiviral or immunosuppressive therapy have been largely unsuccessful with the exception of treatment with interferon-alpha. Candidates for interferon therapy should have detectable markers of viral replication (HBeAg and HBV DNA). They should not have histologic evidence of cirrhosis or decompensated liver disease. Interferon therapy for HBV requires 5 million units delivered subcutaneously every day for at least 3 months. With this therapy, the virus in 30% of cases will sustain the transition from the active replication phase to the nonreplication phase. One-fourth of these patients will lose circulating HBsAg, suggesting complete viral clearance. Side effects are substantial; there is an almost universal occurrence of an influenza-like illness, with myalgia, fever, chills, and headache. Other adverse reactions include depression, bone marrow depression, alopecia, and autoimmune thyroiditis. Patients should be selected with this side effect profile in mind, especially if there are pre-existing psychiatric conditions and cytopenias.

Prevention of HBV has widespread public health implications. Several medical organizations have recommended a program of universal vaccination of infants with the recombinant hepatitis B vaccine. This vaccine is indicated as pre-exposure prophylaxis in health care workers, patients on hemodialysis, intravenous drug users, those with sexual contact with HBV carriers, those with household contact with HBV carriers, and travelers who reside in an endemic area for >6 months. The three-dose regimen is given at time 0, 1 month, and 6 months. It is >90% effective at producing protective anti-HBs. Response rates may be lower in immunosuppressed individuals. Although titers may decrease over time, the protective effect is long-lived owing to the amnestic response at the time of exposure.

Postexposure prophylaxis requires the use of hepatitis B immune globulin (HBIG) (0.06 mg per kg) in addition to the recombinant vaccine. Patients with sexual or parenteral exposures to persons with active HBV infection should receive HBIG within 2 weeks of exposure. Infants born to mothers with HBsAg should receive HBIG at birth. All exposed persons should receive the vaccine in the usual dosing schedule.

HEPATITIS C

Incidence and Epidemiology

Molecular cloning techniques have identified an RNA virus, termed *hepatitis C virus* (HCV), which has been shown to be responsible for most cases of non-A, non-B post-transfusion hepatitis. This advance also permitted the development of serologic and polymerase chain reaction assays for screening and diagnosis. Because most infections with HCV assume a chronic phase, blood donor screening is critical. Along with HIV, anti-HBc, and ALT screening of the blood supply, screening for antibodies to HCV has dramatically reduced the incidence of post-transfusion hepatitis to <1% of all transfusions.

Given that the main mode of transmission is parenteral, the epidemiology of HCV mirrors that of HBV. The worldwide incidence of antibodies to HCV (anti-HCV) is 0.3% to 1.7%, with higher rates in developing countries and lower socioeconomic groups. Within the United States, there is variation between racial groups: a 7% to 8% seropositive rate among inner-city black and Hispanic populations compared with 0.5% among inner-city whites. Based on the homology of RNA sequences, several genotypes of HCV have been described. In the United States, 70% of HCV infections are caused by genotypes Ia and Ib; the remaining 30% of infections are caused by genotypes II and III. Regional variations in these genotypes may explain regional differences in the clinical behavior of HCV.

Although parenteral exposure is the primary means of contracting HCV, 40% of sporadic cases have no identifiable source of infection. Groups at high risk for infection with HCV include intravenous drug users and persons requiring transfusions or other blood products. The risk of sexual transmission is poorly defined but appears to be low. The risk of vertical transmission from mother to fetus is 5% to 10%. The risk is higher if the mother is seropositive for human immunodeficiency virus 1 (HIV-1).

Etiology and Pathogenesis

Based on the observation that HCV infection follows a slightly more aggressive course with immunosuppression secondary to medications or HIV infection, HCV does not appear to rely on immune-mediated injury to the same degree as HBV. Therefore, unlike HBV, the primary mechanism of hepatocellular injury is presumed to be a direct cytopathic effect, although a contribution from immune-mediated injury cannot be excluded. In fact, the immune response in HCV infection is responsible for the syndrome of mixed cryoglobulinemia observed in a small fraction of chronic HCV infections. In this disorder, HCV antigens associated with monoclonal IgM and polyclonal IgG antibody complexes are deposited in the end organ and activate complement, producing dependent purpura, glomerulonephritis, arthritis, and vasculitis.

The incubation period after exposure is usually 6 to 10 weeks, but it may be as long as 4 to 5 months. Similar to HBV infection, antibodies develop against several viral proteins and are the criteria of enzyme-linked immunosorbent assays (ELISAs) and immunoblot diagnostic assays. Anti-HCVs may not be detectable for up to 3 months after the onset of acute hepatitis, however. These antibodies are neither neutralizing nor protective and 70% to 90% of HCV infections assume a chronic phase.

Clinical Features

Most patients infected with HCV never develop a clinical syndrome of acute hepatitis. One-fourth of transfusion-related HCV infections result in jaundice, malaise, fever, and right upper quadrant pain typical of viral hepatitis. Most episodes are mild; thus, HCV does not appear to be the agent responsible for the large number of fulminant hepatic failure cases attributed to non-A, non-B hepatitis.

Irrespective of the patient's age at acquisition and the mode of viral transmission, 70% to 90% of HCV infections enter a chronic phase. Many patients remain asymptomatic for years and are only detected on health screening or at the time of blood donation. The most common symptoms of chronic HCV are nonspecific malaise, fatigue, insomnia, and abdominal discomfort. Some patients may remain asymptomatic even as the disease progresses to cirrhosis.

Findings on Diagnostic Testing

Patients with acute hepatitis caused by HCV usually have aminotransferase levels of <1000 IU per liter; <10% have levels of >2000 IU per liter. Serum bilirubin levels rarely exceed 10 to 15 mg per dl. Severe liver dysfunction with abnormal coagulation variables is uncommon.

As with other forms of acute viral hepatitis, the cornerstone of diagnosis is serologic testing. The main obstacle to diagnosing acute infection is the variable delay in the appearance of anti-HCV. Only 65% of patients have anti-HCV within 2 weeks of symptom onset, but 90% are seropositive after 3 months. The remaining 10% usually develop anti-HCV over several months.

Second-generation ELISAs recognize structural (C22, C33, and C100) and nonstructural (NS3, NS4, and NS5) viral proteins with a 90% sensitivity. The specificity of ELISAs is low. Therefore, when the pretest probability is low, as in blood donor screening, a confirmatory test is required. One confirmatory test is the second-generation radioimmunoblot assay (RIBA-2), in which antibodies to the individual structural and nonstructural proteins are detected. The presence of antibodies to two or more target proteins is indicative of HCV exposure. The most sensitive and specific means of detecting active HCV infection is the serum-based polymerase chain reaction (PCR). PCR can be used to detect HCV if serologic assays produce negative results in a patient with a high probability of having HBV. Similarly, PCR may confirm a positive serologic test result or document clearance of HCV after therapy. Unfortunately, the test's substantial cost prohibits its use for widespread screening.

Liver biopsy is generally not useful for diagnosis of acute HCV infection, but it plays an essential role in the diagnosis and management of chronic HCV. In chronic HCV, there is a variable degree of periportal chronic inflammation, often with discrete lymphoid aggregates. The severity may vary from a minimal increase in periportal lymphocytes to the confluent destruction of hepatocytes in bridging necrosis. There also is a variable degree of fibrosis, ranging from no fibrosis to cirrhosis. The severity of histologic injury correlates poorly with symptoms and elevations in levels of aminotransferases, indicating the importance of liver biopsy in the management of these patients. Liver biopsy should always be performed if patients are being considered for therapy.

Management and Course

With supportive therapy, most patients with acute HCV experience a gradual resolution of symptoms over weeks to months. The infection is self-limited in 10% to 30% of cases and the virus is cleared, but in the remaining 70% to 90% of cases, the infection assumes a chronic course. Asymptomatic HCV infection carries the same probability of chronicity as symptomatic acute HCV infection.

Chronic HCV infection is an indolent disease. Complications generally occur >10 years after acquisition. There are often significant fluctuations in levels of serum aminotransferases. Factors that predict the probability of disease progression are poorly defined, but histologic evidence of severe inflammation and the HCV genotype Ib seem to predict a poor prognosis. When all patients with chronic HCV are followed for 10 years, 25% develop cirrhosis. Similar to chronic HBV, long-term infection with HCV increases the risk of hepatocellular carcinoma, which is greater than the risk imposed by cirrhosis alone.

Although initially approved for HBV treatment, interferon-alpha is currently the only effective therapy for chronic HCV infection. In contrast to interferon's immunomodulatory effects in the treatment of infection with HBV, its mechanism of action in treating infection with HCV is mainly through its antiviral properties. Therapy with 3 million units subcutaneously 3 days per week for 6 months produces normalization of aminotransferase levels in 50% of patients. One-half of these responders relapse, however, and the overall rate of long-term clearance of HCV as defined by PCR is 20% to 25%. Whether higher doses or longer courses of therapy can improve the long-term response rates will be determined by the results of ongoing trials. Predictors of a poor response include histologic evidence of cirrhosis, iron overload, and severe inflammation. Patients with genotype Ib and patients with aminotransferase levels persistently near normal also respond poorly to interferon. Side effects are similar to those associated with interferon therapy for HBV. Patients with cirrhosis, active psychiatric disorders, and cytopenias generally are not candidates for interferon therapy because of the substantial risk of decompensation on therapy.

Liver transplantation should be considered in all patients with symptomatic cirrhosis or complications of portal hypertension (e.g., encephalopathy, refractory ascites, variceal hemorrhage). In general, patients with cirrhosis who meet the criteria for Child-Turcotte-Pugh class B or C cirrhosis are best served by transplantation, whereas patients with Child-Turcotte-Pugh class A cirrhosis should be supported with medical therapy. As with HBV, reinfection of the allograft is the rule, but post-transplant HCV is indolent and rarely results in allograft dysfunction.

The primary means of preventing HCV infection has been blood donor screening. There is no effective vaccine or passive immune therapy against HCV infection.

HEPATITIS D

The hepatitis D virus (HDV), also termed the *delta agent*, is a defective RNA virus that requires the presence of HBV to replicate. Only patients with acute or chronic HBV infection are susceptible to infection with HDV. HDV is present worldwide, with high incidences in regions of Africa, South America, and the Mediterranean, but a relatively low incidence in the United States. Transmission appears to be contact-mediated and possibly through insect vectors.

HDV may increase the severity of acute hepatitis caused by HBV. Diagnosis may be difficult in this setting because there are no clinical or histologic features specific to HDV infection, and commercial antibody assays may not detect the transient IgM response.

Infection with HDV in chronic HBV carriers may result in an acute phase of hepatitis and clinical decompensation of patients with cirrhosis. Many patients develop chronic HDV infection, which may accelerate the progression of chronic HBV hepatitis to cirrhosis. There is no effective therapy, but the risk of recurrent HBV after liver transplantation may be lower in patients coinfected with HDV.

HEPATITIS E

The hepatitis E virus (HEV) is an RNA virus epidemiologically and clinically similar to HAV. It is endemic in developing countries, especially Mexico, Africa, Central Asia, and Southern Asia. Reports in the United States are rare and usually represent infection acquired while traveling in endemic regions. Transmission is mainly by the fecal-oral route. Outbreaks caused by contaminated water or food are common in developing countries.

The incubation period and clinical syndromes of acute hepatitis E are identical to those for HAV. For reasons that remain poorly defined, HEV infection in pregnancy is associated with a fulminant course and a 10% to 20% mortality rate. Diagnosis relies on detection of IgM antibodies to HEV, but the assays are only available in selected centers. Treatment is supportive, and with the exception of the high rate of fulminant hepatitis in pregnancy, full recovery from HEV infection is the rule.

NON A–E HEPATITIS

A small percentage of acute and chronic hepatitis appears to be caused by viruses not detectable by currently available diagnostic assays. A novel agent, designated hepatitis G virus (HGV), has been cloned and appears to be transmitted parenterally. There is no serologic assay and detection requires PCR of serum to detect viral RNA. The virus has been detected in 1% to 2% of blood donors, but the clinical significance of this agent remains unclear. Although rare episodes of acute hepatitis have been observed, most patients with HGV have normal aminotransferase levels. Further clinical experience will clarify the importance of HGV as a cause of acute and chronic hepatitis.

Other nonhepatotropic viruses may produce hepatitis. Cytomegalovirus, Epstein-Barr virus, and varicella-zoster virus may produce acute hepatitis. Herpes simplex virus rarely causes hepatitis, but a few cases of fulminant hepatitis caused by this virus have been reported. Similarly, a fulminant giant cell hepatitis has been associated with infection with paramyxovirus. Although these viruses cause acute hepatitis, none have been proved to cause chronic hepatitis.

NONALCOHOLIC STEATOHEPATITIS

A form of liver injury histologically indistinguishable from alcoholic hepatitis is often observed in patients who do not have a history of ethanol abuse. This syndrome of steatosis with lobular hepatitis has been termed *nonalcoholic steatohepatitis*. Initial reports suggested that nonalcoholic steatohepatitis was more common in obese females and was frequently associated with hyperlipidemia and diabetes mellitus. Subsequent studies reported a higher incidence in males, and diabetes, obesity, and hyperlipidemia were present only in a minority of patients. Mild elevations in levels of serum aminotransferases are often observed, and nonspecific symptoms of fatigue, anorexia, and abdominal discomfort are present in a minority of patients. There is no specific treatment for nonalcoholic steatohepatitis, but clinicians often advise weight loss for obese patients and aggressive treatment of hyperlipidemia and diabetes. Although reports suggest up to 40% of cases progress to fibrosis or cirrhosis, further clinical experience will help define the natural history of this disorder.

ISCHEMIC HEPATITIS

An acute form of ischemic liver injury, termed *ischemic hepatitis* or *shock liver*, often complicates the course of critical illness. The portal vein provides approximately two-thirds of the hepatic blood supply; the residual one-third comes from the hepatic artery. Ischemic injury usually requires reduced flow in both systems. Most patients with ischemic hepatitis have circulatory shock as a result of cardiovascular disease, sepsis, or profound hypovolemia.

In the hours to days after the hemodynamic insult, levels of serum aminotransferases, lactate dehydrogenase, and bilirubin increase to variable degrees. Severe injury is associated with aminotransferase levels in the thousands and marked prolongation of the prothrombin time. The treatment of ischemic hepatitis is largely supportive. Systemic hemodynamics should be optimized, and any coexistent infections should be treated with broad-spectrum antibiotics. Despite apparent severe biochemical dysfunction, most of the laboratory abnormalities improve over 1 to 2 weeks. If the patient survives, liver function usually returns to normal. The overall prognosis usually is poor because of the underlying critical illness.

WILSON'S DISEASE

Incidence and Epidemiology

Wilson's disease, or hepatolenticular degeneration, is an autosomal recessive disorder characterized by excessive accumulation of total body copper. It is a rare disorder, with a worldwide incidence of 3 cases per 100,000 population. Higher incidences may be noted in populations prone to inbreeding. The incidence of heterozygotes is 1 in 90. Abnormal copper metabolism is established from birth. Patients usually are diagnosed in adolescence, although rarely cases manifest after age 50 years.

Etiology and Pathogenesis

The gene for Wilson's disease has recently been cloned and appears to be a copper-transporting P-type ATPase expressed exclusively in the liver. Defective structure or function of the transporter results in impaired biliary excretion and increased hepatic stores of copper. Free copper is also released into the serum and deposited in end organs. Accumulations in the brain, kidneys, bones, and eyes are responsible for the extrahepatic complications of Wilson's disease.

Clinical Features

Patients with Wilson's disease almost universally present between 5 and 50 years of age, with the second decade of life being the peak time of onset. Fifty percent of patients have liver disease. Potential hepatic manifestations include chronic active hepatitis with associated malaise, fatigue, and anorexia. Alternatively, patients present with complications of cirrhosis or a syndrome of fulminant hepatic failure with marked jaundice and encephalopathy. The diagnosis might be suggested by asymptomatic elevations of serum aminotransferase levels in an adolescent or young adult.

Because this primary metabolic defect is localized to the liver, all symptomatic patients with Wilson's disease have some degree of liver disease, but 50% of patients present with extrahepatic manifestations. In 40% of patients, neuropsychiatric complications dominate. For unclear reasons, Wilson's disease never leads to sensory deficits, but spasticity, choreiform movements, dysarthria, ataxia, and intention tremor are the result of copper accumulation in the lenticular nuclei. Patients also usually have subtle behavioral or psychiatric changes. The diagnosis should be suspected in adolescents with a marked decline in scholastic or social performance. Patients with neuropsychiatric manifestations universally have Kayser-Fleischer rings, which are deposits of copper in the peripheral cornea. Other extrahepatic manifestations include Fanconi's syndrome and proximal renal tubular acidosis, osteoporosis with spontaneous fractures, and copper-induced hemolytic anemia.

Findings on Diagnostic Testing

In addition to young persons with abnormal liver chemistry profiles or clinical symptoms suggestive of Wilson's disease, all siblings of Wilson's disease patients should undergo diagnostic testing. Screening for Wilson's disease in a young patient with elevated levels of aminotransferases should include measurement of serum ceruloplasmin, which is decreased in >95% of homozygotes. Ceruloplasmin may also be low in 20% of heterozygotes and in patients with malnutrition, protein-losing enteropathy, and other forms of hepatic failure. Therefore, low ceruloplasmin levels should be confirmed by demonstration of 24-hour urinary copper excretion of >100 mg. The diagnosis cannot be excluded on the basis of a normal ceruloplasmin level. If Wilson's disease is strongly suspected, further diagnostic evaluation with 24-hour urinary copper measurement should be performed. Detection of Kayser-Fleischer rings may require slit-lamp examination. Although the presence of Kayser-Fleischer rings helps to confirm the diagnosis in the appropriate clinical setting, they may be absent in early Wilson's disease. The standard for diagnosis is quantitation of hepatic copper levels in liver biopsy specimens. Histologic findings include steatosis, glycogenated nuclei, and variable degrees of periportal mononuclear infiltrates and fibrosis.

Management and Course

The critical factor in the management of Wilson's disease is establishing a definitive diagnosis early in its clinical course. Untreated, the disease is universally fatal. When treated, patients have a normal life expectancy, but because treatment is life-long, the diagnosis should be established with certainty. The cornerstone of treatment is copper chelation with oral penicillamine (1 g per day). The major obstacle is a 20% incidence of hypersensitivity reactions (e.g., neutropenia, thrombocytopenia, rash, and arthritis). Patients may require dose reduction because of drug-induced nephrotic syndrome. With the exception of neutropenia, a 2- to 3-week withdrawal followed by a stepwise increase in the dose may be attempted in patients who manifest evidence of drug toxicity. Patients intolerant to D-penicillamine should be treated with trientine. Although neurologic symptoms may not resolve completely, patients with cirrhosis may experience long-term survival if they comply with therapy. Fulminant hepatic failure is not responsive to copper chelation and is universally fatal unless liver transplantation is performed. Transplantation should also be considered in the small fraction of patients with advanced cirrhosis who develop complications of progressive portal hypertension despite therapy.

HEMOCHROMATOSIS

Incidence and Epidemiology

Hemochromatosis is characterized by the pathologic accumulation of toxic levels of iron in the cells of various organs and tissues, including the liver. Because hepatic inflammation is not a prominent feature of the disease, hemochromatosis technically is not a form of hepatitis, but the iron-induced hepatocellular injury leads to clinical and biochemical features similar to chronic hepatitis. Hemochromatosis may be caused by a genetic disorder of iron homeostasis termed *hereditary hemochromatosis* (HHC), or it may be caused by a secondary disorder, such as transfusional iron overload (e.g., sickle cell anemia) or dyserythropoiesis (e.g., thalassemia major). The hepatic manifestations of hemochromatosis are similar to those in HHC and secondary hemochromatosis, but differentiation is usually made apparent by the clinical features of the disorders associated with secondary hemochromatosis. Several hepatic disorders including alcoholic liver disease may be associated with uncomplicated iron overload, and differentiation from HHC may be challenging.

HHC is inherited as an autosomal recessive trait, with the responsible gene localized to chromosome 6. It is one of the most common inborn errors of metabolism; the homozygote frequency is 1 in 300 and the heterozygote frequency is 1 in 9. The disease appears to be more common in persons of Northern European ancestry, but the precise incidence among other racial or ethnic groups is unknown.

Etiology and Pathogenesis

The basic pathophysiologic mechanism in HHC is increased intestinal absorption of iron in the setting of normal dietary iron intake. A normal adult absorbs 1 to 2 mg of iron per day, whereas patients with HHC absorb 3 to 4 mg of iron per day. This increased absorption results in an excess accumulation of 700 to 1000 mg total body iron per year. The mechanism of enhanced absorption and intestinal cell transport of iron remains poorly defined.

The clinical features of HHC are produced by intracellular accumulation of toxic levels of iron, which causes hepatocellular destruction and fibrosis in the liver. Although the mechanism of iron toxicity remains poorly understood, damage to cellular and organelle membranes by increased lipid peroxidation has been proposed as an important factor. Iron deposition in the heart, pituitary, pancreas, skin, and gonads is responsible for the extrahepatic manifestations of HHC.

Clinical Features

Liver disease is the most common clinical feature of HHC. Most patients remain asymptomatic until complications of cirrhosis develop, but many patients with precirrhotic HHC are diagnosed after detection of asymptomatic hepatomegaly or mild elevations in levels of serum aminotransferases. Advanced liver disease may present with jaundice, weight loss, fatigue, variceal hemorrhage, ascites, and encephalopathy.

The most common extrahepatic manifestation is diabetes mellitus, which occurs in >50% of patients with HHC. An additional 50% of patients develop other endocrinopathies, including hypogonadism as a result of pituitary and primary gonadal iron overload. Most patients with advanced disease have a bronze or slate gray discoloration of exposed skin as a result of increased melanin production and iron deposition in the basal layers. A degenerative arthropathy with a characteristic predilection for the second and third metacarpophalangeal joints occurs in 25% of patients.

Findings on Diagnostic Testing

Serum aminotransferase levels rarely exceed 100 IU per liter, and in many cases they are normal. Serum measurements of total body iron levels are almost invariably elevated in HHC. The serum ferritin level is usually >500 ng per ml and often is measured in the thousands. However, the serum ferritin level is elevated in any inflammatory disorder or iron overload condition such as in alcoholism. Although a transferrin saturation of >55% is more specific for HHC, the predictive accuracy is <90% and the sensitivity is <80%. Therefore, patients with abnormal iron indices should have the diagnosis confirmed by liver biopsy. The standard for the diagnosis of HHC is hepatic iron quantification and determination of the hepatic iron index. The hepatic iron index is calculated as micromoles of iron per gram of dry liver divided by the patient's age. An index of >2.0 is diagnostic of hemochromatosis, whereas an index of <2.0 essentially excludes HHC. Patients with alcoholic liver disease and those who are heterozygous for HHC often have markedly abnormal serum iron indices, but the hepatic iron index is always <2.0. Histologic evaluation with Prussian blue staining usually demonstrates impressive stores of intracellular iron in >50% of hepatocytes, but this finding may occur in advanced alcoholic liver disease. Noninvasive imaging with CT or magnetic resonance imaging scans may suggest iron overload, but attempts to quantify iron stores with these methods have been disappointing.

Management and Course

The mainstay of HHC treatment is phlebotomy. The usual regimen removes 1 unit (250 mg of iron) every 1 to 2 weeks. Patients may require a total of 75 to 100 sessions over 2 to 3 years before iron stores return to normal levels. Once the transferrin saturation falls to <45% and the serum ferritin level is <50 ng per ml, patients can be maintained on a regimen of phlebotomy every 3 to 4 months. If diagnosed before the onset of cirrhosis or diabetes, patients with HHC compliant with a phlebotomy program can expect a normal survival. Although phlebotomy does not reverse cirrhosis, it does seem to improve survival and should be considered at all stages of HHC. In patients with dyserythropoiesis or other causes of anemia intolerant of phlebotomy, chelation therapy with desferoxamine is an alternative. Desferoxamine requires parenteral infusion and removes only 50 to 75 mg of iron per dose.

In patients with cirrhosis, the 10-year survival rate is 70%. Most deaths caused by HHC are related to complications of liver disease. Up to 30% of patients with HHC will develop hepatocellular carcinoma, and screening patients with established cirrhosis with biannual α-fetoprotein and ultrasound may result in early detection. Patients with advanced cirrhosis should be considered for liver transplantation, but post-transplantation survival in patients with HHC is lower than in patients with other forms of chronic liver disease, possibly because of a higher incidence of diabetes and cardiac disease.

α_1-ANTITRYPSIN DEFICIENCY

Individuals inheriting the ZZ phenotype of α_1-antitrypsin may manifest various liver disorders as a result of the accumulation of abnormal Z α_1-antitrypsin in the endoplasmic reticulum of hepatocytes. Patients usually present in infancy with cholestatic hepatitis or cirrhosis, but some present in adulthood with chronic hepatitis, cirrhosis, or hepatocellular carcinoma. Only 20% of persons with ZZ phenotype will develop clinical liver disease. The other phenotypes, including those commonly associated with emphysema, are not associated with liver disease. Diagnosis is usually suspected in a patient with liver disease who exhibits decreased levels of the α_1 band on serum protein electrophoresis. Determining the specific phenotype of patients and both parents can provide more direct evidence of the diagnosis. Liver biopsy specimens can confirm the diagnosis by the presence of intracellular periodic acid–Schiff (PAS)-positive globules. There is no specific treatment for α_1-antitrypsin deficiency, and liver transplantation should be considered in patients with complications of cirrhosis. In addition to treating complications of cirrhosis, transplantation cures the underlying metabolic defect.

CHAPTER 64

Autoimmune Liver Disease

INCIDENCE AND EPIDEMIOLOGY

The immune system plays a substantial role in the pathogenesis of a diverse group of liver diseases. The severity and chronicity of many variants of viral hepatitis are influenced by the associated immune response. Similarly, a growing body of evidence suggests immune mechanisms contribute to the liver injury in alcoholic liver disease. Some forms of medication-induced liver disease exhibit histologic and clinical characteristics suggestive of immune mediation. Some patients present with autoimmune hepatitis, a chronic inflammatory liver disorder with clinical and serologic features of autoimmunity. Autoimmune hepatitis classically occurs in young women, but it may be seen in children and older adults. The female-to-male ratio is 4:1, which is less than the corresponding ratio for primary biliary cirrhosis. When autoimmune hepatitis occurs in men, it often presents later in life.

Autoimmune hepatitis has been classified according to autoantibody markers (Table 64-1). Several variants appear to have divergent epidemiologic features: Type I is the classic form of autoimmune hepatitis and occurs primarily in young girls and women; type II autoimmune hepatitis is mainly a disease of young children and represents <5% of autoimmune hepatitis in adults; the type IIa variant occurs in young women, whereas type IIb predominates in older men. Type III autoimmune hepatitis is rare and follows an epidemiologic pattern similar to that of type I.

ETIOLOGY AND PATHOGENESIS

Although the precise etiology of autoimmune hepatitis remains poorly defined, current evidence suggests that a genetic predisposition to aberrant immunologic responses is the fundamental pathogenic mechanism. Unaffected relatives of patients with autoimmune hepatitis often have autoantibodies. In addition, the association with the antigens HLA-B8, HLA-DR3, and HLA-DR4 suggests a potential genetic component to autoimmune hepatitis. It is possible that an environmental agent, such as a hepatotropic virus, triggers an immune response that

TABLE 64-1
Classification of Autoimmune Hepatitis

FEATURE	TYPE I	TYPE IIa	TYPE IIb	TYPE III
Autoantibodies	ANA, ASMA, anti-actin	Anti-LKM, anti-liver cytosol I	Anti-LKM (low titer)	Anti-soluble liver antigen, ASMA
Frequency in adults	75–85%	<5%	<5%	10%
Age/sex	Young and middle-aged women	Children and young women	Older men	Young and middle-aged women
Other autoimmune disorders	~20%	~40%	Uncommon	~20%
Associated with hepatitis C infection	Rare	No	Yes	Rare

ANA = antinuclear antibodies; anti-LKM = anti–liver-kidney microsomal antibodies; ASMA = anti–smooth muscle antibodies.

becomes misguided in persons with this putative genetic susceptibility, but this hypothesis has not been proved.

The circulating autoantibodies in autoimmune hepatitis are not specific to the liver and do not appear to be pathogenic. They are probably epiphenomena of a more fundamental immunologic derangement. Abnormal suppressor T-lymphocyte function and associations with many other immunoregulatory disorders are also markers of this poorly defined immunologic defect. Perhaps the most convincing evidence in favor of the role of immunopathogenic factors in autoimmune hepatitis is the near complete resolution of the necroinflammatory response with immunosuppressive therapy. Further understanding of the complex interaction of the immune system with possible environmental triggers may clarify the etiology of autoimmune hepatitis and help identify curative strategies.

CLINICAL FEATURES

Patients with autoimmune hepatitis come to medical attention with a diverse range of presentations ranging from asymptomatic aminotransferase elevations to subfulminant hepatitis. Patients usually present with nonspecific malaise, anorexia, fatigue, and weight loss. Young women often develop amenorrhea. Jaundice occurs in severe cases. Occasionally, complications of portal hypertension (e.g., ascites, encephalopathy, or variceal hemorrhage) are the initial manifestations of autoimmune hepatitis.

Physical examination findings often are normal in early autoimmune hepatitis, but up to 80% of patients have hepatomegaly. Advanced disease is signified by jaundice, splenomegaly, and ascites. Spider angiomata and palmar erythema are present in 50% of cases. There is no one clinical feature of autoimmune hepatitis that distinguishes it from other forms of chronic hepatitis.

Associated autoimmune disorders dominate the clinical presentation in some patients, particularly those with the type I and type IIa variants of autoimmune hepatitis. Autoimmune disorders often associated with autoimmune hepatitis include autoimmune thyroiditis, ulcerative colitis, pleuropericarditis, rheumatoid arthritis, glomerulonephritis, Sjögren's syndrome, and Coombs-positive hemolytic anemia. The most common extrahepatic manifestations are arthritis and rash. A number of other systemic disorders may rarely complicate the course of autoimmune hepatitis, including myocarditis, fibrosing alveolitis, panniculitis, and uveitis.

FINDINGS ON DIAGNOSTIC TESTING

Laboratory Studies

Before the initiation of treatment, essentially all patients with autoimmune hepatitis have elevated serum aminotransferase levels. Typically, aminotransferase levels are 3- to 10-fold above normal, but occasionally, levels as high as 1000 IU per liter are encountered. Variable degrees of hyperbilirubinemia are present in patients with advanced disease. Similarly, prolongation of the prothrombin time, hypoalbuminemia, thrombocytopenia, leukopenia, and anemia may be present in patients with cirrhosis or portal hypertension.

Autoantibody Testing

The cornerstone of diagnosing autoimmune hepatitis is documentation of the presence of circulating autoantibodies. Four subclassifications of autoimmune hepatitis have been described based on serologic and clinical features (see Table 64-1). Type I autoimmune hepatitis is the most commonly encountered and represents the classic form of the disease. Patients have high titers of antinuclear antibodies (ANAs), anti–smooth muscle antibodies (ASMAs), or both. Most patients also have a polyclonal hypergammaglobulinemia, and when first-generation assays for antibodies to hepatitis C virus (anti-HCV) are performed, there is a high rate of false-positive reactions caused by the nonspecific increase in globulins. Only 5% of patients with type I autoimmune hepatitis test positive on second-generation anti-HCV assays and a significant fraction of these test results may also be false-positive. Type II autoimmune hepatitis is most commonly encountered in children, accounting for only 5% of autoimmune hepatitis in adults. It has been subdivided into types IIa and IIb. Type IIa occurs in young women. It is associated with high titers of antibodies to liver-kidney microsomes (anti-LKMs), a low incidence of HCV infection, and an extraordinarily high incidence of associated immune disorders. Type IIb, which occurs in older men, is characterized by a high incidence of HCV infection and low titers of anti-LKMs. Both forms of type II autoimmune hepatitis typically lack ANAs and ASMAs, but hypergammaglobulinemia often is pronounced. Type III autoimmune hepatitis probably represents a variant of type I, because the clinical and epidemiologic features are the same. Patients with type III autoimmune hepatitis have antibodies to a soluble liver antigen, and they often have ANAs and ASMAs. Patients with autoimmune hepatitis may have other autoantibodies, including anti-liver cytosol I, anti-actin, anti-neutrophil cytoplasmic, and low titers of antimitochondrial antibodies. Conversely, other chronic liver diseases may have low titers of ANAs and ASMAs, but titers of >1:320 and >1:40, respectively, are unusual. A small group of patients with the typical clinical features of autoimmune hepatitis have no detectable viral serologic features or autoantibodies. Whether this represents infection with an unknown viral agent or a form of autoimmune hepatitis without autoantibodies remains unclear. Some of these patients demonstrate a complete response to corticosteroids; a feature that some consider to be diagnostic of autoimmune hepatitis.

Liver Biopsy

Percutaneous liver biopsy is required to establish the diagnosis of autoimmune hepatitis and assess the severity and stage of the necroinflammatory response. Autoimmune hepatitis may be histologically indistinguishable from chronic viral hepatitis, with a pattern of periportal mononuclear infiltrate extending into the hepatic lobules termed *piecemeal necrosis*. Some patients have a predominantly plasma cell infiltrate. Severe cases are marked by hepatocellular necrosis extending from portal tract to central vein, which is termed *bridging necrosis*. Although autoimmune hepatitis typically spares the bile ducts, the histologic features of autoimmune hepatitis occasionally are indistinguishable from those of primary sclerosing cholangitis or primary biliary cirrhosis. A variable degree of fibrosis may be present. Up to 25% of type I patients and 80% of type II patients have cirrhosis at the time of presentation. Patients presenting with jaundice and marked aminotransferase elevations predictably have bridging of confluent necrosis with variable degrees of fibrosis. The histologic picture correlates poorly with symptoms in patients with mild clinical disease.

MANAGEMENT AND COURSE

Without immunosuppressive therapy, patients with autoimmune hepatitis usually progress to liver failure, with a mean survival of 5 years. Therefore, immunosuppressive therapy should be initiated in any patient with bridging necrosis on biopsy, gamma globulin levels elevated more than twofold, aminotransferase levels elevated more than fivefold, and hepatitis-related symptoms. It is unknown if asymptomatic patients with minimal histologic injury benefit from therapy. Therapy may be divided into an induction phase and a maintenance or withdrawal phase. Therapy is initiated with prednisone alone or in combination with azathioprine. Both regimens are equally effective in inducing remission. Azathioprine alone is not effective for induction. If prednisone is used alone, the initial dose is 40 to 60 mg per day for severe inflammation, and 20 to 30 mg per day for moderate inflammation. The dose is tapered by 10 mg per week until a dose of 20 mg per day is achieved. The dose is maintained at 20 mg per day until the patient enters remission. Remission is defined as resolution of symptoms, reduction of aminotransferase levels to less than twofold above normal, lowering of gamma globulin levels to <2 g per dl, and improvement to minimal inflammation on liver biopsy. Biochemical remission occurs in 1 to 6 months, but histologic improvement may be delayed for 12 to 36 months. Combination therapy is initiated with 20 to 30 mg per day of prednisone and 1 mg per kg per day of azathioprine. Many clinicians elect to achieve remission with prednisone alone before initiating azathioprine because of a small risk of azathioprine hepatitis. The main advantage of combination therapy is a decreased incidence of adverse corticosteroid side effects. Azathioprine also has serious side effects, and patients must be counseled on the risks of bone marrow suppression, immune suppression, pancreatitis, and the increased risk of malignancy with long-term use. Clinicians must regularly monitor blood counts, especially if higher doses are given.

When remission is achieved, the corticosteroids should be tapered to the lowest possible maintenance dose. There is no consensus on the need to repeat the liver biopsy to establish histologic improvement. The risk of repeating the biopsy should be weighed against an empirical trial of tapering to a maintenance dose. Patients occasionally can be tapered completely off immunosuppressants, but most patients eventually relapse. For any patient, the risk of life-long therapy must be weighed against the risk of disease recurrence. Most patients can be maintained on a low dose of prednisone alone (<10 mg per day) or in combination with azathioprine (1 mg per kg per day). Recent evidence suggests that high-dose azathioprine (2 mg per kg per day) alone may be just as effective at maintaining remission.

Twenty percent of patients with autoimmune hepatitis fail to respond to immunosuppressive medications. Patients with cirrhosis and those with features of autoimmune hepatitis type IIb are less likely to respond. Patients with refractory disease who test positive for HCV on a second-generation assay or by polymerase chain reaction should be considered for interferon therapy. This group should be monitored closely, as interferon may exacerbate autoimmune hepatitis.

At the time of diagnosis, one-third of patients with autoimmune hepatitis will have established cirrhosis. Patients with bridging necrosis appear to progress to cirrhosis in 5 years without therapy. Immunosuppressive regimens have postponed the progression to end-stage liver failure, even in patients with established cirrhosis. A significant number of patients do progress and develop complications of portal hypertension. These patients should be evaluated for liver transplantation. Although recurrent autoimmune hepatitis has been reported in the liver allograft, the overall post-transplant survival rate is excellent. The risk of hepatocellular carcinoma in autoimmune hepatitis–related cirrhosis does not appear to be as high as the corresponding risk for cirrhosis caused by chronic viral hepatitis.

CHAPTER 65

Alcoholic Liver Disease

INCIDENCE AND EPIDEMIOLOGY

The regular consumption of excessive quantities of ethanol is the most common cause of liver disease in the United States. Alcohol-related liver disease is pathologically classified into three forms: fatty liver (steatosis), alcoholic hepatitis, and cirrhosis. There is considerable overlap among these entities. A liver biopsy may have evidence of all three forms of alcoholic liver disease. Steatosis and hepatitis represent varying degrees of injury but are not requisite for the development of cirrhosis. Steatosis is generally benign, asymptomatic, and reversible with abstinence. Most morbidity and mortality from alcohol-related liver disease are caused by hepatitis and cirrhosis.

Ten percent of men and 5% of women meet the diagnostic criteria of alcoholism or regular ethanol consumption that interferes with health status or social and economic function. Lesser degrees of liver injury occur in most alcoholics—only 20% develop severe chronic liver disease. Clinically significant liver disease is more common in men than women by a 3:1 ratio, and the peak incidence is in the fifth and sixth decades, usually after at least 10 years of heavy alcohol consumption. The amount of alcohol required to produce hepatitis or cirrhosis varies among individuals, but as little as 40 g per day (equivalent to four 12-ounce beers, four 4-ounce glasses of wine, or four 1-ounce servings of 80-proof liquor) for 10 years has been associated with cirrhosis. There is considerable evidence to suggest women require less total alcohol consumption to produce clinically significant liver disease. The regional incidence of alcoholic liver disease correlates with the per capita consumption of alcohol. Therefore, countries such as the United States and France, where excessive alcohol consumption is common, have high rates of alcoholic liver disease.

ETIOLOGY AND PATHOGENESIS

Ethanol Metabolism

The mechanisms by which ethanol and its metabolites induce liver injury remain poorly understood, but current evidence suggests several modes of injury. After ingestion, ethanol undergoes partial first-pass metabolism in the stomach and

TABLE 65-1
Effects of Alcohol on Responses to Administered Medications

Increased drug metabolism
    Barbiturates
    Warfarin
    Sulfonylureas
    Phenytoin
    Methadone
Increased drug tolerance
    Benzodiazepines
    Anesthetics
    Barbiturates
Increased drug toxicity
    Acetaminophen
    Isoniazid
    Halothane
    Carbon tetrachloride
    Methotrexate

liver and is subsequently distributed throughout the extracellular and intracellular water space. Most ethanol is metabolized by hepatic alcohol dehydrogenase (ADH) to acetaldehyde, which is subsequently converted by acetaldehyde dehydrogenase (ALDH) to acetate. ADH is the rate-limiting enzyme, and its activity is decreased in the setting of fasting, protein malnutrition, and chronic liver disease. ADH is not inducible with chronic ethanol ingestion, but several isoforms with disparate rates of ethanol metabolism have been associated with differences in the risk of alcoholism and alcoholic liver disease between different ethnic groups. There are also several ALDH isoforms with differing metabolic rates. Disulfiram (Antabuse) acts by blocking ALDH; the accumulation of acetaldehyde leads to the clinical syndrome of flushing, nausea, and vomiting. Isoforms of ALDH with low activities are common among Asian populations. These patients experience a similar flushing syndrome after consuming ethanol and have low incidences of alcoholism and alcoholic liver disease. A smaller portion of ethanol is oxidized by the cytochrome P-450 2E1 (CYP2E1). This enzyme is inducible by chronic ethanol ingestion and may contribute to the increased rate of ethanol elimination in alcoholics. More important, because CYP2E1 is responsible for the metabolism of other drugs, ethanol can increase or decrease the rate of elimination of some medications (Table 65-1).

The oxidation of ethanol results in increased oxygen consumption and an increased $NADH/NAD^+$ ratio. As a consequence, fatty acid oxidation is inhibited, leading to fat accumulation, which, along with altered protein trafficking and excretion, produces hepatocyte swelling. Increased oxygen demand and compromised sinusoidal blood flow in the setting of hepatocyte swelling may produce relative ischemia, particularly in the pericentral zones. Oxygen free radicals formed as a result of cytochrome P-450 induction may contribute to cellular injury. Acetaldehyde may alter membrane and cytoskeletal elements. It has also been associated with increased collagen production. All of these metabolic alterations probably interact with cytokines (e.g., platelet-derived growth factor, tumor necrosis factor, and interleukins) to produce cell necrosis and fibrosis.

Contributing Mechanisms

Excessive ethanol consumption clearly plays a primary role in the development of alcoholic liver disease, but other factors are important as well. Animal studies and clinical observations of high incidences of malnutrition in alcoholics with liver disease suggest that protein and calorie malnutrition predisposes to alcohol liver disease. Moreover, protein and calorie repletion improves the biochemical profile and possibly survival in patients with alcoholic hepatitis. Despite this evidence, the mechanism of enhanced alcohol injury in the setting of malnutrition is unclear.

Immunologic, hormonal, and other environmental factors may also modulate individual susceptibility to alcohol-induced liver disease. Sex-related differences in susceptibility to ethanol toxicity suggest that estrogens and androgens may play a role. Alcohol may induce immune-mediated injury through influences on suppressor T-lymphocyte function, and acetaldehyde adducts may promote autoantibody production. Up to 30% to 40% of alcoholics with liver disease have chronic viral hepatitis, suggesting that some patients have liver injury that is produced by various causes.

CLINICAL FEATURES

The clinical manifestations of alcoholic liver disease cover a wide spectrum, from the asymptomatic mild hepatomegaly of fatty liver to the hepatic failure of fulminant alcoholic hepatitis or cirrhosis. Although a rare patient may be asymptomatic, patients with alcoholic hepatitis generally experience fever, anorexia, malaise, and abdominal pain. Most have physical examination findings of icterus, tender hepatomegaly, and spider angiomata. Severe cases are accompanied by evidence of portal hypertension, including splenomegaly, ascites, encephalopathy, and enlarged collateral abdominal veins. Although 60% to 70% of patients admitted to the hospital with alcoholic hepatitis have simultaneous cirrhosis on biopsy, portal hypertension may be present in the absence of histologic evidence of cirrhosis.

Patients may present with alcoholic cirrhosis without progressing through the stages of steatosis or clinically significant alcoholic hepatitis. At the time of diagnosis, 10% to 20% of patients with cirrhosis are asymptomatic, but most present with nonspecific complaints of weight loss, malaise, failure to thrive, or complications of portal hypertension (e.g., ascites, spontaneous bacterial peritonitis, variceal hemorrhage, and hepatic encephalopathy). Patients with all forms of alcoholic liver disease, especially alcoholic hepatitis and cirrhosis, often have stigmata of alcoholism, including palmar erythema, Dupuytren's contracture, testicular atrophy, gynecomastia, and loss of the male pattern of body hair.

FINDINGS ON DIAGNOSTIC TESTING

Laboratory Studies

Alcoholic liver disease is characterized by distinctive alterations in serum biochemical profiles. Even in the most severe episodes of alcoholic hepatitis with extensive hepatocyte necrosis and hepatic failure, the serum aminotransferase levels are only modestly elevated, typically to <300 IU per liter. Peak levels of >500 IU per liter should prompt the search for alternative or confounding causes of liver disease, such as viral hepatitis, acetaminophen toxicity, or ischemia. The pattern of elevation is also helpful in distinguishing alcohol injury in >90% of patients whose aspartate aminotransferase (AST) levels exceed alanine aminotransferase (ALT) levels. A ratio of AST to ALT of >2 is highly predictive of ethanol liver disease but may occur only in 60% to 80% of patients. A small subset of alcoholic hepatitis patients may demonstrate a predominantly cholestatic biochemical profile, with marked elevations of bilirubin and alkaline phosphatase levels and normal to minimally elevated aminotransferase levels. Although most patients with cirrhosis have abnormal liver chemistry values, patients with well-compensated cirrhosis who abstain from ethanol may have near normal laboratory values.

Patients with alcoholic liver disease often have abnormalities of other laboratory profiles that are caused by liver disease or the toxic effects of ethanol. Macrocytosis is common. It usually is caused by the toxic effects of ethanol, and occasionally by deficiencies of folate or vitamin B_{12}. Anemia and thrombocytopenia may be manifestations of ethanol toxicity, vitamin deficiency, or sequestration caused by splenomegaly. A prolonged prothrombin time and decreased serum albumin level may indicate severe liver dysfunction with compromised synthetic capacity, but nutritional deficiencies can produce similar abnormalities. Active alcoholics may exhibit ketoacidosis, hypophosphatemia, and hypomagnesemia.

Liver Biopsy

The classification of alcoholic liver disease into fatty liver, alcoholic hepatitis, and cirrhosis is based on clinical and pathologic correlations; therefore, confirmation of these abnormalities and exclusion of alternative causes of liver disease require liver biopsy. In patients with only mild steatosis or in patients with coagulopathy, the risk of biopsy may outweigh the benefit of obtaining pathologic confirmation. The decision to proceed with a biopsy should be individualized. Fatty liver or steatosis is characterized by large intracytoplasmic fat droplets often concentrated in the pericentral zone or zone 3 of Rappaport. By definition, simple steatosis is not accompanied by significant inflammation or necrosis, but pericentral fibrosis, a network of collagen surrounding the central vein, may be observed and is possibly a precursor of cirrhosis. In contrast, inflammation and hepatocellular necrosis is the hallmark of alcoholic hepatitis. The inflammatory infiltrate is primarily neutrophilic, and necrosis may range from ballooning degeneration of isolated hepatocytes to confluent centrilobular necrosis. Pericentral fibrosis is common, and up to 60% to 70% of hospitalized patients have associated cirrhosis. The diagnosis of cirrhosis, the final stage alcoholic liver disease, requires documentation of the presence of bands of fibrosis extending between portal tracts and central veins as well as regenerative nodules.

There is no pathognomonic histologic feature of alcoholic liver disease. The diagnosis requires the synthesis of clinical and pathologic information. Mallory's hyaline bodies are aggregates of perinuclear eosinophilic material once thought to be diagnostic of alcohol-induced injury. They are present in at least 30% of patients with alcoholic hepatitis or cirrhosis, but they are also present in other liver disorders, including Wilson's disease, nonalcoholic steatohepatitis, postintestinal bypass hepatitis, and chronic hepatitis C. Alcoholic cirrhosis may be difficult to differentiate from primary hemochromatosis because of the high levels of hepatic iron in alcoholics. These disorders can be distinguished by calculating the iron index: the micromoles of iron per gram of dry liver divided by the patient's age. In hemochromatosis, the iron index is >2, and in alcoholic cirrhosis, it is invariably <2. Alcoholic cirrhosis may be compounded by the coexistence of other liver disorders, particularly hepatitis C, which is present in up to 40% of alcoholics with liver disease.

Structural Studies

Hepatobiliary imaging is often necessary to exclude biliary obstruction or mass lesions as a cause of cholestasis or hepatomegaly. Ultrasound and computed tomographic scanning may demonstrate diffuse or focal fatty infiltration in the setting of steatosis. Alcoholic liver disease often produces nonspecific inhomogeneous ultrasonographic or tomographic patterns, but cirrhosis may exhibit a characteristic nodular pattern. Endoscopic retrograde cholangiopancreatography or percutaneous transhepatic cholangiography may be necessary to exclude bile duct obstruction in patients with a cholestatic pattern of liver chemistry values. Alcoholic liver disease generally does not produce significant bile duct abnormalities, but gallstones are present in up to 30% of patients with alcoholic cirrhosis.

MANAGEMENT AND COURSE

The prognosis of alcoholic liver disease is mainly determined by the pathologic stage at presentation and the patient's ability to abstain from ethanol consumption. The single most important therapeutic intervention is the complete avoidance of ethanol consumption. This often requires a multidisciplinary approach, involving social workers, psychiatrists, primary care physicians, hepatologists, and, most important, social support groups. No therapy for alcoholic liver disease has any proven benefit in the setting of continued heavy drinking.

Alcoholic Steatosis

Alcoholic fatty liver is generally benign and completely resolves after 3 to 6 weeks of abstinence. Patients with pericentral fibrosis may be more likely to develop cirrhosis. The major clinical importance of fatty liver lies in the clinician's ability to recognize significant alcohol-related end-organ damage and to counsel patients to abstain before more severe or irreversible damage ensues.

Alcoholic Hepatitis

In the first 2 weeks after hospitalization for alcoholic hepatitis, there is often a decline in hepatic function and an increase in serum bilirubin levels despite enforced abstinence from ethanol. Hospital mortality rates range from 15% to 28%. Patients with encephalopathy, renal failure, ascites, and variceal bleeding exhibit higher mortalities. Several methods of predicting disease severity and survival have incorporated clinical and laboratory findings, but the most accurate and widely used is Maddrey's discriminant function:

$$\text{serum bilirubin (mg/dl)} + [4.6 \times (\text{patient's prothrombin time} - \text{control prothrombin time})]$$

A discriminant function of >32 identifies patients with severe alcoholic hepatitis who have a mortality rate of >50%.

The management of alcoholic hepatitis centers on abstinence. Eighty percent of patients who continue to drink will develop cirrhosis, with a 5-year survival rate of <50%. In contrast, 70% of patients abstinent from alcohol will have resolution of hepatitis, and only 15% will progress to cirrhosis. Patients and clinicians should recognize that clinical improvement occurs gradually over several months to 1 year before a plateau or new steady state is reached.

The possible contribution of protein and calorie malnutrition to alcohol toxicity has led to several trials of enteral and parenteral nutritional supplementation for the treatment of patients with alcoholic hepatitis. These supplements result in accelerated biochemical improvement, but only one study demonstrated improved survival. Patients do not have higher incidences of encephalopathy. Specialized formulas of branched-chain amino acids are not superior to standard formulas. Patients with alcoholic hepatitis should at least have their calorie intake monitored and supplemented if deficient. Aggressive enteral or parenteral supplementation may be warranted if oral intake is inadequate.

Corticosteroids have been used to reduce the inflammatory response associated with alcoholic hepatitis. Several studies have demonstrated improved survival in patients with a discriminant function of >32 or with spontaneous encephalopathy. One study used prednisone, 40 mg per day for 4 weeks, which produced a 2-month survival rate of 88%, compared with 45% for placebo. These studies usually exclude patients with ongoing bacterial infection or gastrointestinal hemorrhage. In addition, there is often a 1- to 2-week interval between hospitalization and initiation of treatment, suggesting that these populations represent a selected group.

Anabolic steroids and propylthiouracil have shown some promise in treating alcoholic hepatitis, but these medications are not widely used. Further controlled studies may prove their efficacy.

Alcoholic Cirrhosis

As with all forms of alcoholic liver disease, long-term survival of patients with alcoholic cirrhosis is directly related to the stage of the disease and the patient's ability to abstain from ethanol consumption. In cirrhotic patients without jaundice, ascites, or gastrointestinal hemorrhage, 5-year survival rates are 85% with abstinence and 60% with continued heavy drinking. In patients with jaundice or ascites, the 5-year survival rates are 50% with abstinence and 30% with continued drinking. Cirrhotic patients with variceal hemorrhage have the worst prognosis: 5-year survival rates of 35% and 20% in nondrinkers and drinkers, respectively.

Similar to other forms of cirrhosis, treatment is largely supportive. Chronic diuretics are often necessary to correct the total body sodium overload that contributes to ascites and edema formation. Patients with prior variceal hemorrhage have lower risks of rebleeding with endoscopic obliteration of varices. The β-adrenergic antagonist propranolol reduces the risk of bleeding in patients with large varices or portal gastropathy. Encephalopathy is best treated with lactulose, titrated to produce two to three stools per day.

Therapy directed at halting the fibrotic and regenerative processes of cirrhosis has been disappointing. Corticosteroids do not improve survival and have a high incidence of side effects. There is evidence suggesting colchicine improves outcome in alcoholic cirrhosis.

Liver transplantation should be considered for patients who have abstained for several months but continue to suffer from complications of portal hypertension. Although guidelines vary from center to center, at least several months of abstinence are usually required before a transplantation is performed. This period of abstinence serves to select candidates who will probably have low rates of recidivism. Also, it allows for potential improvement in liver function to a condition that may not warrant transplantation. Patients may be referred to a transplant center before completing this prolonged period of abstinence. The many months of waiting on a list of potential recipients often serves as the abstinence period. With appropriate patient selection, the 2-year survival rate after transplantation is 70% to 80%; <10% of patients return to alcoholism.

CHAPTER 66

Cirrhosis, Portal Hypertension, and End-Stage Liver Disease

The treatment of cirrhosis is largely supportive. Interventions mainly target the complications of portal hypertension. The use of orthotopic liver transplantation has grown exponentially. It has become a more definitive therapeutic option for patients and clinicians. The decision to pursue liver transplantation is complex and requires a multidisciplinary approach. Complications of cirrhosis and portal hypertension are the most common indications for orthotopic liver transplantation.

ETIOLOGY AND PATHOGENESIS

Cirrhosis

Cirrhosis represents the final common pathway of many hepatic disorders characterized by chronic cellular destruction. An intervening stage of increased fibrosis is followed by formation of parenchymal regenerative nodules. It is the nodular distortion of the lobules and vascular network that defines cirrhosis and ultimately plays a critical role in the development of portal hypertension. The cellular and biochemical events leading to this altered growth response and resulting architectural distortion are not well characterized.

TABLE 66-1
Causes of Cirrhosis

Common
    Ethanol
    Chronic hepatitis C
    Chronic hepatitis B with or without hepatitis D
Infrequent
    Primary biliary cirrhosis
    Primary sclerosing cholangitis
    Secondary biliary cirrhosis
    Autoimmune hepatitis
    Hemochromatosis
    Cryptogenic cirrhosis
Rare
    Wilson's disease
    α_1-Antitrypsin deficiency
    Small bowel bypass
    Methotrexate
    Amiodarone
    Methyldopa
    Cystic fibrosis
    Sarcoidosis
    Glycogen storage disease
    Hypervitaminosis A

Cirrhosis is often classified according to the gross pattern of architectural distortion: micronodular cirrhosis and macronodular cirrhosis. Alcoholic cirrhosis is typically micronodular; uniformly sized parenchymal nodules are separated by thin bands of connective tissue. The cirrhosis that evolves from the bridging necrosis of severe chronic viral hepatitis is often macronodular, characterized by nodules measuring up to several centimeters separated by asymmetric, thick bands of connective tissue. This classification has limited clinical use because many disease processes present with either variant. Also, micronodular cirrhosis may transform into macronodular cirrhosis. It is not known if there is a difference in the natural history of these pathologic variants of cirrhosis.

A more clinically relevant method of classifying cirrhosis is based on the primary disease processes responsible for hepatocellular injury (Table 66-1). In the United States, most cases of cirrhosis are related to alcoholic liver disease and chronic viral hepatitis. In urban settings, 75% of cirrhosis is alcohol related. Other common causes of cirrhosis include hereditary hemochromatosis, primary and secondary biliary cirrhosis, and autoimmune hepatitis. Several rare disorders that frequently are complicated by cirrhosis should always be considered in the differential diagnosis. These include Wilson's disease, α_1-antitrypsin deficiency, and hypervitaminosis A. In certain clinical settings, a metabolic or toxic form of cirrhosis may develop. For example, cirrhosis may occur years after small bowel bypass surgery, possibly secondary to increased serum concentrations of bacterial endotoxins or toxic bile acids resulting from bacterial overgrowth. Medications such as nitrofurantoin, amiodarone, and methotrexate may produce chronic hepatitis and cirrhosis. Cirrhosis in childhood can be caused by tyrosinemia, galactosemia, α_1-antitrypsin deficiency, Wilson's disease, glycogen storage disease, cystic fibrosis, arteriohepatic dysphasia, and idiopathic neonatal hepatitis. When all of the causes of cirrhosis listed above are excluded, the patient probably has idiopathic (cryptogenic) cirrhosis. This disorder may be the result of an immunologic or viral disease process that cannot be detected by serologic assays. Cryptogenic cirrhosis may account for 10% to 20% of all patients with cirrhosis; it is clinically indistinguishable from the other common causes.

Portal Hypertension

Pressure gradients in the portal circulation follow Ohm's law, which states the pressure gradient is equal to the product of flow and resistance. Portal hypertension occurs if there is increased splanchnic flow or increased resistance in the hepatic vasculature. In cirrhosis, both mechanisms contribute to the development of portal hypertension. Nodular regeneration and fibrosis in the space of Disse increase postsinusoidal and sinusoidal resistance, respectively. Cirrhosis is also accompanied by increased splanchnic flow resulting from decreased tone in the splanchnic arterioles. The mechanisms responsible for splanchnic arteriolar vasodilation are poorly understood but may involve glucagon or nitric oxide. With extrahepatic causes of portal hypertension, such as portal vein thrombosis or massive splenomegaly, either increased resistance or increased flow is the principal mechanism of increased portal pressures. The anatomic site of increased flow or resistance has been used to classify portal hypertension into prehepatic, intrahepatic, and posthepatic portal hypertension (Table 66-2). Intrahepatic causes are often further subdivided into presinusoidal, sinusoidal, and postsinusoidal according to the site of increased resistance. This subclassification is limited because many forms of cirrhosis may involve more than one site of vascular distortion in relationship to the sinusoids.

CLINICAL FEATURES

Although patients with early cirrhosis may be asymptomatic, the most ubiquitous feature of cirrhosis is a general decline in health with nonspecific complaints of anorexia, weight loss, malaise, fatigue, and weakness. More advanced disease may present with one of the complications of portal hypertension.

Endocrine Manifestations

Patients with cirrhosis may manifest several endocrine disturbances. The prevalence of diabetes mellitus is increased in all forms of cirrhosis but particularly in patients with hemochromatosis and alcoholic liver disease. Hypogonadism in males and females is also common in hemochromatosis and alcoholic liver disease, primarily because of the direct gonadal toxicities of iron and alcohol, respectively. In addition, androgenic steroids may bypass metabolism in the liver and subsequently undergo conversion in adipose tissue to the estrogenic steroid estrone. Increased plasma estrogen levels may lead to gynecomastia and palmar erythema.

TABLE 66-2
Classification and Differential Diagnosis of Portal Hypertension

Prehepatic causes
    Portal vein thrombosis
    Splenic vein thrombosis
    Arterioportal fistula
    Splenomegaly
Intrahepatic causes
    Cirrhosis
    Fulminant hepatitis
    Veno-occlusive disease
    Budd-Chiari syndrome
    Schistosomiasis
    Metastatic malignancy
Posthepatic causes
    Right ventricular failure
    Constrictive pericarditis
    Inferior vena cava web

Pulmonary Manifestations

End-stage liver disease is often accompanied by pulmonary disorders. Chronic hyperventilation is probably caused by the same central nervous system alterations responsible for hepatic encephalopathy. Patients may have hypoxemia because of mismatches of ventilation and perfusion induced by ascites, which restricts the ventilation of dependent lung spaces. Alternatively, arteriovenous malformations in the lung may result in right-to-left shunting with associated hypoxia. Rarely, patients present with pulmonary hypertension or a distinct form of right-to-left shunting termed the *hepatopulmonary syndrome* that is potentially reversible with transplantation. Patients with or without ascites may develop a transudative pleural effusion termed *hepatic hydrothorax,* which may embarrass respiratory function. Hydrothorax probably develops from ascites traversing pores in the diaphragm. The onset of hepatic hydrothorax often signals a rapid clinical deterioration.

Renal Manifestations

Although numerous disturbances of sodium and water homeostasis are observed in cirrhosis, the most devastating complication is renal failure caused by the hepatorenal syndrome. Hepatorenal syndrome refers to rapidly progressive oliguric renal failure unrelated to other known causes. It is associated with extreme intrarenal vasoconstriction that leads to sodium retention. Potential precipitants include intravascular volume depletion from hemorrhage, diuretics, or paracentesis. Alternative causes of renal failure include acute tubular necrosis caused by hypovolemia, aminoglycosides, or radiocontrast agents. These disorders can often be distinguished from hepatorenal syndrome on the basis of a normal or elevated urine sodium concentration. Pulmonary artery catheter placement should be considered because it facilitates optimal management of volume status. Hepatorenal syndrome usually is irreversible without transplantation.

FINDINGS ON DIAGNOSTIC TESTING

Laboratory Studies

Liver chemistry values are obtained in essentially all patients with suspected liver disease or portal hypertension, but the patterns and degrees of abnormality are variable and are determined by the primary disorder. Notably, patients with pathologic evidence of cirrhosis may have a normal biochemical profile. Coagulation profiles, complete blood counts, electrolytes, and albumin should all be obtained. Patients with advanced cirrhosis will have prolongation of the prothrombin time and a decrease in serum albumin levels because of impaired hepatic synthetic function. Protein malnutrition and vitamin K deficiency, which are particularly common in alcoholics, may also produce these abnormalities. Patients with portal hypertension may have thrombocytopenia, anemia, or leukopenia on the basis of congestive hypersplenism. Thrombocytopenia resulting from splenic sequestration rarely is <50,000 per µl; lower levels suggest an alternative diagnosis, such as drug-induced, immune-mediated, or disseminated intravascular coagulation–associated thrombocytopenia. In addition to splenic sequestration, anemia may result from gastrointestinal hemorrhage, nutritional deficiencies (e.g., folate, iron, or vitamin B_{12}), or hemolysis. Hyponatremia, hypokalemia, and renal insufficiency are common complications of the altered renal hemodynamics and sodium and water homeostasis observed in cirrhosis.

An accurate determination of the cause of cirrhosis requires a serologic evaluation, the extent of which is largely dictated by the clinical setting. The initial screen should include serum assays for antibody to hepatitis C, antibodies to hepatitis B core antigen and surface antigen, hepatitis B surface antigen, antimitochondrial antibodies, antinuclear antibodies, anti–smooth muscle antibodies, ferritin, transferrin, total iron-binding capacity, and serum protein electrophoresis to measure the α_1 band. Patients younger than age 50 years should be screened for Wilson's disease with an assay of serum ceruloplasmin. In the second stage, selected patients may require specialized studies—for example, polymerase chain reaction can detect hepatitis C viral RNA, serum hepatitis B DNA, α_1-antitrypsin phenotyping, or anti–liver-kidney microsomal antibodies.

Structural Studies

Imaging procedures are often helpful in providing evidence of cirrhosis or portal hypertension. Upper gastrointestinal endoscopy permits detection of varices or portal hypertensive gastropathy but does not allow differentiation of cirrhosis from other causes of portal hypertension. Ultrasound and computed tomographic (CT) studies may demonstrate a lobular, heterogeneous hepatic parenchyma or findings attributable to portal hypertension, including ascites, splenomegaly, and portosystemic collaterals. Standard ultrasound and CT scanning are insensitive modalities for detecting varices, but Doppler ultrasound may demonstrate portal vein thrombosis or hepatofugal flow. ^{99m}Tc–sulfur colloid scintigraphy is a noninvasive means of assessing liver size and blood flow. A heterogeneous pattern of uptake in the liver and increased uptake in the spleen and bone marrow, which is termed a *colloid shift*, are suggestive of but not diagnostic of cirrhosis. Angiography and magnetic resonance imaging may help exclude primary vascular causes of portal hypertension, including the hepatic vein thrombosis of Budd-Chiari syndrome and portal vein thrombosis. Patients with suspected secondary biliary cirrhosis should undergo endoscopic retrograde cholangiopancreatography.

Liver Biopsy

Liver biopsy is the only definitive means of diagnosing cirrhosis and often provides clues to the underlying cause. Liver biopsy also can be used to quantify iron and copper if hemochromatosis or Wilson's disease is in the differential diagnosis. In the setting of coagulopathy, the risks of biopsy-associated hemorrhage often outweigh the benefit of obtaining information provided on biopsy, but angiographically guided transjugular biopsy may be performed if histologic confirmation is deemed critical.

Portal Venous Pressure Measurement

Although rarely needed in clinical practice, direct and indirect measurements of portal pressure are the definitive means of diagnosing portal hypertension. The indirect method involves angiographically positioning a balloon occlusion catheter in the hepatic vein and, with the balloon inflated, measuring the hepatic vein wedge pressure. Analogous to the pulmonary capillary wedge pressure, the hepatic vein wedge pressure measures sinusoidal pressure and is an estimate of portal pressure. It is inaccurate if the causes of portal hypertension are presinusoidal or prehepatic because the major pressure gradient is upstream from the sinusoids. The difference in hepatic vein wedge pressure and the free hepatic vein pressure provides an estimate of the portosystemic gradient, or the pressure drop across the resistance bed of the liver. A portosystemic gradient of >5 mm Hg is consistent with portal hypertension, whereas a gradient of >12 mm Hg identifies patients at risk for variceal hemorrhage. Direct measurement of pressure in the portal circulation is achieved with transhepatic placement of a pressure transducer in the portal vein. The risk of bleeding from the transhepatic approach prohibits the routine use of this procedure.

MANAGEMENT AND COURSE

Management of Ascites

The approach to patients with ascites is detailed in Chapter 17.

Management of Variceal Hemorrhage

Any form of portal hypertension can lead to the formation of portosystemic collaterals. The major sites of collateral formation are through the umbilical vein, producing abdominal wall collaterals; through the superior rectal vein to the middle and inferior rectal vein, producing rectal varices; and through the coronary and left gastric veins to the azygos vein, producing gastroesophageal varices. Collaterals may form in numerous other sites within the abdomen, but hemorrhage from gastroesophageal varices is the primary cause of morbidity from portosystemic collaterals.

The formation of varices is closely related to portal pressures. Below a threshold portosystemic gradient of 12 mm Hg, varices are not encountered, but for unclear reasons, many patients with pressures above this level never develop varices. Bleeding occurs in 30% of patients with varices, but variables for identifying patients at high risk are less than perfect. Absolute portal pressures above the threshold of 12 mm Hg do not correlate well with the risk of bleeding, but the endoscopic size of varices does seem to indicate the patients at highest risk. Variceal hemorrhage is associated with a 50% mortality rate, and without subsequent preventive treatment, the risk of rebleeding is nearly 70%. These high morbidity and rebleeding rates have led to several interventions for the treatment of acute bleeding as well as the prevention of initial or recurrent variceal hemorrhage.

Primary prevention of acute variceal hemorrhage has been directed to patients with large varices on upper gastrointestinal endoscopy. Nonselective β-adrenergic antagonists (e.g., propranolol and nadolol) reduce the rate of bleeding in alcoholic patients with large varices. Propranolol should be initiated at 10 to 20 mg twice daily and titrated to a 25% decrease in resting heart rate. Contraindications include bradycardia, hypotension, congestive heart failure, reactive airway disease, and peripheral vascular disease. Although other more invasive interventions have been studied, β-adrenergic antagonists are the only therapy recommended for the primary prevention of variceal bleeding.

Acute variceal hemorrhage from esophageal or gastric varices represents a medical emergency. Patients should be managed in the intensive care setting; volume resuscitation and optimizing the hemodynamic status are the first priorities. Nonvariceal hemorrhage may account for up to 50% of gastrointestinal bleeding episodes in patients with known cirrhosis. Therefore, early upper gastrointestinal endoscopy is needed to confirm the source of bleeding. Injection sclerotherapy of varices is the procedure of choice for controlling acute variceal bleeding, with success rates approaching 90%. Complications of sclerotherapy include esophageal ulceration, pneumonia, and bacteremia. The recent development of endoscopic band ligation may replace sclerotherapy in the acute and chronic treatment of gastroesophageal varices. Band ligation seems to have a superior side effect profile and is at least as effective as sclerotherapy.

Continuous infusion of vasopressin (0.1 to 0.4 units per minute) may provide control of acute hemorrhage, but 50% of patients fail to respond and side effects of systemic vasoconstriction, including myocardial and cerebral ischemia, are common. Vasopressin therapy should be limited to less than 24 to 48 hours. Coadministration of nitrates may reduce systemic vasoconstriction and lead to improved control of hemorrhage. Continuous infusion of the somatostatin analog octreotide (25–50 µg per hour for 24 to 48 hours) is equivalent to or superior to vasopressin. It does not cause systemic vasoconstriction. In one trial, octreotide was as effective as endoscopic sclerotherapy in controlling acute hemorrhage. Octreotide probably reduces splanchnic blood flow by inhibiting the vasodilating hormones (e.g., glucagon).

If bleeding persists despite the above measures, balloon tamponade is often used. Balloon tamponade is up to 90% effective in stopping variceal hemorrhage, but it is only a temporizing measure. Adverse effects are common and include esophageal rupture and aspirations. Tamponade should never be continued for longer than 24 to 36 hours. Endotracheal intubation should be performed before balloon insertion to prevent airway compromise.

In refractory or recurrent variceal hemorrhage, portosystemic shunting should be considered by transjugular intrahepatic portosystemic shunt (TIPS) or a surgically created shunt. Although both procedures are highly effective in controlling hemorrhage, encephalopathy results in 10% to 20% of patients. The lower morbidity and less invasive nature associated with TIPS make it the logical choice in this setting, but institutional experience and availability may vary.

After acute variceal bleeding has been stopped, secondary prophylactic interventions lower the risk of rebleeding. The only therapy that improves survival is endoscopic sclerotherapy. Complete obliteration of varices is the goal, and several sessions separated by 1 to 2 weeks are often required. Endoscopic band ligation appears to be equally effective and has a more favorable side effect profile. Once the varices are obliterated, endoscopic surveillance to detect recurrence is usually performed annually or biannually. Pharmacotherapy with the nonselective β-adrenergic antagonists propranolol or nadolol also reduces the rate of rebleeding but does not appear to improve survival. Combination therapy with long-acting nitrates may be as effective as sclerotherapy. Many clinicians use propranolol as an adjuvant means of preventing rebleeding over the interval of several weeks that is usually required to achieve endoscopic obliteration of varices.

Although portosystemic shunt surgery reduces the rate of rebleeding, it has largely been abandoned as a means of secondary prophylaxis because of the high incidence of debilitating encephalopathy and the lack of any survival advantage over less invasive therapies. However, patients with normal or near normal hepatic function may be better served with definitive surgical therapy. The distal splenorenal shunt is the favored procedure owing to lower rates of encephalopathy.

The development of TIPS has added a new dimension to the armamentarium of therapies for secondary prophylaxis of variceal bleeding. Although TIPS clearly has a role in patients with hemorrhage refractory to endoscopic therapy, its role as an initial means of secondary prophylaxis remains to be established. Reports suggest that TIPS improves rebleeding rates compared with endoscopic therapy, but high resource utilization, frequent high rates of encephalopathy, limited availability, and a lack of improved survival may prohibit the widespread use of this procedure.

Management of Hepatic Encephalopathy

The mechanism for the development of encephalopathy in severe liver disease remains ill defined. A possible explanation may be a disturbance of central neurotransmission resulting from an accumulation of false neurotransmitters that activate γ-aminobutyric acid receptors. Although serum ammonia is often elevated in hepatic encephalopathy, some cases exhibit normal ammonia levels.

Hepatic encephalopathy is often graded according to the patient's level of consciousness. Grade I is defined as subtle cognitive deficits with a normal level of arousal. In grade II, asterixis appears, speech is slow, and lethargy is present. Grade III is characterized by an obtunded but arousable patient, whereas grade IV is represented by a comatose, unarousable patient.

New-onset hepatic encephalopathy or acute decompensation of chronic hepatic encephalopathy should always prompt a search for precipitating causes. Common causes include gastrointestinal hemorrhage, psychotropic medications, electrolyte disturbances, infection, new-onset renal insufficiency, constipation, and medical or dietary noncompliance. In addition to providing specific therapy for hepatic encephalopathy, the clinician should always attempt to correct the precipitating factors.

Because many of the responsible neurotoxins appear to be produced by intestinal flora, therapy is directed at altering the colonic microenvironment. Lactulose, titrated to produce two to three soft stools per day, is the first-line therapy. Higher doses serve only to cause diarrhea, with possible fluid and electrolyte disturbances. The antibiotics metronidazole or neomycin may be added to treat refractory hepatic encephalopathy. Given the high incidence of protein malnutrition in cirrhotics, protein restriction should be reserved for grade III and IV encephalopathies.

Orthotopic Liver Transplantation

The decision to perform orthotopic liver transplantation mostly depends on the expected survival of the patient with end-stage liver disease. Several prognostic indicators have been developed, but the most commonly used method is the Child-Turcotte-Pugh classification (Table 66-3), which was initially developed to predict survival after variceal hemorrhage. The 3-year survival rate for patients with Child-Turcotte-Pugh class C disease is 30%, whereas the corresponding survival rate for patients in Child-Turcotte-Pugh class A may exceed 90%. Three-year survival rates for class B patients are intermediate and average 50% to 60%. Because orthotopic liver transplantation has a 1-year mortality rate of 10% to 20%, patients at Child-Turcotte-Pugh stage A are better served with medical therapy. Conversely, the post-transplant 3-year survival is >60% in several centers. Patients in Child-Turcotte-Pugh class C clearly benefit from transplantation. Appropriation of patients in stage B is less well defined and is largely determined by individual circumstances. The benefit of orthotopic liver transplantation for any person must be weighed against specific clinical indications such as spontaneous bacterial peritonitis, intractable ascites, refractory encephalopathy, recurrent variceal bleeding, or debilitating fatigue.

Pretransplant evaluation should include an assessment for contraindications and an evaluation for factors that may complicate the post-transplant period. Absolute contraindications include human immunodeficiency virus infection, extrahepatic or metastatic malignancy, active infection, and severe cardiopulmonary disease. Relative contraindications include active ethanol abuse, active hepatitis B infection, previous malignancy, and diabetes mellitus with end-organ damage. Chronologic age is not a contraindication, but patients older than 70 years are rarely acceptable candidates for orthotopic liver transplantation. The evaluation usually includes ultrasound with portal vein Doppler examination, cardiac stress testing, serologic testing for herpes viruses (e.g., cytomegalovirus, herpes simplex virus, varicella-zoster virus), serum α-fetoprotein, and tuberculosis skin testing. Women require a Papanicolaou smear. Women older than 40 years should undergo mammography. Investigation of a patient's social support system is critical and requires the input of a trained social worker. Dental and psychiatric evaluation may be necessary in select patients. The complex decision to approve a patient for orthotopic liver transplantation requires the input of several disciplines. This multidisciplinary approach should consider the medical and social implications of transplantation as well as the limited availability of donor organs and the long pretransplant waiting period.

TABLE 66-3
Child-Turcotte-Pugh Classification System

PROTHROMBIN TIME	BILIRUBIN	ALBUMIN	ASCITES	ENCEPHALOPATHY	SCORE
0–4 seconds above control	0–2.0 mg/dl	>3.5 mg/dl	Absent	Absent	1
4–6 seconds above control	2.0–3.0 mg/dl	2.8–3.5 mg/dl	Nontense	Grade I–II	2
>6 seconds above control	>3.0 mg/dl	0–2.8 mg/dl	Tense	Grade III–IV	3

Class A = 5–6 points; class B = 7–9 points; class C = 10–15 points.

CHAPTER 67

Primary Hepatic Neoplasms

HEPATOCELLULAR CARCINOMA

Incidence and Epidemiology

Worldwide, hepatocellular carcinoma is among the most common causes of cancer death. There is tremendous regional variation in incidence of hepatocellular carcinoma. Extremely high rates are seen in sub-Saharan Africa, Southeast Asia, Japan, and Korea. Intermediate rates are observed in Singapore, Native Americans, and portions of South America. Hepatocellular carcinoma is uncommon in the United States; the incidence is one-tenth the rate of many countries in Southeast Asia. Nonetheless, hepatocellular carcinoma accounts for 12,000 deaths per year in the United States. This regional variation in the incidence of hepatocellular carcinoma is closely related to regional variations in the prevalence of chronic hepatitis B infection and circulating hepatitis B surface antigen (Table 67-1). Hepatocellular carcinoma also has an epidemiologic link with chronic hepatitis C infection. All forms of cirrhosis are associated with an increased risk of hepatocellular carcinoma, but the risk is particularly high in patients with cirrhosis secondary to chronic viral infection. Hepatocellular carcinoma has occasionally been observed to complicate chronic viral hepatitis before the development of cirrhosis. Of the 90% of patients with hepatocellular carcinoma who have coexistent cirrhosis, there is consistently a male predominance, and in the United States, the male-to-female ratio is >2:1.

Other environmental exposures associated with hepatocellular carcinoma include Thorotrast, the radioactive contrast medium used in radiologic procedures between 1920 and 1950. Long-term exposure to vinyl chloride and estrogenic and androgenic steroids have also been associated with an increased incidence of hepatocellular carcinoma. The epidemiologic association with anabolic steroids appears more sound than the association with estrogen use and may partially explain the male-to-female ratio in hepatocellular carcinoma. Aflatoxin B1, a toxic metabolite of an *Aspergillus* species that often contaminates grains and nuts, has been demographically linked to hepatocellular carcinoma.

TABLE 67-1
Risk Factors for Development of Hepatocellular Carcinoma

Chronic hepatitis B infection
Chronic hepatitis C infection
Hemochromatosis
Tyrosinemia
All causes of cirrhosis
Thorotrast
Vinyl chloride
Anabolic steroids
Estrogens
Aflatoxin B1

At least a portion of the geographic variation in hepatocellular carcinoma rates may be related to differences in levels of aflatoxin B1 in food.

Etiology and Pathogenesis

Although the precise molecular mechanisms of hepatocellular carcinogenesis are not fully understood, hepatocellular carcinoma probably results from activation of proto-oncogenes and deactivation of tumor suppressor genes. Genetic injury may result from a variety of sources. Perhaps the best described is random integration of the hepatitis B virus (HBV) genome into the host genome. Although hepatitis C virus is an RNA virus and does not have the same direct mutagenic capacity as HBV, any chronic inflammatory state can generate free radicals capable of inducing genetic injury. Similarly, the regenerative response in cirrhosis may lead to chromosomal rearrangements that foster unrestrained proliferation. For reasons that remain poorly defined, some forms of cirrhosis, such as hemochromatosis and tyrosinemia, have exceptionally high incidences of hepatocellular carcinoma, whereas other diseases, such as Wilson's disease and autoimmune hepatitis, have exceptionally low incidences of hepatocellular carcinoma. Further characterization of the cellular and genetic events leading to hepatocellular carcinoma may clarify these discrepancies.

Clinical Features

Ninety percent of patients with hepatocellular carcinoma have superimposed cirrhosis. The clinical presentations of hepatocellular carcinoma may be subtle; many of the presenting signs and symptoms are often mistakenly attributed to coexisting cirrhosis. Nonspecific symptoms of fatigue, anorexia, weight loss, and jaundice are common. Patients may complain of right upper quadrant pain or increasing abdominal girth. Hepatocellular carcinoma may cause well-compensated cirrhosis to become decompensated, with progressive ascites, encephalopathy, jaundice, or hemorrhage. Occasionally, patients with poorly differentiated tumors present with protracted fever and, rarely, with the paraneoplastic syndrome of hypertrophic osteoarthropathy. On physical examination, most patients exhibit hepatomegaly or a discrete mass. As many as 10% of patients with hepatocellular carcinoma present with an acute abdomen resulting from tumor rupture and hemoperitoneum. This has led to the recommendation that clinicians exercise caution in examining the abdomen of patients who may have hepatocellular carcinoma. Most patients have sequelae of chronic liver disease, including spider angiomata, gynecomastia, and palmar erythema.

Findings on Diagnostic Testing

Laboratory Studies

Patients presenting with hepatocellular carcinoma as their first manifestation of chronic liver disease should have a complete serologic evaluation to determine the cause of cirrhosis. Aminotransferase levels are often mildly elevated but they can be normal; levels are determined by the underlying liver disease. Alkaline phosphatase levels may be particularly elevated if the tumor assumes an infiltrative pattern. In advanced tumors, serum bilirubin levels may be markedly elevated owing to compromised hepatocellular reserve or, less commonly, extrahepatic bile duct obstruction. Other laboratory abnormalities observed in hepatocellular carcinoma include rare instances of paraneoplastic hypercalcemia and erythrocytosis. Large tumors have been associated with hypoglycemia of uncertain cause.

Tumor Markers

Hepatocellular carcinoma is associated with several serum tumor markers. The marker most often used is serum α-fetoprotein (AFP), the glycosylated protein expressed in proliferating fetal hepatocytes. After the first year of life, AFP levels decrease to <10 ng per ml, but several chronic inflammatory states, including viral hepatitis, are associated with AFP elevations to 10 to 100 ng per ml. Although chronic hepatitis in the setting of cirrhosis may be associated with levels in the hundreds, levels of >400 ng per ml usually are caused by hepatocellular carcinoma. A level of AFP of >1000 ng per ml associated with a liver mass is essentially diagnostic of hepatocellular carcinoma. Unfortunately, AFP is only elevated in 60% to 70% of patients with hepatocellular carcinoma. Levels are directly proportional to tumor size, compromising the measurements of sensitivity of AFP as a screening test for early hepatocellular carcinoma. Other tumors (e.g., testicular, ovarian, gastric) and gallbladder carcinoma are also associated with increased serum levels of AFP. Carcinoembryonic antigen is rarely elevated; marked elevations in the setting of a liver mass suggest metastatic adenocarcinoma.

Structural Studies

Several imaging modalities can be used to identify and stage hepatocellular carcinoma. The challenge is to distinguish a small tumor from the regenerative changes associated with cirrhosis. Ultrasound is sensitive for detecting small hepatocellular carcinomas (<2 cm). The hyperechoic pattern in these small tumors differentiates them from hypoechoic metastatic lesions. Ultrasound may be less reliable in distinguishing a small hepatocellular carcinoma from a benign hemangioma, which is also typically hyperechoic. Larger hepatocellular carcinomas are often hypoechoic and may be difficult to differentiate from metastatic lesions, but coexisting cirrhosis or elevated levels of AFP may provide additional diagnostic evidence. A computed tomographic (CT) scan is 80% to 90% sensitive for detecting hepatocellular carcinoma. A spiral CT scan obtains arterial and venous phase contrast images with a single dose of contrast agent. Hepatocellular carcinoma typically is a vascular tumor with marked arterial phase enhancement; the rapid washout of contrast agent leads to the appearance of a hypodense lesion during the venous phase. A hemangioma can be distinguished by a characteristic peripheral-to-central filling pattern and prolonged contrast enhancement. Ultrasound and CT scans demonstrate various patterns of hepatocellular carcinoma growth and extension. One-third of hepatocellular carcinomas are infiltrating, with poorly defined borders. Another one-third are expanding tumors that are well defined and encapsulated. A small percentage of them manifest as multicentric, space-occupying lesions or large pedunculated masses extending from the liver surface. CT scans are especially useful in defining the tumor capsule and invasion of the portal vein.

Other imaging procedures may be required in special circumstances. The accuracy of magnetic resonance imaging (MRI) is similar to that of CT scanning and avoids the potential adverse effects of intravenous contrast agents. MRI is the procedure of choice for differentiating hemangioma from hepatocellular carcinoma. A focal area of increased uptake of ^{99m}Tc-sulfur colloid on an image is virtually diagnostic of the benign lesion, focal nodular hyperplasia, but an unenhanced, or "cold mass," does not differentiate hepatocellular carcinoma from metastatic disease or hepatic adenoma. Angiography is used primarily to define the vascular anatomy in patients being considered for resection. If there is a high index of suspicion for hepatocellular carcinoma and all other imaging tests fail to localize a mass, CT scans after lipiodol injection may be useful. Lipiodol is an iodinated preparation of poppy seed oil that hepatocellular carcinoma cells preferentially concentrate and retain. Intra-arterial injection of lipiodol is followed 2 weeks later by CT scanning. Hepatocellular carcinoma appears as a focal area of enhancement. The most sensitive means of detecting hepatocellular carcinoma is intraoperative ultrasound. Given the invasiveness of these last two procedures, repeat ultrasound or CT scanning after an interval of several months is an alternative means of identifying hepatocellular carcinoma in patients in whom hepatocellular carcinoma is suspected but not detected on initial noninvasive imaging.

Histologic Studies

When a patient with cirrhosis develops a liver mass associated with marked elevation of serum AFP levels, a biopsy to confirm hepatocellular carcinoma may not be necessary. The risk of bleeding induced by ultrasound- or CT-guided biopsy of hepatocellular carcinoma is significant, although small-gauge needle aspiration can often be performed safely. Histologic examination usually reveals cords of undifferentiated hepatocytes, but some tumors are well differentiated and may be difficult to differentiate from a benign hepatic adenoma.

Management and Course

Surgical Therapy

The only option for long-term survival with hepatocellular carcinoma is complete surgical excision of the tumor. Unfortunately, resectability rates range from 5% to 20%. In determining the suitability of a patient for resection, the extent of the tumor and postresection residual hepatic function need to be considered. Any patient with jaundice or complications of portal hypertension will not tolerate further loss of hepatic function. Similarly, any patient with distant metastasis or diffuse hepatic involvement will not benefit from surgery. After successful resection, measurement of serum AFP levels is a useful means of detecting disease recurrence. Although the 5-year survival rate for patients with resectable tumors is 30% to 50%, only 5% to 20% of tumors are resectable. The overall 5-year survival rate for patients with hepatocellular carcinoma is 5%.

Nonsurgical Therapy

Intralesional injection of 100% ethanol has been associated with a decrease in tumor size and prolonged survival. Cryosurgery ablates tumors with intraoperatively placed probes that freeze and destroy surrounding tumor, significantly reducing tumor burden. Intra-arterial embolization and intra-arterial chemoembolization involve placing an intra-arterial catheter surgically or angiographically in the hepatic artery. Particles or coils are used to embolize the vessels feeding the tumor, and in the case of chemoembolization, antineoplastic agents are delivered with the embolizing particles. Intra-arterial therapy may decrease tumor size, but it does not appear to affect survival rates and may precipitate hepatic failure. All of these therapies are ideally suited for patients who cannot undergo surgery and who have only a few hepatic lesions. Intra-arterial embolization is contraindicated if there is significant portal vein thrombosis. Radiation therapy and systemic chemotherapy have limited roles in the management of hepatocellular carcinoma. The role of transplantation is controversial because of the high rate of disease recurrence. Transplantations should be performed only at centers with ongoing protocols.

Screening Protocols for Hepatocellular Carcinoma

The poor prognosis of hepatocellular carcinoma has led to efforts to diagnose the malignancy early in its course with screening programs that target populations at greatest risk for developing the tumor. In the United States, patients with long-standing HBV infection and all patients with established cirrhosis should be considered for screening. There are few data on efficacy to support any one screening strategy, but a reasonable program is annual or biannual ultrasound and serum AFP measurements. Any new mass or incremental rise in AFP levels should be investigated.

FIBROLAMELLAR HEPATOCELLULAR CARCINOMA

Fibrolamellar hepatocellular carcinoma is clinically and pathologically distinct from the hepatocellular carcinoma that complicates cirrhosis. Fibrolamellar hepatocellular carcinoma is not typically associated with cirrhosis. It often occurs in young adults; there is no sex predominance. Patients usually present with abdominal pain, weight loss, hepatomegaly, and an abdominal mass. Serum AFP levels are characteristically normal and imaging procedures often demonstrate intralesional calcification or, rarely, a central scar. Prognosis is favorable relative to the more common variant of hepatocellular carcinoma. Fifty percent to 75% of patients have resectable tumors, and long-term survival is common. Transplantation should be considered in this group given the decreased propensity of fibrolamellar hepatocellular carcinoma to metastasize and the younger age of the patient population.

HEPATOBLASTOMA

Less than 1% of primary liver tumors are derived from fetal hepatocytes and are termed *hepatoblastomas*. Most cases occur in young children, but adults may be affected. Patients present with abdominal pain, weight loss, and a palpable right upper quadrant mass. Unlike fibrolamellar tumors, serum AFP levels usually are elevated, but similar to fibrolamellar tumors, calcification is often evident on ultrasound or CT images. At the time of presentation, a hepatoblastoma often is massive in size. Complete surgical excision is the optimal treatment, but chemotherapy may be beneficial for unresectable tumors. Long-term survival averages 25%.

MESENCHYMAL TUMORS

Mesenchymal tumors account for <1% of primary malignant liver neoplasms. Angiosarcoma is associated with exposure to Thorotrast, arsenic, and vinyl chloride. Patients present later in life. Other histologic variants include rhabdomyosarcoma, leiomyosarcoma, and liposarcoma. Disease is usually advanced at presentation and survival is limited.

BENIGN LIVER MASSES

Hepatic Adenomas

The incidence of benign hepatic adenomas has increased with the use of oral contraceptives. Isolated adenomas occur mainly in women who are of reproductive age. These lesions can grow to large sizes before symptoms occur; most patients present with abdominal pain or a palpable abdominal mass. Intratumor hemorrhage and rupture are frequent complications, especially if the adenoma is associated with contraceptive use. Rarely, patients present with hepatic adenomatosis, characterized by multiple adenomas throughout the liver. These patients frequently have glycogen storage disorders, and malignant degeneration is a well-described complication. Opinion is divided whether isolated hepatic adenomas are at risk for malignant degeneration. Well-differentiated hepatocellular carcinoma may be difficult to distinguish from adenomas, and histologic misclassification of hepatocellular carcinoma as adenoma may later be interpreted as malignant transformation. Adenomas typically appear as hypodense areas on CT scans and as "cold lesions" on ^{99m}Tc–sulfur colloid images. Discontinuing oral contraceptives may result in resolution, but if the lesion persists or hepatocellular carcinoma is suspected, surgical excision is recommended.

Focal Nodular Hyperplasia

Focal nodular hyperplasia is a space-occupying lesion composed of all the normal cell populations usually found in the liver, including reticuloendothelial cells. The etiology is unknown. Lesions usually are detected incidentally during imaging procedures performed for unrelated symptoms. Twenty-five percent are multicentric and most are <5 cm. Diagnosis is often possible based on a classic appearance on imaging procedures. CT or MRI scans may demonstrate a central stellate scar that is often calcified. ^{99m}Tc–sulfur colloid imaging often but not invariably demonstrates a focal area of increased signal as a result of the presence of reticuloendothelial cells. Adenomas, hepatocellular carcinoma, and metastatic tumors are characteristically photopenic, appearing as "cold spots" on ^{99m}Tc–sulfur colloid images. Focal nodular hyperplasia is benign, and no treatment is necessary.

Hemangioma

Cavernous hemangiomas are focal collections of dilated vascular channels and are the most common benign space-occupying lesion, with an estimated prevalence of 5% to 10%. Most are asymptomatic and are detected incidentally, but large hemangiomas can produce symptoms such as abdominal pain. The main clinical importance of this lesion lies in differentiating it from more serious disorders. Radiologic procedures play a primary role in diagnosis of hemangioma because percutaneous biopsy is associated with a high risk of hemorrhage. Hemangiomas are typically hyperechoic on ultrasound and retain contrast for prolonged periods on CT scanning. MRI is the most sensitive and specific means of diagnosing hemangioma. Surgical excision is necessary only for symptomatic lesions.

CHAPTER 68

Gastrointestinal Complications of the Acquired Immunodeficiency Syndrome

ESOPHAGEAL DISORDERS

Etiology and Pathogenesis

Odynophagia or dysphagia affects 30% of all patients with acquired immunodeficiency syndrome (AIDS). The most common cause is infection with *Candida albicans*, which is characterized by superficial esophageal erosions and thick, white plaques of exudate coating the esophageal mucosa. *Candida* esophagitis is usually accompanied by oral thrush, and the absence of thrush should raise suspicion of an alternative cause of esophagitis (e.g., cytomegalovirus [CMV], herpes simplex virus [HSV], or an idiopathic pathogen). (See Chapter 27 for additional discussion on esophagitis and esophageal infections.) In the esophagus, CMV usually produces shallow ulcers, but these may coalesce, forming large ulcers with raised edges. CMV is typically a disseminated disease, and at the time esophagitis is diagnosed, patients often have CMV infection in other sites. HSV generally produces multiple, small, discrete ulcerations that also may coalesce to form deep linear ulcerations. Severely immunocompromised patients may develop large, deep ulcers that are not associated with a known pathogen. Given the inability to culture known pathogens, these ulcers have been termed *idiopathic* or *aphthous ulcers*. Human immunodeficiency virus (HIV) has been isolated from these ulcers, but the pathogenic role of HIV remains unknown. Given that AIDS patients often take many medications, pill-induced esophageal ulcers may account for a small number of these idiopathic ulcers.

Mass lesions of the esophagus are uncommon in AIDS, but Kaposi's sarcoma and lymphoma can metastasize to the esophagus and produce dysphagia. Dysphagia can also result from mediastinal adenopathy, inflammation-induced dysmotility, or a stricture complicating a large esophageal ulcer. It is important to differentiate oropharyngeal dysphagia from esophageal dysphagia. Patients with AIDS are susceptible to a number of central nervous system diseases that can manifest as choking or aspiration caused by an uncoordinated oropharyngeal phase of swallowing.

Clinical Features, Diagnosis, and Management

Barium swallow radiography is a sensitive means of detecting esophagitis, but normal findings do not exclude esophagitis. Definitive diagnosis generally requires histopathologic examination and possibly culture of specimens of esophageal mucosa. Therefore, upper gastrointestinal endoscopy with brushing and biopsy of mucosal abnormalities is the standard for diagnosis. *Candida* esophagitis has a typical endoscopic appearance of thick, white plaques coating the esophagus. The plaques may coalesce to form pseudomembranes. Examination of brush cytology and biopsy specimens should be performed to confirm the presence of pseudohyphae. CMV is identified histopathologically as multinucleated cells with characteristic intracytoplasmic inclusions or "owl's-eye" intranuclear inclusions. HSV may also be identified by Cowdry type A intranuclear inclusions in infected squamous cells, but occasionally viral culture of the biopsy material is necessary to confirm HSV infection. Idiopathic ulcers are large, excavating lesions that may have a cobblestone appearance on endoscopy. Biopsy specimens of idiopathic ulcers, by definition, lack virocytes and demonstrate intense inflammation with necrosis and granulation.

In addition to therapy for specific infectious agents, patients with esophagitis may have incapacitating odynophagia and coexisting hypovolemia and malnutrition, all of which require the clinician's attention. A topical anesthetic agent (e.g., viscous lidocaine) may palliate odynophagia. Volume deficits and electrolyte disorders should be corrected. Occasionally, parenteral nutrition is required while awaiting a symptomatic response to therapy directed at the cause of esophagitis.

Confirmation of *Candida* esophagitis should prompt treatment with an oral imidazole (e.g., ketoconazole or fluconazole). Side effects include dose-dependent nausea, hepatotoxicity, and, with prolonged use, adrenal insufficiency. Fluconazole is more costly but has a slightly higher response rate and fewer adverse reactions. Patients usually experience complete resolution of odynophagia within 1 to 2 weeks. Nonresponders may require higher doses. Refractory candidiasis can be treated with low-dose parenteral amphotericin B. Long-term prophylactic antifungal therapy usually is required once a response is obtained.

Given the high incidence of esophageal candidiasis, one acceptable management option is empirical therapy before embarking on an extensive diagnostic evaluation. Candidates for this strategy should have odynophagia and no dysphagia, as the latter is unusual with candidiasis. Therapy with an oral imidazole, such as ketoconazole (200 mg per day) or fluconazole (100 mg per day) is initiated. Failure to achieve a complete response within 1 week should prompt evaluation with upper endoscopy.

CMV esophagitis requires parenteral therapy with ganciclovir. Given the high incidence of adverse reactions, including neutropenia, patients should have pathologic confirmation of CMV as the agent responsible for esophagitis. Uncontrolled studies suggest a high response rate, but low-dose maintenance therapy provided through a long-term central venous catheter is required to prevent relapses. Refractory esophagitis and infections caused by resistant strains of CMV can be treated with the viral DNA polymerase inhibitor foscarnet. Foscarnet also requires parenteral access. A high rate of adverse reactions to foscarnet mandates frequent monitoring for renal failure, congestive heart failure, electrolyte disturbances, and anemia.

HSV esophagitis responds to high-dose oral or parenteral acyclovir. Parenteral therapy is required in severe cases if patients are unable to ingest pills. As with other opportunistic infections, long-term secondary prophylaxis is needed to prevent relapses. Refractory esophagitis or resistant strains can be treated with foscarnet.

Idiopathic esophageal ulcers often respond to intralesional or systemic corticosteroid treatment. Reports to date have been from uncontrolled studies that use high-dose prednisone (40 mg per day) for >4 weeks. Given that beneficial effects have been observed only in uncontrolled studies, the risk of the additional immunosuppression imposed by systemic corticosteroids needs careful consideration.

Once a specific cause of esophagitis is identified and therapy is instituted, most patients respond. Rarely, patients have refractory disease with intractable odynophagia and poor oral intake requiring nutritional support. Patients with CMV and idiopathic ulcers may develop esophageal strictures that require endoscopic dilation to restore swallowing to normal. Other rare complications of AIDS-associated esophageal ulcers include hemorrhage and fistula formation. Patients with CMV esophagitis often have a poor prognosis with a median survival time of 6 to 8 months; patients with esophagitis caused by other agents have a longer median survival time.

DIARRHEA

Etiology and Pathogenesis

Diarrhea complicates the course of disease in more than one-half of patients infected with HIV. The clinical presentation covers a wide spectrum. Many pathogens can potentially cause diarrhea in AIDS. The differential diagnosis often can be determined based on the clinical pattern of diarrhea (Table 68-1).

Patients with colorectal infections generally present with frequent, low-volume, watery stools, often accompanied by occult or frank blood. Systemic signs of fever and anorexia are common. In addition to opportunistic infections, patients infected with HIV have a higher incidence of infection with *Salmonella* species, *Shigella flexneri*, and *Campylobacter jejuni*. These organisms are also the most common causes of acute bacterial colitis in the general population. These bacteria are more likely to produce bacteremia and prolonged or relapsing infections in patients with AIDS. Similarly, given the frequent need for antibiotics in the treatment of AIDS, *Clostridium difficile* and antibiotics should be considered as the cause of AIDS-associated diarrhea.

Several viruses may produce colitis in AIDS. CMV infection can involve any portion of the gastrointestinal tract, but most often it causes a focal or diffuse colitis. CMV is the most common cause of hematochezia in AIDS. The endoscopic appearance ranges from focal erythema to diffuse colitis with deep ulcerations. HSV may also produce diarrhea, but infection is generally limited to the rectum. Patients with HSV proctitis usually suffer from rectal pain and tenesmus, rather than diarrhea. Increased HIV expression in colonocytes has been associated with chronic colitis, but the pathogenic role of HIV remains unclear.

TABLE 68-1
Clinical Patterns of Acquired Immunodeficiency Syndrome–Associated Diarrhea

FEATURE	SMALL BOWEL TYPE	COLONIC TYPE
Frequency	3–8 stools/day	3–30 stools/day
Volume	Often large	Small
Consistency	Formed to watery	Loose to watery
Blood in stools	No	Frequent
Tenesmus	No	Sometimes
Fever	Rare	Frequent
Anorexia	Mild to absent	Mild to severe

Organisms responsible for small bowel–type diarrhea are mainly protozoa and mycobacteria; the resulting tissue injury and malabsorption produces diarrhea. The protozoan *Cryptosporidium* causes self-limited diarrhea in immunocompetent hosts, but in patients with AIDS, *Cryptosporidium* infection is associated with severe chronic diarrhea and wasting. Although the organism may rarely involve the biliary tract and colon, cryptosporidiosis usually affects the small intestine, producing radiographic and histologic findings similar to celiac sprue. Microsporidia are also protozoa and produce a clinical syndrome indistinguishable from cryptosporidiosis. The two Microsporidia species, *Enterocytozoon bieneusi* and *Septata intestinalis*, are recognized more often and may be responsible for up to one-third of AIDS-associated diarrhea. *Isospora belli* and *Cyclospora* organisms are protozoans related to *Cryptosporidium* and have been associated with chronic diarrhea and malabsorption in AIDS, especially in undeveloped countries.

Mycobacterium tuberculosis rarely infects the gastrointestinal tract in AIDS, but *Mycobacterium avium-intracellulare* complex (MAC) is a common cause of disease in the small intestine. Patients often present with profound wasting, fever, and diarrhea. Bulky abdominal adenopathy may be associated with abdominal pain. Infiltration of the small intestine with infected macrophages results in obstruction of lymphatic flow and malabsorption.

Some patients with AIDS-associated diarrhea and wasting have extensive histologic changes in the small intestine, including villous atrophy and focal crypt necrosis. However, an identifiable pathogen other than HIV cannot be identified. This syndrome has been termed *AIDS-associated enteropathy*, but as with other idiopathic gastrointestinal disorders in AIDS, the pathogenic role of HIV remains unclear.

The protozoans *Entamoeba histolytica* and *Giardia lamblia* are commonly isolated from the stools of homosexual men, but these pathogens usually do not cause diarrheal illness in AIDS.

Clinical Features, Diagnosis, and Management

There is no consensus on the optimal diagnostic evaluation of diarrhea in AIDS. Although a thorough evaluation including upper gastrointestinal endoscopy and biopsy can identify a pathogen in 85% of patients, many pathogens are unresponsive to currently available antimicrobial agents. Many patients are infected with several organisms, and identification and treatment of a single pathogen may not yield a clinical response. Conversely, some infections are very responsive to therapy, and because there is a substantial risk of toxicity from medications such as ganciclovir, a definitive diagnosis should be obtained before initiating therapy. In any diagnostic approach to diarrhea in patients with AIDS, the overall prognosis of the patient along with the potential risks and benefits of identifying the responsible pathogens should be taken into consideration.

The initial noninvasive evaluation should include an examination of a stool sample for *Salmonella*, *Shigella*, and *Campylobacter* species and a stool assay for *C difficile* toxin. Examination for parasites requires three separate stool samples to be processed with a modified acid-fast stain (*Cryptosporidium*, *Isospora*, *Cyclospora*, MAC), a modified trichrome stain (Microsporidia), and a standard saline wet mount (*G lamblia*). When fever, weight loss, and other systemic symptoms suggest a diagnosis of MAC infection, blood should be cultured with a special transport medium (e.g., Du Pont isolator).

If no pathogen is identified or treatment of identified pathogens fails to result in clinical improvement, endoscopic evaluation and biopsy may be required to identify additional pathogens. An alternative approach is to stop the diagnostic evaluation at this point and administer antidiarrheals, as long as CMV infection is not suspected. The choice of initial endoscopic procedure can be made based on the origin of the patient's symptoms—that is, either the small intestine or the colon (see Table 68-1). Colonoscopy with biopsy should be the initial procedure for patients with colitis; a complete examination to the cecum usually is not necessary if gross abnormalities are encountered in the distal colon. Patients with symptoms of injury to the small intestine and malabsorption should undergo upper gastrointestinal endoscopy with biopsy of the duodenum. Histopathologic examination may demonstrate the viral inclusions of CMV or any of the pathogenic protozoa. Special stains identify Microsporidia. Biopsy specimens should be cultured for viruses and mycobacteria in addition to histologic preparation with acid-fast stains to increase the yield for MAC and CMV. Rarely, electron microscopy is necessary to identify Microsporidia.

Treatment of diarrhea in AIDS combines supportive therapy for symptoms and specific therapy targeting identified pathogens (Table 68-2). Antimicrobial therapy for an isolated pathogen may fail to produce a response because of a simultaneous infection with another pathogen, antimicrobial resistance, or inadequate host defenses that result from profound immunodeficiency. Unlike immunocompetent patients with uncomplicated bacterial colitis, antibiotics should be included in treatment of a patient with AIDS who has bacterial colitis caused by *Salmonella*, *Shigella*, or *Campylobacter* species. *Cryptosporidium* and Microsporidia are usually not responsive to antimicrobial agents, but reports suggest that some patients with cryptosporidiosis respond to the macrolide paromomycin, and some strains of Microsporidia respond to albendazole. When a specific therapy produces a clinical response, long-term maintenance therapy is usually required to prevent relapses.

Given the high rate of treatment failures with antimicrobial agents, symptom-based therapy often plays a primary role. Opiates (e.g., diphenoxylate, codeine, paregoric, tincture of opium) may help reduce stool volume. In patients with refractory AIDS-associated diarrhea, the somatostatin analog octreotide can also reduce stool frequency and volume. Whereas fiber supplements are rarely helpful, ingestion of a low-fat, low-lactose, high-protein, high-calorie diet can minimize symptoms of malabsorption and help maintain the patient's nutritional

TABLE 68-2
Treatment of Acquired Immunodeficiency Syndrome–Associated Diarrhea

PATHOGEN	ANTIMICROBIAL THERAPY	COMMENTS
Bacterial		
Salmonella and *Shigella* species	Trimethoprim-sulfamethoxazole double strength, 1 tablet bid; or ampicillin, 500 mg qid; or ciprofloxacin, 500 mg bid	Maintenance therapy often required; parenteral therapy may be required for patients with bacteremia
Campylobacter species	Erythromycin, 500 mg qid; or tetracycline, 500 mg qid; or ciprofloxacin, 500 mg bid	Parenteral aminoglycoside may be necessary for patients with bacteremia
Clostridium difficile	Vancomycin, 125 mg qid; or metronidazole, 250 mg qid	Relapse requires repeat course of therapy, often with prolonged taper or with addition of cholestyramine
Mycobacterial		
Mycobacterium avium-intracellulare complex	Multidrug therapy with 4–5 agents (clarithromycin, clofazimine, ciprofloxacin, ethambutol, amikacin, rifampicin)	Therapy is suppressive and life-long
Protozoan		
Cryptosporidium species	No reliable therapy	Paromomycin and azithromycin are investigational and may benefit some patients
Microsporidia	No reliable therapy	Albendazole is investigational
Isospora belli	Trimethoprim-sulfamethoxazole double strength, 1 tablet qid; or pyrimethamine, 25 mg qd, + sulfadiazine, 1 g qid, + leucovorin, 5 mg qd	Maintenance therapy with trimethoprim-sulfamethoxazole or pyrimethamine often necessary
Cyclospora species	Trimethoprim-sulfamethoxazole double strength, 1 tablet qid	Maintenance therapy often necessary
Giardia lamblia	Quinacrine, 100 mg tid × 7 days; or metronidazole, 750 mg tid × 7 days	Relapse requires repeat courses of therapy
Viral		
Cytomegalovirus	Ganciclovir, 5 mg/kg IVSS bid × 14 days; or foscarnet	Maintenance therapy required to prevent relapses
Herpes simplex virus	Acyclovir, 400 mg per os qid; or acyclovir, 5 mg/kg IV, q8h	Maintenance therapy required to prevent relapses

status. Occasionally, elemental supplements or even total parenteral nutrition (TPN) are necessary. The decision to use invasive therapy such as TPN or enteral feedings through a gastrostomy tube should be based on the disease prognosis and on the potential to control the acute illness.

The most common complication in patients with AIDS-associated diarrhea is wasting and the associated nutritional deficiencies. Nutritional repletion can be achieved with aggressive use of enteral supplements, and rarely, a short-term trial of TPN is required to relieve profound malabsorption. Electrolyte abnormalities and hypovolemia often accompany severe diarrhea and should be corrected with oral or parenteral supplements.

Some pathogens may have a particularly complicated course. CMV infection may be complicated with severe hemorrhage, usually with hematochezia secondary to CMV colitis. Patients with CMV colitis or enteritis may present with severe abdominal pain and perforation as a result of penetration of a CMV ulcer. Patients with MAC infections may present with abdominal pain caused by bulky adenopathy. This adenopathy can cause intestinal obstruction with associated crampy pain and vomiting. Alternatively, the adenopathy may undergo liquefaction necrosis and mimic the clinical presentation of an acute abdomen.

HEPATOBILIARY DISEASES

Etiology and Pathogenesis

Patients with AIDS commonly develop biochemical evidence of hepatobiliary injury. Many of the medications used to control the disease produce cholestasis (e.g., sulfonamides, rifampicin) or hepatitis (e.g., isoniazid, imidazoles). Chronic infection with hepatitis B virus (HBV) or hepatitis C virus (HCV) is also prevalent in HIV-seropositive patients owing to shared routes of exposure. A granulomatosis hepatitis characterized by a progressive rise in alkaline phosphatase levels is usually caused by MAC infection, systemic fungal infection, and, occasionally, miliary tuberculosis. Patients with granulomatous hepatitis usually have systemic symptoms of fever, sweats, and weight loss. AIDS cholangiopathy, a syndrome of sclerosing cholangitis often with associated papillary stenosis, has been linked to infections with *Cryptosporidium* species, Microsporidia, *I belli*, and CMV. Some patients have papillary stenosis without bile duct strictures. The usual presentation is pruritus, abdominal pain, and progressive cholestasis. Infiltrative liver disease secondary to Kaposi's sarcoma and lymphoma may also produce cholangiopathy. Bacillary angiomatosis is a form of sinusoidal dilation, also termed *peliosis hepatitis*, which has been associated with the bacillus *Rochalimaea henselae*. Patients usually present with abdominal pain, elevated liver chemistry values, and a disproportionate increase in serum alkaline phosphatase levels.

Clinical Features, Diagnosis, and Management

Serologic analysis for HBV and HCV and blood cultures for MAC are noninvasive initial studies. Further diagnostic evaluation of elevated liver chemistry values is generally reserved for patients with significant symptoms or a progressive rise in liver chemistry profiles. Ultrasound may reveal biliary dilation in patients with papillary stenosis or sclerosing cholangitis. Endoscopic retrograde cholangiopancreatography (ERCP) is required to confirm this diagnosis. Computed tomographic scans may demonstrate the dilated sinusoids characteristic of bacillary angiomatosis and may also provide ancillary evidence of infiltrative diseases—for example, adenopathy associated with MAC, or lymphoma. Exclusion of granulomatous hepatitis requires liver biopsy, and in addition to histologic examination with special stains, care must be taken to culture the biopsy specimen for mycobacteria and fungi.

Although treatment of hepatobiliary disorders is largely supportive, any disease-specific therapy requires definitive diagnosis with liver biopsy or ERCP. The role of interferon therapy for chronic HCV is limited, as patients are far more likely to succumb to other AIDS-related illnesses and drug toxicity may exacerbate disease or other drug-induced cytopenias. Granulomatous hepatitis caused by mycobacterial or fungal infection and peliosis hepatitis caused by *R henselae* require long-term antimicrobial therapy. Although AIDS cholangiopathy has been associated with numerous pathogens, patients usually do not experience biochemical or clinical improvement with antimicrobial therapy. Patients with papillary stenosis often experience relief of abdominal pain with endoscopic sphincterotomy, but cholestasis usually progresses. Kaposi's sarcoma and lymphoma require systemic chemotherapy and radiation therapy. Patients should be selected on the basis of their long-term prognosis.

Although the course of chronic viral hepatitis has been reported to be more aggressive in AIDS, patients often succumb to other AIDS-related complications. Similarly, the other hepatobiliary complications of AIDS usually are not lethal, but granulomatous hepatitis or drug-induced hepatitis may rarely lead to fulminant hepatic failure. AIDS cholangiopathy can be complicated by cholangitis and has been associated with acalculous cholecystitis, which requires surgical intervention or transcutaneous cholecystotomy.

GASTROINTESTINAL HEMORRHAGE

Severe gastrointestinal hemorrhage is not common in AIDS, but several diseases associated with AIDS may lead to hemorrhage. Large esophageal ulcers and CMV ulcers throughout the gastrointestinal tract may bleed significantly. Other potential causes include ulcers associated with lymphoma and extensive mucosal Kaposi's sarcoma. For reasons that remain unclear, peptic ulcer disease caused by *Helicobacter pylori* is rare in patients with AIDS.

ACUTE ABDOMINAL PAIN

Patients with HIV infection may present with acute abdominal pain caused by diseases prevalent among immunocompetent patients, such as calculous cholecystitis and appendicitis, but some disease processes are specific to AIDS. Acalculous cholecystitis has been associated with AIDS cholangiopathy and has a clinical presentation indistinguishable from that of calculous cholecystitis. Although peptic ulcer disease is uncommon in AIDS, CMV ulcers or ulcers associated with lymphoma throughout the gastrointestinal tract may perforate and produce peritonitis. MAC may present with necrotic bulky adenopathy that mimics peritonitis, with guarding and rebound tenderness. Tuberculosis and fungal peritonitis are potential causes of acute abdomen in patients with AIDS. Other opportunistic infections, such as those produced by CMV, *Cryptococcus neoformans*, and *Toxoplasma gondii*, can cause acute pancreatitis, as can certain medications (e.g., pentamidine, dideoxyinosine, sulfonamides). The mass lesions of Kaposi's sarcoma and lymphoma may present with intussusception or bowel obstruction, with subsequent development of strangulation and perforation. Although a high operative mortality rate has led some to question the utility of surgical intervention in the treatment of AIDS, laparotomy should be considered for patients with an acute abdomen, particularly if a perforated viscus is confirmed or the patient is in the early stages of HIV infection.

CHAPTER 69

Parasitic Diseases: Protozoa and Helminths

PROTOZOA

Entamoeba histolytica

Etiology and Pathogenesis

Human disease from infection with *Entamoeba histolytica* includes asymptomatic colonization, invasive colitis, liver abscess, intestinal perforation, and peritonitis. The life cycle of *E histolytica* begins with ingestion of fecally contaminated matter containing *E histolytica* cysts. Small bowel or colonic excystation in the small intestine or colon is followed by cell division to form eight trophozoites that colonize the colon, produce cysts, and in some cases invade the colonic epithelium. *E histolytica* produces proteases, collagenases, and an extracellular enterotoxin that may disrupt mucosal barriers and induce inflammation. The migration of amebae from the colon to the liver is by way of the portal vein. Areas of amebic invasion in the colonic and hepatic tissues contain amorphous eosinophilic debris and lack an exuberant inflammatory response because of lysis of neutrophils and monocytes.

Primates and humans are the only known reservoirs of the organism, which is most prevalent in Central and South America, Africa, and India. Groups with more severe amebiasis include malnourished individuals, very young and old persons, pregnant women, and patients on corticosteroids. In developed nations, immigrants from

---

TABLE 69-1
Clinical Manifestations of *Entamoeba histolytica* Infection

Intestinal disease
    Noninvasive intestinal colonization
    Diarrhea in patients with acquired immunodeficiency syndrome
    Acute amebic proctocolitis
    Chronic nondysenteric intestinal amebiasis
    Ameboma
    Toxic megacolon
    Amebic peritonitis secondary to perforation
    Amebic strictures
Extraintestinal disease
    Liver abscess, rarely with extension to thorax, pericardium, or peritoneum
    Brain abscess
    Cutaneous amebiasis
    Venereal infection

---

endemic areas, long-term visitors to endemic areas, promiscuous male homosexuals (because of oral-anal contact), patients with acquired immunodeficiency syndrome (AIDS), and institutionalized persons are at increased risk of developing infection.

Other enteric amebae are mostly nonpathogenic and include *E gingivalis* (associated with poor dental hygiene), *E hartmanni* (smaller cysts and trophozoites than *E histolytica*), *E coli* (multinucleate cysts), *E polecki* (infects pigs and monkeys), *Endolimax nana* (nonpathogenic colonic commensal), and *Iodamoeba bütschlii* (nonpathogenic commensal). *Dientamoeba fragilis*, which does not have a cyst form, may cause prolonged diarrhea.

Clinical Features, Diagnosis, and Management

Most patients infected with *E histolytica* do not develop colitis or liver abscess; rather, they report mild diarrhea with cramping or no symptoms (Table 69-1). These patients do not have trophozoites or blood in the stool. Endoscopic examinations appear normal. Patients with acute amebic proctocolitis report 1 to 3 weeks of an increasing frequency of bloody diarrhea with abdominal pain and tenderness. One-third of patients are febrile. Weight loss is common. Fecal leukocytes may not be present in this form of disease. Chronic nondysenteric intestinal amebiasis is characterized by long-standing (>5 years in some cases) abdominal pain, flatulence, diarrhea, fecal mucus, weight loss, and colonic ulcers containing amebae visible on colonoscopy. An ameboma is a tender abdominal mass originating in the cecum or ascending colon. It is usually associated with amebic dysentery. Barium enema radiography may reveal one or more "apple-core" lesions. Colonoscopy with biopsy is diagnostic. Toxic megacolon and amebic peritonitis are life-threatening complications of amebic infection and may develop insidiously. Amebic strictures occur in <1% of patients with amebic dysentery. Strictures may develop with or without concurrent dysentery.

Amebic liver abscess develops in 10% of patients who have had invasive amebiasis, usually within the last year. Active colonic disease usually is not present when hepatic involvement is diagnosed. Patients who have had acute symptoms for <10 days often report fever and abdominal pain and exhibit multiple amebic abscesses, whereas chronic presentations are characterized by hepatomegaly and weight loss. Lung infection may result from direct extension of a liver abscess into the thorax. Atelectasis, elevation of the diaphragm, and pleural effusions are common and do not by themselves represent pulmonary disease. Peritonitis from rupture of amebic liver abscess is less severe than amebic peritonitis from a bowel perforation because there usually is no concurrent bacterial infection. Other extraintestinal manifestations include pericarditis, cutaneous amebiasis, brain abscess, and amebic penile or cervical ulceration.

Three stool samples should be examined to make the diagnosis of intestinal amebiasis, including a wet preparation to look for motile trophozoites containing erythrocytes and a formalin-ethyl acetate step to identify cysts. Colonoscopy is preferred to sigmoidoscopy because disease involvement is predominantly right-sided. The colonic mucosa may be hemorrhagic and exhibit shallow, discrete ulcers with raised edges. Wet preparations of ulcer aspirates and biopsy specimens may detect amebae. Serologic tests, in particular the indirect hemagglutination assay, produce positive results in 88% of patients with amebic dysentery and in 99% of those with liver abscess. The results of this assay remain positive for years; therefore, it is not useful to assess clearance of the organism. The diagnosis of *E histolytica* liver abscess often relies on serologic testing because abscess aspirates are often negative for the amebae. Ultrasound demonstrates the abscess and excludes other disorders (e.g., cholecystitis). In contrast to an echinococcal cyst, which, if aspirated, can produce anaphylaxis, aspiration of a suspected amebic liver abscess should be performed in febrile patients with right upper quadrant pain to exclude pyogenic abscess.

Asymptomatic persons in developed nations who are at low risk of reinfection should be treated to prevent future invasive disease and spread of infection to others. Poorly absorbed agents that maximize drug delivery to the colon with minimal systemic effects include diloxanide, furoate, iodoquinol, and paromomycin. Metronidazole is the drug of choice for invasive colonic disease or liver abscess. A poorly absorbed agent should be taken with metronidazole to clear the colon of *E histolytica*. Second-line drugs for invasive disease include emetine, dehydroemetine, and chloroquine. Aspiration of an amebic liver abscess usually is not needed. Colonic surgery is avoided, except for megacolon or perforation, owing to its technical difficulty in this setting.

Giardia lamblia

Etiology and Pathogenesis

Giardia lamblia is the most common infectious agent identified in water-borne outbreaks of diarrhea in the United States. There are two stages to the life cycle of *G lamblia*: the trophozoite and the cyst. The trophozoite has a convex dorsal surface and flat ventral surface, with four pairs of posteriorly directed flagella and two nuclei, each with a central karyosome, which give a facelike appearance on stained preparations. After exposure to secondary bile salts, a neutral pH, and other intestinal factors, the trophozoites encyst to form oval, smooth, thin-walled cysts. Ingestion of as few as 10 to 25 cysts is pathogenic. Excystation to the trophozoite form in the small intestine is followed by enterocyte adherence. Damage to the brush border develops with deficiencies of lactase and other enzymes. Simultaneous colonization with bacteria or yeast may contribute to malabsorption. An immune response develops that provides partial immunity

TABLE 69-2
Symptoms of Infection with *Giardia lamblia*

SYMPTOM	PERCENTAGE OF PATIENTS (RANGE)
Diarrhea	90 (64–100)
Malaise	86 (72–97)
Flatulence	75 (35–97)
Foul-smelling, greasy stools	75 (57–87)
Abdominal cramps	71 (44–85)
Bloating	71 (42–97)
Nausea	69 (59–79)
Anorexia	66 (41–82)
Weight loss	66 (56–76)
Vomiting	23 (11–36)
Fever	15 (0–24)
Constipation	13 (0–26)
Urticaria	10 (5–14)

Source: Adapted with permission from DR Hill. Giardiasis. In Mandell GR, Douglas RG, Bennett J (eds), Principles of Infectious Diseases. New York: Churchill-Livingstone, 1990;2113.

against reinfection, contributes to organism clearance by production of secretory antibodies, and contributes to disease by initiation of inflammation.

G lamblia can infect sheep, beavers, cattle, dogs, and cats, but it is uncertain if these species are important reservoirs for human infection. Water-borne outbreaks have occurred in the Northeast, Northwest, and Rocky Mountain regions of the United States and British Columbia in Canada. Person-to-person transmission is the second most common mode of acquisition and may occur in children in day care centers, sexually active male homosexuals, and institutionalized individuals. Food has been documented as a vehicle for *G lamblia* transmission in commercial food establishments. Conditions that predispose to giardiasis include common variable immunodeficiency, X-linked agammaglobulinemia, previous gastric surgery, achlorhydria, and, possibly, AIDS.

Clinical Features, Diagnosis, and Management

G lamblia infection produces a range of presentations, including asymptomatic cyst passage (up to 6 months); acute, self-limited diarrhea; and chronic diarrhea, malabsorption, and weight loss (Table 69-2). After cyst ingestion, there is a 1- to 2-week incubation period before symptoms develop. Acute symptomatic giardiasis is characterized by diarrhea (usually for several weeks), cramps, bloating, flatulence, eructation, malaise, nausea, and anorexia. Stools are initially watery but later are greasy, foul-smelling, and may float. Weight loss of >4.5 kg occurs in >50% of cases. Chronic intermittent diarrhea for months may be associated with malaise, lassitude, lactose intolerance, and malabsorption of fat, protein, D-xylose, and vitamins A and B_{12}.

The traditional method for diagnosis of giardiasis is stool examination for trophozoites or cysts. Collection of three stool samples increases the diagnostic sensitivity to as high as 90%. Antigen detection assays for stool (enzyme-linked immunosorbent assay [ELISA], immunofluorescence) can be used to assist in diagnosis. In cases where stool testing produces negative findings, duodenal aspiration, duodenal biopsy, or the Entero-Test string may demonstrate the organism. Biopsy specimens of the small intestine may show spruelike changes in some but not all affected patients. The serum may be positive for anti-*Giardia* IgM antibodies in current infection, whereas the level of IgG antibodies may remain elevated for years.

Quinacrine is considered the therapy of choice worldwide; however, it is not manufactured in the United States. Quinacrine has an efficacy of 90% but causes nausea, vomiting, and cramping, especially in children. In the United States, metronidazole is the most commonly used agent, with an efficacy of 80% to 95%. Side effects of metronidazole include a metallic taste, nausea, dizziness, headache, neuropathy, a disulfiram-like effect if taken with alcohol, and, rarely, neutropenia. Metronidazole should be avoided if possible during pregnancy (especially the first trimester) because of potential teratogenicity. Oral paromomycin may be considered for treatment of pregnant women; however, its efficacy is only 60% to 70%. Furazolidone has been advocated as an alternative drug for the treatment of giardiasis in children. The role of treatment for asymptomatic cyst passers is controversial. Prevention of giardiasis includes water purification and good personal hygiene.

Cryptosporidium *Species*

Etiology and Pathogenesis

Cryptosporidium species are most commonly associated with life-threatening diarrhea in patients with AIDS. As water-borne pathogens, *Cryptosporidium* species also cause large-scale outbreaks of diarrhea in healthy individuals as well as diarrhea in malnourished children in developing areas, children in day care centers, travelers, and veterinary and health care workers. *C parvum* is the primary mammalian pathogen infecting humans, calves, piglets, foals, mice, and goats. Infection begins with ingestion of small numbers of oocysts, which excyst in the small intestine after exposure to gastric acid, bile, and digestive enzymes. The sporozoites infect the mucosal epithelium, causing villous atrophy, crypt elongation, and lamina propria inflammation, especially in immunocompromised individuals. *Cryptosporidium* infections cause malabsorption or secretory diarrhea by unknown mechanisms.

In addition to AIDS, risk factors for acquisition of *Cryptosporidium* infections include weaning, crowding, summer and autumn months, contact with infected persons or animals, day care centers, hospitals, and ingestion of contaminated water. The reservoir for *Cryptosporidium* infections appears to be animals, including calves, piglets, goats, and lambs. Person-to-person spread may be the major means of transmission in hospitals, day care centers, and families.

Clinical Features, Diagnosis, and Management

In immunocompetent hosts, *Cryptosporidium* infections cause self-limited diarrhea (usually for 10 to 14 days), cramping, anorexia, malaise, myalgias, weight loss, and fever (<39°C) after an incubation of 3 to 14 days. In immunocompromised patients, the organism causes severe diarrhea that may be in excess of 17 liters per day and may contribute to malnutrition or death. The most widely used method for diagnosis is acid-fast staining of stool specimens. Direct immunofluorescence staining may add sensitivity by detecting smaller numbers of oocysts.

Elevated serum IgM or IgG antibody titers are detected in 95% to 100% of patients within 2 weeks of symptom onset; increased IgG titers may persist for long periods. Intestinal biopsy specimens are positive in some cases, but usually biopsy is not necessary if stool samples have been properly collected.

No antimicrobial or antiparasitic agent has been convincingly shown to eradicate *Cryptosporidium* organisms in most patients. Spiramycin, paromomycin, azithromycin, hyperimmune bovine colostrum, and immunoglobulin concentrate have shown promise in some studies. Prevention of infection involves careful hand washing, avoidance of contaminated water, and avoidance of infected persons for 1 to 2 weeks after their symptoms resolve.

Other Enteric Protozoa

Cyclospora Species

Cyclospora organisms produce a clinical syndrome similar to cryptosporidiosis. Diarrhea occurs after ingestion of contaminated fruit or water, and travelers to Nepal, children in Peru, and hospital personnel in Chicago have been affected. A large outbreak in the United States was associated with contaminated raspberries. Acid-fast stains of stool samples or duodenal aspirates can diagnose the organism.

Isospora belli

Isospora belli is a coccidian protozoan that causes a prolonged diarrheal illness in AIDS patients, other immunocompromised individuals, and, rarely, in travelers. Once ingested, sporulated oocysts excyst and invade the intestinal epithelium. The organism produces severe diarrhea (similar to *Cryptosporidium*), cramping, nausea, and weight loss. Cysts are detected in stool by acid-fast staining, whereas intracellular parasites may be detected in biopsy specimens of the small intestine. Trimethoprim-sulfamethoxazole given for 10 days is effective treatment, although relapses are common in patients with AIDS.

Blastocystis hominis

Blastocystis hominis is a protozoan commonly detected in the stool of patients with diarrhea. Its pathogenic role is controversial. The organism is frequently detected in asymptomatic individuals. In symptomatic individuals, eradication is not always associated with symptom improvement. Symptoms attributed to *B hominis* infection include diarrhea, abdominal pain, anorexia, weight loss, and flatulence. The parasite is detected on stool examination. Treatment with metronidazole and iodoquinol has variable success.

Trypanosoma cruzi

Trypanosoma cruzi, acquired from the bite of the reduviid bug, produces Chagas' disease. The organism differentiates into epimastigotes and then infective metacyclic trypomastigotes in the intestine of the insect. Insect feces containing trypomastigotes infect human hosts through cutaneous puncture sites or mucous membranes. Acute infection is usually asymptomatic, but some patients exhibit unilateral periorbital edema (Romaña's sign), fever, adenopathy, hepatosplenomegaly, myocarditis, and constitutional symptoms. Chronic disease occurring years later is characterized by cardiac or gastrointestinal manifestations. Progressive loss of visceral innervation, especially in the esophagus and colon, produces dysphagia, regurgitation, and constipation. The diagnosis of Chagas' disease is made by detecting parasites in Giemsa-stained blood, cultivating organisms in specialized media, performing xenodiagnosis with reduviid bugs, or using serologic tests. There are no effective treatments for chronic disease.

Miscellaneous

Microsporidian protozoa, predominantly *Enterocytozoon bieneusi*, and *Septata intestinalis*, most frequently cause diarrhea in AIDS patients. Diagnosis requires intestinal biopsy with electron microscopic examination of the specimens. *Balantidium coli* is a ciliate protozoan that causes rectosigmoid colon ulcerations with dysentery or secondary bacteremia.

HELMINTHS

Nematodes

Trichuris trichiura (Whipworm)

Etiology and Pathogenesis. Humans become infected with the whipworm, *Trichuris trichiura*, after ingestion of embryonated eggs. After excystation, larvae penetrate the intestinal mucosa, molt, mature, and reattach as adults to the colonic wall. Mature female worms release 2000 to 6000 eggs into the stool daily for several years. Ova require warm, moist soil for development. Infection is most frequent in areas without latrines and in communities where human feces are used as fertilizer.

Clinical Features, Diagnosis, and Management. The diagnosis is confirmed by finding ova in the stool or adult worms in the colonic mucosa. Mebendazole is the recommended therapy. Albendazole is also effective.

Enterobius vermicularis (Pinworm)

Etiology and Pathogenesis. *Enterobius vermicularis* (pinworm) is encountered among school-age children living in areas of high population density in both temperate and tropical climates. Ingested ova hatch in the small intestine; larvae mature as they migrate to the ileum. Adult females migrate out through the anus to lay eggs on the perianal or perineal skin. Poor personal hygiene and exposure to infected peers contribute to infection in children 5 to 10 years of age. Anilingus may also lead to person-to-person transmission.

Clinical Features, Diagnosis, and Management. *E vermicularis* infections produce perianal pruritus, local skin trauma, secondary bacterial dermatitis, vulvovaginitis, urinary tract infection, and secondary enuresis. Peritoneal nodules may form in patients who develop intestinal perforation secondary to appendicitis, diverticulitis, or malignancy. Granulomatous inflammation may occur in the female genital tract as well as in the liver and epididymis. The diagnosis is most effectively made by applying transparent adhesive tape to the perianal skin early in the morning. The tape is transferred to a microscope slide. Eggs are prominent at low magnification. Three swabs provide a diagnostic sensitivity of 90%, whereas stool examination for ova and parasites detects only 10% to 15% of cases. Pinworm can be treated with pyrantel pamoate, mebendazole, or albendazole. Prevention of spread requires handwashing, laundry of contaminated clothing, and possibly treatment of the entire household to interrupt transmission.

Capillaria philippinensis

Etiology and Pathogenesis. *Capillaria philippinensis* infects persons in the Philippines, Thailand, Indonesia, Japan, Taiwan, Egypt, and Iran after ingestion of raw freshwater fish that contain infectious larvae. Adult organisms invade the mucosa of the small intestine and cause inflammation of the lamina propria. Ova are released into the lumen; some are passed in the stool, and others excyst in the intestine and produce an autoinfection.

Clinical Features, Diagnosis, and Management. Patients present with chronic diarrhea, abdominal pain, borborygmi, constitutional symptoms, malabsorption, weight loss, and, in rare cases, death. The diagnosis is made by detection of ova, larvae, or adult worms after multiple stool examinations. Mebendazole, albendazole, or flubendazole is effective therapy, along with fluid and electrolyte replacement.

Trichostrongylus Species

Etiology and Pathogenesis. *Trichostrongylus* species are parasites of herbivorous animals that infect humans in the Middle East and Asia. Ingestion of food or water contaminated by animal feces that contain larvae usually is the cause of infection, although larvae may invade through the skin. Adult worms live in the proximal small intestine.

Clinical Features, Diagnosis, and Management. Some patients present with mild epigastric pain, diarrhea, flatulence, anemia, eosinophilia, and emaciation. The diagnosis is made by identification of ova in the stool. Pyrantel pamoate, mebendazole, or albendazole is an effective treatment.

Ascaris lumbricoides

Etiology and Pathogenesis. *Ascaris lumbricoides* is the most prevalent intestinal nematode, infecting 1.2 billion people worldwide in tropical and temperate areas. After contaminated food or water is ingested, eggs hatch in the duodenum and larvae penetrate the intestinal wall; enter the venous circulation; and migrate to the lungs, where they ascend the trachea to the pharynx, are reswallowed, and complete their development in the small intestine. Female ascarids produce 200,000 eggs per day, 10 to 12 weeks after the ingestion of ova.

Clinical Features, Diagnosis, and Management. Patients present with pulmonary manifestations (bronchospasm, mucus hypersecretion, bronchiolar inflammation, and production of sputum that contains Charcot-Leyden crystals and larvae), urticaria, and gastrointestinal findings (abdominal pain, nausea, anorexia, diarrhea, and, possibly, growth retardation in children). Serious complications of *A lumbricoides* infection include partial or complete intestinal obstruction, an abdominal mass, intussusception, volvulus, perforation, and localized abscesses. Biliary complications result from migration of the adult *A lumbricoides* into the common bile duct and include cholecystitis, ascending bacterial cholangitis, secondary liver abscess, bile peritonitis, biliary calculi, and acute pancreatitis. Chest radiographs may show pulmonary infiltrates. Radiographs of the abdomen may show adult worms in the gastrointestinal tract or bile duct. Blood testing is remarkable for eosinophilia. The diagnosis usually is made by identifying ova in feces. *A lumbricoides* responds to mebendazole, pyrantel pamoate, or albendazole. Intestinal obstruction may require surgery. Biliary obstruction may need surgical or endoscopic extraction of dead worms after anthelmintic chemotherapy.

Trichinella spiralis

Etiology and Pathogenesis.   Humans become infected with *Trichinella spiralis* after ingestion of incompletely cooked meat containing larvae. *T spiralis* is widespread among carnivorous animals (pigs, wild boars, bears, walrus, horses). Encysted larvae are released in the small intestine, molt to become adults, and mate. After mating, females remain embedded in the mucosa. The females release larvae, which invade the mucosa, enter the lymphatics or bloodstream, and encyst in skeletal muscle cells.

Clinical Features, Diagnosis, and Management.   The initial intestinal phase of trichinosis is characterized by nausea, vomiting, pain, and diarrhea. The systemic phase begins 1 to 3 weeks later and manifests as fever, myalgia, facial or periorbital edema, headache, conjunctivitis, and occasionally a rash. Cardiac involvement or meningoencephalitis may be fatal. Laboratory abnormalities include eosinophilia and elevations in creatine phosphokinase levels in 50% of cases. The diagnosis is confirmed by serologic testing (bentonite flocculation test, indirect immunofluorescence test, or ELISA), which may take 3 or more weeks to become positive. Muscle biopsies are rarely needed. Mebendazole is the recommended treatment. NSAIDs and corticosteroids may control symptoms. Trichinosis can be prevented by cooking potentially contaminated meat to at least 76.6°C.

Hookworms

Etiology and Pathogenesis.   Hookworms (*Ancylostoma duodenale*, *A ceylanicum*, *Necator americanus*) anchor to the mucosa of the small intestine and produce an anticoagulant that facilitates blood loss. Ova are excreted in the feces and excyst in soil, ultimately becoming filariform larvae that can invade the human host through cutaneous fissures or hair follicles in the feet or hands. Larvae then pass to the lungs, ascend the trachea to the pharynx, and are swallowed. Hookworms are widely distributed worldwide but are rare in the United States. Poor sanitation is central to transmission. Persons who do not wear shoes are at higher risk of infection.

Clinical Features, Diagnosis, and Management.   Skin penetration by the larvae produces an edematous, pruritic, papulovesicular eruption, whereas migration of the larvae through the lung causes coughing, wheezing, pulmonary infiltrates, and eosinophilia (Löffler's syndrome). Acute intestinal symptoms include epigastric pain, tenderness, flatulence, and, rarely, acute hemorrhage. Chronic disease produces iron deficiency anemia and hypoalbuminemia, growth retardation, and impaired intellectual development in children and fetal and maternal death during pregnancy. Infection may be diagnosed by detection of ova in stool samples. Treatment of hookworm relies on iron supplementation and therapy with mebendazole, pyrantel pamoate, or albendazole.

Strongyloides stercoralis

Etiology and Pathogenesis.   *Strongyloides stercoralis* enters the skin from fecally contaminated soil, then migrates to the lungs, and ultimately reaches the small intestine. Adults reside in the mucosa and release ova into the lumen. The ova hatch quickly, releasing larvae that autoinfect the host through penetration of the intestinal mucosa or perianal skin. *S stercoralis* infections may persist for decades because of low levels of autoinfection. The organism is endemic in tropical Africa, Asia, and Latin America, but is also present in Eastern Europe and the southern United States.

Clinical Features, Diagnosis, and Management.   In some cases, cutaneous penetration produces a maculopapular rash or linear urticaria (larva currens). Respiratory manifestations range from no symptoms to coughing, shortness of breath, wheezing, fever, pulmonary infiltrates, and eosinophilia. Intestinal infection can lead to abdominal pain, diarrhea, vomiting, malabsorption, steatorrhea, weight loss, and, rarely, obstruction. Life-threatening hyperinfection with bacterial superinfection may present in immunosuppressed individuals. Clinical presentations in these populations include sepsis, meningitis, peritonitis, and endocarditis. Eosinophilia may be absent in immunocompromised patients. The diagnosis is made by identifying larvae in stool samples, duodenal aspirates, or biopsy specimens of the small intestine. Serologic tests provide presumptive evidence of infection. Thiabendazole is the treatment of choice; ivermectin and albendazole are alternatives.

Cutaneous Larva Migrans

Etiology and Pathogenesis.   Dog and cat hookworms (*Ancylostoma braziliense, A caninum*) cannot complete their life cycles in humans but can infect the skin through contact with contaminated soil in the Caribbean, Africa, South America, and the Gulf and southern Atlantic coasts of North America.

Clinical Features, Diagnosis, and Management.   Patients present with creeping eruption, a dermatitis characterized by serpiginous, papulovesicular, erythematous, pruritic lesions. Topical thiabendazole is the treatment of choice; oral albendazole is an alternative.

Visceral Larva Migrans

Etiology and Pathogenesis.   Infection with larvae of dog and cat ascarids (*Toxocara canis, T cati*) results from ingestion of ova originating in animal feces. Larvae are released in the intestine but cannot complete their life cycle in humans.

Clinical Features, Diagnosis, and Management.   Patients may be asymptomatic or present with fever, cough, abdominal pain, urticaria, hepatomegaly, dermatitis, ocular involvement, eosinophilia, and hypergammaglobulinemia. An ELISA is available to detect anti-*Toxocara* antibodies. High levels of isohemagglutinins against AB blood group antigens are often seen. Thiabendazole or diethylcarbamazine are effective treatments.

Anisakiasis

Etiology and Pathogenesis.   Anisakiasis results from ingestion of raw or incompletely cooked seafood (e.g., squid, cod, herring, salmon, mackerel, Pacific pollock,

Pacific red snapper). In human hosts, larvae attempt to penetrate the stomach, small intestine, or colon, producing local inflammation but usually no eosinophilia.

Clinical Features, Diagnosis, and Management. In acute gastric anisakiasis, abdominal pain, nausea, vomiting, and occasionally hemorrhage develop 12 to 24 hours after ingestion of contaminated fish. Several days later, intestinal involvement produces symptoms mimicking appendicitis, Crohn's disease, obstruction, or perforation. Abdominal radiographs may demonstrate thumbprinting, lumenal narrowing, or a mass lesion. The diagnosis is often made by upper gastrointestinal endoscopic extraction of worms from the stomach or duodenum. Surgery may be necessary to relieve obstruction or to repair perforation.

Angiostrongylus costaricensis

Etiology and Pathogenesis. *Angiostrongylus costaricensis* typically resides in rodent mesenteric arteries but may infect the same site in humans. Eggs hatch in the arteries and larvae migrate through the intestinal wall, are passed in the feces, and invade slugs. Human infection results from ingestion of slug-infested vegetation.

Clinical Features, Diagnosis, and Management. Adult worms and ova elicit a granulomatous arteritis in the ileocecal region, which can produce arteritis, thrombosis, infarction, and perforation. Clinical presentations include nausea, vomiting, right lower quadrant pain, a palpable mass, fever, an acute abdomen, eosinophilia, and leukocytosis. Surgery is often necessary, and the diagnosis is made by identification of organisms on surgical specimens. Thiabendazole has been used for treatment, but its efficacy is unproven.

Cestodes (Tapeworms)

Taenia saginata

Etiology and Pathogenesis. The beef tapeworm, *Taenia saginata*, may be several feet in length. Human infection results from ingestion of beef or meat from camels or other herbivores that contains cysticerci, the larval form of *T saginata*. After digestion of the infected meat, the cysticercus breaks down, and a scolex is released that attaches in the jejunum. Worm development is followed by passage of fecal proglottids and ova in the stool. Cattle ingest ova from human feces. Larvae migrate to the muscle, completing the life cycle.

Clinical Features, Diagnosis, and Management. Most infected persons are asymptomatic; however, some report abdominal discomfort, anxiety, vertigo, nausea, vomiting, diarrhea, and weight loss. The diagnosis of *T saginata* infection is made by finding ova or proglottids in the stool. Niclosamide is the treatment of choice.

Library Resource Center
Renton Technical College
3000 N.E. 4th St.
Renton, WA 98056

Taenia solium

Etiology and Pathogenesis. Humans become infected with the pork tapeworm, *Taenia solium*, after ingestion of infective *Cysticercus cellulosae*, which release scoleces in the small intestine. Proglottids and ova are released in the stool. Hogs are infected when they ingest ova. Infection is common in Latin America.

Clinical Features, Diagnosis, and Management. *T solium* produces cysticercosis, a disease caused by encystment of cysticercus larvae in the brain (which can be fatal), subcutaneous tissue, skeletal muscle, eyes, or other organs. Intestinal infection is diagnosed by detection of ova or proglottids in the stool. Computed tomographic (CT) or magnetic resonance imaging (MRI) studies may demonstrate cysticerci in involved areas. Antibodies in the serum or cerebrospinal fluid are detected in some cases. Niclosamide or praziquantel treat intestinal infection, whereas praziquantel and albendazole are effective therapy for neurocysticercosis. Corticosteroids may prevent cerebral edema.

Diphyllobothrium latum

Etiology and Pathogenesis. The fish tapeworm, *Diphyllobothrium latum*, infects humans after ingestion of raw or incompletely cooked fish that contains the tapeworm in its procercoid stage. *D latum* is found in pike, salmon, trout, whitefish, and turbot in northern regions of Europe, Asia, and North America and temperate regions of South America. The life cycle is completed when coracidia are released in fresh water from human feces. Coracidia subsequently infect crustaceans, which are then eaten by freshwater fish.

Clinical Features, Diagnosis, and Management. Patients present rarely with vitamin B_{12} deficiency caused by tapeworm competition for the vitamin. The diagnosis is made by identification of ova or proglottids in stool samples. Niclosamide is recommended for treatment.

Hymenolepis nana

Etiology and Pathogenesis. Infection with the dwarf tapeworm, *Hymenolepis nana*, follows ingestion of ova. Transmission is hand-to-mouth or by ingestion of fecally contaminated food or water. An oncosphere is liberated that penetrates the intestinal mucosa and forms a cercocystis. The cercocystis releases a scolex at maturity, which anchors in the small intestine.

Clinical Features, Diagnosis, and Management. Some patients present with anorexia, abdominal pain, diarrhea, flatulence, or weight loss. The diagnosis is made by identifying eggs in the feces. Praziquantel is the treatment of choice.

Echinococcus Species

Etiology and Pathogenesis. Humans are infected with ova of *Echinococcus granulosus* after ingestion of fecally contaminated food or water. After excystment, larvae invade the intestinal mucosa and disseminate through the lymphatics and blood circulation to form cysts in the liver, lungs, bones, brain, muscles, eyes, heart, and other organs. Infection is endemic in areas of poor sanitation in Australia, New Zealand, North Africa, the Middle East, and South America. The typical echinococcal or hydatid cyst contains an external hyaline cuticula, an inner germinal membrane with brood capsules, protoscoleces, and daughter cysts. Infection from another organism, *E multilocularis*, is acquired by ingesting plants contaminated by canine feces.

Clinical Features, Diagnosis, and Management.   Most hydatid cysts grow slowly. Tissue damage is secondary to pressure from an enlarging cyst or rupture into the biliary tract (rarely producing obstructive jaundice or ascending cholangitis), peritoneum (producing anaphylaxis or peritoneal seeding), or lung. The diagnosis is based on identification of a hydatid cyst on CT, MRI, or ultrasound studies. Serologic tests are available, but results are not always positive in affected patients. Surgical excision is a common approach to therapy. Some clinicians report successful percutaneous aspiration and drainage of liver cysts despite the potential risk of anaphylaxis. Administration of mebendazole or albendazole has been advocated before surgery. A scolicide (20% sodium chloride) should be injected into the cyst at the time of surgery or drainage. High-dose albendazole is recommended as suppressive therapy in patients who cannot undergo surgery.

E multilocularis produces an alveolar hepatic cyst with a jellylike matrix. Patients present with hepatomegaly, abdominal pain, obstructive jaundice, and evidence of invasion of contiguous structures. The diagnosis is made by typical findings on ultrasound, CT, or MRI studies. The presence of antibodies against *Echinococcus*-specific antigen 5 has high specificity for *E multilocularis* infection. Surgery is the only reliable treatment for *E multilocularis*. Mebendazole or albendazole is used to treat inoperable disease.

Trematodes

Schistosomiasis

Etiology and Pathogenesis.   Adult worms of *Schistosoma* species live as pairs within venules in their human host. The ova produce lytic enzymes that allow penetration of the intestinal wall and permit ova excretion in the stool. Miracidia, released from hatching ova, penetrate snails. After maturation into cercariae, the organisms penetrate human skin during water-related exposures and make their way to the portal circulation. After 3 weeks, the organism migrates to the superior mesenteric veins (*S mansoni*) or inferior mesenteric veins (*S japonicum*). *S mansoni* is endemic in Africa, Latin America, and the Middle East. *S japonicum* is found in China, Japan, the Philippines, and Indochina. *S intercalatum* occurs in Western and Central Africa, and *S mekongi* is found along the Mekong River in Indochina.

Clinical Features, Diagnosis, and Management.   Invasion of skin by cercariae of *Schistosoma* species may produce a mild pruritic dermatitis. Systemic onset of acute schistosomiasis (Katayama fever) occurs 3 to 8 weeks after invasion. Fever, malaise, urticaria, abdominal discomfort, diarrhea, weight loss, cough, hepatosplenomegaly, adenopathy, and eosinophilia may last for months. Chronic intestinal disease is characterized by mucosal congestion, hypertrophy, and ulceration of the mucosa. Patients present with abdominal pain, bloody diarrhea, intestinal polyps, and strictures. Liver disease manifests as periportal fibrosis, which may progress to Symmers' clay pipestem (portal) fibrosis with presinusoidal portal hypertension. The pathologic picture in the liver is predominantly mesenchymal; the parenchyma and liver function are preserved until late in the disease. Esophageal variceal hemorrhage and ascites may complicate liver involvement. Pulmonary manifestations of schistosomiasis include obliterative arteritis, pulmonary hypertension, and cor pulmonale. Other sites of involvement include the gallbladder (cholecystitis, cholelithiasis), spinal cord, brain, and kidneys (glomerulonephritis, nephrotic syndrome).

The diagnosis of schistosomiasis is confirmed by identifying ova in stool or biopsy specimens. Colonoscopic findings include hyperemia, friability, and polyps. Praziquantel is recommended for treatment of all *Schistosoma* species, but treatment does not reverse certain sequelae of chronic infection (e.g., liver disease, esophageal varices). Oxamniquine is a therapeutic alternative. Portal hypertension and bleeding esophageal varices may require endoscopic sclerotherapy or surgical decompression.

Liver Flukes

Etiology and Pathogenesis.   The liver flukes *Clonorchis sinensis* and *Opisthorchis viverrini* are found in the Far East in persons who eat raw fish. Adult flukes can live in the biliary tract for up to 30 years, releasing eggs into the bile and eventually into the stool. Humans may become infected with *Fasciola hepatica* after ingestion of watercress contaminated with encysted metacercariae. The larvae excyst, penetrate the gut wall, migrate through the peritoneum, and invade the liver before penetrating the bile ducts, where they spend their adult lives.

Clinical Features, Diagnosis, and Management.   Hepatomegaly and liver tenderness, dyspepsia, anorexia, icterus, edema, and diarrhea may be observed at the onset of infections with *C sinensis* and *O viverrini*. Long-term complications include pyogenic cholangitis, cholelithiasis, chronic cholecystitis, pancreatitis, and cholangiocarcinoma. The diagnosis is confirmed by demonstrating ova in the stool or bile. Ultrasound may show liver enlargement; sludge, dilation, and thickening of the wall of the gallbladder; and bile duct dilation or cholangiocarcinoma. Endoscopic retrograde cholangiopancreatography may show biliary dilation and filling defects, tortuosity and irregular dilation of the intrahepatic ducts, and blunting of the terminal branches of the biliary tree. Praziquantel is the only drug that is active against liver flukes.

Patients with *F hepatica* develop fever, hepatomegaly, right upper quadrant pain, weight loss, anemia, eosinophilia, and diarrhea >6 weeks after infection. The diagnosis is suggested by serologic testing and confirmed by demonstration of ova in the stool, duodenal aspirates, or bile. Bithionol is the recommended treatment.

Intestinal Flukes

Etiology and Pathogenesis.   The intestinal fluke, *Fasciolopsis buski*, is acquired by ingestion of cercariae on water plants (e.g., water caltrop, water hyacinth, water chestnut, water bamboo). Adult organisms attach to the mucosa of the upper small intestine and release ova into the feces. Heterophyidae are trematodes that infect human hosts who ingest infected, raw, or incompletely cooked fish in the Middle East or Asia. *Nanophyetus salmincola* is found in the Pacific Northwest and Siberia and is acquired from ingestion of incompletely cooked salmon. Infection with *Echinostoma* species occurs after ingestion of contaminated raw snails, fish, and amphibians.

Clinical Features, Diagnosis, and Management.   Infection with *F buski* may cause intestinal inflammation, ulceration, and mucosal abscesses. Some patients present with epigastric pain, nausea, and diarrhea. Heterophyidae infections produce colicky abdominal pain, tenderness, diarrhea, and eosinophilia. *N salmincola* infections are characterized by abdominal pain, diarrhea, nausea, vomiting, and eosinophilia. Praziquantel is the drug of choice for treatment of these infections.

CHAPTER 70

Gastrointestinal Manifestations of Systemic Diseases

CARDIOVASCULAR DISEASES

Aortic Stenosis

Fifteen percent to 41% of patients with gastrointestinal angiodysplasias also have aortic stenosis. Most angiodysplasias in patients with aortic stenosis occur in the right colon. The association between the two conditions remains controversial. Aortic valve replacement may result in cessation of bleeding, but the angiodysplasias usually persist.

Congestive Heart Failure

Congestion of the splanchnic bed may complicate congestive heart failure, producing anorexia; nausea; abdominal pain; distention; and, rarely, ischemic injury, diarrhea, malabsorption, or protein-losing enteropathy. There is an increased incidence of peptic ulcer disease and upper gastrointestinal hemorrhage with heart failure. Hepatic congestion may produce jaundice, right upper quadrant pain, transudative ascites, abnormal liver chemistry values, prolonged prothrombin time, and, rarely, cirrhosis (if congestion is prolonged). Medications for heart failure produce gut toxicity, including anorexia, nausea, vomiting, and intestinal ischemia (with digoxin); nausea, anorexia, and diarrhea (with antiarrhythmics); electrolyte disturbances and constipation (with diuretics); mucosal damage (with potassium); and pancreatitis (with diuretics).

Other Cardiac Diseases

Dysphagia may result from left atrial enlargement. Intestinal infarction may be caused by embolism from cardiac thrombi or myxomas and endocarditis. Complications of cardiac surgery include peptic ulcer, cholecystitis, pancreatitis, intestinal infarction, and hepatic necrosis.

CHROMOSOMAL AND GENETIC ABNORMALITIES

Anderson-Fabry Disease

Anderson-Fabry disease, an X-linked glycosphingolipidosis, is caused by impaired function of α-galactosidase A. Deposition of ceramide trihexose produces episodic constipation, diarrhea, nausea and vomiting, abdominal pain, intestinal ischemia, and perforation, as well as renal failure, peripheral paresthesias, and cerebrovascular events. Biopsy specimens from the intestine show foamy or electron-dense deposits in the vascular endothelium and unmyelinated neurons.

Down's Syndrome

Down's syndrome (trisomy 21) is associated with duodenal stenosis and atresia, malrotation, annular pancreas, tracheoesophageal fistula, esophageal stenosis, hiatal hernia, esophageal reflux, imperforate anus, and Hirschsprung's disease. Acquired hepatitis B infection is more common in institutionalized persons.

Familial Mediterranean Fever

Familial Mediterranean fever, an autosomal recessive disorder mapped to chromosome 16, produces recurrent fever, synovitis, serositis, and dermatitis. Attacks may be precipitated by stress and infections.

Gaucher's Disease

Gaucher's disease is characterized by sphingolipid deposition in the reticuloendothelial system, including the liver and spleen. Patients present with hepatosplenomegaly, hepatic fibrosis, or cirrhosis (with ascites and esophageal varices).

Hepatic Porphyrias

Acute intermittent porphyria, hereditary coproporphyria, and variegate porphyria are autosomal dominant conditions characterized by recurrent abdominal pain, nausea, vomiting, constipation, disorientation, seizures, and peripheral neuropathy. Drugs (e.g., barbiturates, steroids, sulfonamides, ethanol), surgery, and pregnancy are precipitating causes (Table 70-1). The diagnosis is established by demonstration of excess porphobilinogen and δ-aminolevulinic acid in the urine.

Hereditary Angioedema

Hereditary angioedema is an autosomal dominant deficiency of C1 esterase that leads to recurrent swelling of the orofacial region, extremities, and gut. The swelling may be provoked by stress or trauma. Abdominal manifestations include

TABLE 70-1
Characteristics of the Hepatic Porphyrias

DISORDER	NEUROPSYCHIATRIC SYMPTOMS	SKIN LESIONS	HEPATIC DISEASE	BIOCHEMICAL ABNORMALITIES		
				Erythrocytes	Urine	Feces
Acute intermittent porphyria	+	–	–	–	Increased PBG, ALA	–
Variegate porphyria	+	+	–	–	Increased coproporphyrin, PBG, ALA	Increased protoporphyrin and coproporphyrin
Hereditary coproporphyria	+	+	–	–	Increased coproporphyrin, PBG, ALA	Increased coproporphyrin
Porphyria cutanea tarda	–	+	+	–	Increased uroporphyrin	–
Protoporphyria	–	+	+	Increased protoporphyrin	–	Increased protoporphyrin
Secondary porphyrinuria	–	–	+	–	Increased coproporphyrin	–

ALA = aminolevulinic acid; PBG = porphobilinogen.

Source: From JR Bloomer. The hepatic porphyrias. Gastroenterology 1976;71:689.

pain, tenderness, bloating, nausea, and vomiting. "Thumbprinting" and other signs of mucosal edema are evident on barium radiography. Synthetic androgens (e.g., danazol, methyltestosterone) may ameliorate attacks. Analgesics and epinephrine are used to treat acute abdominal symptoms. Premedication with fresh frozen plasma or antifibrinolytic agents should be considered before upper gastrointestinal endoscopy.

Familial Hyperlipidemias

Hyperlipidemia type I and type V are associated with recurrent pancreatitis. An increased incidence of gallstone formation occurs in type IV.

Niemann-Pick Disease

Niemann-Pick disease is an inherited disorder of sphingomyelinase activity occurring mostly in people of Jewish ancestry. Patients manifest hepatosplenomegaly and hepatic failure in infancy as a result of an accumulation of sphingomyelin.

Tangier Disease

Tangier disease is an autosomal recessive deficiency of α-lipoprotein characterized by the deposition of cholesterol in the reticuloendothelial system, leading to hepatosplenomegaly, enlarged tonsils, adenopathy, peripheral neuropathy, and yellow-orange patches in the colonic mucosa.

Turner's Syndrome

Turner's syndrome (X chromosome monosomy) is associated with gastrointestinal hemorrhage caused by intestinal vascular malformations.

CONNECTIVE TISSUE DISEASES

Ehlers-Danlos Syndrome

Ehlers-Danlos syndrome is a group of inherited diseases of collagen formation. Gastrointestinal manifestations include gastrointestinal bleeding from mucosal lesions, mesenteric ischemia or intra-abdominal bleeding from splanchnic artery thrombosis or rupture, megaesophagus, intestinal dilation, bacterial overgrowth, colonic hypomotility, and perforation.

Pseudoxanthoma Elasticum

Pseudoxanthoma elasticum, an inherited disorder of connective tissue synthesis, may be complicated by gastrointestinal bleeding caused by ineffective vasoconstriction and vessel retraction after injury resulting from elastic fiber degeneration in visceral blood vessels. Some patients respond to angiographic embolization.

Progressive Systemic Sclerosis

More than 50% of patients with progressive systemic sclerosis or scleroderma have gastrointestinal complications. These include tightening of the perioral skin, gingival inflammation, impaired taste, diminished esophageal body contractions and reduced lower esophageal sphincter pressure, delayed gastric emptying, acid hypersecretion, intestinal hypomotility and dilation, small bowel and colonic pseudodiverticula, bacterial overgrowth, and telangiectasias.

Polymyositis and Dermatomyositis

Polymyositis and dermatomyositis are characterized by inflammation of striated muscle and, to a lesser degree, smooth muscle. The gastrointestinal tract may be involved along its entire length, but the proximal esophagus is most commonly affected, producing dysphagia, regurgitation, and aspiration. Other gut manifestations include esophageal reflux, small bowel and colonic dysmotility, colonic pseudodiverticula, and pneumatosis intestinalis. Malignancy, especially gastric cancer, is found in 25% of patients with dermatomyositis.

Rheumatoid Arthritis

Gastrointestinal manifestations of rheumatoid arthritis include temporomandibular joint arthritis (impairing chewing), sicca syndrome, stomatitis, gingivitis, esophageal dysmotility, secondary amyloidosis (affecting any portion of the gastrointestinal tract), mesenteric vasculitis (leading to hemorrhage, ischemia, infarction), cholecystitis, appendicitis, perisplenitis, splenic infarction, pancreatitis, and hepatic arteritis. Patients with Felty's syndrome are prone to intra-abdominal sepsis. Chronic use of NSAIDs may produce gastrointestinal mucosal damage. Therapy with methotrexate can cause hepatic fibrosis and cirrhosis. Gold preparations can cause colitis.

Sjögren's Syndrome

Sjögren's syndrome is associated with impaired saliva production, impaired esophageal motility, pancreatic insufficiency, primary biliary cirrhosis, and chronic active hepatitis.

Systemic Lupus Erythematosus

Systemic lupus erythematosus may affect the gastrointestinal tract in several ways. Serosal inflammation may produce lupus peritonitis and ascites. Mesenteric vasculitis may result in intestinal ischemia or perforation. Gastritis, mucosal ulcers, pancreatitis, hepatic vasculitis, intussusception, enteritis, esophageal and gastric dysmotility, and pneumatosis intestinalis may be seen.

Seronegative Spondyloarthropathies

The seronegative spondyloarthropathies include ankylosing spondylitis, psoriatic arthritis, the reactive arthritides (e.g., Reiter's syndrome), arthritis associated with inflammatory bowel disease, and Whipple's disease.

DERMATOLOGIC DISEASES

Ataxia-Telangiectasia

Ataxia-telangiectasia is an autosomal recessive condition with marked immunoglobulin deficiency and defective cell-mediated immunity. It is associated with development of adenocarcinoma of the stomach and colon and intestinal lymphoma at early ages. Elevations in levels of smooth muscle antibody, antimitochondrial antibody, and α-fetoprotein may occur without clinically relevant disease.

Blue Rubber Bleb Nevus Syndrome

Blue rubber bleb nevus syndrome is associated with gastrointestinal bleeding secondary to rubbery visceral angiomas.

Cowden's Syndrome

Cowden's syndrome is an autosomal dominant disease characterized by ectodermal, mesodermal, and endodermal hamartomas. Multiple hamartomatous polyps may develop from the esophagus to the colon, causing blood loss and intestinal obstruction. They have low potential for malignant degeneration.

Epidermolysis Bullosa

Epidermolysis bullosa is a group of diseases in which the cohesion of the epidermis and dermis is disrupted by minor trauma. Epidermolysis bullosa lethalis is a fatal autosomal recessive disease of infancy associated with oral, anal, and esophageal blistering and pyloric atresia. Epidermolysis bullosa dystrophica is a disorder characterized by the formation of thin-walled esophageal bullae, which may progress to erosions, ulcers, pseudodiverticula, webs, strictures, and obstruction.

Pemphigus

Pemphigus is a group of diseases characterized by acantholysis resulting in bullae formation, occasionally involving the esophagus.

Hereditary Hemorrhagic Telangiectasia

Hereditary hemorrhagic telangiectasia is an autosomal dominant disorder associated with formation of telangiectasias, aneurysms, and arteriovenous malformations throughout the body. Gastrointestinal hemorrhage develops in 10% to 40% of patients. Large vascular ectasias may occasionally form a mass lesion. Hepatic vascular malformations can lead to hepatomegaly, hematobilia, portal hypertension, esophageal varices, and hepatic encephalopathy.

Neurofibromatosis

Neurofibromatosis is an autosomal dominant disease that involves the gastrointestinal tract in 25% of cases. Rarely, the gallbladder and liver are also involved. Complications include gastrointestinal hemorrhage, obstruction, and development of leiomyomas, sarcomas, and neurogenic neoplasms.

Stevens-Johnson Syndrome

Stevens-Johnson syndrome is a severe hypersensitivity reaction with fever, mucositis, and a diffuse rash that may progress to an exfoliative dermatitis. The oropharyngeal mucosa often exhibits erosions and sloughing. The entire gut may be affected in severe cases. Mucosal injury may produce dysphagia, odynophagia, esophageal strictures, and gastrointestinal hemorrhage.

Tylosis

Tylosis is an autosomal dominant disorder characterized by thickening of the skin on the palms and soles. Papillomas form in the esophageal mucosa. The disease is associated with a 95% probability for development of esophageal carcinoma.

Urticaria

Patients with chronic urticaria may develop abdominal pain, gastroduodenitis, peptic ulcer, and mucosal edema secondary to histamine release. Urticaria may also be a manifestation of systemic vasculitis, systemic mastocytosis, a familial complement deficiency, or infection.

ENDOCRINOLOGIC DISORDERS

Acromegaly

Acromegaly is a disorder of excess growth hormone production that leads to enlargement of the tongue and organs of the digestive system. Patients have a proclivity for development of colonic adenomas and cancer.

Addison's Disease

Addison's disease results from an underproduction of mineralocorticoids and corticosteroids by the adrenals. It is associated with steatorrhea, anorexia, nausea, vomiting, weight loss, abdominal pain, gastritis, antibodies against the gastric proton pump and intrinsic factor, and, rarely, achlorhydria and pernicious anemia.

Diabetes Mellitus

Nausea, vomiting, anorexia, abdominal pain, gastritis, and acute fatty liver are complications of diabetic ketoacidosis. Long-standing diabetes may produce esophageal dilation, delayed esophageal emptying, esophageal reflux, and weak esophageal peristalsis with nonperistaltic contractions. Symptoms of esophageal dysfunction are rare. *Candida* esophagitis may cause odynophagia in patients with diabetes. Gastroparesis is defined as delayed gastric emptying. It may produce early satiety, bloating, heartburn, nausea, vomiting, bezoars, and contribute to poor glycemic control. Diarrhea may occur with or without steatorrhea and is multifactorial (i.e., bacterial overgrowth, secretion, motility disturbance, anal neuropathy, bile acid malabsorption, associated celiac sprue, and pancreatic insufficiency). Constipation results from colonic motor dysfunction and depression, whereas fecal incontinence results from neuropathic damage to the anal sphincter. Thoracic radiculopathy may produce severe abdominal pain. Intestinal angina, malabsorption, diarrhea, and hemorrhage may result from mesenteric atherosclerosis or microvascular disease. Impaired gallbladder contractility predisposes to gallstone formation. Hepatomegaly, steatosis, and, rarely, hepatitis may develop secondary to poor control of blood sugar.

Hyperparathyroidism

Hyperparathyroidism may be characterized by anorexia, nausea, vomiting, constipation, and abdominal pain, which probably are symptoms of hypercalcemia. Hypercalcemia may lead to pancreatitis and possibly may predispose to peptic ulcer formation.

Hypoparathyroidism

Gastrointestinal manifestations of hypocalcemia secondary to hypoparathyroidism include abdominal pain, intestinal tetany, diarrhea, steatorrhea, and intestinal pseudo-obstruction as well as esophageal candidiasis caused by associated immune dysfunction.

Hyperthyroidism

Gastrointestinal symptoms of hyperthyroidism include anorexia, nausea, vomiting, increased stool frequency, mild steatorrhea, and a high incidence of gastritis and hypochlorhydria. Moderate to severe hyperthyroidism may cause heart failure and subsequent dysfunction and passive congestion of the liver. Primary biliary cirrhosis and chronic active hepatitis are associated with autoimmune thyroid disease. Goiters may produce esophageal displacement and dysphagia in the absence of hyperthyroidism.

Hypothyroidism

Hypothyroidism may lead to delayed esophageal emptying, constipation, distention, diarrhea caused by bacterial overgrowth, intestinal pseudo-obstruction, megacolon, and poor gallbladder contractility. Other manifestations include impaired salivary, gastric, intestinal, and pancreatic secretion; ascites; and histologic changes in liver architecture suggestive of central congestive fibrosis.

Pregnancy-Related Disorders

Common gastrointestinal symptoms in pregnancy include altered appetite, pica, ptyalism, gingivitis, nausea, vomiting, heartburn, constipation, and hemorrhoids. Gastroesophageal reflux occurs in 40% of pregnancies and is worse during the third trimester, whereas nausea occurs in >50% of pregnancies and is most severe during the first trimester. Constipation results from mechanical compression of the colon, motor inhibitory effects of circulating hormones, and lack of exercise. Delayed gallbladder emptying is reported, and the incidence of cholecystitis is slightly increased during pregnancy. Jaundice is most often secondary to benign intrahepatic cholestasis. Toxemia may produce indirect hyperbilirubinemia secondary to hemolysis. The HELLP (hemolysis, elevated liver enzyme levels, low platelet levels) syndrome is a potentially catastrophic variant of toxemia. Its features suggest a thrombotic microangiopathic process. Acute fatty liver of pregnancy occurs in young primigravidas in their third trimester. Vomiting, jaundice, encephalopathy, and acute renal failure are often present. Microvesicular fat deposition in the central zone is seen in liver biopsy specimens. Splenic artery rupture is a rare, life-threatening complication of pregnancy that manifests as acute abdominal pain and shock.

GRANULOMATOUS DISEASES

Many infectious and noninfectious diseases are associated with granuloma formation in the liver and intestine. In the developed world, the etiologic factors most frequently responsible for hepatic granulomas are sarcoidosis, tuberculosis, primary biliary cirrhosis, and other primary liver diseases (Table 70-2). Crohn's disease and tuberculous enteritis are the most common causes of granulomatous inflammation of the intestine.

HEAVY METAL TOXICITY

Lead Poisoning

Lead poisoning may result from ingestion or removal of lead-based paints, battery or jewelry manufacture, welding, automobile radiator repair, or eating from painted dishes acquired abroad. Presentations include recurrent, severe abdominal pain (i.e., lead colic, which may mimic acute abdomen), oral ulcers, constipation, paresthesia and peripheral neuropathy, a metallic

TABLE 70-2
Causes of Hepatic Granulomas

	PERCENTAGE OF CASES
Sarcoidosis	35
Tuberculosis	20
Undetermined	11
Primary biliary cirrhosis	5
Other cirrhosis	5
Schistosomiasis	2
Lymphoma	2
Brucellosis	2
Medication-induced or toxic hepatitis	1
Acute viral hepatitis	1
Fungal infections	1
Other infections	5
Other noninfectious causes	9

Source: Adapted from PT Harrington, JT Gutierrez, CH Ramirez-Ronda, et al. Granulomatous hepatitis. Rev Infect Dis 1982;4:639.

taste in the mouth, a gingival lead line, anemia, renal dysfunction, mild hepatitis, and secondary porphyria. The diagnosis is established by 72-hour urine lead measurement after administration of calcium disodium edetate.

Arsenic Poisoning

Arsenic poisoning may occur in persons who are involved in wood preservation and glass and metal manufacturing and in those who are victims of intentional poisoning. Doses of 100 to 300 mg can cause acute symptoms and death. Acute arsenic poisoning produces abdominal pain, vomiting, diarrhea, garlicky breath, dysphagia, hepatomegaly, jaundice, and circulatory collapse as a result of blockade of cellular oxidative processes. The diagnosis is made by Gutzeit's or Reinsch's test or by measuring arsenic levels in a tissue sample (e.g., hair or nails). Chronic arsenic toxicity is more insidious. Symptoms include weakness, nausea, diarrhea, constipation, macular skin pigmentation, leukoderma, palmar and plantar keratoses, pancytopenia, edema, peripheral vascular disease, neuropathy, cirrhosis, portal hypertension, and possibly an increased tendency to development of cutaneous, hematologic, respiratory, and hepatic malignancies.

Gold Toxicity

Gold-induced enterocolitis can affect both the small intestine and colon. The clinical course is protracted and often fatal. Colonoscopy reveals an erythematous, friable, ulcerated mucosa that resembles ulcerative colitis.

HEMATOLOGIC DISORDERS

Hemolytic Uremic Syndrome

Hemolytic uremic syndrome is characterized by hemolysis, thrombocytopenia, and acute renal failure. A common cause is enteric infection with *Salmonella*, *Shigella*, or *Campylobacter* species or *Escherichia coli* (especially O157:H7). Endothelial cell injury, perhaps mediated by endotoxins or immune complexes, is followed by intravascular coagulation and then thrombotic microangiopathy in the glomerulus and gastrointestinal mucosa.

Thrombotic Thrombocytopenic Purpura

Thrombotic thrombocytopenic purpura is similar to hemolytic uremic syndrome, except that it occurs in older persons (30 to 40 years of age) and manifests as fever, neurologic findings, and an association with cholecystitis.

Hypercoagulability

Oral contraceptives, pregnancy, inflammation, and surgery reduce antithrombin levels. Paroxysmal nocturnal hemoglobinuria is an acquired hemolytic disorder associated with a thrombotic diathesis, whereas antithrombin III deficiency and protein C deficiency are inherited hypercoagulable disorders. In these conditions and in polycythemia rubra vera (see below), mesenteric and portal vein involvement can lead to intestinal ischemia and portal or hepatic vein thrombosis, respectively.

Coagulation Factor Deficits

Gastrointestinal hemorrhage may complicate the course of disease in patients with coagulation factor deficits, whether the condition is inherited (e.g., factor VIII deficiency in hemophilia A, factor IX deficiency in hemophilia B, factor XI deficiency) or whether it is an acquired or iatrogenic condition (e.g., in the presence of lupus anticoagulant, vitamin K deficiency, liver disease, or warfarin therapy).

Platelet Defects

Gastrointestinal bleeding may occur with platelet defects. Inherited diseases associated with platelet defects include von Willebrand's disease, Bernard-Soulier syndrome, and Glanzmann's thrombasthenia. Aspirin and NSAIDs may also interfere with platelet function.

Plummer-Vinson (Paterson-Kelly) Syndrome

Plummer-Vinson (Paterson-Kelly) syndrome produces dysphagia (caused by hypopharyngeal or esophageal webs), iron deficiency anemia, glossitis, cheilosis, dyspepsia, diarrhea, flatulence, hoarseness, paresthesias, pyorrhea, koilony-chia, atrophic gastritis, splenomegaly, and an increased risk of development of hypopharyngeal and esophageal malignancies. The significance of iron deficiency anemia in the pathogenesis of the syndrome is not understood. A hereditary predisposition as well as deficiencies of riboflavin, thiamine, and pyridoxine have been implicated as etiologic factors.

Sickle Cell Anemia

Acute sickle cell crisis may produce abdominal pain, ileus, mucosal ulcers, and gastrointestinal hemorrhage. Multiple air-fluid levels are evident on abdominal radiographs. Hepatobiliary findings include jaundice, hepatomegaly, cholelithiasis, cholecystitis, and transfusion-related hemosiderosis. Splenomegaly is prevalent in early disease, but recurrent splenic infarctions lead to autosplenectomy and hyposplenism.

Hemoglobin C Disease

Hemoglobin C disease has manifestations similar to those of sickle cell anemia, but attacks are milder and splenomegaly persists into adulthood.

Hereditary Spherocytosis

Hereditary spherocytosis is an autosomal dominant disorder characterized by fragile erythrocytes. Patients present with indirect hyperbilirubinemia (as a result of hemolysis), jaundice, pigment gallstones, splenomegaly, and relapsing pancreatitis.

METABOLIC DISEASES

Systemic Amyloidosis

Because of widespread extracellular deposition of amyloid, amyloidosis produces macroglossia, disrupted esophageal contractions, reduced lower esophageal sphincter pressure, prominent gastric and intestinal folds, gastric outlet obstruction, gastric ulcer, gastrointestinal hemorrhage, mesenteric retraction, intestinal obstruction, pseudo-obstruction, bacterial overgrowth, intestinal ischemia, hepatosplenomegaly, and pancreatic exocrine insufficiency.

Capillary Leak Syndrome

Gastrointestinal manifestations of the capillary leak syndrome, an episodic illness characterized by increased small vessel permeability and fluid shifts, include nausea, vomiting, and diarrhea secondary to impaired fluid absorption in the gastrointestinal tract.

NEOPLASTIC DISORDERS

Acute and Chronic Leukemias

Gastrointestinal involvement with acute and chronic leukemia is common. Leukemic infiltration of the gums, tonsils, esophagus, stomach, intestine, and colon can cause oral pain and bleeding, dysphagia, obstruction, hemorrhage, and enterocolitis. Hepatosplenomegaly, portal hypertension, subcapsular splenic hemorrhage, and splenic rupture may also result from leukemic infiltration. Various chemotherapies can cause mucositis, nausea, vomiting, diarrhea, constipation, ileus, hemorrhage, and even an acute abdomen. Necrotizing enterocolitis (sometimes called *typhlitis*) may complicate chemotherapy-induced neutropenia. Immunosuppressed leukemic patients are at risk for opportunistic infections caused by *Candida* organisms, herpesvirus, or cytomegalovirus.

Multiple Myeloma and Waldenström's Macroglobulinemia

If multiple myeloma involves the gastrointestinal tract, the formation of plasmacytomas can produce abdominal pain, gastrointestinal ulceration, hemorrhage, and obstruction. Hyperviscosity may result in intestinal ischemia and mesenteric thrombosis. Multiple myeloma may also be complicated by amyloidosis. Waldenström's macroglobulinemia, an IgM-secreting variant of myeloma, is associated with hepatosplenomegaly and malabsorption caused by plasma cell infiltration of the liver, intestine, and lymph nodes.

Heavy-Chain Diseases

α-Heavy-chain disease, the most common of the heavy-chain diseases, may result in the infiltration of the intestine and abdominal lymph nodes with malignant B lymphocytes and α-chains. Symptoms and complications include abdominal pain, palpable masses, vomiting, weight loss, malabsorption, hypocalcemia, obstruction, intussusception, and perforation.

Hodgkin's Disease

Presinusoidal portal hypertension results from increased intrahepatic blood flow resulting from splenomegaly or intrahepatic infiltration with malignant Hodgkin's lymphoma cells. Rarely, enlarged mesenteric lymph nodes manifest as an abdominal mass or cause obstruction.

Non-Hodgkin's Lymphoma

Up to 10% of patients with non-Hodgkin's lymphoma exhibit symptoms of gastrointestinal tract involvement: obstruction, hemorrhage, abdominal masses, and perforation. Hepatic and splenic invasion is frequent.

Polycythemia Vera

Gastrointestinal manifestations of the erythrocytosis and hyperviscosity associated with polycythemia vera include peptic ulcer disease, Budd-Chiari syndrome, splanchnic circulatory insufficiency, gastrointestinal hemorrhage, hepatosplenomegaly (caused by extramedullary hematopoiesis), and cheilosis and glossitis (caused by iron deficiency anemia).

Essential Thrombocytosis

Essential or primary thrombocytosis predisposes to gastrointestinal bleeding, mesenteric thrombosis, and hepatosplenomegaly (caused by extramedullary hematopoiesis or Budd-Chiari syndrome).

Malignant Melanoma

Malignant melanoma metastasizes to the stomach in 26%, the small intestine in 58%, and the colon in 26% of all cases. In some cases, the liver, pancreas, and gallbladder are also involved. Symptomatic manifestations include abdominal pain, anorexia, hemorrhage, obstruction, intussusception, perforation, jaundice, and cholecystitis.

Ovarian Cancer

Ovarian cancer often encases the abdominal viscera, producing intestinal obstruction that leads to malnutrition and intestinal infarction.

Paraneoplastic Syndromes

The major clinical gastrointestinal manifestations of paraneoplastic syndromes are anorexia, dysphagia, nausea, vomiting, bloating, constipation, and diarrhea. Impaired gastrointestinal motility may result from paraneoplastic visceral neuropathy and from tumor-induced hypercalcemia.

Cancer Cachexia

Cancer cachexia is characterized by progressive involuntary weight loss, anorexia, and metabolic disturbances. The circulating humoral factors responsible for this paraneoplastic syndrome are unknown. Tumor necrosis factor released by macrophages may be one determinant.

Mastocytosis

Gastrointestinal dysfunction occurs in 25% of patients with mastocytosis. Symptoms are probably caused by the release of mast cell products (e.g., histamine). Patients present with abdominal pain, nausea, diarrhea, malabsorption, gastritis, and peptic ulcer disease.

Diffuse Esophageal Leiomyomatosis

Diffuse esophageal leiomyomatosis is an autosomal dominant disorder. Patients present with achalasia caused by entrapment of ganglia secondary to esophageal leiomyomas. Other manifestations include mastocytosis, intestinal leiomyomas or neurofibromas, and urticaria pigmentosa.

NEUROMUSCULAR DISORDERS

Brain Injury

Acute brain injury secondary to stroke, trauma, tumor, or surgery produces gastric erosions, ulcerations (Cushing's ulcer), and hemorrhage, whereas chronic sequelae of brain injury include oropharyngeal and cricopharyngeal dysfunction, constipation, and fecal incontinence.

Dementia Syndromes

Dementia syndromes are associated with failure to thrive as a result of reduced oral intake, esophageal foreign bodies, peptic ulcer disease, and other intra-abdominal processes.

Migraine

Gastrointestinal manifestations of migraine headaches include nausea, vomiting, abdominal pain, and diarrhea. Abdominal migraines are characterized by recurrent identical attacks of abdominal pain, no abdominal symptoms between attacks, a family history of migraine headache, and response to migraine therapy.

Multiple Sclerosis

Multiple sclerosis is associated with anorectal dysfunction, gastroparesis, abnormal colonic motor activity, and oropharyngeal motor disturbances. Patients present with incontinence, nausea, vomiting, constipation, megacolon, and dysphagia.

Muscular Dystrophies

Duchenne's muscular dystrophy, an X-linked recessive disorder that occurs in childhood, may be associated with nausea, vomiting, abdominal distention, constipation, acute gastric dilation, and pseudo-obstruction. Myotonic dystrophy, an autosomal dominant disease, has prominent gastrointestinal symptoms, including oropharyngeal dysphagia, aspiration, nausea, abdominal distention and pain, ileus, diarrhea, constipation, and symptomatic cholelithiasis. Oculopharyngeal muscular dystrophy is associated with oropharyngeal dysphagia and pharyngo-oral and pharyngonasal regurgitation.

Parkinsonism

Gastrointestinal manifestations of parkinsonism include oropharyngeal dysphagia (caused by involvement of the swallowing centers), esophageal hypomotility, constipation, megacolon, and pseudo-obstruction. These effects may be exacerbated by administration of anticholinergic medications that treat parkinsonism.

Spinal Cord Lesions

Spinal cord transection often leads to constipation and fecal incontinence as a result of loss of rectal sensation, reduced control of defecation, and anal dysfunction. High spinal cord lesions can impair gastric and small bowel motility, resulting in gastric distention, esophageal reflux, and adynamic ileus. Acute abdominal emergencies may be mimicked by pain referred aberrantly because neural pathways are dysfunctional; in this setting, there is increased abdominal muscle spasticity, but no abdominal rigidity or tenderness.

Other Neuromuscular Diseases

Stiff man syndrome may lead to dysphagia as a result of cricopharyngeal and upper esophageal spasm. Oropharyngeal dysfunction also occurs with amyotrophic lateral sclerosis, myasthenia gravis, and Kearns-Sayre syndrome. Familial visceral neuropathies and myopathies and pure dysautonomia are associated with intestinal pseudo-obstruction. Hereditary internal anal sphincter myopathy, an autosomal disorder, is characterized by a hypertrophic sphincteric muscle, constipation, and proctalgia fugax.

NUTRITIONAL DISTURBANCES

Malnutrition

Kwashiorkor-marasmus syndromes are caused by protein-calorie undernutrition. Vitamin and mineral deficiencies, diarrhea (resulting from intestinal and pancreatic atrophy), and infectious complications (resulting from malnutrition-induced immunodeficiency) can accompany this type of illness. Hepatomegaly, fatty liver, and chronic calcific pancreatitis may develop. Rapid refeeding with carbohydrate-rich solutions produces hypophosphatemia, hypokalemia, hypomagnesemia, and, in some cases, death.

Obesity

Obesity predisposes to cholelithiasis, esophageal reflux, and fatty liver. Gastric surgery for obesity may lead to cholecystitis and deficiencies of vitamin B_{12}, folate, and iron, whereas jejunoileal bypass is associated with significant intestinal and hepatic (cirrhosis) complications.

ORGAN TRANSPLANT COMPLICATIONS

Bone Marrow Transplantation

Gastrointestinal complications of bone marrow transplantation result from induction regimens (lethal doses of chemotherapy and radiation therapy), immunosuppression, and graft-versus-host disease. Induction regimens can lead to oropharyngeal pain, nausea, vomiting, abdominal pain, diarrhea, and hemorrhage. Immune system dysfunction predisposes to bacterial and fungal (usually *Candida albicans*) infections in the initial 30 days after transplant, and viral and parasitic infections thereafter. Infection with *Clostridium difficile* can cause severe and prolonged diarrhea without pseudomembrane production in patients with neutropenia. Graft-versus-host disease may be acute (onset <100 days post-transplant) or chronic (onset >100 days post-transplant). It is less likely to occur if syngeneic or T-lymphocyte–depleted marrow is transplanted. Early clinical signs include watery diarrhea, anorexia, nausea, vomiting, abdominal pain. Radiographic findings include thickening of the bowel wall, rapid intestinal transit time, and loss of distal small bowel mucosal folds. Rectal biopsy specimens show epithelial necrosis, crypt abscesses, and crypt obliteration.

Renal Transplantation

In a patient who has had a renal transplantation, oral and esophageal thrush result from immunosuppression and antibiotic use, whereas gastrointestinal bleeding is secondary to gastritis, stress, or peptic disease. Intestinal ischemia, diverticulitis, cytomegalovirus (CMV)-induced colitis, and intra-abdominal abscesses may affect some patients postoperatively. Pancreatitis may result from azathioprine or prednisone therapy. Lymphomas, Kaposi's sarcoma, and other malignancies are associated with prolonged immunosuppressive therapy.

Cardiac Transplantation

After cardiac transplantation, gastrointestinal hemorrhage may result from hemorrhagic gastritis or peptic disease. Other gastrointestinal complications include pancreatitis, cholecystitis, ileus, bowel perforation, gastric outlet obstruction, and perirectal abscess.

Liver Transplantation

In addition to the problems of liver rejection and common bile duct ischemia postoperatively, liver transplant patients can present with CMV colitis or enterocolitis, pancreatitis, and gastrointestinal bleeding.

Blood Transfusion

Rarely, graft-versus-host disease occurs when blood is transfused from a first-degree relative to an immunocompromised recipient.

PSYCHOLOGICAL DISORDERS

Anorexia Nervosa and Bulimia

The complications of anorexia nervosa are mostly those of starvation. Bulimia can produce acute gastric dilation with rupture, dental enamel erosion, esophagitis, Mallory-Weiss tears, and esophageal rupture.

Anxiety and Stress

Emotional factors may cause or contribute to globus symptoms: noncardiac chest pain, nonulcer dyspepsia, and irritable bowel syndrome.

Major Depression or Conversion Disorder

Psychogenic vomiting, constipation, and other gastrointestinal complaints are manifestations of major depression or conversion disorder.

Munchausen's Syndrome

Patients with Munchausen's syndrome often feign gastrointestinal illnesses, including abdominal emergencies, hematemesis, and inflammatory bowel diseases.

Schizophrenia

Schizophrenics may present after ingesting a foreign body. Also, antipsychotic medications have significant anticholinergic activity that may cause gastric retention, megacolon, and constipation.

PULMONARY DISEASES

Gastroesophageal Reflux Disease

Gastroesophageal reflux may lead to chronic cough, hoarseness, and nocturnal asthma.

Respiratory Failure

Respiratory failure and mechanical ventilation may be complicated by gastrointestinal hemorrhage from erosive gastritis and peptic ulcer disease. Chronic respiratory failure may also predispose to development of pneumatosis intestinalis.

α_1-Antitrypsin Deficiency

The ZZ phenotype of α_1-antitrypsin deficiency, an autosomal recessive disorder, is associated with development of hepatic cirrhosis. Liver biopsy specimens show characteristic periportal granules containing α_1-antitrypsin.

Aspiration of Gastroenteric Contents

Life-threatening respiratory distress or pneumonia may result from aspiration of gastroenteric contents. Aspiration may be detected using scintigraphic studies or by addition of methylene blue to the feeding solutions. Small-volume feeds, postpyloric feeding tubes, and elevating the head during feeding may reduce the incidence of this complication.

Cystic Fibrosis

Affected infants with cystic fibrosis may present with meconium ileus, intussusception, intestinal atresia, volvulus, and perforation. Chronic constipation, small bowel obstruction, and rectal prolapse may develop in older children. Gastroesophageal reflux results from reduced saliva production, gastrointestinal hypomotility, chronic coughing, and postural drainage of pulmonary secretions. Pancreatic insufficiency leads to malabsorption of fat and nonfat nutrients. Glucose intolerance is common, but development of frank diabetes is unusual with cystic fibrosis. Chronic biliary obstruction often occurs but rarely has significant clinical sequelae.

RENAL FAILURE

Uremia is associated with dysgeusia, oral inflammation, parotitis, sicca syndrome, abdominal pain, anorexia, nausea, vomiting, constipation, pseudo-obstruction, and intussusception. Gastrointestinal hemorrhage results most commonly from hemorrhagic gastritis or angiodysplasia. Abnormal bile acids may produce "uremic diarrhea." Pancreatic exocrine insufficiency is described with uremia and may contribute to malnutrition. Duodenal pseudomelanosis, a pigmentation of the proximal duodenum with iron sulfide or hemosiderin, occurs with renal failure. Metastatic calcifications may be deposited in the mesenteric vessels, resulting in ischemia, hemorrhage, or infarction. Chronic ambulatory peritoneal dialysis may predispose to bacterial peritonitis as well as development of refractory exudative ascites. Hemodialysis may predispose to acquisition of hepatitis infections or to hemosiderosis.

SUBSTANCE ABUSE

Ethanol

Ethanol consumption can produce dysphagia and promote esophageal reflux by delaying esophageal emptying and decreasing the frequency of peristaltic contractions. Heavy acute ingestion of alcohol may result in gastric erosions, but there is no proven association of chronic ethanol ingestion with peptic ulcer disease. Alcoholism may result in diarrhea and malabsorption because of enhanced small bowel transit, reduced brush border enzyme activity, impaired absorption, pancreatic insufficiency, liver disease, and malnutrition. Other complications include pancreatitis, hepatic steatosis, hepatitis, cirrhosis, and carcinoma of the larynx, nasopharynx, esophagus, and liver.

Cocaine

Anorexia and diarrhea are common with cocaine use, whereas intestinal ischemia and hepatocellular necrosis are rare complications. The practice of smuggling cocaine in swallowed condoms can result in intestinal obstruction or death if a condom ruptures internally.

Opiates

Gastrointestinal symptoms of opiate abuse include anorexia, nausea, vomiting, abdominal pain, and constipation. Intravenous use may lead to viral hepatitis, cirrhosis, hepatic abscess, or talc granulomas.

Tobacco

Complications of tobacco smoking include carcinoma of the oropharynx, esophagus, and pancreas. Smokers are also at increased risk for the development of peptic ulcer disease and Crohn's disease.

VASCULITIDES

Behçet's Disease

Gastrointestinal manifestations of Behçet's disease, a systemic illness of unknown etiology characterized by necrotizing vasculitis, include oral lesions resembling aphthous ulcers, esophageal ulcers (which may bleed, perforate, or lead to stricture), and intestinal involvement resembling Crohn's disease (which may result in bleeding or perforation).

Giant Cell Arteritis

Disseminated fibrinoid necrosis of smaller arteries that occurs in giant cell arteritis can result in intestinal ischemia, abdominal pain, nausea, anorexia, weight loss, hemorrhage, and perforation.

Henoch-Schönlein Purpura

The gastrointestinal tract is affected in 50% of cases of Henoch-Schönlein purpura, a systemic small vessel vasculitis. Symptoms include abdominal pain, diarrhea, vomiting, obstruction, and intussusception. The bowel may exhibit edema, submucosal or subserosal hemorrhage, and thickened folds on radiographic or endoscopic evaluation.

Köhlmeier-Degos Disease

Köhlmeier-Degos disease is a vasculitis of small to medium-sized arteries that is characterized by renal failure, intestinal ischemia, bleeding, and perforation.

Polyarteritis Nodosa

Polyarteritis nodosa is a systemic necrotizing vasculitis of small to medium-sized arteries, often caused by hepatitis B infection. Two-thirds of patients present with gastrointestinal complaints. Epigastric pain, nausea, anorexia, mucosal ulceration, bleeding, diarrhea, appendicitis, cholecystitis, pancreatitis, obstruction, hepatic infarction, pseudomembranous colitis, pneumatosis intestinalis, peritonitis, and intra-abdominal abscess may develop.

Churg-Strauss Disease

Churg-Strauss is a systemic vasculitis that may lead to nausea, vomiting, hemorrhage, perforation, and cholecystitis.

Wegener's Granulomatosis

Vasculitis associated with Wegener's granulomatosis can result in intestinal or colonic ischemia, hemorrhage, and perforation. The presence of antineutrophil cytoplasmic antibodies may assist in diagnosis.

Cryoglobulinemia

Circulating immune complexes characteristic in cryoglobulinemia may initiate a vasculitis that involves the gut in 20% of cases, producing cramping, enterocolitis, and, rarely, ischemia of the small intestine or colon.

CHAPTER 71

Gastrointestinal Manifestations of Immunologic Disorders

IMMUNODEFICIENCY DISEASES OF THE GUT

B-Lymphocyte (Antibody) Defects

X-Linked Hypogammaglobulinemia

Etiology and Pathogenesis. X-linked (congenital or Burton's) hypogamma-globulinemia occurs predominantly in males and is characterized by low serum levels of all immunoglobulins (<200 mg per dl). An intrinsic B-lymphocyte defect with a maturation block in B-cell differentiation is present. Pre-B cells are present in bone marrow, but circulating B cells are absent.

Clinical Features, Diagnosis, and Management. Patients present in infancy or early childhood (after loss of maternal IgG) with recurrent pyogenic infections that affect the gastrointestinal tract in 30% of cases. Diarrhea caused by *Campylobacter* organisms is the most common infectious condition. Perirectal abscesses, bacterial overgrowth in the small bowel, and viral infections (hepatitis, enterovirus) also occur. Giardiasis is surprisingly uncommon. An increased incidence of lymphomas and leukemias has been reported. Examination of rectal biopsy specimens reveals a neutrophilic lamina propria infiltrate, crypt abscesses, and an absence of plasma cells. Treatment is with parenteral immunoglobulin replacement.

Selective Immunoglobulin A Deficiency

Etiology and Pathogenesis. Selective IgA deficiency is the most prevalent primary immune deficiency. It usually occurs sporadically, although familial cases are reported and drugs (e.g., phenytoin, penicillamine, sulfasalazine) can

TABLE 71-1
Disorders that May Occur in Association with Immunoglobulin A Deficiency

Gastrointestinal associations
   Celiac sprue
   Pernicious anemia
   Vitamin B_{12} deficiency secondary to bacterial overgrowth
   Intrinsic factor deficiency
   Nodular lymphoid hyperplasia
   Food allergy
   Crohn's disease
   Disaccharidase deficiencies (unproven)
Extraintestinal associations
   Collagen vascular diseases
   Atopy
   Malignancy (lymphoma, carcinoma [?])

produce reversible deficiency. Most patients lack serum and secretory IgA1 and IgA2. IgA deficiency also is associated with celiac sprue (Table 71-1).

Clinical Features, Diagnosis, and Management.   Most IgA-deficient persons are asymptomatic, but some people develop recurrent bacterial and viral sinopulmonary infections. The frequency of giardiasis is not greater in IgA-deficient patients than in the general population. Jejunal biopsy specimens usually appear normal, but immunofluorescence reveals few or no IgA-producing cells and increased numbers of cells secreting IgM, which can bind to secretory component. There is no specific treatment for IgA deficiency.

Common Variable Hypogammaglobulinemia

Etiology and Pathogenesis.   Common variable hypogammaglobulinemia is a heterogeneous group of disorders that usually are sporadic but can be familial. It is characterized by an intrinsic defect in terminal B-cell differentiation and variable alterations in T-cell function. One-third of patients exhibit atrophic gastritis and pernicious anemia. In contrast to the classic symptoms of pernicious anemia and gastric atrophy, however, patients with common variable hypogammaglobulinemia exhibit an absence of mucosal plasma cells, a lack of autoantibodies, involvement of the entire gastric mucosa, and normal gastrin levels with defective gastrin release in response to meal or bombesin stimulation. Nodular lymphoid hyperplasia may affect the small intestine as well as the colon, rectum, and stomach. The nodules consist of lymphoid follicles with germinal centers within the lamina propria. Plasma cells are absent or reduced in number. The lymphoid hyperplasia is thought to reflect B-lymphocytes unable to undergo full differentiation and is not a premalignant condition.

Clinical Features, Diagnosis, and Management.   Patients with common variable hypogammaglobulinemia present at a later age (second or third decade of life) with less severe infections than those associated with X-linked hypogammaglobulinemia. Recurrent respiratory infections or diarrhea (60% of cases) and steatorrhea are the most prevalent complications. Giardiasis is an especially common cause of symptoms and may cause extensive mucosal damage with malabsorption. Cryptosporidiosis, strongyloidiasis, and bacterial overgrowth with anaerobic species also occur but are less common. Infections caused by *Campylobacter* species may mimic ulcerative colitis. Intestinal biopsy specimens often show villous atrophy, but the lesion differs from celiac sprue in that there is a paucity of lamina propria plasma cells, and the condition rarely responds to dietary gluten exclusion. Chronic liver disease occurs in 10% to 15% of patients, in many cases secondary to viral hepatitis acquired from intravenous immunoglobulin preparations; other causes include cholelithiasis, autoimmune hepatitis, sclerosing cholangitis, and biliary cryptosporidiosis.

T-Lymphocyte Defects

Congenital Thymic Hypoplasia

Etiology and Pathogenesis. Congenital thymic hypoplasia (DiGeorge syndrome) results from defective embryonic formation of the third and fourth pharyngeal pouches. It is characterized by absent T-lymphocyte function, hypoparathyroidism, and cardiovascular abnormalities.

Clinical Features, Diagnosis, and Management. Neonates present with tetany or seizures and other congenital anomalies. Other gastrointestinal manifestations include candidiasis, chronic diarrhea, and malabsorption.

Chronic Mucocutaneous Candidiasis

Etiology and Pathogenesis. Chronic mucocutaneous candidiasis is a group of five syndromes characterized by increased susceptibility to *Candida* infections. The disease has variable association with Addison's disease, diabetes, hypothyroidism, and hypoparathyroidism.

Clinical Features, Diagnosis, and Management. Patients typically present with recurrent oropharyngeal or esophageal candidiasis, which may be complicated by stricture formation. Therapy is with ketoconazole or amphotericin B.

Combined B- and T-Lymphocyte Defects

Severe Combined Immunodeficiency Syndromes

Etiology and Pathogenesis. Severe combined immunodeficiency syndromes are a group of disorders with defective B- and T-lymphocyte function. These syndromes may be autosomal or X-linked recessive and result from adenosine deaminase deficiency or defective expression of major histocompatibility complex antigens. The variant syndrome of reticular dysgenesis has a coexisting granulocyte deficiency.

Clinical Features, Diagnosis, and Management. Infants present with life-threatening infection (cytomegalovirus, rotavirus), diarrhea, malabsorption, and failure to thrive. Graft-versus-host disease may develop because of exposure to maternal lymphocytes during delivery. Intestinal biopsy specimens show an absence of plasma cells, partial villous atrophy, and macrophages in the lamina propria that stain positive to periodic acid–Schiff stain. Bone marrow transplantation is needed to prevent a fatal outcome.

Wiskott-Aldrich Syndrome

Etiology and Pathogenesis.   Wiskott-Aldrich syndrome is an X-linked recessive condition that is caused by defective T-lymphocyte function and poor antibody response to polysaccharide antigens.

Clinical Features, Diagnosis, and Management.   Patients present with eczema, thrombocytopenia, recurrent infections, and development of lymphoma as well as gastrointestinal manifestations (i.e., hemorrhage, diarrhea, malabsorption, colitis). Bone marrow transplantation is the treatment of choice.

Ataxia-Telangiectasia

Etiology and Pathogenesis.   Ataxia-telangiectasia is an autosomal recessive disorder of defective DNA repair mechanisms, with frequent chromosomal abnormalities and increased sensitivity to radiation. Defects in cellular and humoral immunity, including IgA deficiency, are prominent.

Clinical Features, Diagnosis, and Management.   Clinical manifestations include ataxia, oculocutaneous telangiectasia, recurrent sinopulmonary infections, and high incidences of lymphoreticular malignancies and adenocarcinoma. Mild abnormalities of liver function may be noted, and levels of α-fetoprotein are elevated.

Phagocytic Cell Defects

Chronic Granulomatous Disease

Etiology and Pathogenesis.   Chronic granulomatous disease represents a group of X-linked or autosomal recessive disorders of defective phagocytic cell oxidative metabolism. Microbicidal activity is defective because toxic oxygen metabolites (e.g., hydroxyl radical, hydrogen peroxide) are not generated. This leads to increased susceptibility to pyogenic (*Staphylococcus* species, *Serratia marcescens*, *Salmonella* species, gram-negative enterococci) and fungal (*Candida* and *Aspergillus* species) infections, especially if the organisms are positive for catalase.

Clinical Features, Diagnosis, and Management.   Patients usually present in infancy with infection, granuloma formation throughout the body, and pigmented, lipid-bearing tissue histiocytes. Hepatomegaly is common. Liver abscesses form in about one-third of cases and often require surgery. Gastrointestinal manifestations include gingivitis, stomatitis, antral strictures, perianal abscesses, *Salmonella* gastroenteritis, diarrhea, and malabsorption.

Complement Deficiency

Etiology and Pathogenesis

The most common complement deficiency syndrome is hereditary angioedema, an autosomal dominant disorder with decreased levels (85% of cases) or impaired function (15% of cases) of C1 esterase inhibitor. The condition is believed to result from increased vascular permeability that is mediated by kinins, the production of which is inhibited by C1 esterase inhibitor. Lymphoproliferative disorders and collagen vascular diseases may produce an acquired deficiency of C1 esterase inhibitor. Familial Mediterranean fever, characterized by defective C5a inhibitor protein in serosal fluid, is the other complement deficiency state with gastrointestinal symptoms.

Clinical Features, Diagnosis, and Management

Patients present with painless, nonpitting, subepithelial edema of the skin and mucous membranes. Attacks develop over the course of hours and are often precipitated by trauma, infections, or surgery. Gastrointestinal manifestations include abdominal pain, vomiting, diarrhea, tenderness, intussusception, fever, hypotension, and increased bowel sounds. Barium radiographs may show mucosal edema, whereas biopsy specimens show an absence of inflammatory infiltrates. The diagnosis is confirmed by quantitative and qualitative analysis of C1 esterase inhibitor. C4 levels may also be reduced. Anabolic steroids (e.g., danazol, stanozolol) can prevent attacks.

IMMUNODEFICIENCY SECONDARY TO GUT DISEASE

Protein-Losing Enteropathy and Intestinal Lymphangiectasia

Etiology and Pathogenesis

Protein loss caused by protein-losing enteropathy or intestinal lymphangiectasia may produce hypogammaglobulinemia, which usually reduces IgG levels most severely but also reduces the number of lymphocytes, particularly T cells.

Clinical Features, Diagnosis, and Management

The hypogammaglobulinemia associated with these conditions rarely has clinical significance; however, the lymphopenia may produce anergy and increased susceptibility to infection. The diagnoses are suggested by increased fecal α_1-antitrypsin levels or increased ^{51}Cr-albumin clearance.

Other Secondary Immunodeficiencies

Protein-calorie malnutrition impairs cell-mediated immunity. Sulfasalazine, penicillamine, and phenytoin produce reversible IgA deficiency. Corticosteroids increase susceptibility to a broad range of infections.

FOOD HYPERSENSITIVITY

Etiology and Pathogenesis

Food hypersensitivity or allergy refers to reactions that are mediated by the immune system, whereas food intolerance describes nonimmunologically mediated adverse reactions. True food hypersensitivity is rare (0.3% to 7.5% in children), declines with age, and is more prevalent in atopic individuals. Uptake of ingested antigens and presentation to the mucosal immune system may occur by three routes: M cells overlying lymphoid follicles; intestinal enterocytes that absorb antigens and stimulate suppressor T cells; and paracellular antigen absorption with presentation to the immune system by lamina propria macrophages and dendritic cells. A local IgA secretory response may follow ingestion of dietary antigens, but a systemic immune response rarely develops because of immune tolerance. Food hypersensitivity represents a breakdown in oral tolerance, and usually results from ingestion of milk, eggs, nuts, fish, shellfish, soybeans, and wheat. There are two major categories of food hypersensitivity: immediate (IgE-mediated, type I) and delayed (late-phase IgE-mediated, immune complex–mediated, and cell-mediated). Plasma histamine levels rise in patients who have gastrointestinal symptoms elicited by food challenge, which is indicative of a central role for mast cell degranulation in food hypersensitivity.

Clinical Features, Diagnosis, and Management

Patients present with eczema, urticaria, rhinitis, asthma, abdominal symptoms, and even anaphylaxis within minutes to hours of food ingestion. Cofactors such as aspirin ingestion or exercise may profoundly increase the clinical expression of food allergy. The diagnosis of food hypersensitivity relies on the following criteria: demonstration that ingestion of the implicated food can reproducibly induce symptoms, and evidence that an immunologic mechanism is involved. Because food challenges and skin testing may trigger anaphylactic reactions, diagnostic testing should be performed only in a facility that can deal with serious allergic reactions. Direct skin testing with the prick technique with food extract is a simple and sensitive method for detecting mast-cell–bound IgE antibodies. A positive test result (i.e., a wheal >3 mm larger than a control solution wheal) indicates the presence of sensitizing antibodies but does not confirm food hypersensitivity. In patients with known anaphylaxis, skin testing should not be performed. Rather, assays for IgE antibodies to food allergens (e.g., radioallergosorbent test, enzyme-linked immunosorbent assay) may be used. Systematic elimination of different foods may identify foods that induce allergic reactions. The most restrictive elimination diet is an elemental diet. It can provide diagnostically useful information if patients report allergies to multiple foods or if patients cannot identify a specific food to which they might be allergic. Double-blinded, placebo-controlled oral food challenges are the most reliable method of confirming food hypersensitivity but should be avoided if the patient has a history of anaphylaxis.

The only acceptable treatment of food hypersensitivity is avoidance of the offending food, but antihistamines and corticosteroids may play a secondary role in management of symptoms. Oral or parenteral immunization (hyposensitization) has not been shown to reduce food allergy, but breast feeding until the age of 6 months may have a protective effect against its development.

EOSINOPHILIC GASTROENTERITIS

Etiology and Pathogenesis

Eosinophilic gastroenteritis is probably not a single entity but rather a heterogeneous group of disorders with similar clinicopathologic features, including eosinophilic infiltration of a portion of the gut wall. Allergic phenomena have been proposed as a cause for eosinophilic gastroenteritis; however, some patients have no atopic symptoms, the response to dietary elimination is usually disappointing, and many patients have no family history of allergy.

Clinical Features, Diagnosis, and Management

With mucosal involvement, patients present with symptoms similar to those of inflammatory bowel disease, including diarrhea, cramping, nausea, vomiting, abdominal pain, malabsorption, weight loss, protein-losing enteropathy, occult fecal bleeding, anemia, growth retardation in children, and, rarely, perforation. Charcot-Leyden crystals secondary to lumenal eosinophil extrusion may be seen on examination of the stool. A low level of peripheral eosinophilia occurs in most cases. Barium radiographs may show diffuse mucosal nodularity, intralumenal narrowing, widening of small bowel segments, and antral cobblestoning. Biopsy of the small intestine may reveal the diagnostic finding of diffuse infiltration of the mucosa with eosinophils. Eosinophilic gastroenteritis is distinguished from hypereosinophilic syndrome, periarteritis nodosa, lymphoma, Crohn's disease, and intestinal parasitism by the clinical history and the lack of systemic inflammation. When the muscular propria is involved, eosinophilic gastroenteritis produces intestinal obstruction. Barium radiography of the upper gastrointestinal tract demonstrates irregular narrowing of the antrum or small intestine, but biopsy of the gastric mucosa may not be helpful. Eosinophilic infiltration of the serosa produces eosinophilic ascites or pleural effusions.

Prednisone (20 to 40 mg per day for 7 to 10 days) is effective therapy for most patients with eosinophilic gastroenteritis, although repeat courses or prolonged administration is often necessary. The long-term prognosis is favorable, although the disease follows a waxing and waning course. Some patients require total parenteral nutrition.

GRAFT-VERSUS-HOST DISEASE

Intestinal Disease Secondary to Induction

Etiology and Pathogenesis

The combination of chemotherapy and radiation therapy before bone marrow transplantation produces immediate intestinal necrosis. Regeneration of the mucosa can takes up to 3 weeks (Table 71-2).

Clinical Features, Diagnosis, and Management

Anorexia, cramping, abdominal pain, and diarrhea result from damage to the small intestine and colon. Stool cultures should be obtained to exclude infection. Rectal biopsy specimens show no evidence of graft-versus-host disease or opportunistic infection. Treatment includes supportive measures and total parenteral nutrition.

TABLE 71-2
Gastrointestinal Complications of Bone Marrow Transplantation

VARIABLE	SECONDARY TO INDUCTION PROTOCOL	ACUTE GVHD	CHRONIC GVHD
Onset after transplantation	0–20 days	20–80 days	>80 days
Clinical features	Anorexia, abdominal pain, diarrhea	Large-volume diarrhea, abdominal pain, ± rash, ± liver disease	Dysphagia, oral ulcers, diarrhea
Radiography	Not helpful	Mucosal edema, mucosal ulcers, pneumatosis	Esophageal strictures and webs
Endoscopy and manometry	Nonspecific	Normal → erythema → sloughing; stomach and rectum are spared	Upper esophageal bands and webs, lower third of esophagus is spared
Histology	Rectal mucosa shows nuclear atypia and crypt cell regeneration	Early: rectal tissue shows crypt cells apoptosis; late: mucosal disintegration	Esophageal tissue shows infiltration of neutrophils and necrosis of basal layer

GVHD = graft-versus-host disease.

Acute Graft-Versus-Host Disease

Etiology and Pathogenesis

Acute graft-versus-host disease, occurring 3 to 4 weeks after bone marrow transplantation, consists of dermatitis, mucositis, enteritis, and hepatic dysfunction. There are three theories of the mechanism leading to acute graft-versus-host disease: (1) donor cell destruction of host immune cells with tissue damage secondary to infection; (2) activation of cytotoxic pathways and release of cytotoxins and cytokines, which then cause tissue damage; and (3) direct recognition of alloantigens on recipient epithelial cells by donor cytotoxic cells, leading to destruction of epithelial cells.

Clinical Features, Diagnosis, and Management

The typical gastrointestinal manifestation of acute graft-versus-host disease is profuse, watery diarrhea (up to 10 liters per day) 3 weeks after transplantation. The severity of the gastrointestinal symptoms usually parallels the severity of skin (erythematous, maculopapular rash on the palms, soles, and trunk) and liver involvement. Other symptoms include anorexia, vomiting, buccal mucositis, abdominal pain, hemorrhage (esophagitis, gastric erosions), protein loss, and discrete ulcers caused by secondary cytomegalovirus infection. Barium radiographs may show bowel wall edema, pneumatosis cystoides intestinalis, and mucosal ulcerations. These acute radiographic features may normalize or, in some cases, take on a chronic, segmental, ribbonlike appearance. Endoscopy shows erythema or mucosal sloughing, which is most prominent in the ileum, cecum, and ascending colon. The earliest histologic change is necrosis of individual intestinal crypt cells. This finding, known as apoptosis, is diagnostic if observed in normal-appearing tissue 20 days after transplantation. Later changes, including total denudation of the mucosa, are not as specific. Management consists of nutritional support, fluid and electrolyte resuscitation, administration of steroids (prednisone in doses up to 2 mg per kg for 1 to 2 weeks) and immunosuppressants (cyclosporine, antithymocyte globulin, anti–T-cell monoclonal antibodies), and vigilance for secondary infections. Octreotide may reduce high-output diarrhea.

Chronic Graft-Versus-Host Disease

Etiology and Pathogenesis

Chronic graft-versus-host disease occurs 80 to 400 days after bone marrow transplantation, most often in patients who have had prior acute graft-versus-host disease. It predominantly involves the skin, liver, and gastrointestinal tract.

Clinical Features, Diagnosis, and Management

Gastrointestinal involvement affects the mouth (mucositis), esophagus (dysphagia, gastroesophageal reflux), and small intestine (patchy fibrosis of the lamina propria and submucosa and bacterial overgrowth secondary to dysmotility). Esophageal disease is often associated with skin involvement (hyperpigmentation and scleroderma-like changes). Upper gastrointestinal endoscopic findings range from generalized desquamation of the upper and middle esophagus to weblike fibrous bands. Esophageal manometry and pH testing may reveal nonspecific motor abnormalities and prolonged acid exposure. Histologic changes in the esophagus include infiltration with neutrophils and lymphocytes, necrosis of individual cells of the basal mucosa, and fibrosis of the submucosa. Prednisone alone or in combination with azathioprine is often effective. Antireflux therapy should be initiated, but esophageal dilation may be needed to treat progressive web and stricture development.

Graft-Versus-Host Disease in Transplantation of the Small Intestine

Graft-versus-host disease may develop after transplantation of the small intestine. Occurrence of the disease may be dependent on the extent of the graft, but animal and clinical studies suggest that graft rejection is a more prevalent phenomenon. Natural killer cells also have been hypothesized to contribute to the development of graft-versus-host disease after small bowel grafts.

CHAPTER 72

Vascular Lesions: Ectasias, Tumors, and Malformations

ANGIODYSPLASIA

Incidence and Epidemiology

Sporadic mucosal vascular ectasias of the gastrointestinal tract that are not associated with cutaneous lesions, systemic vascular lesions, or a familial syndrome are termed *angiodysplasias* (Table 72-1). Vascular ectasias that occur in association with lesions of the skin or other organs are termed *telangiectasias*. Angiodysplasia and telangiectasia are endoscopically and histologically identical; the terminology serves only to distinguish the disparate clinical syndromes.

Angiodysplasia is the most common vascular abnormality in the gastrointestinal tract. Endoscopic surveys have demonstrated prevalence rates of 1% to 2% in the stomach and duodenum and 3% to 6% in the colon. The prevalence of angiodysplasia increases with age; most patients are older than 60 years of age. These lesions are one of the most common causes of lower gastrointestinal hemorrhage in the elderly.

Etiology and Pathogenesis

The increased prevalence of angiodysplasia in the elderly has led to the theory that it results from aging-associated degeneration of vascular integrity. Pathologically, angiodysplasias are dilated, thin-walled clusters of capillaries associated with dilated, tortuous, submucosa veins. Dilated submucosal veins appear to be the earliest lesions, and chronic obstruction of venous outflow at the level of the muscularis appears to be the initial pathophysiologic defect.

Early reports suggested that angiodysplasia was associated with aortic stenosis. This prompted theories that angiodysplasia might be the result of hypoperfusion and mucosal ischemia. There is little evidence to support this notion, and

TABLE 72-1
Vascular Lesions of the Gastrointestinal Tract

Vascular ectasia disorders
  Angiodysplasia
  Gastric antral vascular ectasia ("watermelon stomach")
  Telangiectasia associated with multisystem disease (e.g., hereditary hemorrhagic
    telangiectasia, CREST syndrome, Turner's syndrome)
Vascular tumors
  Hemangiomas
  Multiple-hemangioma syndromes (e.g., intestinal hemangiomatosis, universal
    hemangiomatosis, blue rubber bleb nevus syndrome, Klippel-Trénaunay-Weber
    syndrome)
  Malignant vascular tumors (e.g., angiosarcoma, hemangiopericytoma, Kaposi's sarcoma)
Other vascular lesions
  Dieulafoy's lesion
  Miscellaneous (e.g., multiple phlebectasia, pseudoxanthoma elasticum, Ehlers-
    Danlos syndrome)

CREST syndrome = syndrome of calcinosis, Raynaud's phenomenon, esophageal dysmotility, sclerodactyly, telangiectasia.

any association of cardiac disease and angiodysplasia is probably related to the increased clinical recognition of bleeding from pre-existing angiodysplasias. Similarly, the association of chronic renal failure with bleeding angiodysplasia may be related to platelet dysfunction rather than any etiologic relationship.

Clinical Features

Gastrointestinal hemorrhage is the only clinical complication of angiodysplasia. Bleeding may be occult or overt and may occur in the upper or lower gastrointestinal tract. Angiodysplasia within one region of the gastrointestinal tract is associated with a 15% to 20% risk of angiodysplasia in other sites. Up to 60% of patients have multiple angiodysplasias within the same portion of the intestinal tract. Most colonic lesions are located in the right colon and are associated with low-grade chronic bleeding, but up to 15% of patients present with acute massive hemorrhage. Patients with colonic lesions may present with iron deficiency anemia, melena, or hematochezia. Patients with upper tract lesions may present with iron deficiency anemia, melena, or hematemesis. Although the percentage of angiodysplastic lesions that bleed is unknown, autopsy series suggest that most do not produce clinically evident bleeding.

Findings on Diagnostic Testing

The more widespread application of endoscopy to evaluate patients with gastrointestinal hemorrhage has increased the detection of mucosal lesions of angiodysplasia. Upper gastrointestinal endoscopy, enteroscopy of the small intestine, and colonoscopy are the primary methods of identifying angiodysplasia in the gastrointestinal tract. The lesions typically appear as discrete, bright red, flat, or slightly raised lesions that range in size from 0.2 to 1.0 cm. They blanch when touched with a biopsy forceps, which distinguishes the condition from intramucosal hemorrhage. Angiography may identify colonic angiodysplasia overlooked on colonoscopy and angiodysplasia lesions in the small intestine not accessible by enteroscopy. The characteristic angiographic findings include dilated, slowly emptying veins in the intestinal wall, a vascular tuft during the arterial phase of the study, and rapid filling of the dilated vein. Angiography demonstrates active bleeding in only 10% to 20% of patients with acute bleeding from colonic angiodysplasia. ^{99m}Tc-labeled erythrocyte scintigraphy is more sensitive in detecting acute hemorrhage. Patients with acute lower tract bleeding should undergo emergency colonoscopy or erythrocyte scintigraphy as the initial imaging procedure. Positive erythrocyte scans should be followed by angiography or colonoscopy.

Management and Course

One-half of patients with bleeding angiodysplasia have persistent or recurrent bleeding, whereas the other 50% do not experience further bleeding. Any therapeutic intervention in these patients must consider this natural history of angiodysplasia. Patients with mild, chronic blood loss who do not require transfusion are best managed conservatively with oral iron supplements. Several reports have suggested a benefit for estrogen alone or in combination with progesterone, especially for patients with renal failure or hereditary hemorrhagic telangiectasia. Other series have failed to demonstrate a decrease in transfusion requirements. Although the efficacy of hormonal therapy for sporadic angiodysplasias remains in question, an empirical trial of oral contraceptives containing low-dose estrogen is often worthwhile in selected patients. Gynecomastia in males and recurrent menstruation in postmenopausal females may limit compliance. Hormonal therapy should be avoided in patients with a history of thromboembolism, atherosclerotic disease, or hormone-sensitive neoplasms.

More invasive interventions should be reserved for patients with acute bleeding or chronic bleeding who require transfusion. Several techniques of endoscopic obliteration are used to manage chronic blood loss from the upper and lower gastrointestinal tract. For gastric and duodenal angiodysplasia, monopolar electrocautery, bipolar electrocautery, and heater probe coagulation are used, but only argon and Nd:YAG laser therapy has been shown to decrease the transfusion requirement. The same techniques are used to manage colonic angiodysplasia, but there is only limited evidence suggesting they decrease transfusion requirement. Laser therapy in the colon has been associated with more frequent complications, probably because tissue penetration is deeper. In all series evaluating endoscopic therapy, multiple sessions are often necessary, and 50% of patients experience persistent or recurrent bleeding (presumably from angiodysplasia at other sites).

For acute upper and lower gastrointestinal bleeding, heater probe coagulation and electrocautery techniques are often used because they are widely available and effective for managing gastrointestinal hemorrhage. Occasionally, bleeding from colonic angiodysplasia can be severe enough to obscure the endoscopic view. In these cases, angiography may help identify the source of acute blood loss and selective intra-arterial infusion of vasopressin may control it. Subsequent endoscopic obliteration or angiographic embolization is often used to prevent rebleeding, but the latter is frequently complicated by abdominal pain and fever and occasionally bowel infarction, necessitating emergency colectomy.

When all medical and endoscopic therapies fail to control bleeding, surgical resection should be considered. Preoperative angiography can often define the extent of angiodysplasia in the small intestine and the colon. Rebleeding rates seem to be lower in the immediate postoperative period, but in patients followed for 3 to 4 years, rebleeding rates are 40% to 50%.

GASTRIC ANTRAL VASCULAR ECTASIA

Incidence and Epidemiology

Gastric antral vascular ectasia (GAVE), also known as "watermelon stomach," is a distinctive syndrome of vascular ectasias localized to the gastric antrum. Most patients are elderly, and there is a female-to-male ratio of 4:1. Although endoscopic surveys have been limited, the disorder appears to be rare and is observed in <0.03% of upper endoscopic examinations.

Etiology and Pathogenesis

The etiology of GAVE remains unknown. A strong association with hypochlorhydria has led to theories that hypergastrinemia has a role. Gastrin-induced vasodilation and spindle cell proliferation may explain the distinctive pathologic findings. Antral folds are often hypertrophic and contain tortuous, thin-walled submucosal veins. Ectatic vascular channels associated with spindle cell proliferation extend into the lamina propria. The lesion is also associated with cirrhosis, leading to speculation that vascular congestion may promote these vascular abnormalities.

Clinical Features

Although acute upper gastrointestinal hemorrhage has been reported in patients with GAVE, most bleeding is chronic and low grade. Iron deficiency anemia is the most common presenting feature of GAVE. This disorder has only recently been recognized; therefore, the percentage of cases not affected by clinically significant bleeding is unknown.

Findings on Diagnostic Testing

Upper gastrointestinal endoscopy is the only definitive means of diagnosing GAVE. The lesions appear as bands of intense erythema along longitudinal antral folds; it is this striped pattern that prompted use of the term "watermelon stomach." Differentiating GAVE from the erythema of gastritis is based on visualization of dilated vessels on high-resolution endoscopic images or by noting that the vascular channels blanch when compressed with biopsy forceps. Although rarely necessary, biopsy is safe. Biopsy specimens reveal the distinctive dilated vascular channels and fibromuscular hyperplasia within the lamina propria. Angiography and barium radiography are generally of limited diagnostic value for this condition.

Management and Course

Patients with iron deficiency anemia often fail to respond to iron supplements alone. Estrogen-progesterone therapy and other medical therapies have been largely anecdotal and are of uncertain clinical benefit. As patients with GAVE only rarely have vascular ectasias elsewhere in the gastrointestinal tract, endoscopic and surgical therapy is often definitive. Electrocoagulation, heater probe coagulation, and laser therapy are all successful in controlling bleeding, but multiple sessions usually are required. Laser therapy requires fewer sessions, but availability can be limited. Endoscopic therapy usually is well tolerated, but symptomatic ulceration and delayed acute hemorrhage may occur. If patients do not respond to endoscopic therapy, antrectomy is essentially curative.

SYSTEMIC TELANGIECTASIA SYNDROMES

When vascular ectasias occur in conjunction with vascular lesions of the skin or other organs, they are termed *telangiectasias.* Hereditary hemorrhagic telangiectasia (HHT), also known as *Osler-Weber-Rendu syndrome,* is an autosomal dominant disorder associated with vascular ectasia of the skin, mucous membranes, and internal organs. Patients usually present in childhood with recurrent and severe epistaxis. Gastrointestinal hemorrhage may not occur until the fourth decade of life, and it occurs in 15% of cases. Bleeding from a source in the upper intestinal tract, characterized by melena and hematemesis, is more common than lower tract bleeding. Occult bleeding from a posterior nasal or pharyngeal source may mimic upper gastrointestinal hemorrhage and should be considered in the differential diagnosis. The diagnosis of hereditary hemorrhagic telangiectasia is suggested by lesions on the oral and nasopharyngeal membranes, tongue, face, hands, and chest. Most patients have a family history of HHT or family members with chronic epistaxis. Gastrointestinal lesions are identified by endoscopic examination, and most are located in the stomach and duodenum. Estrogen-progesterone therapy improves epistaxis and may reduce the rate of gastrointestinal bleeding. Endoscopic laser therapy is effective in controlling bleeding. The role of surgery is limited because of the diffuse nature of the disorder.

Bleeding gastrointestinal telangiectasias also occur in the CREST (calcinosis, Raynaud's phenomenon, esophageal dysmotility, sclerodactyly, telangiectasia) variant of progressive systemic sclerosis. These patients have vascular lesions on the hands, lips, face, and tongue, as well as other signs of systemic sclerosis. Gastrointestinal hemorrhage is not a dominant feature of this disorder but has been reported from telangiectasias in the colon, stomach, and small intestine. The therapeutic approach is similar to that for sporadic angiodysplasia.

HEMANGIOMAS

Incidence and Epidemiology

Hemangiomas are benign vascular growths that usually are detectable at birth or shortly after birth, but often do not produce symptoms until young adulthood (often in the third decade of life). Hemangiomas are uncommon. Although their true prevalence is unknown, they represent a rare source of gastrointestinal hemorrhage.

Etiology and Pathogenesis

Hemangiomas are hamartomas that result from abnormal vascular development in the intestinal wall. There are two distinct histologic types: capillary and cavernous. The two types also differ in their clinical behavior. Capillary hemangiomas are usually located in the small intestine and are composed of discrete clusters of thin-walled, tiny vessels, the caliber of normal capillaries. Cavernous hemangiomas are mainly found in the colon. They can be polypoid (circumscribed) or expansive (diffuse). Histologically, cavernous lesions are clusters of dilated, thin-walled vascular channels separated by scant stromal tissue. Growth characteristics, especially of cavernous hemangiomas, suggest that hemangiomas are benign neoplasms rather than congenital hamartomas.

Clinical Features

Many hemangiomas are asymptomatic, but the most common clinical presentation is gastrointestinal hemorrhage. Capillary hemangiomas tend to cause low-grade chronic bleeding, but cavernous lesions may produce massive bleeding. As most cavernous lesions are located in the rectosigmoid region, hematochezia is a common presenting symptom. Polypoid and expansive lesions may cause nausea, vomiting, and abdominal pain as a result of obstruction or intussusception. Multiple hemangiomas throughout the digestive tract is a condition termed *intestinal hemangiomatosis,* which affects 10% of patients. In the rare neonatal syndrome of universal hemangiomatosis, cavernous lesions are disseminated to other organs, including the brain and skin. Two other rare disorders associated with diffuse cutaneous and gastrointestinal hemangiomas are the blue rubber bleb nevus syndrome and Klippel-Trénaunay-Weber syndrome. In the former, cutaneous lesions affect the limbs, trunk, and face. Their blue color and rubbery consistency are the source of the syndrome's descriptive name. Lesions also occur throughout the gastrointestinal tract and usually produce occult bleeding. In the latter syndrome, patients have distinctive soft tissue and bony hypertrophy of one limb. Gastrointestinal lesions are cavernous and usually located in the rectum.

Findings on Diagnostic Testing

Endoscopy readily identifies most hemangiomas in the stomach, proximal duodenum, and colon. Capillary lesions appear as punctate red nodules, whereas cavernous lesions vary in appearance from blue polyps to expansive, flat, mass lesions. On barium radiography, these larger lesions can be mistaken for adenomatous polyps or carcinoma. Angiography is useful for detecting hemangiomas in the small intestine. The characteristic puddling of contrast in the venous phase is a typical finding in angiographic images of large cavernous lesions, but may be absent in small lesions.

Management and Course

Symptomatic sporadic hemangiomas are best managed with surgical resection. Occasionally, small capillary hemangiomas are amenable to endoscopic obliteration, but large cavernous lesions have high rates of massive hemorrhage or perforation with this therapy. In disorders with multiple gastrointestinal hemangiomas, conservative therapy with iron supplementation is recommended initially. Persistent hemorrhage or obstruction at a defined site requires surgical resection.

DIEULAFOY'S LESION

Incidence and Epidemiology

Dieulafoy's lesion is an arterial malformation associated with massive gastrointestinal hemorrhage, accounting for 1% to 2% of acute upper gastrointestinal bleeding episodes. Lesions may occur at any age, but the peak incidence is in the sixth decade of life. Men are affected twice as often as women.

Etiology and Pathogenesis

Dieulafoy's lesion appears to be a developmental abnormality in a submucosal artery. The vessel fails to decrease in caliber as it approaches the mucosa, and a small mucosal defect may expose the artery. The artery is injured and bleeding results. The pathologic events producing the mucosal defect and vessel rupture are unclear, but acid-peptic mechanisms do not appear to be involved.

Clinical Features

Most Dieulafoy's lesions are located in the proximal stomach, but there are rare reports of lesions in the small intestine and colon. Bleeding is usually abrupt and massive. Patients characteristically have no previous gastrointestinal symptoms. A Dieulafoy's vessel is a sporadic lesion and is not associated with other systemic signs or symptoms.

Findings on Diagnostic Testing

As with all other mucosal vascular lesions, upper gastrointestinal endoscopy is the primary means of diagnosing Dieulafoy's lesion. The lesion appears as a discrete 1- to 3-mm visible vessel that is often surrounded by a punctate erosion. Because the lesion is <5 mm in size, the endoscopist must consciously search for this lesion in patients with upper gastrointestinal hemorrhage. Active bleeding may obscure endoscopic visualization. Angiography may identify a bleeding vessel in this setting.

Management and Course

Endoscopic therapy is used to treat Dieulafoy's lesion: heater probe coagulation, electrocautery, epinephrine injection, sclerotherapy, or a combination of cautery and injection therapy. Up to 80% of patients achieve long-term control with this approach. If massive bleeding prevents adequate delivery of endoscopic therapy or if the patient rebleeds after a trial of endoscopic therapy, surgical wedge resection is the procedure of choice. Mortality averaged 25% in the past, but diagnostic and therapeutic advances have dramatically improved the survival of patients with this condition.

MISCELLANEOUS VASCULAR LESIONS

There are several rare mucosal vascular tumors of the gastrointestinal tract. Angiosarcoma, epithelioid hemangioendothelioma, and hemangiopericytoma are malignant neoplasms of the cellular components of blood vessels. All may be complicated by gastrointestinal hemorrhage or obstruction. Kaposi's sarcoma frequently disseminates to the gastrointestinal tract and is among the most common causes of gastrointestinal bleeding in patients with acquired immunodeficiency syndrome.

Ehlers-Danlos syndrome is a group of inherited disorders of collagen synthesis. Patients characteristically have hyperelastic skin, easy bruising, and hyperextensible joints. Patients with type I Ehlers-Danlos syndrome may have severe gastrointestinal bleeding as a result of compromised vascular integrity in mucosal capillaries. Abnormal vascular structure also contributes to the hemorrhage observed in patients with pseudoxanthoma elasticum. Abnormal elastin fibers in blood vessels prevent the normal vasoconstriction and retraction of injured vessels. This results in impaired hemostasis, and minor mucosal trauma may lead to significant gastrointestinal hemorrhage.

CHAPTER 73

Mesenteric Vascular Insufficiency

ISCHEMIA OF THE SMALL INTESTINE

Incidence and Epidemiology

Mesenteric ischemia usually affects the elderly, especially those with atherosclerotic and cardiovascular disease. Among the most common causes of acute intestinal ischemia is vascular occlusion by an embolus that originates from the heart of a patient who is in atrial fibrillation or who has an akinetic ventricular wall (Table 73-1). Similarly, occlusion caused by thrombosis usually occurs in mesenteric vessels that are atherosclerotic, whereas nonocclusive mesenteric ischemia occurs in association with the low-flow state often seen in patients with cardiovascular disease. The significance of atherosclerosis as a cause of chronic mesenteric insufficiency is emphasized by its association with diabetes, hyperlipidemia, and other complications of peripheral vascular disease. Mesenteric ischemia can affect young persons, but the underlying cause usually is penetrating trauma, strangulation obstruction of the small intestine, vasculitis, or celiac artery compression syndrome.

Etiology and Pathogenesis

Mesenteric ischemia occurs when splanchnic blood flow is insufficient to maintain adequate nutrient delivery to the small intestine. The microvascular network of the splanchnic circulation embodies several anatomic and physiologic adaptive mechanisms to maintain oxygen delivery. An acute reduction in the arterial perfusion pressure of the intestinal tract results in a compensatory dilation of the resistance arterioles. This autoregulation serves to maintain adequate tissue perfusion in the setting of acute mesenteric artery occlusion. In the setting of systemic hypotension, however, the more efficient autoregulatory mechanisms in other organs and activation of the autonomic nervous system and the renin-angiotensin axis result in disproportionate decreases in splanchnic blood flow. This systemic response also increases tone in venous capacitance vessels, which augments systemic venous return

TABLE 73-1
Clinical Factors That Predispose to Mesenteric Ischemia

Arterial embolism
    Prior embolic event
    Atrial fibrillation (recent cardioversion)
    Rheumatic heart disease
    Prosthetic valve
    Recent myocardial infarction
    Recent vascular instrumentation
        Cardiac catheterization
        Angioplasty
        Angiography
Arterial thrombosis
    Known vascular disease
        Atherosclerosis
        Aortic dissection
        Vasculitis
    Trauma
    Hypercoagulable states
    Dehydration
Vasospasm
    Dehydration
    Shock
    Congestive heart failure
    Pericardial tamponade
    Cardiopulmonary bypass
    Dialysis
    Vasoconstrictive medications
        Digoxin
        α-Adrenergic agonists
        β-Adrenergic antagonists
        Vasopressin
        Cocaine
Venous thrombosis
    Hypercoagulable states
        Hormones or pregnancy
        Carcinoma
        Polycythemia
        Coagulopathies
        Protein S deficiency
        Protein C deficiency
        Dehydration
    Venous obstruction
        Portal hypertension
        Budd-Chiari syndrome
        Carcinoma
    Low splanchnic blood flow
        Congestive heart failure
        Shock
    Intestinal obstruction
    Trauma
    Sclerotherapy

to the heart and serves to maintain cardiac output. The net result is a redistribution of blood flow from the gastrointestinal tract to the brain, heart, kidney, and skeletal muscle. The angiotensin-mediated relative vasospasm of the splanchnic resistance arterioles in response to systemic hypotension is the primary pathophysiologic insult in nonocclusive mesenteric ischemia and most cases of ischemic colitis.

Even when the autoregulatory capacity of the splanchnic circulation is overwhelmed, the intestinal tract has the capacity to increase oxygen extraction. Relative tissue hypoxia creates a steeper gradient for oxygen extraction. In addition, recruitment of unperfused capillary beds increases the perfused capillary density, which decreases the diffusion distance of oxygen.

An extensive network of collaterals between the systemic and splanchnic circulation and between the three major splanchnic vascular beds provides additional protection from ischemia caused by segmental occlusion. The celiac axis communicates with the superior mesenteric vessels through the pancreaticoduodenal cascade, and the superior mesenteric vessels connect with the inferior mesenteric vessels by way of marginal vessels connecting the middle colic and left colic arteries. In chronic ischemia, these collaterals can become quite large; therefore, the clinical syndrome of intestinal angina does not occur unless at least two of the three major mesenteric arteries are diseased. It is important to understand that collateral flow is established by vasodilation of resistance arterioles in the ischemic segment. Therefore, vasodilating agents used to treat intestinal ischemia caused by nonocclusive vasospasm may preferentially dilate other vascular beds, compromising collateral flow in the spastic segment.

Mesenteric ischemia occurs when the insult that compromises splanchnic flow overwhelms these adaptive mechanisms. The earliest manifestations of ischemia are increased capillary permeability followed by impaired epithelial function. Impaired mucosal function compromises normal absorptive mechanisms and permits the leakage of large molecules to pass through a normally selective barrier. If ischemia persists, epithelial cells are shed from the villous tip, and eventually, mucosal necrosis leads to ulceration. When the ischemic insult is prolonged, infarction of the submucosa and muscularis propria results in transmural necrosis, at which point the bowel is no longer viable. Early reversal of the ischemic insult leads to epithelial regeneration and restoration of the bowel to a normal state.

Ischemia causes cellular injury through a complex interaction of several mechanisms. The initial insult is invariably caused by tissue hypoxia, but recent evidence suggests that other events perpetuate the injury even after blood flow is restored. Reperfusion injury is mediated by oxygen free radicals generated by xanthine oxidase after the sudden influx of oxygen. These free radicals can damage tissues directly and by means of neutrophil recruitment and activation. Once epithelial integrity has been compromised, digestive enzymes and hydrochloric acid also perpetuate intestinal injury. This process is critical in the pathogenesis of stress gastritis. Loss of the gut barrier permits entry of enteric bacteria. Bacterial endotoxins and exotoxins may play an important role in the systemic and hemodynamic complications of mesenteric ischemia.

Clinical Features

Strangulation Obstruction

Obstruction of the small intestine coexists with segmental ischemia caused by strangulation in 20% to 40% of patients. Ischemia is caused by dilation of the bowel wall and volvulus of the dilated segment, both of which impair venous and arterial flow. Patients present with the usual signs of obstruction: abdominal distention, pain, and vomiting. Although constant pain, fever, and signs of peritoneal irritation have been heralded as indicators of strangulation, these symptoms are not always encountered. It must be emphasized that it is not possible to differentiate uncomplicated obstruction from obstruction with strangulation based on the clinical signs and symptoms. Urgent surgical exploration is essential to minimize the risk of transmural infarction and peritonitis.

Acute Mesenteric Arterial Embolization

Arterial embolization to the superior mesenteric artery accounts for 5% of all peripheral emboli events and is the cause of 15% to 40% of all acute mesenteric ischemic events. Because emboli originate from the heart and atherosclerotic plaques in the aorta, most patients have underlying atrial fibrillation, ventricular wall dyskinesia, or atherosclerotic vascular disease. Also, patients often have a history of embolic events. Patients typically present with a sudden onset of diffuse, severe, colicky abdominal pain that evolves into a constant, steady pain. Vomiting and explosive diarrhea are common in the initial phases owing to ischemia-stimulated peristalsis. Occult or overt gastrointestinal hemorrhage usually indicates mucosal necrosis and is a late finding. Initially, the abdominal examination is notable for hyperactive bowel sounds and minimal tenderness despite the presence of excruciating pain. With prolonged ischemia, the abdomen becomes distended, bowel sounds become scarce, and abdominal tenderness increases as a result of transmural infarction. Sequestration of fluid into the bowel wall and superimposed bacteremia may lead to hemodynamic instability and fever. These late findings are associated with bowel wall necrosis and portend a poor prognosis. The clinician must maintain a high index of suspicion, especially if patients have underlying cardiovascular disease, in order to recognize the early symptoms of intestinal ischemia when the condition is still reversible.

Acute Mesenteric Arterial Thrombosis

Acute mesenteric thrombosis usually occurs at the site of pre-existing atherosclerotic disease. Low-flow states secondary to hypovolemia and cardiac failure promote thrombus formation. Consequently, most patients with acute mesenteric thrombosis have pre-existing cardiac or atherosclerotic vascular disease. A small number of patients develop thrombosis of the superior mesenteric artery as a result of aortic dissection or a hypercoagulable state. In some cases, the clinical presentation is often indistinguishable from that of acute embolic occlusion of the superior mesenteric artery. However, the onset of pain caused by thrombus formation may be more gradual than the onset of pain related to embolic occlusion. The clinical severity of the syndrome usually depends on the presence or absence of collateral flow from the celiac axis and inferior mesenteric circulation. If collaterals are well developed, thrombotic occlusion may not produce significant morbidity.

Mesenteric Venous Thrombosis

Acute mesenteric venous thrombosis often is the consequence of an intra-abdominal inflammatory process such as appendicitis, inflammatory bowel disease, or diverticulitis. Although many cases are idiopathic, a large proportion of these patients have underlying hypercoagulable conditions. Conditions associated with low-flow states such as congestive heart failure also predispose to venous thrombosis. As with arterial thrombosis, the onset of clinical symptoms is usually insidious. The severity of symptoms varies from unrecognized, self-limited abdominal discomfort to fulminant bowel infarction with peritonitis. Venous thrombosis frequently leads to massive fluid sequestration, resulting in hemodynamic compromise. As with other causes of mesenteric ischemia, abdominal tenderness, overt gastrointestinal hemorrhage, and circulatory collapse are late events. Recognizing this syndrome before the onset of infarction is difficult given the nonspecific symptoms (e.g., vague abdominal pain, diarrhea, and vomiting) that characterize the initial clinical presentation.

Nonocclusive Mesenteric Ischemia

Nonocclusive mesenteric ischemia almost invariably occurs in the setting of profound hypotension caused by hemorrhagic or cardiogenic shock. The manifestations of nonocclusive mesenteric ischemia are similar to those of occlusive insults, but the condition causing shock usually dominates the clinical presentation. In addition, many patients are obtunded and unable to report abdominal pain. In a conscious patient, crampy abdominal pain evolves into dull, constant, periumbilical pain. Hemorrhage is an indication of mucosal necrosis, whereas abdominal guarding and rigidity suggest progression to transmural infarction.

Chronic Mesenteric Ischemia

Chronic mesenteric ischemia, also called intestinal angina, is a rare clinical syndrome distinct from the occlusive and nonocclusive forms of acute mesenteric ischemia. Intestinal angina occurs primarily in patients with atherosclerotic peripheral vascular disease and in those with associated risk factors such as hyperlipidemia, diabetes mellitus, and tobacco use. Because of the extensive collateral network within the splanchnic circulation, intestinal angina almost always requires high-grade obstruction of at least two of the three major splanchnic arteries. A small number of patients with chronic mesenteric ischemia may have obstruction of the celiac axis as a result of extrinsic compression by the median arcuate ligament of the diaphragm. Most patients with celiac axis compression syndrome are women; presentation occurs at a younger age than with ischemia caused by atherosclerosis. Although controversy exists over the true pathophysiologic mechanism of this chronic pain syndrome, 50% of patients have intestinal angina, and surgical correction of the vascular obstruction improves symptoms. Intestinal angina is defined by the classic triad of postprandial abdominal pain, chronic weight loss, and sitophobia (fear of eating). The abdominal pain is analogous to angina pectoris and lower extremity claudication. Pain typically develops 30 to 90 minutes postprandially and may last several hours. Physical examination usually reveals evidence of peripheral vascular disease. Abdominal findings are nonspecific, although many patients have abdominal vascular bruits. Despite the diffuse reduction in splanchnic arterial flow, acute mesenteric infarction rarely complicates the course of intestinal angina.

Findings on Diagnostic Testing

Laboratory Studies

Patients with acute ischemic injury to the small intestine usually have numerous laboratory abnormalities. Patients with intestinal infarction have leukocytosis, lactic acidosis, and hyperamylasemia. Other nonspecific abnormalities include elevations of serum alkaline phosphatase and creatine phosphokinase levels. Elevations in the hematocrit are indicative of fluid sequestration, which is particularly severe in mesenteric venous thrombosis. Laboratory tests have limited diagnostic value, however, because most results are normal in the early phases of ischemia when the bowel wall is still viable. In addition, the abnormalities are nonspecific and simply reflect the systemic inflammatory response or tissue necrosis.

Structural Studies

Abdominal radiographs should be obtained to exclude obstruction of the small intestine. In the absence of obstruction, ischemia usually manifests as a nonspecific bowel gas pattern or ileus. Occasionally, thickened mucosa will appear as a "thumbprinting" pattern on the bowel wall. As intestinal infarction sets in, air may dissect the bowel wall, producing pneumatosis cystoides intestinalis. Although free intraperitoneal air indicates perforation, this finding is not always present. Ultrasound with Doppler evaluation of the splanchnic vessels is especially useful in documenting multivessel stenosis in chronic intestinal angina. Dynamic contrast-enhanced computed tomographic scans may demonstrate lack of filling in a thrombosed mesenteric vein as well as nonspecific thickening of the bowel wall. In contrast to ischemic colitis, endoscopy is not useful in the evaluation of patients with suspected mesenteric ischemia.

Angiography

The cornerstone of evaluating patients with mesenteric ischemia is angiography. In addition to its diagnostic and therapeutic capacity, angiography is often critical in planning operative reconstruction. In arterial embolic occlusion, there is usually an abrupt obstruction in a tributary of the superior mesenteric artery. A lack of associated collaterals provides ancillary evidence that the obstruction is acute. It may be difficult to distinguish arterial thrombosis from embolic occlusion, but atherosclerotic narrowing of the superior mesenteric artery usually is prominent and collaterals often are well developed. The venous phase of angiography can identify the site of mesenteric thrombosis. In nonocclusive mesenteric ischemia, there is evidence of vasospasm and absence of the typical arterial blush in the bowel wall. Patients with intestinal angina invariably have high-grade stenosis of at least two vessels, whereas patients with celiac axis compression syndrome demonstrate a discrete narrowing at the origin of the celiac axis. Because most patients with mesenteric ischemic syndromes have associated cardiovascular and atherosclerotic disease, many patients have coexisting atherosclerotic stenosis of the splanchnic arteries. Distinguishing clinically significant lesions from incidental atherosclerosis requires the synthesis of historic, physical, and radiologic information.

Surgery for Diagnosis

Diagnostic laparoscopy or laparotomy is indicated for patients with suspected intestinal infarction or suspected obstruction and strangulation of the small intestine. Both complications require definitive surgical therapy.

Management and Course

The initial therapeutic priority in all patients with acute mesenteric ischemia is fluid resuscitation and restoration of hemodynamic stability. Hypovolemia caused by sequestration of fluids compounds ischemic injury by activating angiotensin-mediated splanchnic vasoconstriction. Monitoring of central venous and pulmonary artery pressure helps ensure that the volume status is optimized. Patients with intestinal infarction often have lactic acidosis, which, if profound, requires bicarbonate replacement and, possibly, mechanical ventilation. Broad-spectrum antibiotics should be administered in anticipation of bacteremia resulting from breakdown of the mucosal defense barrier.

In patients with nonocclusive mesenteric ischemia, vasodilators can be administered by angiographic catheterization. If repeat contrast injection demonstrates a response, a continuous infusion of papaverine can be administered through the angiographic catheter for 12 to 24 hours. This often results in clinical improvement, but surgical intervention may be required if transmural necrosis develops.

Patients in the early phase of mesenteric venous thrombosis can be treated with anticoagulation therapy, but the primary treatment of all other patients with acute mesenteric ischemia is surgical. For an arterial embolism, blood flow can be restored by extracting the clot with a balloon embolectomy catheter. Re-establishing flow after arterial thrombosis is more difficult and usually requires bypass with a synthetic graft or a saphenous venous segment. At the time of surgery, any obstruction is relieved and any necrotic tissue is resected. Intravascular injection of fluorescein dye is helpful in defining bowel viability. The extent of necrotic tissue is highly variable and depends largely on the anatomic site of vascular compromise. Sudden occlusion of the only remaining patent vessel may lead to infarction of the entire small intestine and colon, whereas occlusion of a superior mesenteric artery tributary usually causes segmental necrosis. After the initial resection, a second-look operation often is performed to further assess bowel viability, but there is no consensus on the value of this strategy.

The prognosis of acute mesenteric ischemia largely depends on the extent of intestinal injury at the time of diagnosis. Unfortunately, in most patients, acute mesenteric ischemia is recognized after infarction has occurred, and the comorbid conditions often present in these syndromes contributes to mortality rates as high as 50% to 90%. The prognosis for mesenteric venous thrombosis is slightly better.

The treatment of chronic intestinal angina is revascularization with bypass or reimplantation of the diseased vessels to the aorta. Percutaneous translumenal angioplasty has been associated with a high rate of complications and technical failure. Most patients who undergo successful revascularization achieve long-term relief of symptoms.

ISCHEMIC COLITIS

Incidence and Epidemiology

As with all forms of visceral ischemia, ischemic colitis occurs primarily in middle-aged and elderly persons. The overall incidence is unknown because many cases resolve spontaneously and are unrecognized. Ischemic injury to the colon usually occurs in association with aortic bypass surgery or acute systemic hypotension.

Etiology and Pathogenesis

The same adaptive mechanisms protecting the small intestine from ischemic injury are operative in the colon. Autoregulation, capillary recruitment, increased oxygen extraction, and collateral flow all help maintain the oxygen supply in the setting of compromised arterial inflow. The cecum, right colon, and transverse colon are served primarily by tributaries of the superior mesenteric artery, whereas the left colon receives flow from tributaries of the inferior mesentery artery. The splenic flexure is in the watershed region of the superior and inferior mesenteric arteries and is the most susceptible to ischemic insult. The rectum is well protected by an overlapping vascular supply from tributaries of the inferior mesenteric artery and the internal iliac artery. In contrast to acute mesenteric ischemia, spontaneous occlusion of the inferior mesenteric artery is an uncommon cause of ischemic colitis. Most cases are caused by systemic hypoperfusion or surgical disruption of blood flow in the inferior mesenteric artery after aortic surgery. Systemic hypoperfusion is often accompanied by angiotensin-mediated vasoconstriction similar to the pathophysiologic events of nonocclusive mesenteric ischemia.

Clinical Features

Many cases of mild colonic ischemia are not recognized because patients are unable to report symptoms in the immediate postoperative period or in the setting of a critical illness that compromises splanchnic blood flow. The most common presentation is crampy lower abdominal pain, nausea, vomiting, and bloody diarrhea several hours to days after an episode of hemodynamic instability. The low-flow state is transient and not recognized in many patients. A small percentage of patients with chronic colonic ischemia present with obstructive symptoms caused by a segmental ischemic stricture. Physical findings of acute ischemic colitis are nonspecific and include fever, abdominal tenderness, and occult or overt rectal blood.

Findings on Diagnostic Testing

With the exception of a rare patient with colonic infarction, laboratory abnormalities are usually mild and nonspecific in patients with ischemic colitis. Abdominal radiography may demonstrate thickening of the bowel wall or "thumbprinting" of the mucosa. In contrast to mesenteric ischemia, angiography is rarely informative in ischemic colitis because most spontaneous episodes are the result of systemic low-flow states rather than acute occlusion of the inferior mesenteric artery. Sigmoidoscopy is very useful in confirming the diagnosis. Because the systemic and splanchnic vascular supply overlap, the rectum usually is spared, and abnormal mucosa is first encountered in the rectosigmoid region. The mucosa is usually edematous and friable in the early stages of ischemic colitis and frankly ulcerated in the late stages. The distribution of injury is variable, but usually involves the left colon. Endoscopic biopsy reveals nonspecific inflammation and, occasionally, a characteristic pattern of superficial epithelial sloughing and subepithelial hemorrhage.

Management and Course

Most patients with ischemic colitis improve with conservative measures that optimize cardiovascular function. Unlike for nonocclusive mesenteric ischemia, vasodilator agents have not proved useful in treating ischemic colitis. Vasoconstricting agents and volume depletion should be avoided. If patients deteriorate clinically or demonstrate frank peritonitis, emergency surgical exploration is required, and all necrotic segments should be resected. Similarly, patients with symptomatic colonic strictures should undergo elective resection. Revascularization is not indicated for ischemic colitis. Although a small percentage of patients succumb to complications of ischemic colitis, survival is most often limited by the acute illness precipitating the compromised colonic perfusion.

CHAPTER 74

Radiation Injury

ETIOLOGY AND PATHOGENESIS

Ionizing radiation is delivered in units; the accepted SI (Système International d'Unités) unit of dose is the gray (Gy), which is equivalent to 100 rad or 1 joule of energy distributed over 1 kg of tissue. Most modern radiation therapy regimens use megavoltage photons that disperse high-energy electrons in targeted tissues. These high-energy electrons create breaks in double-stranded DNA by directly interacting with the DNA and by fostering the formation of volatile oxygen free radicals. Such DNA damage disturbs cell replication and, if significant enough, causes cell death.

The cytotoxicity of a given dose of radiation therapy depends on the form of radiation. In general, alpha particles are more damaging than gamma rays, and beta particles produce an intermediate degree of injury. The deeper penetration and more widespread use of gamma irradiation makes this modality the most common modality associated with visceral injury. The toxicity of a given dose can be altered by the coadministration of chemotherapy. The agents most often associated with radiosensitizing effects include 5-fluorouracil, doxorubicin, bleomycin, and actinomycin D.

The gastrointestinal injury from radiation therapy is separated into acute and chronic forms based on distinct pathophysiologic mechanisms and clinical presentations. In acute injury, radiation-induced cellular toxicity destroys existing epithelial cells and interferes with proliferation. Small doses of radiation can cause villous blunting and minor alterations in mucosal function, but larger doses can denude extensive regions of mucosa. The result is massive fluid and electrolyte losses and bacteremia caused by disruption of the mucosal defenses. Simultaneous damage to vascular endothelial cells produces increased vascular permeability and edema. The natural history of the injury also depends on the dose of radiation administered. Most injuries caused by lower doses are self-limited, but higher cumulative doses can lead to persistent or progressive disease.

Patients with chronic radiation damage often present months or years after exposure primarily because of small vessel ischemic injury. Endothelial inflammation coupled with smooth muscle and fibroblast proliferation compromise blood flow in the small vessels. Excessive fibrosis and the presence of atypical fibroblasts characterize chronic radiation injury. Progressive ischemic injury and fibrosis may lead to stricturing, ulceration, fistulization, and perforation.

CLINICAL FEATURES, DIAGNOSIS, AND MANAGEMENT

Radiation Injury to the Esophagus

Radiation esophagitis is a frequent complication of therapy directed at tumors of the lung, mediastinum, and hypopharynx. Acute injury invariably occurs at doses of 6000 cGy given in fractions of 1000 cGy per week. Lower doses or longer schedules are associated with lower rates of esophagitis. The most common symptoms—odynophagia and chest pain—usually develop during the second week of treatment. The chest pain is usually substernal, constant, and exacerbated by swallowing. Esophagitis can interfere with esophageal motility. Therefore, dysphagia also is a common symptom in the acute setting.

The diagnosis of acute radiation esophagitis is usually apparent from the clinical setting. Rarely is upper gastrointestinal endoscopy required to confirm the diagnosis. Most patients are treated with supportive measures. Adjusting the radiation treatment by dose reduction or modification of the radiation field usually facilitates healing. In severe cases, therapy may need to be withheld for several days, in spite of the fact that, for the patient, the tumoricidal effect of the therapy may be compromised. Viscous lidocaine and prokinetic agents often alleviate odynophagia and dysphagia, respectively. The nutritional status of the patient should be monitored closely. Although most patients with acute radiation esophagitis can be maintained on oral supplements, patients with prolonged and severe episodes may require enteral feeding by nasoenteric or gastrostomy tube.

Chronic radiation injury to the esophagus may occur up to 5 years after exposure and usually manifests as dysphagia caused by fibrotic strictures. The risk of stricture formation correlates with the dose: Studies predict that 1% to 5% of patients receiving 6000 cGy and 50% of patients receiving 7500 cGy develop radiation-induced esophageal injury. Several weeks after the start of therapy, patients may present with recurrent aspiration and pneumonia as a result of a tracheoesophageal fistula. Rarely, an aortoesophageal fistula occurs, resulting in massive and fatal hemorrhage. Fistulae are usually caused by tumor necrosis of primary esophageal or lung neoplasms. The vasculitis of chronic radiation injury may also contribute to fistula formation. Barium swallow radiography is helpful in defining a stricture or fistula. Upper gastrointestinal endoscopy with brushing and biopsy of strictures is necessary to exclude malignancy. This is especially important if the patient presents with dysphagia >10 years after radiation exposure, given the increased risk of secondary squamous cell carcinoma. If a stricture is short and straight, endoscopic dilation may alleviate dysphagia. Strictures with large diverticula or excessive angulations are at high risk of perforation and are best managed with surgical resection. Patients who are not candidates for surgery require conservative therapy with enteral feedings. Patients with tracheoesophageal fistulae may also require enteral feeding to reduce the complications of aspiration, but oral secretions often cause persistent problems. Endoscopically placed, silicone-coated, expandable metal stents may palliate these patients; however, the risk of intractable chest pain, hemorrhage, and displacement is significant.

Radiation Injury to the Stomach

The stomach is relatively resistant to radiation damage. Ulceration and stenosis are rarely seen at doses of <4500 cGy, but transient hypochlorhydria is common, even at low doses. The large lumen of the stomach may be responsible for this resistance because the two narrow regions—the antrum and the cardia—are the most common sites of radiation-induced stricture formation. Therapy for gastric radiation injury is usually supportive; obstruction, hemorrhage, and perforation are extremely rare.

Radiation Injury to the Small Intestine

The small intestine is the most radiosensitive organ in the gastrointestinal tract. The high turnover rate of the mucosa of the small intestine makes it particularly susceptible to radiation injury. Radiation enteritis occurs most commonly after pelvic or retroperitoneal radiation therapy. There is an obvious dose-response relationship: clinically significant acute toxicity occurs in 20% of patients receiving 1000 cGy, in 40% of patients receiving 1000 to 3000 cGy, and in 90% of patients receiving >3000 cGy. Fixed loops of bowel resulting from adhesions are particularly susceptible. Similarly, patients with a thin body habitus or chronic mesenteric vascular insufficiency as well as patients receiving radiosensitizing chemotherapy are at increased risk for development of radiation enteritis. Sucralfate given during radiation exposure may reduce acute injury by coating denuded areas of mucosa. Barium radiography before initiating radiation therapy can assess the location of bowel loops and may help define fields that will minimize bowel exposure. Similarly, maintaining a full bladder at the time the dose is delivered may displace the small intestine out of the radiation field. More aggressive maneuvers to exclude loops of bowel from the field include operative fixation of the bowel to a site removed from the targeted organ. This is useful when radiation is delivered as adjuvant therapy after a primary surgical resection.

Acute injury is characterized by loss of regenerative epithelium, malabsorption, diarrhea, and abdominal pain. Patients usually respond to a 10% reduction in the radiation dose. Supportive therapy begins with antispasmodics, bulk-forming agents, and antidiarrheals. Most cases are self-limited, but with high doses of radiation, the injury may be severe and persistent. Rarely, perforation complicates the course of acute enteritis.

Chronic injury occurs in 5% of treated patients and presents months to years after the exposure. Progressive small-vessel vasculitis leads to ischemia-mediated fibrosis, ulceration, and fistulization. Fibrotic stricturing may cause signs or symptoms of obstruction. In addition, the associated stasis in the small intestine may promote bacterial overgrowth. Patients frequently present with diarrhea, which may be caused by bile salt malabsorption, bacterial overgrowth, impaired mucosal absorptive capacity, or an enteric fistula. Fistulae may also communicate with the genitourinary system. Rarely, patients present with acute gastrointestinal hemorrhage or peritonitis caused by ulceration or infarction.

Treatment of diarrheal symptoms usually is supportive. Dietary manipulation, including avoidance of fats and lactose, may improve malabsorptive symptoms. Cholestyramine and antibiotics are often given empirically for bile salt malabsorption and bacterial overgrowth, respectively. There is no convincing evidence that 5-aminosalicylates and corticosteroids provide any benefit. Nutritional status should be monitored closely. Patients with severe disease require parenteral nutrition. These conservative measures should be attempted in all patients with strictures and fistulae. If severe symptoms persist or the course is complicated by refractory obstruction or bleeding, surgical resection may be necessary. Because of a high rate of anastomotic failures and adhesions that can further complicate the clinical course, surgical intervention should be reserved as a last resort. Unless there is extensive fistulization, resection of the diseased segment is preferred over a bypass procedure. After surgical resection, 50% of patients remain disease-free, whereas the other 50% develop recurrent strictures or fistulae and often require further surgery.

Radiation Injury to the Colon

Radiation injury to the colon is a common complication of treatments targeting the cervix, uterus, prostate, bladder, and testes. Radiation therapy for testicular cancer often involves an extensive field that may include the transverse colon. Most cases of radiation colitis develop in the rectosigmoid colon after pelvic irradiation. The combination of radiation implants and external beam irradiation increases the risk of colitis.

Acute injury occurs in the first 6 weeks after exposure and manifests as tenesmus, urgency, and diarrhea. Lower gastrointestinal endoscopy usually demonstrates minimal nonspecific mucosal injury. Treatment is primarily supportive, and symptoms resolve within 2 to 6 months.

Chronic radiation colitis usually occurs several months to years after therapy. The most common symptom is recurrent rectal bleeding, but rectal pain and diarrhea also occur. Rarely, patients develop a rectovaginal or rectovesical fistula and present with symptoms related to the genitourinary tract. Radiation colitis has a characteristic endoscopic appearance of scattered telangiectasias on a background of pale, friable mucosa. Biopsy is not necessary to make the diagnosis unless there is a coexisting stricture, in which case recurrent malignancy must be excluded. Barium enema radiography is often necessary to define the extent of complicating strictures or fistulae.

If symptoms are minimal and bleeding does not require transfusions, the prognosis of chronic radiation colitis is excellent; there is a 70% spontaneous remission rate. Patients with high-grade strictures, refractory symptoms, or severe hemorrhage that requires transfusion rarely achieve spontaneous remission and usually require intervention. Response rates to medical therapy have been disappointing. Uncontrolled trials suggest that sucralfate enemas (2 g in 20 ml water) with or without steroid enemas may improve symptoms. Most trials evaluating 5-aminosalicylates and steroid enemas have demonstrated no response. Chronic rectal bleeding is best managed initially with endoscopic laser photocoagulation or electrocautery. Although several sessions are necessary, ablation of mucosal telangiectasias reduces transfusion requirements and hospitalization rates. Endoscopic dilation is also effective in relieving symptoms caused by short, discrete, colonic strictures. Surgical resection is reserved for patients with long, tortuous strictures or refractory bleeding.

Radiation Injury to the Hepatobiliary System

The recent proliferation of bone marrow transplantation has been accompanied by an increase in the frequency of liver toxicity caused by cytoreductive therapy. Veno-occlusive disease is a complication of certain chemotherapeutic agents as well as radiation therapy. It occurs more often when these two modalities are combined for bone marrow ablation. The disease results from thrombotic and fibrotic obliteration of small central veins, which leads to centrilobular congestion. The clinical syndrome occurs 1 to 4 weeks after exposure and presents with jaundice, weight gain, ascites, right upper quadrant pain, and, occasionally, encephalopathy. Treatment is usually supportive with fluid restriction and cautious use of diuretics. The mortality rate is 30% to 50%.

The incidence of hepatotoxicity from radiation therapy directed to liver neoplasms has been reduced by innovative three-dimensional multiplanar delivery techniques. Focusing the radiation field to one lobe of the liver allows delivery of higher cumulative doses without increasing toxicity. Radiation liver damage can manifest as Budd-Chiari syndrome, with progressive weight gain, ascites, and jaundice. Primary parenchymal injury results in focal necrosis and, eventually, bridging fibrosis. There is no specific therapy other than correction of fluid and electrolyte disorders. Patients with jaundice have a poor prognosis. The overall mortality rate is 10% to 20%.

CHAPTER 75

Endoscopy

PRINCIPLES OF ENDOSCOPIC EVALUATION OF THE GASTROINTESTINAL TRACT

Utility of Endoscopy

Gastrointestinal endoscopy has transformed all aspects of the diagnosis and treatment of patients with diseases of the gastrointestinal tract. Each endoscopic procedure has a specific set of indications and contraindications. In general, an endoscopic procedure is indicated only when the results are expected to influence the course of patient management. In some cases, however, the attendant risks of endoscopy may outweigh the benefits. Before proceeding with endoscopic intervention, patients should give a complete history and have a complete physical examination to establish the indication for the study and exclude the presence of any contraindications. Many procedures require bowel cleansing or prolonged fasting; therefore, the clinician must be aware of comorbid conditions, such as diabetes, heart failure, or renal dysfunction, which may require adjustments in patient preparation instructions. All patients should be counseled on the risks and benefits of endoscopy; written and verbal informed consent is mandatory.

Principles of Conscious Sedation

Most endoscopic procedures require conscious sedation to permit a safe and complete examination. The optimal agents and dosages vary, but all carry the risk of cardiopulmonary complications. All patients should be monitored for changes in blood pressure, heart rate, and respiratory rate throughout the course of sedation. Many centers use pulse oximetry and electrocardiographic monitoring, but it is uncertain if routine use of these more expensive monitoring procedures improves treatment outcomes. No electronic monitoring can replace clinical judgment. Therefore, if significant cardiopulmonary signs or symptoms arise, the procedure should be aborted. The benzodiazepine antagonist flumazenil and the opiate antagonist naloxone can be used to reverse the effects of benzodiazepines and narcotics, respectively, in patients with complications of oversedation, but they should not be used routinely to reverse sedation. Slow titration of the initial dose of the sedative agent is the best way to avoid oversedation.

Antibiotic Prophylaxis

The role of preprocedure antibiotics to prevent endocarditis or bacteremia in patients with vascular or other prostheses is undefined. Based on the documented risks of bacteremia with given procedures and the risks of establishing an infection in certain pre-existing conditions, the American Society of Gastrointestinal Endoscopy promotes guidelines for the use of antibiotic prophylaxis before endoscopic procedures (Table 75-1). In many circumstances, no definitive recommendations can be made and the decision is made at the clinician's discretion. Antibiotics can be costly, and many have a substantial risk of allergic reactions. These issues must be considered when contemplating the use of prophylactic antibiotics. The standard regimen includes parenteral ampicillin (1 to 2 g) and gentamicin (1.5 mg per kg, up to 80 mg) 30 minutes before the procedure, followed by oral amoxicillin (1.5 g) 6 hours after the procedure. Amoxicillin may be replaced by a repeat dose of the parenteral regimen 8 hours after the procedure. Intravenous vancomycin (1 g) is substituted for ampicillin in patients with penicillin allergies.

Coagulation Disorders

Although coagulation abnormalities are not absolute contraindications to the performance of endoscopy, the use of endoscopic biopsy can be associated with an increased risk of bleeding. Before any therapeutic intervention, including percutaneous gastrostomy tube placement and electrocoagulation for polypectomy or hemostasis, attempts should be made to correct coagulation disorders. Prolongation of prothrombin time unrelated to the administration of warfarin may require parenteral vitamin K therapy. If there is no response to vitamin K or if emergency therapy is necessary, coagulation factors should be supplemented with fresh frozen plasma. Antiplatelet agents (e.g., aspirin) should be withheld for 7 to 10 days before and after these therapeutic measures. Depending on the underlying medical condition, warfarin can often be withheld for 5 to 7 days before the procedure and reinstituted 1 to 2 days after therapy. If medical conditions prohibit discontinuation, the patient is hospitalized, warfarin is discontinued, and heparin is initiated. When the prothrombin time normalizes, the patient is prepared for the procedure, and heparin is discontinued 4 hours before the intervention. Heparin can be restarted 4 hours after the procedure, and warfarin can be reinstituted 12 to 24 hours after heparin if no procedure-related hemorrhage occurs.

UPPER GASTROINTESTINAL ENDOSCOPY

Indications and Contraindications

Many symptoms attributable to diseases of the esophagus, stomach, and duodenum are best assessed by esophagogastroduodenoscopy (EGD) or upper gastrointestinal endoscopy. The American Society of Gastrointestinal Endoscopy has

TABLE 75-1
Recommendations for Antibiotic Prophylaxis

RISK GROUP	PROCEDURE	ANTIBIOTIC PROPHYLAXIS
High risk for endocarditis (prosthetic valve, prior endocarditis, systemic pulmonary shunt, synthetic vascular graft <1 yr old)	Stricture dilation, sclerotherapy	Recommended
	Esophagogastroduodenoscopy or colonoscopy	Insufficient data (endoscopist discretion)
Moderate risk for endocarditis (rheumatic valvular disease, mitral valve prolapse with insufficiency, hypertrophic cardiomyopathy, most congenital malformations)	Stricture dilation, sclerotherapy	Insufficient data (endoscopist discretion)
	Esophagogastroduodenoscopy or colonoscopy	Not recommended
Low risk for endocarditis (coronary bypass surgery, pacemakers, implantable defibrillators)	All endoscopic procedures	Not recommended
Prosthetic joints	All endoscopic procedures	Not recommended
Obstructed biliary system or pancreatic pseudocyst	Endoscopic retrograde cholangiopancreatography	Recommended
Cirrhosis and ascites	Stricture dilation, sclerotherapy	Insufficient data (endoscopist discretion)
	Esophagogastroduodenoscopy or colonoscopy	Not recommended
All patients	Percutaneous gastrostomy	Recommended

TABLE 75-2
Indications for Upper Gastrointestinal Endoscopy

Diagnostic
    Upper abdominal distress despite an appropriate trial of therapy
    Upper abdominal distress associated with signs or symptoms of organic disease
        (weight loss, anorexia)
    Refractory vomiting of unknown cause
    Dysphagia or odynophagia
    Esophageal reflux symptoms unresponsive to therapy
    Upper gastrointestinal bleeding
    When sampling of duodenal or jejunal tissue or fluid is indicated
    To obtain a histologic diagnosis for radiographically demonstrated gastric or
        esophageal ulcers, upper intestinal tract strictures, or suspected neoplasms
    To screen for varices so that patients with cirrhosis can be identified as possible
        candidates for possible prophylactic medical or endoscopic therapy
    To assess acute injury after caustic ingestion
    When management of other disease processes is affected by the presence of
        upper gastrointestinal pathologic conditions (e.g., use of anticoagulants)
Therapeutic
    Treatment of variceal and nonvariceal upper gastrointestinal bleeding
    Removal of foreign bodies
    Removal of selected polypoid lesions
    Dilation of symptomatic strictures
    Palliative treatment of stenosing neoplasms
    Placement of percutaneous feeding gastrostomy tube
Surveillance
    Follow-up of selected gastric, esophageal, or stomal ulcers to document healing
    Barrett's esophagus
    Familial adenomatous polyposis
    Adenomatous gastric polyps
    Follow-up of varices eradicated with endoscopic therapy

---

established consensus guidelines for the appropriate use of EGD (Table 75-2). Therapeutic endoscopy is often indicated for control of variceal and nonvariceal bleeding, dilation of strictures, removal of some foreign bodies, palliation of advanced malignancies with stents or tumor ablation, and placement of a percutaneous gastrostomy tube. The advent of longer endoscopes has expanded the capability of upper gastrointestinal endoscopy in the diagnosis and potential treatment of diseases of the small intestine. Enteroscopy is indicated when investigating chronic bleeding presumed to be secondary to a source in the small intestine or if visualization or sampling the small intestine is warranted on the basis of radiologic abnormalities.

The major contraindications to the performance of upper gastrointestinal endoscopy include perforation, hemodynamic instability, cardiopulmonary distress, and inadequate patient cooperation. Coagulation disorders are relative contraindications to therapeutic interventions. Percutaneous gastrostomy tube placement is contraindicated if the stomach is inaccessible because of a prior gastrectomy or interposed bowel, liver, or spleen.

Patient Preparation and Monitoring

Patients should not ingest solid food for 6 to 8 hours or liquids for 4 hours before elective upper gastrointestinal endoscopy. If delayed gastric emptying is suspected, a liquid diet can be instituted 24 hours before the procedure and the fasting interval increased to 8 to 12 hours. For complete gastric outlet obstruction, evacuation of the stomach with a nasogastric tube is usually necessary. If an emergency endoscopic procedure is required for gastrointestinal bleeding, measures should be taken to avoid aspiration. Evacuation of the stomach with an orogastric tube before the procedure, attentiveness to oral suction during the procedure, and prophylactic endotracheal intubation in an obtunded patient all serve to protect the patient's airway.

Immediately before the procedure is begun, the posterior pharynx is anesthetized with a topical spray or a gargle anesthetic. The clinical benefit of these agents has been called into question; their use should be avoided in patients with acute hemorrhage or delayed gastric emptying given the increased risk of aspiration. A short-acting benzodiazepine (e.g., midazolam) usually provides a sufficient level of conscious sedation for diagnostic upper gastrointestinal endoscopy. Some endoscopists add intravenous opiates, although the synergistic cardiopulmonary depressant effects of this combination may increase the rate of complications. Longer therapeutic procedures, including percutaneous gastrostomy tube placement, require the administration of opiates for patient comfort. Throughout the procedure, a trained assistant should work in concert with the endoscopist to monitor the oral secretions as well as the overall clinical condition of the patient.

Performance of the Procedure

The endoscope is introduced blindly or under direct visualization by passing the instrument into the posterior pharynx and instructing the patient to swallow. Direct visualization is the preferred method because it is less traumatic and provides a view of the larynx. A standard EGD involves a complete inspection of the esophagus, stomach, and the first two portions of the duodenum. A pediatric colonoscope or push enteroscope can be advanced into the proximal jejunum. Enteroscopy can also be performed with the sonde enteroscope, which relies on peristaltic movement to propel the instrument into the distal jejunum or ileum, but this instrument does not provide biopsy or therapeutic capabilities.

Endoscopic biopsy or brush cytology studies may provide a pathologic diagnosis. For some disease processes (e.g., infections caused by *Helicobacter pylori* and causes of malabsorption in the small intestine), random biopsies of normal-appearing mucosa may be indicated. Upper gastrointestinal endoscopy also provides the capability of therapeutic intervention. Dysphagia resulting from esophageal strictures or achalasia can be relieved with endoscopic dilation using pneumatic balloon or sequential bougienage techniques. The safest means of bougienage dilation involves passage of the dilator over a guidewire that is placed endoscopically into the distal stomach. Although fluoroscopy reduces the complication rate of dilation, radiation exposure and resource limitations have precluded its routine use in many centers. Acute or chronic nonvariceal hemorrhage can be controlled with electrocoagulation, heater probe application, injection therapy, or laser photocoagulation. Large or bleeding esophageal varices may be treated with injection sclerotherapy or band ligation. Mucosal polyps can be excised with electrocoagulation using hot biopsy forceps or with snare polypectomy. Large stenosing esophageal or gastric malignancies can be ablated with laser photocoagulation or electrocoagulation. Esophageal malignancies can also be palliated with deployment of metallic expandable stents.

Complications

Diagnostic upper gastrointestinal endoscopy is usually very safe, with low rates of serious complications. Most complications are related to oversedation, emphasizing the need for preprocedural patient assessment and vigilant patient monitoring throughout the period of sedation. The high rate of wound infections associated with gastrostomy tube placement can be substantially reduced with the use of prophylactic antibiotics. The benefit of prophylactic antibiotics for other indications remains unproven.

LOWER GASTROINTESTINAL ENDOSCOPY

Indications and Contraindications

Diseases or symptoms referable to the colon and rectum are best evaluated with colonoscopy or flexible sigmoidoscopy. Flexible sigmoidoscopy is useful as a screening test for colorectal neoplasia in asymptomatic, normal-risk persons older than 50 years. Sigmoidoscopy is also used to complete the examination of the colon in conjunction with barium enema radiography and to investigate rectosigmoid symptoms in young persons who are at extremely low risk of colorectal neoplasia. In general, sigmoidoscopy is preferred to colonoscopy when the clinical setting suggests that the disease is localized to the rectosigmoid region. However, all patients older than 40 years with symptoms referable to any portion of the colon are best evaluated with total colonoscopy. The American Society of Gastrointestinal Endoscopy has established recommendations for the use of colonoscopy (Table 75-3) that are intended as guidelines. They should not replace the clinical judgment of the clinician.

As with any endoscopic procedure, colonoscopy is contraindicated if a perforation is suspected or if the patient is uncooperative. Lower gastrointestinal endoscopy specifically is contraindicated in the setting of fulminant colitis and the suppurative phase of acute diverticulitis. Recent myocardial infarction is a relative contraindication to colonoscopy and should delay elective procedures for several weeks.

Patient Preparation and Monitoring

Most lower gastrointestinal endoscopic procedures require cleansing of the colon. A limited preparation of the left colon is usually sufficient for flexible sigmoidoscopy and can be achieved with two tap water or small volume sodium phosphate enemas administered 1 hour before the examination. This limited preparation precludes the use of electrocautery because of the hazard of residual explosive gases. Colonoscopy or any lower gastrointestinal endoscopic procedure employing electrocautery requires full preparation of the colon. The two most commonly used agents are sodium phosphate and balanced electrolyte

TABLE 75-3
Indications for Colonoscopy

Diagnostic
    Fecal occult blood
    Hematochezia in the absence of a convincing anorectal source
    Melena, if an upper intestinal source is excluded
    Unexplained iron deficiency
    Abnormality on barium enema that is probably significant (filling defect, stricture)
    To exclude the presence of synchronous cancer or polyps in a patient with confirmed
        colorectal neoplasia
    Chronic, unexplained diarrhea
    Selected patients with altered bowel habits at risk for colonic neoplasia
    Inflammatory bowel disease if establishing a diagnosis or determining the extent
        of disease will alter management decisions
Therapeutic
    Excision of polyps
    Bleeding from vascular ectasias, neoplasia, polypectomy site, or ulceration
    Foreign body removal
    Decompression of acute colonic pseudo-obstruction or volvulus
    Balloon dilation of stenotic lesions
    Palliative treatment of inoperable stenosing or bleeding neoplasms
Surveillance
    Prior history of colorectal cancer or adenomatous polyps
    Family history of hereditary nonpolyposis colon cancer
    Family history of colorectal cancer in a first-degree relative (<55 yrs) or in several
        family members
    Long-standing (>7–10 yrs) chronic ulcerative pancolitis with biopsies to detect dysplasia;
        colitis limited to the left side may require less intensive surveillance

solutions containing polyethylene glycol (PEG). Sodium phosphate is given orally in 45-ml aliquots the evening before and 3 hours before colonoscopy, whereas PEG solutions are administered in 1- to 2-gallon volumes over a period of 4 to 6 hours the evening before colonoscopy. Mannitol and other carbohydrate purgatives should be avoided if electrocoagulation is anticipated because bacterial fermentation produces explosive hydrogen gas. Both sodium phosphate and PEG solutions yield adequate bowel cleansing, but patients often prefer the small-volume sodium phosphate solution to the unpleasant tasting, large-volume PEG solutions. However, sodium phosphate may lead to dangerous fluid and electrolyte shifts in patients with heart failure or renal insufficiency; PEG solutions are the preferred agents for patients with these conditions.

Sedation and monitoring are similar to the practices used with upper gastrointestinal endoscopy. Colonoscopy, however, almost invariably requires the addition of opiates to standard benzodiazepine sedation to minimize the visceral pain associated with colonic distention and stretching. This combination of a benzodiazepine and an opiate has a synergistic depressant effect on the cardiopulmonary system, emphasizing the need for standard cardiopulmonary monitoring. Unlike colonoscopy, flexible sigmoidoscopy to the splenic flexure is often accomplished without sedation. A skilled endoscopist can often perform this procedure with minimal discomfort to the patient. The lack of sedation adds to the convenience and efficiency of the procedure, which improves patient compliance, particularly in screening large populations of asymptomatic persons.

Performance of the Procedure

Flexible sigmoidoscopy involves introduction of the instrument to the descending colon or splenic flexure, whereas total colonoscopy involves passage of the instrument to the cecum. Although experienced endoscopists may reach the cecum in 90% to 98% of examinations, there are a significant number of patients with a colonic anatomy that precludes safe completion of the procedure. Therefore, the well-trained endoscopist should be willing to abandon a colonoscopic study that appears unreasonably traumatic.

As with upper gastrointestinal endoscopy, colonoscopy provides the capability to obtain biopsy specimens to establish the diagnosis of endoscopic abnormalities and to sample normal-appearing mucosa if occult conditions (e.g., microscopic colitis) are suspected. Therapeutic colonoscopy techniques include polypectomy with hot biopsy forceps or with snare polypectomy using electrocoagulation to promote hemostasis. Acute and chronic bleeding from angiodysplasias can be treated with electrocoagulation, heater probe application, and laser photocoagulation. Less common procedures include through-the-scope pneumatic balloon dilation of discrete benign strictures, decompressive colonoscopy with tube placement for acute pseudo-obstruction, and palliative laser ablation of inoperable neoplasms.

Complications

The overall risk of serious complications, including perforation and uncontrolled hemorrhage, is approximately 1 in 500 for diagnostic colonoscopy. Therapeutic maneuvers increase the risk of complications, although there are wide variations in reported rates. Hemorrhage after polypectomy is common and may occur in up to 1% to 2% of patients and often occurs up to 7 to 10 days after the procedure when residual necrotic tissue and scar tissue are sloughed. The risk of perforation is also increased in therapeutic maneuvers. The transmural burn syndrome represents a localized, contained perforation that may be associated with localized pain, fever, and leukocytosis 6 to 24 hours after polypectomy or after any therapy that uses electrocoagulation. Many patients can be treated conservatively with parenteral broad-spectrum antibiotics, but any patient with signs of frank perforation should undergo surgical exploration.

ENDOSCOPIC RETROGRADE CHOLANGIOPANCREATOGRAPHY

Indications and Contraindications

Endoscopic retrograde cholangiopancreatography (ERCP) is indicated in the evaluation of patients with suspected biliary or pancreatic disorders when noninvasive imaging with ultrasonography or computed tomographic (CT) scanning is

TABLE 75-4
Indications for Endoscopic Retrograde Cholangiopancreatography

Suspected biliary disorders
    Unexplained jaundice or cholestasis
    Postcholecystectomy complaints
    Postbiliary surgery complaints
    Acute cholangitis
    Acute gallstone pancreatitis
    Evaluation of bile duct abnormalities on other imaging studies
    Sphincter of Oddi manometry
Suspected pancreatic disorders
    Chronic upper abdominal pain consistent with pancreatic origin
    Unexplained weight loss
    Steatorrhea
    Unexplained recurrent pancreatitis
    Evaluation of pancreatic abnormalities on other imaging studies
    To obtain pancreatic duct brushings or pure pancreatic juice
Before therapeutic intervention
    Endoscopic sphincterotomy
    Endoscopic biliary drainage
    Endoscopic pancreatic drainage
    Balloon dilation of pancreaticobiliary strictures
    Preoperative mapping for pancreatic or biliary resections

equivocal and when therapeutic intervention is necessary (Table 75-4). Various abdominal symptoms can be attributed to the pancreaticobiliary system, and the decision to proceed with ERCP should be made by a clinician experienced in the care of patients with these disorders. ERCP has a role in the preoperative evaluation of selected patients undergoing laparoscopic cholecystectomy, pancreatic resection, or surgical pseudocyst drainage. Many of the available therapeutic options, including endoscopic sphincterotomy, stone extraction, and biliary or pancreatic stent placement, also require the availability of surgical support. Thus, the treatment of patients undergoing ERCP often requires the combined expertise of the endoscopist and the surgeon.

In addition to the standard contraindications for all endoscopic procedures, ERCP is relatively contraindicated in the presence of an obstructed biliary system or documented pancreatic pseudocyst unless immediate endoscopic or surgical drainage is planned. Any procedure performed under these conditions should be accompanied by administration of prophylactic antibiotics (see Table 75-1). Therapeutic interventions, particularly endoscopic sphincterotomy, are contraindicated in patients with severe coagulopathy.

Patient Preparation and Monitoring

All patients undergoing ERCP should be prepared in the same manner as patients undergoing EGD. Attention should be given to several factors specific to ERCP. First, because the endoscope used for ERCP is equipped with side-viewing rather than with forward-viewing optics, special attention should be given to patients with dysphagia. Passage of the instrument through the esophagus is done blindly, increasing the risk of perforation in the setting of a Zenker's diverticulum or esophageal stricture. The ductal injection of contrast material can result in significant systemic absorption, as demonstrated occasionally by the appearance of a postinjection nephrogram. Although anaphylactic reactions have not been reported, erythema and rash can occur, and some clinicians choose to pretreat patients who have a history of reactions to contrast agents with antihistamines and corticosteroids 12 and 2 hours before the procedure. Because ERCP involves radiographic imaging of the upper abdomen, any residual gastrointestinal contrast agent should be evacuated with purgatives. Immediately before sedating the patient, abdominal radiographs should be obtained to ensure that all contrast material is gone and to establish the location of soft tissue shadows and calcifications.

The sedation of patients undergoing ERCP is similar to the procedure used for patients undergoing upper gastrointestinal endoscopy. Because biliary manipulation and injection are often associated with visceral pain, opiates are frequently added. Patient movement should be minimized to obtain optimal imaging. Because the patient is in the prone position on the fluoroscopic table rather than in the left decubitus position used for upper gastrointestinal endoscopy, special attention should be given to removing oral secretions.

Performance of the Procedure

ERCP involves passage of the side-viewing endoscope into the second portion of the duodenum and visualization of the ampulla of Vater. Both the pancreatic and biliary system can be cannulated with specialized catheters that are advanced through the duodenoscope. After selective cannulation of the pancreatic or biliary system is achieved, radiologic contrast dye is injected under fluoroscopic guidance until the entire ductal system is visualized. Care should be taken to avoid injecting air, because bubbles may be mistaken for biliary or pancreatic stones. Overinjection of dye into the pancreas leads to staining of the parenchyma, a pattern termed *acinarization*, which is associated with an increased risk of ERCP-induced pancreatitis. Abdominal radiographs are obtained during the injection and periodically as the contrast dye drains from the duct. After one ductal system is examined, the alternative system is cannulated and injected. For some disorders, only cholangiography or pancreatography is necessary. In specialized centers, biliary manometry can be performed as part of the ERCP examination with a specialized water-perfused manometry catheter positioned across the sphincter of Oddi. The ampulla of Vater may not be easily accessible in patients whose anatomy has been altered by a Billroth II or Roux-en-Y gastrojejunostomy.

ERCP is a nonoperative method of treating many pancreaticobiliary disorders. Endoscopic sphincterotomy is often performed to facilitate biliary stone extraction. The procedure involves cannulation of the common bile duct with a papillotome, a specialized catheter with an exposed wire that extends across the most distal portion of the catheter. Positioning the wire across the papilla and applying electrical current produces a cut through the papilla. After sphincterotomy, stones may pass spontaneously, but extraction with balloon catheters or baskets placed through the endoscope and into the bile duct is often necessary. If endoscopic stone extraction fails, a nasobiliary tube or endoscopic stent can be placed while the patient awaits definitive surgical therapy. Sphincterotomy also relieves obstruction caused by sphincter of Oddi dyskinesia or papillary stenosis. Specialized centers may perform sphincterotomy of the minor papilla for treatment of pancreas divisum.

Biliary or pancreatic strictures can also be treated with ERCP. Inoperable malignant obstruction of the extrahepatic bile ducts is best relieved with endoscopic placement of a plastic or metallic stent, in many cases after the performance of sphincterotomy. Occasionally, patients with primary sclerosing cholangitis will have dominant strictures of the extrahepatic bile ducts, which are amenable to pneumatic balloon dilation followed by stent placement. For most benign biliary strictures, however, surgical therapy is preferred because of the superior long-term patency. Transpapillary placement of a pancreatic stent has been used to treat symptomatic pancreatic ductal strictures and pseudocysts in patients with chronic pancreatitis.

Complications

Acute pancreatitis is the most common complication of ERCP. Sixty percent to 80% of patients undergoing ERCP develop asymptomatic elevations in serum amylase and lipase levels, but clinically overt pancreatitis is much less common. Retrospective series report an incidence of 1% to 2%, but prospective series suggest that symptomatic acute pancreatitis occurs in up to 4% to 7% of patients undergoing ERCP. The risk is increased by acinarization of the pancreas, repeated attempts at cannulation, and sphincter of Oddi manometry. Conservative management leads to resolution for most patients, but severe necrotizing pancreatitis occurs in a small subset of patients.

Endoscopic sphincterotomy has an overall complication rate of 5% to 8%, equally divided between bleeding, perforation, cholangitis, and pancreatitis. One percent to 2% of patients undergoing sphincterotomy require surgical intervention for related complications; the mortality rate for sphincterotomy is 0.5% to 1%. Attempted biliary drainage with endoprosthesis placement is associated with an 8% risk of cholangitis, but most of these episodes occur when drainage is unsuccessful or incomplete. Stent occlusion and cholangitis are delayed complications that occur in 40% of patients a mean of 5 to 6 months after endoprosthesis insertion.

ENDOSCOPIC ULTRASOUND

Indications and Contraindications

Endoscopic ultrasound (EUS) provides the capability to obtain high-resolution ultrasound images from within the upper and lower gastrointestinal tract. Specialized endoscopes with an ultrasound probe at the tip and oblique-viewing optics can generate acoustic images of gastrointestinal wall layers and surrounding strictures. Increased availability of the instruments and clinical experience with the technique have expanded the list of clinical indications for EUS (Table 75-5). Focal intramural and extramural mass lesions and wall thickening are easily identified with EUS. The localization to a specific wall layer (i.e., mucosa, submucosa, muscularis, serosa, extralumenal) often helps to identify the histologic origin of the lesion. EUS is also of value in identifying and staging several tumors, including esophageal carcinoma, gastric carcinoma, gas-

---

TABLE 75-5
Indications for Endoscopic Ultrasound

Tumor staging (esophageal, gastric, pancreatic, ampullary, distal bile duct, rectal, non–small cell lung)
Neuroendocrine tumor localization
Evaluation of submucosal mass lesions
Suspected chronic pancreatitis
Detection of distal bile duct stones
Fine-needle aspiration of adjacent lymph nodes or mass lesions

---

tric lymphoma, ampullary carcinoma, distal bile duct carcinoma, pancreatic carcinoma, and rectal carcinoma. EUS is both sensitive and specific in determining the local extent of the tumor (T stage) and the presence of regional lymph nodes (N stage), but it is not a reliable means of establishing distant metastatic disease (M stage). EUS is superior to CT and magnetic resonance imaging studies and to transabdominal ultrasound for pancreatic imaging, and it is the most accurate means of defining vascular invasion by tumors in the peripancreatic bed. Similarly, EUS is able to localize pancreatic islet cell tumors not detected by conventional imaging studies. Evidence suggests that the sensitivity of EUS is equivalent to that of ERCP for detecting common bile duct stones and chronic pancreatitis.

The introduction of instruments to obtain ultrasound-directed fine-needle aspiration has further expanded the role of EUS. Sampling of pancreatic mass lesions has proved useful, particularly in patients with unresectable disease who are candidates for palliative radiation therapy or chemotherapy protocols. EUS-directed transesophageal aspiration of mediastinal lymph nodes has proved superior to other nonsurgical methods of staging non–small cell lung cancer and often provides information critical to the decision to pursue surgical or nonsurgical therapy in these patients. The same instrumentation used in tissue sampling has launched EUS into the realm of therapeutics. EUS-guided needle injection of the celiac ganglia has been used to control chronic pain caused by chronic pancreatitis or pancreatic cancer. Future refinements in endosonographic image quality and performance will probably expand the diagnostic and therapeutic capabilities of EUS.

Because EUS is a specialized form of upper and lower gastrointestinal endoscopy, the contraindications are identical to those of diagnostic endoscopy in their respective locations in the gastrointestinal tract.

Patient Preparation and Monitoring

The patient preparation for EUS of the upper gastrointestinal tract is identical to the process for EGD. Similarly, EUS of the rectum or colon requires bowel cleansing in accordance with the techniques used for flexible sigmoidoscopy or colonoscopy, respectively. The principles of sedation and monitoring are also based on the standard practices for upper and lower gastrointestinal endoscopy.

Performance of the Procedure

There are two principal types of echoendoscopes. The linear or curved array instruments provide 100-degree sector images parallel to the longitudinal axis of the endoscope, whereas radial scanning instruments provide 360-degree images perpendicular to the longitudinal axis of the endoscope. Although upper echoendoscopes usually have oblique-viewing optics, echocolonoscopes are available with forward-viewing optics. The ultrasound frequency can be altered on most of the available instruments; higher-frequency imaging (12 to 20 MHz) provides increased resolution, and lower-frequency imaging (5.0 to 7.5 MHz) provides increased depth of penetration. Because images from linear or curved array instruments are oriented along the axis of the endoscope, specialized needles can be advanced through the working channel and directed under real-time ultrasound guidance into a lesion for tissue aspiration.

EUS provides high-resolution images of the bowel wall and, in most structures, identifies five echolayers that correlate with the mucosa, muscularis mucosae, submucosa, muscularis propria, and serosa or adventitia. Directing the instrument to a focal submucosal mass or an area of wall thickening can identify the layer from which the abnormality originates. The pancreas can be visualized from the duodenum or posterior wall of the stomach, whereas the bile duct and gallbladder can be identified from the duodenum. The major vascular structures of the splanchnic circulation can also be identified from the duodenum or stomach. Flow within these structures can be assessed by the color flow and pulse Doppler modes that are available on curved array instruments.

Complications

EUS has a safety profile similar to that of diagnostic upper and lower gastrointestinal endoscopy. The larger diameter of the echoendoscope makes traversing lumenal strictures more hazardous, which is problematic for esophageal tumors. Patients with significant dysphagia should undergo preliminary forward-viewing endoscopy or barium swallow radiography so that the severity of lumenal narrowing can be assessed. EUS-directed biopsy has also been proved to be safe, with a complication rate of 1% to 2%.

CHAPTER 76

Imaging Procedures

Imaging of the abdomen and gastrointestinal tract is an essential element of the diagnostic evaluation of many patients who exhibit signs and symptoms suggestive of digestive disorders. In some instances, these procedures also provide a means of obtaining histologic diagnoses with image-guided biopsies or needle aspiration. Moreover, radiologic testing plays an important role in facilitating many therapeutic interventions.

CONTRAST RADIOLOGY

Pharynx

Pharyngoesophagography provides structural and functional assessments of patients with swallowing disorders. A cine or video recording of the swallowing of a bolus of liquid or solid barium provides a detailed examination of the activation and coordination of the muscles involved in deglutition. Periodic radiographs are obtained to identify morphologic abnormalities. Single- and double-contrast barium esophagrams are an integral part of this examination and help exclude associated motility or structural abnormalities of the esophagus.

Barium examination of the pharynx and esophagus is the procedure of choice in evaluating patients with oropharyngeal dysphagia or recurrent aspiration. Swallowing dysfunction is particularly common in patients with cerebrovascular disease, neuromuscular disorders, head and neck tumors, and previous head and neck surgery or radiation therapy. Barium swallow radiography is a sensitive means of detecting laryngeal penetration and aspiration. *Penetration* refers to the entry of barium into the larynx during the swallowing process because of abnormal coordination; *aspiration* refers to the entry of barium into the larynx during normal breathing because of poor pharyngeal clearance. Pharyngograms are more sensitive than upper gastrointestinal endoscopy in identifying diverticula and are >95% sensitive in detecting mucosal neoplasms.

Upper Gastrointestinal Tract

Contrast radiography of the upper gastrointestinal tract can provide diagnostic information on patients who exhibit various signs and symptoms referable to the esophagus, stomach, or duodenum. Patients should fast for 6 to 8 hours before the study. A complete examination involves both single- and double-contrast studies. For a double-contrast study, the patient swallows barium and an effervescent agent, and the gaseous distention in conjunction with a series of changes in the patient's position makes it possible to obtain detailed images of the mucosa. The single-contrast study is particularly useful for defining gross lumenal abnormalities (e.g., strictures).

In most settings, upper gastrointestinal barium radiography is less sensitive and specific than upper gastrointestinal endoscopy for detecting mucosal disease, although studies performed by a radiologist who specializes in double-contrast examinations may have an accuracy approaching that of upper gastrointestinal endoscopy. The sensitivity of barium swallow radiography for detecting reflux esophagitis can be as high as 90%, but it is an unreliable means of detecting Barrett's mucosa. Similarly, although double-contrast examinations can detect ulcers and strictures of the esophagus, endoscopic biopsy is necessary to confirm the histologic diagnosis. Double-contrast studies are also sensitive for detecting gastric erosions and ulcers. There are radiographic features that suggest a benign gastric ulcer, including prepyloric location and symmetric radiating folds, but some clinicians advocate endoscopic biopsy of all gastric ulcers. Contrast examination of the duodenum may identify duodenal ulcer disease, and it is superior to endoscopy for defining lumenal strictures. Occasionally, it is difficult to distinguish active from healed gastroduodenal ulcers on barium radiographic studies. Upper gastrointestinal endoscopy is the procedure of choice when examining patients with acute gastrointestinal hemorrhage.

Although there are no absolute contraindications to contrast radiography of the upper gastrointestinal tract, the use of barium is contraindicated in patients with suspected perforation. In these cases, a water-soluble agent (e.g., meglumine [Gastrografin]) should be substituted. Because Gastrografin may trigger an intense inflammatory response if aspirated, however, barium is the agent of choice if a tracheoesophageal fistula or swallowing disorder is suspected. A thorough examination requires extensive maneuvering of the patient, which means that studies of immobile or uncooperative patients are often of limited diagnostic value.

Small Intestine

The small intestine may be examined by dedicated barium radiography or by small bowel enema (enteroclysis), which provides more detail. In dedicated barium radiographic studies of the small intestine, the patient is often given metoclopramide 20 minutes before ingesting 500 ml barium. A brief examination of the upper gastrointestinal tract is performed and the barium is followed through the small intestine with periodic fluoroscopy and abdominal radiography. Enteroclysis requires a skilled and dedicated radiologist. The duodenum is intubated with a balloon occlusion catheter; the injection of barium is followed by the infusion of 1500 to 2000 ml of a 0.5% solution of methylcellulose, which distends the loops of the small intestine and provides a detailed, double-contrast examination of the mucosa. Enteroclysis is more sensitive than dedicated barium radiography of the small intestine for defining small tumors or subtle mucosal abnormalities, but enteroclysis is more time consuming and labor intensive and is more uncomfortable for the patient because of the duodenal intubation and distention. As a result, dedicated barium radiography of the small intestine is often used initially, and if there is a high suspicion of a pathologic condition in the small intestine and the standard examination findings are normal, enteroclysis can be performed.

Contrast studies are the procedures of choice in evaluating patients with symptoms of partial or incomplete obstruction of the small intestine. In addition to defining the level of obstruction, the study may identify the cause of obstruction. Barium radiography of the small intestine is particularly useful for diagnosing and defining the extent of Crohn's disease. Disease complications (e.g., strictures and fistulae) are best identified with barium studies. Benign and malignant tumors of the small intestine can be detected, but the clinician must remember that small tumors can be overlooked on dedicated barium radiography of the small intestine. Enteroclysis is the best test for detecting subtle mucosal abnormalities. Enteroclysis is also the preferred test if a mucosal malabsorptive process or Meckel's diverticulum is suspected. Although barium studies are often used in patients with unexplained gastrointestinal bleeding, the diagnostic yield is extremely low, primarily because barium studies cannot identify vascular ectasias.

Colon

To achieve an adequate examination of the mucosa of the colon, the patient must undergo colonic cleansing before barium enema radiography. Preparative regimens vary, but a common procedure involves a diet of clear liquids for 24 hours followed by ingestion of 300 ml magnesium citrate and 10 mg bisacodyl the evening before the study and a repeat dose of bisacodyl the morning of the procedure. Patients with renal failure should not be given purgatives that contain magnesium. Single-contrast barium enema radiography involves filling the entire colon with low-density barium, whereas double-contrast evaluation uses a small amount of high-density barium followed by insufflation of air, which produces a thin coating of barium over the entire colonic mucosa.

Single-contrast agents provide only limited views of mucosal structures and are primarily indicated if a colonic stricture or diverticular disease is suspected. Double-contrast studies are superior to single-contrast examinations for defining mucosal disease including colorectal polyps. Areas of the rectum and sigmoid colon are often difficult to visualize on barium radiography, and no examination of the colon should be considered complete without flexible sigmoidoscopy. Conversely, the cecum cannot be visualized in up to 10% of patients undergoing colonoscopy, and barium enema radiography is often necessary in these circumstances to achieve a complete examination of the colon.

Although colonoscopy is superior to barium enema radiography for detecting small colorectal polyps and subtle mucosal disease, barium enema radiography is 95% sensitive for detecting colorectal cancer. Double-contrast barium radiography is capable of reliably defining polyps >1 cm in diameter and can detect ulcerations in advanced inflammatory bowel disease. However, the superior sensitivity and specificity of endoscopy as well as the capability to obtain biopsy specimens and perform a polypectomy has established colonoscopy as the procedure of choice for these disorders. Barium enema radiography remains the procedure of choice for defining colonic strictures and complications related to diverticular disease.

Barium enema radiography is less expensive and safer than colonoscopy, but it requires adequate patient mobility. Barium enema radiography is contraindicated in the setting of toxic megacolon, ischemic colitis, or confirmed perforation. If a perforation is suspected, water-soluble contrast agents should be used. Colonic perforation is a rare complication of barium enema radiography.

ULTRASOUND

Diagnostic ultrasound relies on differences in acoustic impedance between distinct tissues. Acoustic impedance determines the speed of sound in a given tissue, and when a sound wave encounters an interface of tissues with different densities, a portion of the sound wave is reflected. As sound travels through acoustically homogeneous substances (e.g., fluid), echoes are minimal or absent. When sound encounters the border of substances with dramatically different acoustic densities (e.g., an air-tissue interface), however, all of the acoustic energy is reflected, producing an intense echo signal. Ultrasound images are generated by transformation of returning echoes into electrical signals with a magnitude proportional to the intensity of sound wave amplitude.

Currently available ultrasound units provide real-time images with a resolution that is based on the frequency of the transducer. Higher-frequency probes increase the resolution but diminish the depth of penetration. Pulse and color-flow Doppler units have the capacity to qualitatively and quantitatively assess the flow in vascular strictures. Despite improvements in instrument standardization, the overall accuracy of ultrasound continues to depend on the skill of the technician and the interpreting radiologist.

Liver

Ultrasound is a noninvasive means of diagnosing several hepatic disorders. The normal hepatic parenchyma appears homogeneous and relatively hypoechoic, but in cirrhosis, the liver usually appears small, lobular, heterogeneous, and relatively hyperechoic. Other diffuse hepatocellular disorders are inconsistently associated with nonspecific changes in parenchymal echo texture. Documenting the dimensions of the hepatic lobes is helpful in establishing the small size. Collateral vessels or ascites caused by portal hypertension can also be identified. Furthermore, Doppler assessment can establish the presence and direction of flow (hepatofugal versus hepatopetal) in the portal vein. Doppler ultrasound should be the initial procedure for patients with suspected occlusion of the portal or hepatic vein.

Ultrasound is also instrumental in examining hepatic mass lesions; several series have documented a sensitivity equivalent to that of computed tomographic (CT) scanning. The lack of intravenous contrast and radiation exposure have prompted recommendations that ultrasound serve as the initial imaging modality to detect liver masses. Ultrasound is particularly accurate in defining cystic lesions of the liver. Moreover, ultrasound has a sensitivity of 90% and a specificity of 93% for detecting hepatocellular carcinoma, and is a more sensitive technique than CT scanning for detecting tumors <3 cm in diameter. Conversely, contrast-enhanced CT scanning is more sensitive than ultrasound for defining liver metastases. Similarly, hemangiomas characteristically appear as peripheral hyperechoic lesions, but confirmation of the diagnosis usually requires contrast-enhanced CT or magnetic resonance imaging (MRI) studies or tagged erythrocyte nuclear scintigraphy. Because ultrasound provides real-time images, it is often the procedure of choice for obtaining image-guided biopsy specimens of hepatic mass lesions.

Biliary Tract

Ultrasound is the noninvasive procedure of choice for examining patients with suspected biliary disorders. The sensitivity and specificity for detecting gallstones are 98% and 95%, respectively. Stones typically appear as focal hyperechoic densities with acoustic shadowing distal to the stone because of near complete reflection of the sound wave. Ultrasound also is a sensitive means of detecting gallbladder sludge, which appears as an amorphous hyperechoic collection, without shadowing, in the dependent portion of the gallbladder. Ultrasound is far less accurate for detecting common bile duct stones, with sensitivities ranging from 15% to 60%; however, the associated biliary dilation is usually evident. CT scanning is superior to ultrasound for identifying distal bile duct stones and other causes of extrahepatic bile duct obstruction.

Ultrasound is often used as the primary diagnostic test for acute cholecystitis. Ultrasound criteria include the presence of increased gallbladder wall thickness, a sonographic Murphy's sign, a distended gallbladder, pericholecystic fluid, and stones or sludge. The sonographic Murphy's sign is defined as maximal tenderness with the ultrasound transducer positioned over the gallbladder. This finding has a sensitivity of 65%, but it is often absent in gangrenous cholecystitis. Based on the above criteria, ultrasound has an overall accuracy of 90% in diagnosing acute cholecystitis. In many centers, radionuclide imaging is used as a complementary test if the results of ultrasound are equivocal.

Pancreas

Ultrasound of the pancreas often is limited by the organ's retroperitoneal location and ultrasound's inability to image through overlying bowel gas. As a result, a CT scan is the noninvasive procedure of choice for excluding pancreatic disease. Ultrasound still has a substantial role in evaluating patients with pancreatic disorders, however. Ultrasound should be the initial imaging procedure for patients with acute pancreatitis, primarily because of its ability to detect gallstones. In addition, when the pancreas is visualized, complications of acute and chronic pancreatitis including fluid collections, abscesses, and pseudocysts may be identified. Ultrasound often is preferable to CT scanning for following a pseudocyst over time because of the lower cost and lack of radiation exposure.

Ultrasound may detect up to 80% to 90% of pancreatic adenocarcinomas and 50% of pancreatic endocrine tumors. Contrast-enhanced CT scanning has a superior sensitivity and provides added staging information, making it the noninvasive procedure of choice for evaluating pancreatic neoplasms. If a mass lesion is identified on ultrasound, however, an image-guided biopsy can establish the diagnosis for up to 90% of tumors.

Miscellaneous Abdominal Structures

Ultrasound is the best imaging technique for establishing the presence of ascites. As little as 30 ml of fluid can be detected in the hepatorenal recess. Acute appendicitis usually is a clinical diagnosis, but ultrasound can provide corroborative evidence for the diagnosis. In acute appendicitis, the appendix is visualized as a thick-walled, noncompressible target lesion. The finding of a complex fluid collection distinct from the ovaries is suggestive of an associated abscess. Ultrasound is also helpful in identifying other intra-abdominal inflammatory processes, including diverticulitis and abdominal abscesses, but CT scanning is a more sensitive method of diagnosing these disorders.

COMPUTED TOMOGRAPHY

CT produces cross-sectional images of the body by reconstructing radiographic images obtained from multiple positions in a fixed arc encircling the patient. Tissues are represented on a gray-scale continuum measured in Hounsfield units. Imaging of abdominal structures requires orally administered contrast agents to identify lumenal structures and intravenous contrast agents to identify vascular structures and focal abnormalities in specific organs. Axial images can be obtained every 1 to 10 mm. The recent introduction of helical or spiral CT scanning has shortened scan times to <1 minute. Arterial phase and venous phase scans can be obtained with a single injection of contrast. As with ultrasound, CT can guide needle biopsies and catheter drainage of collected fluid.

In preparation for abdominal CT scanning, the patient should drink water-soluble contrast material 12 and 2 hours before the procedure. If the contrast agent is given intravenously, the patient should fast or ingest only clear liquids for the 6 hours preceding the test. Anaphylactic reactions are rare, but milder reactions (e.g., rash, urticaria, and vomiting) are more common. The risk of contrast-induced renal failure is increased significantly in patients with diabetes and pre-existing renal dysfunction or if the contrast agent is administered with other nephrotoxins (e.g., aminoglycosides).

Liver

CT findings may be normal in the early stages of cirrhosis, but with advanced architectural changes, there are often characteristic tomographic changes. The liver may be small with irregular edges and demonstrate inhomogeneous contrast enhancement. The right lobe and left medial lobe are often disproportionately smaller relative to the caudate and left lateral lobes. CT scans may demonstrate portosystemic collaterals or ascites, which are suggestive of portal hypertension. Contrast-enhanced scans also can define portal venous and hepatic venous thrombosis. Chronic portal vein thrombosis often is accompanied by an extensive network of porta hepatitis collaterals termed *cavernous transformation of the portal vein.*

A CT scan is of primary importance in diagnosing and defining the cause of hepatic mass lesions. Hepatocellular carcinoma may be characterized by the appearance of a solitary mass, multicentric masses, or an infiltrative pattern on the CT scan. Unfortunately, distinguishing hepatocellular carcinoma from the regenerative changes of cirrhosis is often challenging and the overall sensitivity of CT is <70%. Both hepatocellular carcinoma and hepatic metastases typically have a hypodense appearance on contrast-enhanced scans, but if the scans are obtained early during the arterial phase of enhancement, hepatocellular carcinomas may demonstrate marked contrast enhancement. Hemangiomas produce a characteristic pattern of enhancement that begins peripherally and progresses centrally over time. On non-contrast scans, hemangiomas appear hypodense relative to the surrounding parenchyma. Hepatic adenomas and focal nodular hyperplasia are also often identified by their hypodense appearance on delayed-contrast images. A minority of masses caused by focal nodular hyperplasia demonstrate a central stellate scar. CT is an extremely sensitive technique for detecting hepatic cysts and abscesses. Because the tomographic features of many hepatic mass lesions are similar, CT-guided needle aspiration is often necessary to establish a histologic diagnosis.

Biliary Tract

Although clearly less sensitive than ultrasound for detecting gallbladder stones, CT scanning is equivalent to ultrasound for detecting biliary dilation, and it provides superior imaging of the distal common bile duct. A common bile duct >8 mm in diameter or a common hepatic duct >6 mm in diameter is suggestive of biliary obstruction. CT is more sensitive than ultrasound for detecting distal bile duct stones. However, the absence of stones or biliary dilation on a CT scan does not exclude the presence of choledocholithiasis. Cholangiography remains the procedure of choice for examining the distal bile ducts. CT scanning is often used in conjunction with cholangiography to detect bile duct carcinomas. Although less sensitive than endoscopic retrograde cholangiopancreatography (ERCP), CT scanning may also demonstrate saccular dilation and diffuse stricturing of the biliary tree consistent with primary sclerosing cholangitis.

Pancreas

A CT scan is the preferred noninvasive modality for pancreatic imaging. Intravenous contrast enhancement is necessary to distinguish the major splanchnic vessels in the peripancreatic bed. Adenocarcinoma usually appears as a hypodense mass; the overall sensitivity of CT scanning for detecting these neoplasms approaches 90%. In addition to identifying the primary tumor, a CT scan can provide critical staging information. Demonstration of vascular invasion of the large splanchnic vessels in the peripancreatic bed or of distant metastatic disease establishes the tumor as incurable. A CT scan is highly sensitive for documenting liver metastases, but even with the new-generation spiral scanning techniques, the sensitivity for determining vascular invasion is only 30% to 50%. CT has limited accuracy in detecting small endocrine tumors of the pancreas. Whereas nonfunctioning tumors are often large and easily demonstrated on CT scans, gastrinomas and insulinomas are often <2 cm in diameter and escape detection. Cystic masses of the pancreas are readily identified, but CT-guided needle aspiration may be necessary to distinguish neoplastic cysts from pancreatic pseudocysts.

Although usually reserved for patients with severe disease, contrast-enhanced CT scanning often provides information critical to the management of acute pancreatitis. The extent of pancreatic necrosis, as represented by unenhanced parenchyma, has been closely correlated with the risk of complications (e.g., infected fluid collections and abscesses). CT is the most sensitive means of detecting pseudocysts and peripancreatic fluid collections. CT-guided needle aspiration for Gram's stain and culture can be used if the clinical signs suggest the presence of an infection. CT-guided catheter drainage is one of many therapeutic options for patients with refractory pseudocysts.

Miscellaneous Abdominal Structures

CT has emerged as perhaps the most important preoperative staging procedure for many gastrointestinal malignancies. A CT scan is often used in the staging of esophageal, gastric, small intestinal, and colorectal malignancies. Although it is generally impossible to differentiate gastrointestinal wall thickening caused by inflammatory disorders from thickening caused by a neoplasm on a CT scan, CT is a sensitive technique for detecting distant metastatic disease and invasion of adjacent structures. CT is also useful in the surveillance for tumor recurrence after curative resection.

CT is the most sensitive means of detecting intra-abdominal abscesses. In patients with Crohn's disease or diverticulitis with palpable abdominal masses and systemic signs of infection, CT scans may reveal a localized fluid collection in addition to the nonspecific bowel wall thickening observed in these disorders. Distinguishing an abscess from a fluid-filled loop of bowel demands an adequate preparation with an oral contrast agent. When an intra-abdominal abscess is identified, the initial therapeutic approach often involves CT-guided catheter drainage of the abscess cavity.

Although surgical exploration is recommended for patients with an established obstruction of the small intestine, a CT scan is often helpful in confirming the diagnosis if the findings on an abdominal radiograph are equivocal. In addition, the various causes of obstruction (e.g., adhesions, lumenal mass lesions, extrinsic mass lesions, and inflammatory disorders) can usually be distinguished on CT scans.

MAGNETIC RESONANCE IMAGING

MRI relies on the magnetic properties of hydrogen nuclei in various tissues. MRI scanners apply a magnetic field to the body and radiofrequency pulses disturb the alignment of hydrogen nuclei with the magnetic field. The signal intensity used to generate an image is based on the time required for the hydrogen nuclei to return to the original magnetic orientation (T1 weighted) and the decay of the nuclear orientation imposed by the radiofrequency pulse (T2 weighted). Images can be reconstructed in multiple planes, but anatomic references are easier to establish in the transverse plane. Because acquisition time is often on the order of minutes, image quality is very susceptible to motion artifact. Therefore, MRI has not proved useful for examining lumenal structures. Future advances in scanning techniques and software may decrease the image acquisition time and improve the spatial resolution of the bowel.

MRI primarily has played a secondary role to CT scanning for abdominal imaging. Focal lesions of the liver and pancreas are readily identified with MRI, but there is no evidence that MRI is superior to contrast-enhanced CT scanning. To date, MRI has primarily been used to image these structures in patients who cannot tolerate intravenous contrast agents.

The capability to specifically image fluid-filled and vascular structures is unique to MRI. Gradient echo techniques are used to define the biliary tree, providing images with good resolution. As the quality of these images improves, MRI cholangiography may replace ERCP as a diagnostic modality in some patients with disorders of the biliary system. Gradient echo imaging techniques are also being used to define blood flow in vascular structures. This is particularly useful as a noninvasive means of detecting portal vein or hepatic vein thrombosis or atherosclerotic disease of the splanchnic circulation.

Any ferromagnetic particle may be accelerated toward the scanner's magnet. Therefore, a careful history regarding prior surgical procedures and metal exposures should be obtained. MRI is contraindicated in patients with intraocular metallic fragments or ferromagnetic cerebral aneurysm clips. Most orthopedic and cardiovascular prostheses are safe. The presence of a cardiac pacemaker, however, is a relative contraindication to MRI because the powerful magnetic field can inhibit pacemaker function. Recent studies suggest that MRI can be safely performed in carefully selected patients with pacemakers.

ANGIOGRAPHY

Although MRI and CT scans provide images of the major splanchnic vessels, angiography remains the standard for imaging the gastrointestinal vascular system. Standard techniques involve fluoroscopically guided injection of a contrast agent into the selected vessel followed by sequential radiographs. Digital subtraction techniques have gained popularity because they require smaller amounts of the contrast agent and can be viewed on a video monitor; however, standard fluoroscopic techniques continue to provide superior image resolution. Technical considerations vary with each procedure. Arterial vessels are usually accessed by transfemoral or transaxillary approaches. The systemic venous circulation is usually entered from an internal jugular cannula, whereas portal venous access requires a transhepatic puncture. Most procedures can be performed in an outpatient service. Patient preparation requires clearing any residual lumenal contrast agent, and oral intake should be limited to clear liquids for 6 to 8 hours before the study. A low dose of a benzodiazepine is usually administered immediately before the study, and throughout the procedure the patient is monitored for changes in heart rate, blood pressure, pulse oximetry values, and cardiac rhythm. The overall complication rates vary from 1.75% to 3.3%. The most common complications are puncture site bleeding and catheter-induced hemorrhage or embolization. Reactions to contrast agents occur in <1 in 1000 patients and anaphylaxis is even less common. The risk of renal failure is related to the amount of contrast material used with an overall risk of 1 in 10,000 patients.

Angiography is the cornerstone of diagnosing occlusive and nonocclusive diseases of the splanchnic circulation. Selective injection of the superior mesenteric artery can identify any of the causes of acute mesenteric ischemia, including an arterial embolus, an arterial thrombus, a venous thrombus, and arteriolar vasospasm. Similarly, injection of the celiac, superior mesenteric, and inferior mesenteric arteries demonstrates significant narrowing of at least two of these vessels in patients with intestinal angina. Less common vascular disorders (e.g., mesenteric vasculitis and aneurysms) can also be identified by angiography. Venous phase studies are necessary to detect thrombosis of the portal vein or one of its major tributaries. Hepatic vein balloon occlusion venography is the procedure of choice for identifying the hepatic vein occlusion responsible for the Budd-Chiari syndrome, and translumenal balloon angioplasty can be used to restore hepatic vein patency.

Because many tumors have abnormal vascular patterns, angiography can be used to identify primary or metastatic lesions. The introduction of contrast-enhanced CT and MRI techniques has diminished the role of angiography in the primary diagnosis of tumors, but it remains a valuable tool for detecting vascular invasion. Angiographic techniques also have a role in neuroendocrine tumor localization using selective intra-arterial secretin injections followed by hepatic vein gastrin measurements for gastrinomas and intra-arterial calcium infusion with hepatic vein insulin measurements for insulinomas. Angiography is also

TABLE 76-1
Indications and Contraindications to a Transjugular Intrahepatic
Portosystemic Shunt

Indications
    Control of esophageal, gastric, small intestinal, or colonic variceal bleeding
    Control of bleeding from portal gastropathy
    Treatment of intractable ascites
Contraindications
    Fulminant hepatic failure
    Severe preprocedure hepatic encephalopathy despite medical therapy
    Active hepatic infection or bacteremia
    Decompensated heart failure
    Complete portal vein thrombosis

instrumental in the therapy of a wide variety of hepatic metastases through the use of hepatic artery infusion catheters and chemoembolization techniques.

Angiography is an important supplement to endoscopic intervention for variceal and nonvariceal gastrointestinal hemorrhage. Patients with bleeding gastroesophageal varices who have failed to respond to endoscopic therapy should be considered for a transjugular intrahepatic portosystemic shunt (TIPS) (Table 76-1). A TIPS is created by channeling a needle catheter from a hepatic vein tributary through the liver parenchyma until a branch of the portal vein is encountered. The established tract is dilated, and a stent is positioned across the tract to maintain patency. Ten percent to 20% of TIPS procedures are complicated by encephalopathy, but most cases can be controlled with medical therapy. When the portosystemic gradient is reduced to <12 mm Hg, a TIPS is extremely effective in reducing the risk of further bleeding. However, long-term patency rates have been disappointing, and a TIPS primarily has been viewed as a bridge to liver transplantation.

Nonvariceal upper and lower gastrointestinal hemorrhage occasionally requires angiography to identify or treat the source of blood loss. Although usually not helpful in identifying the source of upper gastrointestinal bleeding, selective arterial embolization is an effective means of controlling arterial bleeding caused by peptic ulcer disease if endoscopic therapy fails and the patient is a poor surgical candidate. Angiography plays a more important role in localizing and treating bleeding below the ligament of Treitz. Bleeding from diverticula, vascular ectasias, tumors, and aneurysms can be identified by angiographic techniques. Intra-arterial vasopressin can be infused to control bleeding once a source is identified. Although sources of chronic lower gastrointestinal blood loss are best treated by endoscopic or surgical interventions, angiography may be helpful in identifying the source of blood loss.

Subject Index

Abdomen
    acute conditions of, 59–67
    examination of
        in abdominal pain, 54–55, 64
        in gas and bloating, 71
        in ileus or obstruction, 79
        in pancreatitis, 54, 475
    pain in, 49–67. *See also* Pain, abdominal
Abdominal cavity, 499–509
    abscess in, 506–508, 687
    anatomy of, 499–500
    developmental anomalies of, 500–502
    embryology of, 499
    fistulae in, 508–509
    hernias of, 501–506
Abetalipoproteinemia, 87, 92, 358–359
Abscess
    abdominal, 506–508, 687
    anorectal, 456–457
    in Crohn's disease, 406, 407, 414, 416, 417
        anorectal, 456, 457
    of liver, amebic, 601, 602–603
    of pancreas, in acute pancreatitis, 478
    pilonidal, 463
    retroperitoneal, 518–519
Acanthosis nigricans, 146
Acetaminophen hepatotoxicity, 546, 548–550
N-Acetylcysteine in acetaminophen hepatotoxicity, 549, 550
Achalasia, 5, 7, 10, 217–220
    botulinum toxin injection in, 10, 220
    cricopharyngeal, 5, 10, 151, 215
    dysphagia in, 5, 7, 10, 218
    in elderly, 151, 220
    esophageal carcinoma in, 240
Achlorhydria, with watery diarrhea and hypokalemia, 88, 494
Acid ingestion, esophageal injury in, 207
Acid secretion, gastric
    and bacterial overgrowth in small intestine, 330
    in dyspepsia, nonulcer, 288
    in elderly, 152–153, 154
    measurement of, 271, 278
    in peptic ulcer disease, 269, 271, 285
    reflux in, 226–234
    in short bowel syndrome, 364
    in VIPomas, 88, 494
    in Zollinger-Ellison syndrome, 276–280

Acidosis, metabolic, 82
    diabetic ketoacidosis, 44, 50, 55, 64
Acrodermatitis enteropathica, 359
Acromegaly, 433, 621
Actinomycosis, retroperitoneal, 519
Acute abdomen, 59–67
Acyclovir in AIDS-associated diarrhea, 598
Addison's disease, 621–622
Adenocarcinoma. *See also* Carcinoma
    anal, 462
    of colon, 445–453
    of esophagus, 243–245
    of pancreas, 474, 486–492
    of small intestine, 367–370, 417, 442
    of stomach, 266, 287, 300–305
Adenoma
    of colon, 431–436
        in familial adenomatous polyposis, 438–442
        malignant, prognostic features in, 435–436
        progression to carcinoma in, 432, 434, 447
        surveillance for adenocarcinoma in, 435, 452–453
    of liver, 591
        drug-induced, 548
    of pancreas, 491–492
    of small intestine, 367–370
    of stomach, 306
Adhesions, intestinal obstruction in, 61, 77, 78
    in pregnancy, 164
Adrenal disorders, 621–622
Aeromonas infections, 201, 340
Aerophagia, gas and bloating in, 68, 71, 73
Aflatoxin B1, and hepatocellular carcinoma, 586–587
Aganglionosis of colon, 377
Agenesis of pancreas, 468
AIDS. *See* HIV infection and AIDS
Alanine aminotransferase serum levels, 125, 127
    in alcoholic liver disease, 573
    in hepatitis, 551–552
    in hyperbilirubinemia and jaundice, 117
Albumin
    in ascitic fluid, 137
    infusion in ascites, 139
    serum levels of, 124, 129, 137

Library Resource Center
Renton Technical College
3000 N.E. 4th St.
Renton, WA 98056